STATISTICS FOR EXERCISE SCIENCE AND HEALTH WITH MICROSOFT® OFFICE EXCEL®

STATISTICS FOR EXERCISE SCIENCE AND HEALTH WITH MICROSOFT® OFFICE EXCEL®

J. P. VERMA
Centre for Advanced Studies,
Lakshmibai National Institute of Physical Education,
Gwalior, India

WILEY

Published by John Wiley & Sons, Inc., Hoboken, New Jersey
Published simultaneously in Canada

Library of Congress Cataloging-in-Publication Data:

Verma, J. P., author.
Statistics for exercise science and health with Microsoft Office Excel / J.P. Verma, Centre for Advanced Studies, Lakshmibai National Institute of Physical Education, Gwalior, India.
pages cm
Includes bibliographical references and index.
ISBN 978-1-118-85521-8 (hardback)
1. Microsoft Excel (Computer file) 2. Sports sciences. 3. Sports sciences–Statistical methods–Computer programs. 4. Exercise–Statistical methods. I. Title.
GV741.V47 2014
613.7′1–dc23

2013047834

ISBN: 9781118855218

10 9 8 7 6 5 4 3 2 1

This book is dedicated to
my mother,
whose loving spirit sustains me still

CONTENTS

PREFACE

Statistics is tough. Statistics is boring. Statistics is dry. These are the preconceived notions of most students about the subject. After considerable experience in my teaching career, I have realized that almost all difficult concepts of statistics can be taught well in a simple manner. This book is primarily meant for students of Exercise Science and Health, as a text book of statistics for their graduate, predoctoral, and doctoral course work. It can be used by students of any of the applied branches of physical education and sports sciences such as sport psychology, sport kinesiology, sport management, sport pedagogy, sport biomechanics, nutrition, and yoga. Since Excel® computing has been discussed in each chapter, this makes the book more useful for all those students who are required to analyze data in their thesis or project.

This book is the result of my experience in teaching statistics for the last three decades at the Lakshmibai National Institute of Physical Education, Gwalior and of my interaction with professionals while conducting workshops in many Indian and foreign universities. Being the only faculty of statistics in India working in the field of physical education and sports, scarcity of study material in statistics in these areas was a hindrance to teaching. This compelled me to produce a much needed text for the students. I strongly believe that if you teach statistics to students of Exercise Science and Health using illustrations from their own domain, they understand it better. Although writing this book took around two years, the contents and concepts included in it have been accrued based on deliberations with my students and research scholars during my entire teaching career.

The purpose of this book is to provide readers with a basic understanding of statistics and to help them in solving a variety of problems in exercise science and health. Besides serving as a textbook for students, this book will also give them a solid foundation for their future research work. One of the main features of this book is that it follows the "simple to complex" approach. Even students with no prior knowledge of statistics can understand the text if they refer its chapters in sequential order.

After writing this book, I think I have become more disciplined in my approach. It was my desire to create a book that students of Exercise Science and Health would love to read, and I worked with the minutest possible detail to enhance the clarity of the topics in each chapter.

As you go through the text, you will find sections such as "Check Your Progress" and "Practice Exercise" that follow the discussion of major topics. There is also an exhaustive list of exercises at the end of each chapter. In order to comprehend the discussed topics and concepts well, students must solve the problems listed in these three sections. This will help them in understanding the intricacies of different concepts discussed in the chapter. The solutions for all the questions in the sections "Check Your Progress," "Practice Exercise," and "Chapter Exercise" given at the end of the chapter can be used by students to check the correctness of their answers. For easy reference, all the important definitions and formulas used have been given in each chapter.

Excel computing for most of the statistical techniques discussed in each chapter has been shown by means of different examples. Students should master the statistical techniques discussed in the chapter by manual process first and may verify the results later by using the Excel methods. The Excel facility of statistical computing discussed in different chapters of the text will enable the masters' degree students, PhD scholars, and research personnel to solve their research problems in the area of statistical inference, regression models, research designs, and applied research.

The faculty who uses this as a textbook will find it useful as it presents many illustrative studies with real or simulated realistic data in different chapters to clarify and illustrate the analytical techniques covered in the text. Some of the examples cited in the text are from my own as well as my colleagues' research studies.

This book has been organized in 12 chapters. Each chapter is self-contained and includes enough solved exercises for students to understand the procedure of computation in a systematic manner.

In Chapter 1, students learn what statistics is, how it is useful in research, and its application in exercise science and health. Deliberations are made about the ways in which research data can be analyzed by using different types of statistics. The readers are introduced to Excel computing in this chapter.

Chapter 2 discusses the characteristics of different data types and the procedure for investigating the nature of data. It discusses the situations where one can identify the suitable measure of central tendency and variability for drawing conclusions. For instance, why the median is preferred over the mean in case of skewed data although the mean is the most suitable measure of central tendency in the case of interval or ratio data. A detailed discussion has been made on developing a profile chart, which invariably forms the part of every thesis. This chapter also discusses procedures to compute various descriptive statistics by means of Excel.

In Chapter 3, the procedure for drawing different graphs and charts has been discussed. The stem and leaf diagram has been discussed to understand the distribution of data. Developing histograms with Excel has been shown for understanding the distribution of data.

Chapter 4 discusses the importance of probability in decision making. Computing probability in different situations has been shown by means of many solved examples. One can learn to compute the probability of various events by using Excel functionality if the data are also normally distributed.

In Chapter 5, students are introduced to some very important distributions such as the binomial, Poisson, and normal distributions. Students may learn how to test the normality of data, which is one of the main assumptions in using any of the statistical tests for hypothesis testing.

In Chapter 6, the importance of sampling over population has been discussed at great length. The chapter includes different types of probability and non-probability sampling techniques. Another important feature of this chapter is discussion on the two different considerations for deciding the sample size in conducting research. Students have been shown why the sample mean follows a normal distribution in case of a large sample irrespective of the population distribution.

Chapter 7 discusses statistical inference, which includes the theory of estimation and testing of hypothesis. Different parametric tests such as the z, t, F, and χ^2 have been discussed in detail. Students are shown why the null hypothesis is rejected if the calculated value of z is greater than its critical value. Using the p-value for testing of hypothesis has been extensively discussed. Besides manual computation by means of examples, the step-by-step procedure of using Excel in computing z, t, and F have been shown as well. This will help the students to analyze their dataset for their thesis work and research articles.

In Chapter 8, the completely randomized design and randomized block design and one factorial experiment have been discussed. The solutions to these designs have been shown by means of the one-way ANOVA, two-way ANOVA with one observation per cell, and two–way ANOVA with n observations per cell. The chapter also includes discussion on the ANCOVA design by means of a solved example. The most important feature of this chapter is that the students can learn to solve these designs by using the Excel functionalities.

Chapter 9 enables the students to understand the relationships among different variables by means of product moment correlation, partial correlation, and multiple correlation. This chapter includes simple and multiple regression. The students can learn to develop a regression model for estimating the criterion variable on the basis of explanatory variables. The chapter also discusses various assumptions in regression analysis and how to test the model as well. The important feature of this chapter is that one can develop the regression model and test its significance as well by using Excel features.

Chapter 10 deals with various types of nonparametric tests for hypothesis testing in a situation where the normality assumption is not satisfied. The researchers can use these tests for testing hypotheses for parametric data also in a situation where assumptions for the parametric tests fail.

In Chapter 11, different types of nonparametric associations have been discussed. Many situations arise in research where such associations are required to be computed.

Finally, Chapter 12 is devoted to the development of norms. A detailed procedure has been discussed for developing a weighted scale for assessing the performance of an individual. This scale can be used in many situations in physical education because human performance improves at a faster rate in the beginning; however, at a higher level, a lot of effort is required for even a slight enhancement in performance. Therefore, a slight improvement at the higher level may be rewarded more by using this weighted scale.

I am indebted to many of my colleagues who have helped me professionally over the years. Particularly, I would like to show my gratitude to Prof. Gupta YP, Prof. Sekhar, Prof. Prasad J, and Prof. Khare D for providing some of the crucial inputs in completing this text. All my research scholars and graduate students deserve special thanks for providing me the food for thought throughout my whole teaching career. Their insightful queries and difficulties in understanding different concepts have helped me to incorporate all those deliberations and solutions in this text.

I am very much thankful to Susanne Steitz-Filler, Senior Editor, John Wiley & Sons, and her team for providing me all the support and encouragement in presenting this book to the audience in its present form. My sincere thanks to Sari Friedman for providing me all the guidance in the publication of this text. She was very prompt and supportive of all my queries during the whole process of publication. At last, I would like to place on record the efforts made by Gowri Vasanth, Project Manager at SPi-Global, and her team in typesetting and editing this book.

I wish to thank my brother, Verma Pankaj, who helped me in resolving certain issues in preparing this manuscript. I must appreciate the effort of my children, Priyam and Prachi, for making available their skill sets and time in helping me to modify the language of the manuscript quite often.

At last, a special mark of appreciation to my wonderful wife, Haripriya, for her patience and good nature in understanding the long hours of work that necessitated my being locked away in my study room at "LNIPE" for endless hours, night after night, and on weekends, working on the manuscript. She is really a remarkable lady.

For each topic, considerable effort has been made to describe each and every step, so that on going through any topic, students can grasp its concept well. I hope that the book will provide students and researchers with a useful material for their course work and research activity. Suggestions and queries from readers are most welcome via email at vermajprakash@gmail.com. A timely response to them shall be ensured.

J. P. Verma, PhD
Professor of Statistics
Director, Centre for Advanced Studies

1

SCOPE OF STATISTICS IN EXERCISE SCIENCE AND HEALTH

1.1 INTRODUCTION

The use of statistics has become very popular in exercise science and health research because of the availability of many statistical packages. Researchers have begun to use advanced statistical techniques to draw meaningful conclusions. Exercise scientists use statistical techniques to refine their exercise schedule for different categories of people. Using a statistical model helps the researcher to fine-tune his research. The assessment of fitness status is based on the statistical model where different components of health-related fitness are given an appropriate weight to develop a fitness index. By using computer software, the exercise scientists can begin to assess the functional fitness of an individual. Knowledge of statistics empowers research scientists to develop customized fitness prescriptions.

Identification of talent in sports is one of the major thrust areas of research. Knowledge of cause-and-effect relationships provides a scientific basis to develop strategies for talent identification at an early age in different sports. Exercise scientists play an important role in nurturing these young players in different sports. By understanding the nature of different sports, these scientists can develop different exercise programs. By understanding statistical techniques, one can test the appropriateness of the developed schedule. Thus, the use of statistics provides a scientific basis for developing any exercise regimen.

Fitness and health are complementary to each other. Hence, health scientists are always engaged in propagating the need for fitness activities along with proper

Statistics for Exercise Science and Health with Microsoft® Office Excel®, First Edition. J. P. Verma.

nutritional intake. The main issue is to identify the optimum level of fitness regimen and the nutritional intake for different categories of people. Such knowledge is created by designing an appropriate research experiment and analyzing its findings. By using advanced statistical techniques, one can understand the fitness status and health deficiency of the people in a particular community. Obesity is a menace; hence, health scientists are always interested in identifying the parameters that cause it in different communities. By using statistical modeling, one can identify the lifestyle parameters that are responsible for the increase in the body mass index (BMI) of individuals.

Statistics plays an important role not only in exercise science and health but also in its applied areas such as physical education, sports biomechanics, sports psychology, and sports sciences. For instance, indices can be developed for assessing different parameters such as flexibility, muscular endurance, and muscular strength by using the regression model. Several researchers have developed a methodology for assessing fat percentage on the basis of a few skin folds or bodily circumference by using statistical techniques. One can also use statistical tests in estimating the accuracy of such an assessment. Similarly, researchers in the area of sports biomechanics can use statistical tools to identify the specific muscles used by high performance players. Sports psychologists can identify the specific psychological traits required for being successful in sports. By using some advanced statistical techniques, one can identify the traits that help an individual win in a particular sport. Sports has become very competitive in nature, and scientists now focus on methods to enhance the performance of the players. The researcher can develop a model for maximizing a sportsman's performance by enhancing other parameters to optimal levels. Thus, it is clear that there is tremendous scope for statistics not only in exercise science and health but also in their applied areas.

1.2 UNDERSTANDING STATISTICS

> **FACTS TO KNOW**
>
> Statistics provides authenticity in research findings

The term statistics is used to denote the data as well as the subject. The important thing is the context in and the purpose for which it is used. This text is about statistics; hence, one should understand its definition first. *Statistics* can be defined as an applied science that deals with the collection, compilation, analysis, and interpretation of data. It is also considered a branch of mathematics because most of the statistical techniques are based on mathematical concepts and derivations. A main purpose of statistics is to understand the characteristics of a large group of subjects or entities based on a small subset drawn from it. In other words, one wishes to investigate population characteristics on the basis of the sample drawn from it. The meaning of population depends on the context in which it is used. For instance, if it is required to estimate the BMI of people over 40 years of age in a locality, then all those whose age is more than 40 years shall constitute the population. On the other hand, if one wishes to understand the fitness culture in the schools of a state, then all the schools will constitute the population. To know the characteristics of the population, one needs to define some parameters on the basis of which its nature can be understood. Two such parameters that are generally used by researchers are mean μ and standard deviation σ, where μ indicates the central value of the dataset and σ is used for understanding the variation of the data in the population. Owing to the large size of the population and various other reasons (as discussed in Chapter 6), these population parameters μ and σ are estimated by the sample statistics and $\overline{x}$, respectively. Thus, the term statistics is also used to denote the function of sample observations.

Research studies on statistics can be broadly classified into descriptive and inferential. In *descriptive* studies, researchers gather data on a group of people or organization to understand their characteristics. For instance, collecting data on the height of the players in a tournament can reveal several interesting features. The mean height can reveal what the average athlete's height is, whereas the range can indicate the maximum variation among the athletes' height. The statistics that are used for descriptive studies are usually mean, standard deviation, variance, coefficient of variation, skewness, kurtosis, and so on.

In inferential studies, a researcher uses those statistical techniques on the basis of which a conclusion about the population characteristics can be drawn from the sample data. Consider a situation where it is necessary to know the impact of a weight training program on back strength. A study may be conducted on a randomly drawn sample of athletes. The data so obtained from the sample may be analyzed by using inferential statistics to draw a conclusion, which can be generalized for the population. The most important aspect of any inferential study is to draw the sample randomly, without which the conclusion drawn about the population characteristics cannot be considered to be authentic. Some statistical techniques used for inferential studies are hypothesis testing, correlation, regression analysis, and so on.

1.3 WHAT STATISTICS DOES?

A main advantage of using statistics in analyzing data is that the reliability of findings can be verified. In addition to this, one can also be sure that the results obtained from the experiment are authentic and, hence, more acceptable to the scientific community. There are ways and means by which one can also test the accuracy of the findings. Let us try and understand what statistics does. A teacher conducts a few statistical tests in which the average performances of the students A and B are given by 55 and 58 marks, respectively. Can it be concluded that the student B is better than student A in statistics. For some it may be, and for others it may not be. But if the difference between their performances is 10 in favor of B, then majority of the people would say that B is better than A but still some may think otherwise. To conclude, all these decisions are subjective in nature and lack authenticity. But if these two averages are compared by using the statistical test, the difference of 3 marks in their averages may provide 95% confidence to the researcher to believe that B's performance is better than A. What does "the researcher is 95% confident in favor of B" mean? It simply indicates that if you conduct 100 such tests of statistics, at least 95 times B's performance would be better than A's.

1.4 STATISTICAL PROCESSES

A statistical process can be defined as the type of statistical analysis that is used by the researcher in his research study. Before discussing the different types of statistical techniques, let us first see how many types of statistical processes can be encountered in research, and what are the appropriate statistical techniques used in these processes. Broadly, the research processes can be divided into the following five categories.

1.4.1 Descriptive Process

The descriptive process refers to describing the characteristics of a group of individuals, an organization, or a group of similar entities. In such studies, one describes various characteristics of the subjects under study. These studies not only provide interesting information but also help in decision-making. Findings in the descriptive studies may at times provide new topics for research and investigation. The statistics that are used in descriptive studies are known as descriptive statistics. Such statistics are the mean, standard deviation, coefficient of variation, range, skewness, kurtosis, and so on. There are many situations in which descriptive studies may be undertaken. For instance, one may take up a study to prepare a profile of Indian wrestlers. In this case, statistics such as the mean, range, standard deviation, skewness, and kurtosis of different parameters such as height, weight, total body fat, endurance, flexibility, and strength may be computed to understand the different characteristics of Indian wrestlers. Another example of a descriptive study can be the case study of any particular celebrity in sports. In such a case, different descriptive statistics are calculated on the data obtained from the same subject at different points of time.

1.4.2 Comparative Process

All those studies where the researcher is interested in comparing two or more groups come under this category. Often there is interest in comparing the effect of two training programs, the anxiety levels among male and female players, or the IQ of high and low performers in sports. Such studies can be categorized as the comparative process. The statistics that are used in comparative studies are known as comparative statistics. Such statistics are *Z*, *t*, *F*, and chi-square. In comparing more than two groups, analysis of variance is used to analyze the data.

1.4.3 Relationship Process

In the relationship process, the researcher is usually more interested in exploring the relationships among different parameters. For instance, one may be interested in the relationship between the leg length, reaction time, and leg strength with that of the 100 m performance. Similarly, one may like to determine the relationship between the fat percentage and age with cardio respiratory endurance. In such studies, the relationship statistics such as correlation coefficient, partial correlation, and multiple correlation are used to investigate the relationship.

> **FACTS TO KNOW**
>
> In the inferential process the phenomenon that is investigated exists but is unknown, whereas in the predictive process the phenomenon is not known and nor does it exists as well.

1.4.4 Inferential Process

In the inferential process, a conclusion about the population characteristics is drawn on the basis of the information from a sample. Techniques such as statistical estimation and testing of hypothesis are used to draw inferences about the population characteristics. Studies such as estimating students' IQ in a college on the basis of a sample of students, or comparing the agility of gymnasts and basketball players on the basis of two samples obtained from the college gymnasts and basketball players, come under the inferential process. Statistical techniques such as point estimation; interval estimation; *s*, *t*, *F*, and *Z* tests; and analysis of variance are used to analyze the data in such studies.

1.4.5 Predictive Process

The predictive process is used in studies where we try to predict a future event on the basis of the information from a sample. There is a difference between the inferential process and the predictive process. In the predictive process, a phenomenon that does not exist as of now is predicted on the basis of the information from a sample. On the other hand, in the inferential process, a phenomenon about the population that exists but is not known is estimated on the basis of the information from a sample. Consider a study in which it is of interest to know whether a particular student would qualify in a competitive examination on the basis of his mathematical ability, reasoning ability, and IQ scores. In such a study, the predictive process is used because the happening of the event, that is, the result of the competitive examination, is not known at the time of predicton. Statistical techniques such as regression analysis, logistic regression, and discriminant analysis are used to analyze the data in such situations.

1.5 NEED FOR STATISTICS

The following are reasons why students should take a course in statistics and develop mastery of this subject.

1.5.1 To Understand Research Literature

One cannot read much of the literature in research journals without encountering statistical concepts, methods, and techniques. Without understanding the concepts and fundamentals of statistics, it becomes difficult to interpret the findings mentioned in research articles, as a result of which one loses interest in research activities and is discouraged from undertaking research problems.

1.5.2 To Construct a Research Problem

There is a huge difference between abstract thinking and rational thinking. A researcher is required to convert an abstract thought into a feasible research study. This requires knowledge of various statistical designs without which it becomes impossible to frame an experimental study. Further, knowledge of advance statistical techniques gives insight to the researcher in developing the hypotheses for investigation in the study. In the absence of knowledge about various statistical techniques, it is just not possible to develop a meaningful research study.

1.5.3 To Develop a Scientific Temper

Using statistics in decision-making helps an individual to inculcate scientific temper. A scientific temper is required at each and every step in life. It helps an individual to think rationally in any situation. For instance, during a match, a player's decision for any move is based purely upon his earlier experience. A coach plans the training schedule for his trainee on the basis of his previous experience. While taking a shot, the batsman always calculates the risk on the basis of his scientific judgment. Thus, the development of a scientific temper helps an individual to take decisions rationally all the time.

1.5.4 To Assess the Authenticity of Research Findings and to Contradict Unjustifiable Claims

> **FACTS TO KNOW**
>
> Learning statistics sharpens your faculties and helps in developing a good research problem

Several researchers publicly announce findings based on their research work. In order to assess the authenticity of their statements, one can read their research report. But to satisfy oneself about the conformity between their statements and the actual fact, one should be able to understand the statistical techniques used in the report. Many companies make a claim about their product by using the research findings of their scientists. These claims may be tested by conducting an experiment under controlled conditions and analyzing the data. For example, if a fitness lab announces that their oral tablets reduce 10 lbs weight in 15 days, this claim may be tested by actually conducting an experiment. Normally while making such claims, companies hide certain facts that are required to justify their claims. For instance, they may not reveal for which age group and weight category the finding is true. Thus, knowledge of designing an experiment and various statistical techniques are essential to write-off the unjustifiable claims.

1.5.5 To Develop Indices for Various Characteristics and Performances

Certain concepts in exercise science cannot be directly measured. For instance, to measure the body strength there is no single test. Instead, one may test arm strength, back strength, leg strength, and shoulder strength separately. One may develop a single index for body strength by giving appropriate weight to these components. Similarly, an index can be prepared to measure the flexibility, health-related fitness, or endurance of an individual. To develop such indices, some advanced statistical techniques such as regression analysis and factor analysis can be used. Thus, knowledge of these techniques equips the researcher to take up such studies in exercise science and health.

1.5.6 To Develop Norms on Various Traits

Norms on different test items provide motivation to an individual. In developing norms for parameters such as sit-ups, pull-ups, push-ups, and so on in different age and sex categories, performance of these parameters needs to be converted into a score by using a scale ranging from 0 to 100. Such norms are easily understood by a lay man and can be used as a selection criteria for certain courses and programs. The norms for the test items are developed by assuming normality of the data. In a situation when the data is not normal, a certain transformation is used before using different scaling techniques. Statistical techniques such as percentile scale, T-scale, and weighted scale are used to develop such norms. Thus, the knowledge of these techniques will equip the researcher to take up normative studies for developing norms for different physical, physiological, and psychological traits in people of different age and sex categories.

1.5.7 To Conduct Research

An important reason to understand the concepts of statistics and learn advanced statistical techniques is to equip an individual for research. The knowledge of sampling techniques allows the researcher to select a representative sample that represents the population. Similarly, knowledge of the different statistical designs helps researchers to choose an appropriate methodology for the experiment and identify the proper statistical test to analyze the data. Thus, it is extremely important to have appropriate knowledge of statistical concepts, methods, and techniques to conduct research in an efficient manner and to draw valid conclusions.

1.6 STATISTICS IN EXERCISE SCIENCE AND HEALTH

No academic discipline can grow without advancement in research; this is true for exercise science and health as well. One of the important dimensions of research is the design of the experiment. Proper statistical design used in a study helps the researcher to isolate the factors responsible for the performance in any event. Further, using appropriate statistical design reduces overall error in the experiment, giving more reliable conclusions. New techniques in different sports can be tested against the existing technique for better results by using an appropriate statistical technique. For instance, in comparing the effectiveness of three different warm-up exercises on a 400 m performance, one may plan a completely randomized design where the subjects may be randomly assigned to three different warm-up exercises. One-way analysis of the variance technique can be used to identify the best warm-up program for the 400 m event. Similar experiments can help to determine the best duration of the warm-up program for the 100 m event. Thus, the development of new techniques and strategies in sports is the result of research experiments conducted over a period of time.

Different statistical techniques are used to solve varieties of research problems in exercise science. For instance, development of test batteries for measuring the concept of motor fitness, athletic fitness, general fitness, and specific fitness in different sports requires factor analysis technique to solve the problem. Similarly, norms construction requires identification of the appropriate scaling procedure. Further, if a coach is interested in the extent of relationships between performance and independent parameters, partial correlation may be used whereas multiple correlation allows him to find the reliability in estimating the performance on the basis of certain known characteristics. To find the optimum training load for different levels of athletes, the experiment can be planned by using the proper statistical design.

To measure qualitative characteristics such as competitive anxiety, attitude toward sports, knowledge of health education, and self concept, questionnaires can be developed. These questionnaires are developed using statistical techniques such as item analysis including difficulty rating and index of discrimination along with the reliability analysis. Further, keys may be developed by using statistical techniques such as factor analysis. Most of the statistical techniques mentioned in this chapter are discussed in detail in different chapters of the book. Thus, we see that any advancement in exercise science and health is not possible without statistical aids.

Every academic discipline has different research requirements; exercise science and health too demand separate attention from a statistical point of view. To give specific focus to the problems in this area this book has been titled *Statistics for Exercise Science and Health with Microsoft® Office Excel®*.

Check Your Progress

Note: Tick the correct answer by using the sign (√)

	True	False
1. Statistics is the function of population values	–	–
2. *t*-statistics is used for testing of hypothesis	–	–
3. Population is an aggregate of all the items	–	–
4. Statistics can be used to denote the distribution used in the analysis of data	–	–
5. If the sample is not random, population characteristics cannot be estimated from the statistics computed from sample observations	–	–
6. Inferential statistics is used for drawing conclusions about population characteristics	–	–
7. Descriptive statistics describes population characteristics	–	–
8. The mean μ and standard deviation σ are known as population statistics	–	–
9. Statistics describes sample characteristics	–	–
10. The mean, $\bar{x}$, and sample standard deviation, s, are known as sample statistics	–	–
11. Statistics provides scientific explanation to research findings	–	–
12. The statistics t, F, and Z are known as comparative statistics	–	–
13. Multiple correlation is a predictive statistics	–	–

1.7 COMPUTING WITH EXCEL

1.7.1 Installing Analysis ToolPak

While using Excel for analyzing data you must check that the Add-ins "Analysis ToolPak" is already installed in your Excel. Without its installation, you cannot use the functionality discussed in various chapters of this book. Follow the steps given while installing this ToolPak in your Excel:

1. After starting the Excel in your system, click the sequence of commands.

Office button ⟶ **Excel Options** ⟶ **Add-Ins**

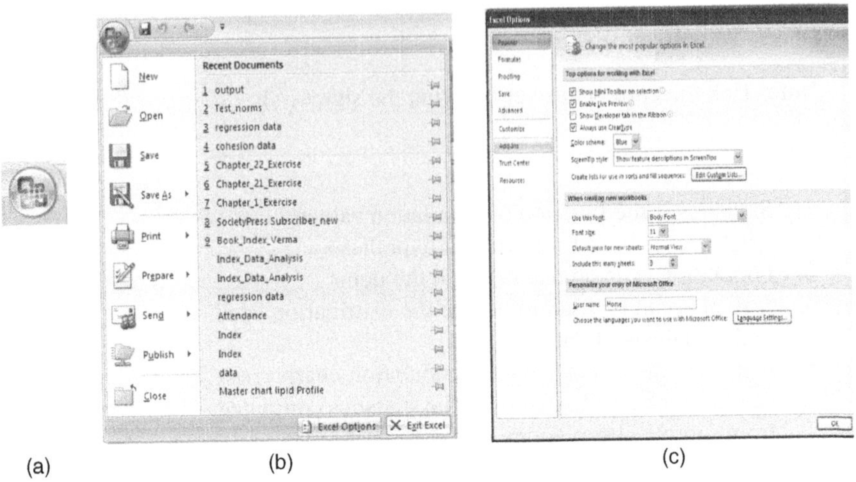

Figure 1.1 (a–c) Sequence of commands in installing Analysis ToolPak.

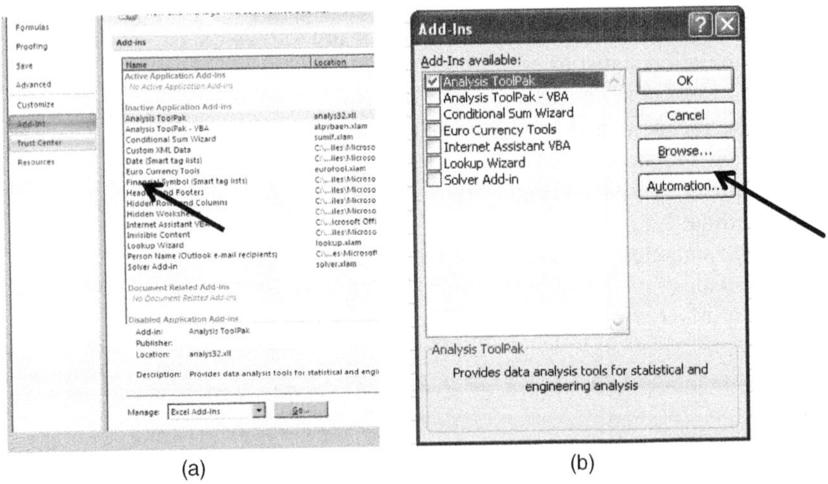

Figure 1.2 (a,b) Options for installing Analysis ToolPak.

While clicking these commands, you will see the following screens in sequence as shown in Figure 1.1(a–c).

2. After clicking the **OK** in Figure 1.1(c) you will get the screen as shown in Figure 1.2(a). By scrolling choose the option **Analysis ToolPak** and then select the option **Excel Add-Ins**. Click **OK** to get the screen as shown in Figure 1.2(b). Select the **Analysis ToolPak** and then click **OK** to get it installed.
3. Restart the Excel to use the functionality of Analysis ToolPak.

	A	B
1	Slong_Jump	
2		
3	Mean	64.5
4	Standard Error	1.087811
5	Median	64.5
6	Mode	65
7	Standard Deviation	3.439961
8	Sample Variance	11.83333
9	Kurtosis	-0.71601
10	Skewness	0.081888
11	Range	11
12	Minimum	59
13	Maximum	70
14	Sum	645
15	Count	10
16	Largest(1)	70
17	Smallest(1)	59

Figure 1.3 Dataset in the column B which is required to be formatted.

1.7.2 Formatting Cell Entries in Excel

Most of the time when you compute various statistics using Excel, it shows you long scores in fraction such as 1.087811258, 3.43996124, 11.83333333, and −0.716014396. This disturbs the whole formatting. You can format the cell entries by the following command sequence. Let us consider the following output generated in Excel while computing descriptive statistics as shown in Figure 1.3.

Let us see how scores in the second column as shown in Figure 1.3 can be formatted.

Select the second column by clicking the mouse on the column label B and right click the mouse to get the option **Format Cells** as shown in Figure 1.4

Clicking the option **Format Cells** in Figure 1.4 will take you to Figure 1.5 to decide on the number of decimal places in your output. Select 2 or anything else as per your requirement. Let other options be selected by default. Click **OK** to get your desired formatted output as shown in Figure 1.6.

After choosing the option in Figure 1.5, the final output looks like what is shown in Figure 1.6.

1.7.3 Initiating Computation with Excel

Excel can be used for simple as well as advanced computing. One must understand its basics to exploit its full potential. The following example will make you learn how to add, subtract, multiply, divide, and compute mathematical expressions.

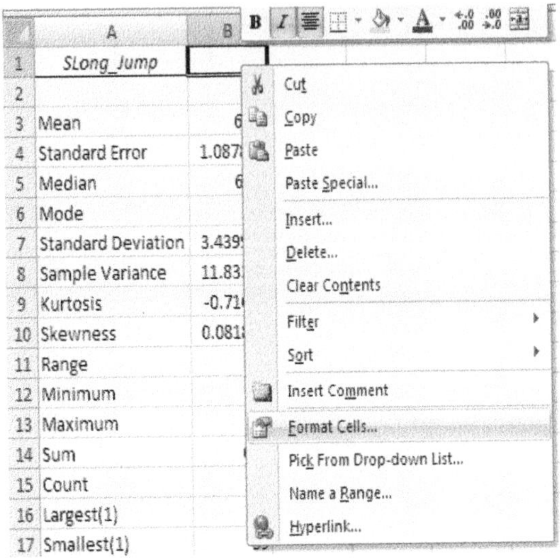

Figure 1.4 Choosing the option for formatting data.

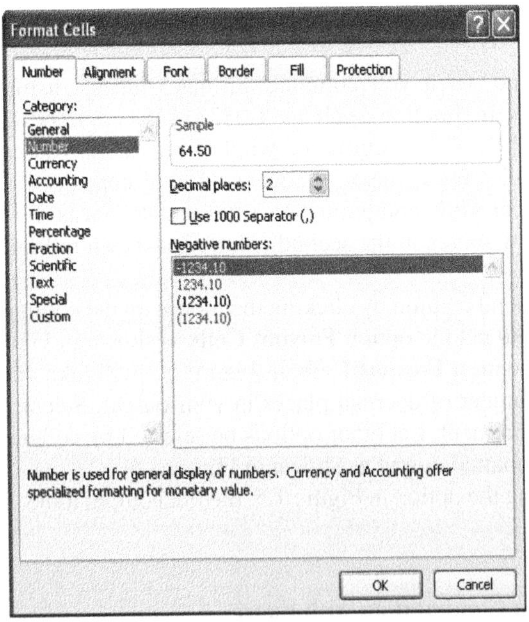

Figure 1.5 Choosing the option for deciding decimal places and other specifications.

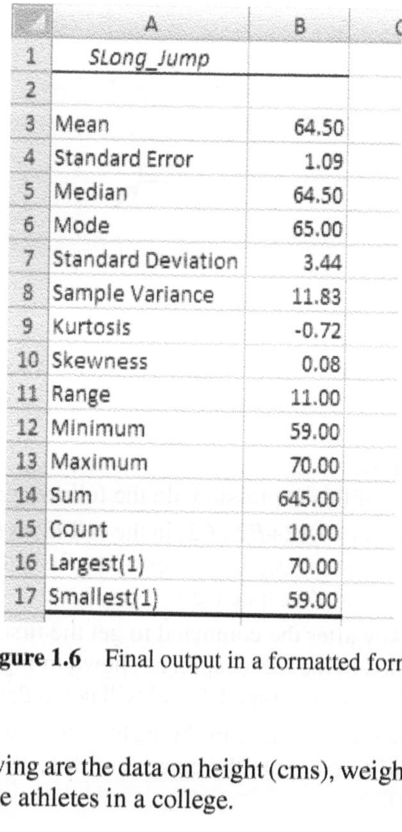

	A	B
1	SLong_Jump	
2		
3	Mean	64.50
4	Standard Error	1.09
5	Median	64.50
6	Mode	65.00
7	Standard Deviation	3.44
8	Sample Variance	11.83
9	Kurtosis	-0.72
10	Skewness	0.08
11	Range	11.00
12	Minimum	59.00
13	Maximum	70.00
14	Sum	645.00
15	Count	10.00
16	Largest(1)	70.00
17	Smallest(1)	59.00

Figure 1.6 Final output in a formatted form.

Example 1.1 Following are the data on height (cms), weight (lbs), and arm length (cms) obtained on male athletes in a college.

Height (*X*)	185	190	188	180	178	172	168
Weight (*Y*)	189	165	169	178	184	169	167
Arm length (*Z*)	82	84	81	83	79	80	78

Compute the following:

i. $X+Y+Z$
ii. $X-Y$
iii. $X \times Y$
iv. $\sum X$, $\sum Y$, and $\sum Z$
v. $\sum X^2$, $\sum Y^2$

Solution: To compute the above-mentioned expression, first, the three sets of scores should be typed column-wise in the Excel sheet.

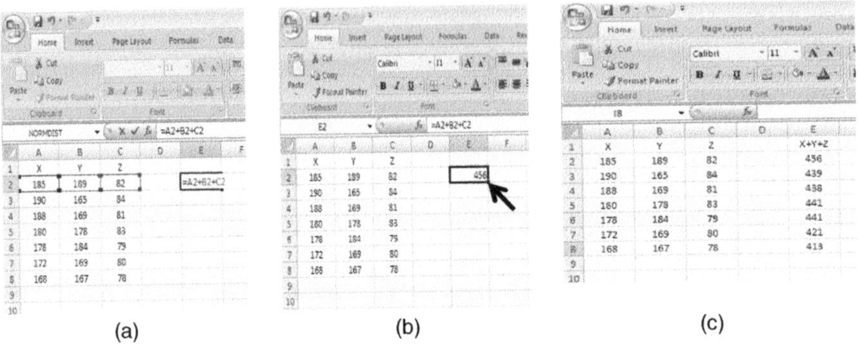

Figure 1.7 (a–c) Steps in computing $X+Y+Z$.

i. Computing $X+Y+Z$
   To find the value of this expression, do the following:
   a. Type the formula = **(*A*2+*B*2+*C*2)** in the cell *E*2 as shown in Figure 1.7(a). *A*2, *B*2, and *C*2 are the cell addresses of the first athlete's data on the three variables *X*, *Y*, and *Z*, respectively.
   b. Click Enter key after the command to get the first subject's data on three variables added in the *E*2 location as shown in Figure 1.7(b). Kindly note that unless the = sign is typed, Excel will not understand this as a formula.
   c. Drag the black dot located in the right corner at the bottom of the cell *E*2 downward to compute the expression for other subjects as shown in Figure 1.7(c).
ii. Computing $X-Y$
   This can be computed by using the formula = ***A*2–*B*2**. Other processes shall remain the same as discussed in the first problem. This computation is shown in column *E* of Figure 1.8.
iii. Computing $X \times Y$
   This can be computed by using the formula = ***A*2****B*2**. In Excel, star(*) is used as the operator for multiplication. Other processes remain the same. This computation is shown in column *F* of Figure 1.8.
iv. Computing $\sum X$, $\sum Y$, and $\sum Z$
   These expressions can be quickly computed by using the $\sum$ command in the header of Excel. To get the sum of the data in a column, place the cursor just below the data set and click $\sum$ command in the header. Clicking the enter key will give you the value of the sum of that variable. This has been shown in Figure 1.8.
v. Computing $\sum X^2$, $\sum Y^2$
   These expressions can be computed by using the following formula = ***A*2^2**. The cap "^" command is used to find the power of the variable and can be

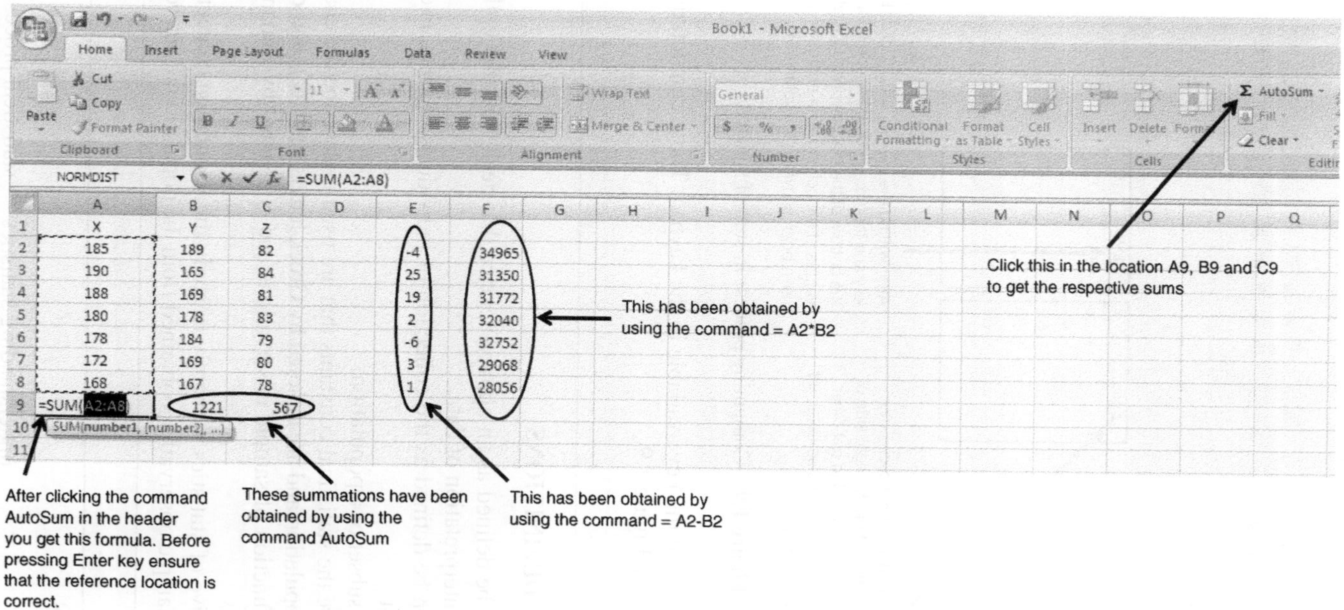

Figure 1.8 Computing process in subtraction, multiplication, and addition.

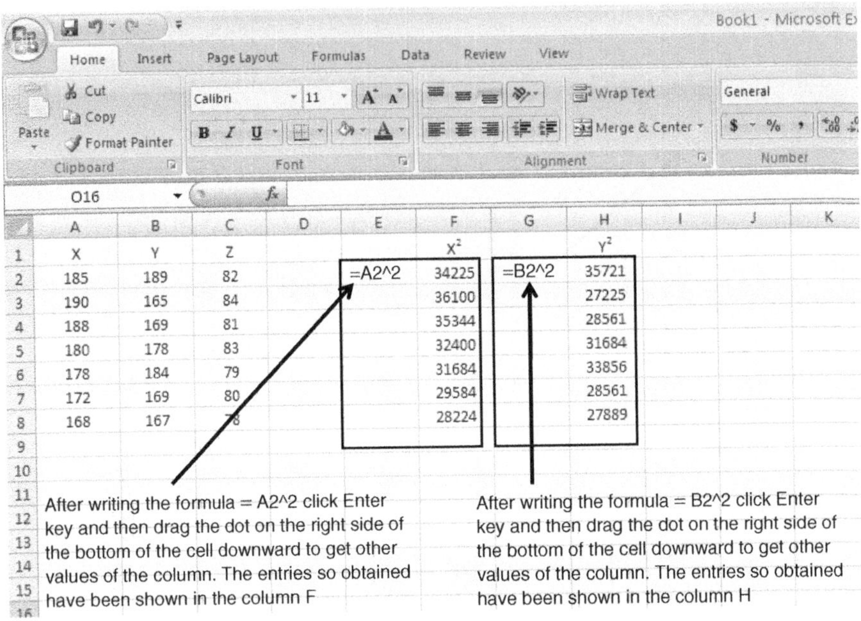

Figure 1.9 Computing process in sum of squares.

created by using the key available in the keypad. These computations have been shown in Figure 1.9.

IMPORTANT DEFINITIONS

Statistics may be defined as an applied science that deals with the collection, analysis, and interpretation of data.

Population can be defined as the collection of individuals, objects, events, or item of interest.

A ***sample*** is a subset of a population.

Parameters are the statistical constants that are used to describe the characteristics of the population and are denoted by Greek letters such as μ and σ.

Statistic is a function of sample observations and is denoted by roman letters such as $\bar{x}$ and s.

The objective of statistics is mainly to study the population characteristics based on the sample observations obtained from the population of interest.

KEY TERMS

statistic
parameters
understanding statistics
population
statistical processes

CHAPTER EXERCISE

1. Give two examples in sports for each of the data types: nominal, ordinal, interval, and ratio.
2. Classify each of the following as nominal, ordinal, interval, or ratio data.
   - i. The time required to score a century in a cricket match.
   - ii. Scores in a basketball match.
   - iii. The ranking of volleyball players by the judges.
   - iv. The marks of students in a class.
   - v. Height of a player.
   - vi. The number of hours a sportsman practices.
   - vii. Student's categories: 1, General; 2, SC/ST; 3, OBC; 4, Handicapped.
   - viii. Rating of players on a five-point scale based on playing ability.
   - ix. The reaction time of an athlete.
   - x. Assessment of anxiety on a five-point scale.
3. Elaborate a situation where a researcher in exercise science may organize a descriptive study.
4. Give a specific example of data that might be gathered from each of the following areas: training methods, coaching, yoga, fitness, and talent identification.
5. Suppose you are the head of a teaching organization that runs exercise science courses. Give an example of how you could use descriptive statistics to make better administrative decisions. Give an example of how you could use inferential statistics to make better management decisions.
6. What do you mean by statistical process? Discuss different types of statistical processes with suitable examples in the field of exercise science.
7. Explain the need for statistics in research.

ANSWERS

Check Your Progress

1. F	3. F	5. T	7. F	9. T	11. T	13. T
2. T	4. T	6. T	8. F	10. T	12. T	

Chapter Exercise

2. i. Ratio
   ii. Ratio

iii. Ordinal
iv. Ratio
v. Ratio
vi. Ratio
vii. Nominal
viii. Interval
ix. Ratio
x. Interval

FURTHER READING

1. Al-Kadi IA. The origins of cryptology: the Arab contributions. Cryptologia 1992;16(2):97–126. DOI: 10.1080/0161-119291866801.
2. Cohen JB. Misuse of statistics. Journal of the American Statistical Association (JSTOR) 1938;33(204):657–674. DOI: 10.1080/01621459.1938.10502344.
3. Dodge M, Stinson C. Microsoft Office Excel 2007 Inside Out. USA: Microsoft Press; 2007. ISBN 0-7356-2321-X.
4. Dodge Y. The Oxford Dictionary of Statistical Terms. UK: OUP; 2006. ISBN 0-19-920613-9.
5. Hays WL. Statistics for the Social Sciences, Holt, Rinehart and Winston. 1973. p xii-ISBN 978-0-03-077945-9.
6. Huff D. How to Lie With Statistics. New York: WW Norton & Company, Inc.; 1954. ISBN 0-393-31072-8.
7. Moses LE. Think and Explain with Statistics. USA: Addison-Wesley; 1986. p 1–3. ISBN 978-0-201-15619-5.
8. Peck R, Olsen C, Devore J. Introduction to statistics and data analysis. 3rd ed. USA: Duxbury Press; 2007. ISBN: 978-0-495-11878-7.
9. Thompson B. Foundations of Behavioral Statistics. USA: Guilford Press; 2006.

2

UNDERSTANDING THE NATURE OF DATA

2.1 INTRODUCTION

Large sets of data are gathered by researchers in the field of exercise science and health to understand the performance of individuals on different parameters. These data become meaningful only if they are reduced to some manageable form. To understand the nature of these data, one needs to perform some form of descriptive analysis. Such an analysis will help researchers to draw conclusions about the nature of the dataset by computing a single indicator.

Consider a situation where a study is conducted on 400 school children to know their body composition. A body fat analyzer is used to assess the fat percentage of the 400 children in a school. By looking at these data, one cannot draw any conclusion about the obesity of the children. One needs to compute an aggregate value of this dataset so as to draw a meaningful conclusion. Such an aggregate value is known as a measure of central tendency. There are three measures of central tendency: the mean, median, and mode. These averages are computed to obtain an idea about the aggregate score of the dataset. These measures of central tendency are useful in different situations. In the above example, the mean is the best measure of central tendency. This is because computation of the mean depends on all the scores. There is a thorough discussion on the different measures of central tendency later in this chapter.

Let us consider another example where the mean fat percentage of the children in two schools is the same. In the first school, the fat percentage does not vary much

Statistics for Exercise Science and Health with Microsoft® Office Excel®, First Edition. J. P. Verma.

from child to child, whereas in the second school, it does. Therefore, simply by looking at the values of the mean of the two schools, one cannot arrive at a conclusion as to the school in which the children are less obese. To resolve this dilemma, in addition to the mean value, one also needs to compute some measures of variability in order to get an idea about the variation of the scores around the mean value. Thus, one would need to compute both the measure of central tendency and the measure of variability to arrive at the correct picture of each school's dataset.

2.2 IMPORTANT TERMINOLOGIES

To understand the concepts and procedures discussed in this chapter, let us first understand the various terminologies that are used.

2.2.1 Raw Scores

Raw scores refer to original data that have been generated in a study and on which no statistical treatment has been done. The data generated in a study that measures the performance in a skill test on basketball players, the runs scored by the players in a cricket tournament, or the anthropometric measurements of swimmers are examples of raw scores. These data are known as raw scores because they have not been processed. On the other hand, if these data are converted into a standard score or arranged in class intervals, then they become processed data and are no longer considered raw data.

2.2.2 Single Scores

Single scores refer to data that have been approximated into whole numbers or integers. If the data have been obtained with scores up to one, two, or three decimal places, then they can be converted into whole number scores by approximating the scores to the nearest whole numbers. The rule of approximation is that if the fractional value is equal to 0.5 or more, then the integer value is increased by 1. For example, the equivalent single score of 6.4 would be 6, whereas for the score of 7.52, it would be 8. This is because in the score of 6.4, the fractional value is 0.4, which is less than 0.5, and hence there is no increase in the whole number part; so the approximate single score is 6. On the other hand, 7.52 has a fractional value of 0.52, which is more than 0.5, and hence the approximate single score is obtained by increasing the whole number part by 1, that is, 7 becomes 8. Let us look at the single scores of the following numbers:

i. $9.3 \sim 9$ (the fraction 0.3 is less than 0.5, hence there is no change in the whole part of the number).
ii. $12.49 \sim 12$ (the fraction 0.49 is less than 0.5, hence there is no change in the whole part of the number).

iii. 19.51 ~ 20 (the fraction 0.51 is more than 0.5, hence the whole part of the number has been increased by 1).

Let us see what happens if the approximation of 12.49 is made in two steps as shown below.

Step 1: 12.49 ~ 12.5 (correct)
Step 2: 12.5 ~ 13 (incorrect)

It then seems that the single score for 12.49 is 13. Logically, both the steps seem to be correct according to the above rule for fraction conversion, but in example (ii), the single score of 12.49 is 12 and hence there is a contradiction. This contradiction can be solved by understanding the rule, which says that an approximation of an approximated figure cannot be taken and therefore the score 12.5, which is already an approximated figure of 12.49, cannot be further approximated to 13.

2.2.3 Variables and Attributes

A *variable* may be defined as a measurable phenomenon that keeps on changing from time to time, place to place, and individual to individual. It follows that anything that can vary can be considered a variable. For example, height is a variable because it varies from person to person. Similarly, weight, reaction time, and fat percentage are all variables. A variable need not necessarily be numerical. For example, name is a variable because it varies from person to person. Similarly, sport specialization, courses, city, and country are all examples of variables.

An *attribute* refers to the characteristics of an individual. For example, gender is an attribute because an individual can be either male or female. Similarly, IQ (high or low), academic achievement (high or low), and color of the eye (black, brown, or blue) are the examples of attributes. Sometimes, attributes can be criteria based. For instance, if an individual is classified as *tall* (if the height is more than 72 in.) or *short* (if the height is less than 61 in.), then height becomes an attribute.

An attribute can be classified as two-class, three-class, or *n*-class attribute depending on the number of classes an attribute is classified into. For instance, if an athlete is classified as a *smoker* or *nonsmoker*, then the smoking status becomes a two-class attribute. Similarly, eye color can be a three-class attribute, with classification into *black*, *brown*, or *blue*.

2.2.4 Independent and Dependent Variables

An *independent variable* can be defined as a variable that an experimenter manipulates to see its effect on other factors. On the other hand, a variable is said to be *dependent* if it depends on the independent variable. This distinction is particularly relevant in investigating cause–effect relationships. For instance, if a researcher is interested in observing the effect of different durations of pranayama on lung capacity, then the pranayama duration becomes the independent variable as it is being manipulated by the researcher to see its impact on lung capacity, whereas lung capacity becomes a dependent variable because it depends on the different intensities of pranayama. In this experiment, pranayama is the cause and lung capacity is an effect. Similarly, in investigating the effect of a conditioning program on a student's fitness, the conditioning program is the independent variable and the student's fitness is the dependent variable. Since the conditioning program has been manipulated by the researcher, it is an independent variable and acts as a cause, whereas the student's fitness is a dependent variable, which is affected by the cause.

2.2.5 Continuous and Discrete Variables

A variable that can assume any real number value is known as a *continuous variable*. The timing of an athlete in a track event can assume any fractional value within a range. A person's height, weight, long jump performance, reaction time, and so on can take any real value within reasonable limits. In all these cases, variables can assume any order of fractional value, for instance, the height of an individual may take any value between 5 and 6 ft., that is, 5.36 or 5.42 ft., and so on. Similarly, weight, age, or performance can also assume any fractional value. These are all examples of continuous variables.

A variable is said to be *discrete* if it takes only whole number or integer values. For example, the score in a cricket match, points scored in a basketball match, the number of goals in a football or hockey match, all of which are whole numbers, are all discrete variables.

2.3 MEASUREMENT OF DATA

Researchers generate enormous amounts of data every day in the field of exercise science and health. All the data so obtained, such as timing an event, gender, athlete's ranking, classification, and so on, require different approaches under statistical analysis. This is because the same data may represent different factors, depending on the trait they indicate. For instance, consider two numbers 20 and 40, which may represent the marks obtained by two students, the ranking of two athletes, or the bib numbers of two athletes. Although 40 is the double of 20, it makes no sense in comparing these values if they indicate the bib numbers of athletes because in this case, they are just two numbers that distinguish the two athletes and do not carry any meaning. Similarly, if these two numbers represent the ranking of two athletes, computing the average becomes meaningless as they are just ranks. However, if they were the marks scored by two students, then the average of the two marks makes sense. The appropriateness of the statistical technique used in data analysis depends on the scale of measurement of the data collected. Thus, the researcher must know the scale of measurement of the data before identifying the statistical technique for data analysis. In general, data are measured on four different scales, namely, *nominal*, *ordinal*, *interval*, and *ratio*.

2.3.1 Nominal Scale

Nominal scale data are obtained by measuring data at the lowest level. The data so obtained are often referred to as *nominal data*. The values representing nominal data are used only to classify or categorize. If in a survey study, "male" is represented by "1" and "female" by "0," then these numbers simply denote the category to which an individual belongs and do not carry any meaning. Similarly, if Christian is coded as "1," Jewish as "2," and Hindu as "3," then these numbers are used only for classifying an individual. The number 3 does not indicate a higher category; in fact, it is used to simply identify an individual as Hindu and no other meaning is attached to it. Some other types of variables that often produce nominal data are participation level sports specialization, smoking status, body types, and so on. There are limited statistical techniques that can be used for analyzing nominal data. The chi-square is the most widely used statistical tool for analyzing such data.

2.3.2 Ordinal Scale

The level of measurement of ordinal data is higher than that of nominal data. Data measured on ordinal scale can be classified into different categories and can also be graded. Thus, ordinal data also possess the characteristics of nominal data. By using ordinal data, a coach can evaluate soccer players by ranking their competencies on playing ability with the numbers from 1 to 5. A player with ranking 1 is an extremely good player, whereas a player with ranking 5 is the least competent. However, in ordinal data, the spacing between any two consecutive numbers may not be uniform. For example, the difference in the competencies between the players ranked 1 and 2 may not be the same as that between the competencies of the players ranked 2 and 3. Another example of ordinal data is the ranking of students on the basis of their intelligence, nature, extroversion, and so on. To analyze the data measured on ordinal scale, nonparametric tests such as the median test, Mann–Whitney test, or Kruskal–Wallis test are used.

Nominal and ordinal data are usually obtained by imprecise measurements. Such data are obtained when there are no objective criteria of assessment. For this reason, nominal and ordinal data are said to be *nonmetric data*. These nonmetric data are also referred as *qualitative data* or *nonparametric data*. To analyze these data, a large number of nonparametric tests are available, which have been discussed in detail in Chapter 11.

2.3.3 Interval Scale

Interval data represent a higher level of measurement compared to ordinal data. For interval data, the difference between any two consecutive numbers makes sense unlike that in ordinal data. Interval data can be graded in ascending or descending order. In addition, the distance between any two consecutive numbers on the scale is uniform. Temperature measurement on the Fahrenheit scale is an example of interval data. The temperature readings on this scale such as 25°, 27°, and 29° can be ranked, and the difference between the consecutive readings is the same. In other words, the quantum of heat between 25° and 27° is equal to the amount of heat between 27° and 29°.

In interval data, there is no real zero. Zero is a matter of convenience in such data, and it does not indicate the absence of phenomenon. For example, the zero on the Fahrenheit scale does not mean the lowest possible temperature. Thus, the ratio of two consecutive numbers is not the same. For instance, a temperature of 40° is not twice that of 20°. In other words, the doubling principle fails in interval data. Other examples of interval data are attitude ratings, levels of body flexibility, and frustration levels.

2.3.4 Ratio Scale

Data obtained on ratio scale represent the highest level of measurement. Ratio data have properties that are similar to those of interval data. The most important feature of ratio data is that there is an absolute zero, and the ratio of two numbers is meaningful. Absolute zero indicates the absence of the phenomenon. For instance, height is a ratio data, for which there is a natural zero. Zero height is the indication of absence of height. If the heights of three persons are 35, 50, and 70 in., then they can be ranked according to their heights and one can say that the person of height 50 in. is taller than the person whose height is 35 in. Thus, unlike nominal data, here the numbers have a meaning. Further, the doubling principle holds as one can infer that the person whose height is 70 in. is twice as tall as the person whose height is 35 in. This was not the case with interval data where no natural zero exists. Thus, ratio data possess the characteristics of all the three levels of data, that is, nominal, ordinal, and interval data. Other examples of ratio data are weight, biceps, chest circumference, skin-fold measurement, and timings.

Since interval and ratio data are obtained through precise measurement, they are termed as *metric data* or *quantitative data*. Metric data are also known as *parametric data*. To analyze metric data, a large number of parametric statistical tests are available, which shall be discussed in different chapters of this book.

2.4 PARAMETRIC AND NONPARAMETRIC STATISTICS

Statistical techniques can be classified as parametric or nonparametric. Parametric statistics are used when the data are measured in either interval or ratio scale, whereas nonparametric statistics are used for data that are measured in either nominal or ordinal scale. Statistics such as the mean, standard deviation, Pearson's correlation, Z, t, and F are known as *parametric statistics*, whereas the median, quartile deviation (QD), runs, Mann–Whitney's U-statistic, and Kruskal–Wallis' H-statistic are known as *nonparametric statistics*. Parametric tests are more powerful than the nonparametric tests, provided the required assumptions about the data are satisfied. One of the major assumptions for using parametric tests is that of normality. The data must be normally distributed in order to use parametric tests. Detailed discussions on these statistics and tests are found in different chapters of this book. The statistical techniques used for data measured at any level of measurement can be used for data measured at a higher level of measurement but cannot be used for data measured at a lower level of measurement. For instance, all statistical techniques that can be used for nominal data can also be used for ordinal data, but the techniques that are applicable for interval data cannot be used for ordinal data. Thus, all those statistical techniques that can be used for interval, ordinal, or nominal data can also be used for ratio data. However, some of the statistical techniques specifically require data to be measured only on the ratio scale. Chapters 10 and 11 are specifically meant for nonparametric statistics, whereas parametric statistics have been discussed in detail in all other chapters.

2.5 FREQUENCY DISTRIBUTION

A *frequency distribution* is the representation of scores and their frequency in a tabular format. A frequency distribution provides a consolidated picture of the data. One can visualize the way frequencies are distributed in different class intervals. The class intervals can be made discrete or continuous.

In discrete class intervals, the limits of the class intervals are distinct such as 11–15, 16–20, and 21–25. Since there is a discontinuity between two consecutive class intervals, the actual lower limit (LL) of any class interval is obtained by subtracting 0.5 from its lower limit. For example, the LL of the class interval 16–20 would be obtained by subtracting 0.5 from 16, that is, $16 - 0.5 = 15.5$. This is because any score that is 15.5 or more would fall into the class interval 16–20.

In continuous class intervals, the limits overlap. For example, 15–20, 20–25, and 25–30 are continuous class intervals. Here, the upper limit of a class interval is the same as the LL of the next higher class interval. For this reason, it may be difficult to identify the class interval for a score that is equal to the lower or higher class limit. For example, if a data item has the score 20, it is difficult to identify whether it belongs to the class interval 15–20 or 20–25. Therefore, in continuous class intervals, it is assumed that the upper limit of the class interval is excluded from that class. Under this assumption, class intervals become mutually exclusive. Owing to this assumption, the score 20 will now belong to the class interval 20–25 and the score 25 will belong to the class interval 25–30. Continuous class intervals are constructed if the data obtained are continuous in nature. Thus, in the above example, as long as the score is less than 25, may be 24.9999, it will belong to the class interval 20–25 but the moment it becomes 25, it would fall into the next class interval, 25–30.

Raw data are referred to as *ungrouped data*, whereas data arranged in the class interval form are known as *grouped data*. Let us see how a frequency distribution table is constructed from raw data. The procedure is explained by means of an example. Consider the following scores, which are the weights of 47 athletes in a college. The steps involved in constructing the frequency distribution are as follows.

Weights in lbs										
103	110	119	121	111	145	160	120	115	139	103
116	125	129	117	154	113	119	125	124	130	128
147	110	108	121	126	129	165	140	130	120	124
122	126	123	157	117	125	106	123	115	116	108
104	131	110								

Steps for Constructing the Frequency Distribution Table

1. *Computing Range*: The first step is to compute the range of the scores by subtracting the lowest score from the highest score in the dataset. Here, the lowest score is 103 and the highest score is 165.

$$\text{Range} = 165 - 103 = 62$$

2. *Deciding the Width of the Class Intervals*: The next step is to find the width of the class intervals. The width of the class intervals is obtained by dividing the range by the number of class intervals required to be constructed. As a convention, the number of class intervals should be between 10 and 20. Less than 10 class intervals will make the computation easier at the cost of accuracy in computing various statistics. On the other hand, a large number of class intervals enhance accuracy in computation but the computation becomes difficult.

   Let us take the number of class intervals to be the minimum of 10. We divide the range by 10 to get the width of the class intervals.

$$\text{Width of the class intervals} = \frac{62}{10} = 6.2$$

   Due to convenience, the width is taken as a whole number, in this case, 6. By taking the width as 6, the number of class intervals shall become 11 in this case.

3. *Constructing the Lowest Class Interval*: One needs to decide the lowest class interval by taking the width calculated in step 2 in such a manner that it includes the lowest score in the dataset. Similarly, the highest class interval must include the highest score of the dataset. To fulfill these conditions, the number of class intervals may be sometimes more than or less than 10.

   Another issue before constructing the class interval is to decide whether it should be discrete or continuous. In general, the decision about constructing discrete or continuous class intervals depends on whether the dataset is discrete or continuous. However, this is merely a convention, and there is no hard and fast rule in this regard. In fact, one may construct discrete class intervals for continuous data also, and vice versa.

Here, the data are discrete, so discrete class intervals can be constructed. The lowest score in the dataset is 103 and the width is 6; hence, the lowest class interval can be any of the four class intervals: 100–105, 101–106, 102–107, or 103–108. All these four class intervals include the lowest score 103. But one should prefer the lowest class interval as 100–105 or 101–106. This is because the lowest score 103 lies close to the middle of the class interval, and therefore the accuracy in computation increases.

4. *Counting Frequencies in Each Class Interval*: Once the lowest class interval is decided, the other class intervals can be constructed by taking the width 6 as shown in Table 2.1. After constructing the class intervals, all the scores in the dataset are placed in the appropriate class intervals by putting a tally mark (a vertical line). After marking four tally marks, the fifth one should be placed diagonally across the four. Count the tally marks to get the frequencies of each class interval. Table 2.1 shows the frequency distribution of the data.

2.5.1 Assumptions in Calculating Statistics from the Grouped Data

In converting raw data into class intervals, the identity of individual scores is lost, owing to which it is not possible to add all the scores and therefore statistics such as the mean and standard deviation cannot be calculated. For instance, in a frequency distribution if a class interval 16–20 has a frequency 5, one can only say that the five scores lie in the range 16–20 but one does not know the actual scores. Since the

TABLE 2.1 Frequency Distribution for the Data on Weights (in lbs) of 50 Athletes

Class Intervals	Tally Marks	Frequency
101–106	IIII	04
107–112	~~IIII~~ I	06
113–118	~~IIII~~ II	07
119–124	~~IIII~~ ~~IIII~~ I	11
125–130	~~IIII~~ ~~IIII~~	10
131–136	I	01
137–142	II	02
143–148	II	02
149–154	I	01
155–160	II	02
161–166	I	01
	Total	47

magnitudes of all the five scores are unknown, it is not possible to add these scores, because of which it is not possible to calculate the mean and standard deviation. To solve this problem, two assumptions are made while calculating different statistics from grouped data.

First Assumption: In computing statistics from grouped data, the first assumption is that the frequencies are concentrated at the midpoint of the class intervals. This assumption is used in calculating the mean and standard deviation. In computing the mean and standard deviation, it is essential to know the magnitude of each and every score; thus if the frequency of class interval 31–35 is 4, it is assumed that all four would be equal to its midpoint, 33. In assuming so, there is more likelihood of committing an error as actual scores may not be all equal to 33. But if in some class intervals, actual scores are less than the midpoint, in others it may be more with the result the net error becomes close to zero. This fact can be seen in Table 2.2.

Second Assumption: The second assumption that is used while computing various statistics from the grouped data is that the scores are evenly distributed in the class intervals. For instance, if the class interval 29–33 has a frequency 5, then it is assumed that the scores are 29, 30, 31, 32, and 33, which are equally spaced. This assumption is used while computing the median and QD. This fact has been shown in Table 2.3. The error in computing these statistics increases if the width of the class interval increases, and that is why the smaller the width of the class intervals, the greater is the accuracy in computation.

2.6 SUMMATION NOTATION

Computing the sum of the scores is very common in statistical calculations. While computing the average score of a batsman, average height of athletes, or average

TABLE 2.2 The Effect of Frequencies Being Concentrated at the Midpoint of the Class Interval

CI	x	f	fx	Actual Scores	Sum of Actual Score	Net Error
31–35	33	4	132	31, 32, 32, 33	128	+4
26–30	28	3	84	28, 29, 30	87	−3

TABLE 2.3 Explanation of Frequencies Being Evenly Distributed in the Class Interval

CI	x	f	Scores Equally Spaced
29–33	31	5	29, 30, 31, 32, 33
24–28	26	3	24, 26, 28

mark of the students in a class, it is required to find the total of all the scores. A Greek letter $\sum$ (pronounced as sigma) is used to denote the summation of a set of values.

Example 2.1 In an experiment, weight training was given for 1 month to six subjects, as a result of which their fat% was reduced to 14, 22, 18, 21, 24, and 28 lbs respectively. Find $\sum_{i=1}^{6} x_i$.

If we denote first value by x_1, second value by x_2, and so on, then we can write

$$x_1 = 14, \quad x_2 = 22, \quad x_3 = 18, \quad x_4 = 21, \quad x_5 = 24, \quad x_6 = 28$$

By using the summation sign, the sum of these six values could be written as $\sum_{i=1}^{6} x_i$. This is read as summation of x_i, where i assumes the values from 1 to 6. The numbers 1 and 6 are the lower and upper limits of the summation. Thus,

$$\sum_{i=1}^{6} x_i = x_1 + x_2 + x_3 + x_4 + x_5 + x_6$$
$$= 14 + 22 + 18 + 21 + 24 + 28 = 127$$

By changing the limits, the value of summation also changes. For example,

$$\sum_{i=4}^{6} x_i = x_4 + x_5 + x_6$$
$$= 21 + 24 + 28 = 73$$

In general, the symbol $\sum_{i=1}^{n} x_i$ means the sum of all the values of x_i, where i ranges from 1 to n. This summation sign can be used if the summation is required to be over all the squares of the scores or the sum of multiplication of x and y as well. Thus, we can write

$$\sum_{i=1}^{4} x_i^2 = x_1^2 + x_2^2 + x_3^2 + x_4^2$$

and

$$\sum_{i=1}^{3} x_i y_i = x_1 y_1 + x_2 y_2 + x_3 y_3$$

Sometimes, the limits of summation are omitted if all the data are to be added and the sum is written as $\sum x_i$. Some authors prefer to drop the subscript also and use $\sum x$ to represent the sum of all the data.

Example 2.2 If $x_1 = 3$, $x_2 = 6$, and $x_3 = 10$, calculate the following.

i. $\sum x_i$, ii. $\sum_{i=1}^{3} x_i^2$, iii. $\sum_{i=2}^{3} (x_i^2 + x_i)$

Solution:

1. $$\sum x_i = x_1 + x_2 + x_3$$
$$= 3 + 6 + 10 = 19$$

2. $$\sum_{i=1}^{3} x_i^2 = x_1^2 + x_2^2 + x_3^2$$
$$= 3^2 + 6^2 + 10^2$$
$$= 9 + 36 + 100 = 145$$

3. $$\sum_{i=2}^{3} (x_i^2 + x_i) = (6^2 + 6) + (10^2 + 10)$$
$$= 42 + 110 = 152$$

Theorem 2.1 The sum of two or more variables is the sum of their summations. Thus,

$$\sum_{i=1}^{n} (x_i + y_i + z_i) = \sum_{i=1}^{n} x_i + \sum_{i=1}^{n} y_i + \sum_{i=1}^{n} z_i$$

Proof

$$\text{LHS} = \sum_{i=1}^{n} (x_i + y_i + z_i)$$
$$= (x_1 + y_1 + z_1) + (x_2 + y_2 + z_2) + \ \dots \ + (x_n + y_n + z_n)$$
$$= (x_1 + x_2 + \ \dots \ x_n) + (y_1 + y_2 + \ \dots \ + y_n) + (z_1 + z_2 + \ \dots \ + z_n)$$
$$= \sum_{i=1}^{n} x_i + \sum_{i=1}^{n} y_i + \sum_{i=1}^{n} z_i = \text{RHS}$$

Hence proved.

Theorem 2.2 If k is a constant, then

$$\sum_{i=1}^{n} kx_i = k \sum_{i=1}^{n} x_i$$

Proof

$$\begin{aligned}\text{LHS} &= \sum_{i=1}^{n} kx_i \\ &= kx_1 + kx_2 + \ldots\ldots + kx_n \\ &= k(x_1 + x_2 + \ \ldots\ + x_n) \\ &= k\sum_{i=1}^{n} x_i = \text{RHS}\end{aligned}$$

Hence proved.

Theorem 2.3 If k is a constant, then

$$\sum_{i=1}^{n} k = nk$$

Proof
In Theorem 2.2, if all the values of x_i are equal to 1, then

$$\sum_{i=1}^{n} k = \underbrace{k + k + \ldots\ldots + k}_{n \text{ terms}} = nk$$

2.6.1 Double Summation

When all the scores arranged in rows and columns are to be added, the double summation is used.

$$\sum_{i=1}^{n}\sum_{j=1}^{m} y_{ij}$$

Here, i represents the row and takes values from 1 to n and j represents the column and takes values from 1 to m.

Consider the following matrix of scores in Table 2.4. The elements represent the number of students belonging to different classes and different age categories.

The addition of all the numbers in this table is denoted by

$$\sum_{i=1}^{3}\sum_{j=1}^{4} y_{ij}$$

where

$$i = 1, 2, 3$$

TABLE 2.4 Number of Students in Different Classes and Age Categories

		Age				
		9	10	11	12	$n = 3$
Class	4	25	5	6	8	
	5	5	20	8	10	
	6	8	12	26	12	
		$m = 4$				

and

$$j = 1, 2, 3, 4$$

The symbol y_{ij} denotes the score in ith row and jth column, where i and j denote the class and age, respectively. Thus, $y_{24} = 10$, $y_{12} = 5$, and so on. Let us see how the double summation is carried out in this problem.

$$\sum_{i=1}^{3}\sum_{j=1}^{4} y_{ij} = \sum_{i=1}^{3}(y_{i1} + y_{i2} + y_{i3} + y_{i4}) = \left[\sum_{j=1}^{4} \text{has been opened first}\right]$$

$$= (y_{11} + y_{12} + y_{13} + y_{14}) + (y_{21} + y_{22} + y_{23} + y_{24}) + (y_{31} + y_{32} + y_{33} + y_{34})$$

$$= (25 + 5 + 6 + 8) + (5 + 20 + 8 + 10) + (8 + 12 + 26 + 12)$$

$$= 44 + 43 + 58 = 145$$

Remark

1. The inner summation is opened first and then the outer summation is expanded.
2. Sometimes, double summation $\sum_{i=1}^{n}\sum_{j=1}^{m} y_{ij}$ is also written as $\sum_{ij} y_{ij}$.

2.6.2 Triple Summation

Triple summation is required to be calculated if all the scores in an $n \times m$ matrix, where each cell has more than one score, are required to be added. This is denoted by

$$\sum_{i=1}^{n}\sum_{j=1}^{m}\sum_{k=1}^{r} y_{ijk}$$

Consider the data in Table 2.5 representing the subject's age in different weight and height categories.

TABLE 2.5 Age of the Subjects in Different Height and Weight Categories

		Height (j)		
		Low	Medium	High
	Below Normal	9 10 12	10 12 14	16 12 13
Weight (i)	Normal	14 16 12	12 10 16	16 18 20
	Above Normal	12 14 13	13 10 11	15 16 20

Here,

i = Weight category, $i = 1, 2, 3, n = 3$

j = Height category, $j = 1, 2, 3, m = 3$

k = Age of the children $k = 1, 2, 3, r = 3$

Here, y_{ijk} represent the kth score in the ith row and jth column.
Thus,

$$\sum_{i=1}^{n}\sum_{j=1}^{m}\sum_{k=1}^{r} y_{ijk} = \sum_{i=1}^{3}\sum_{j=1}^{3}(y_{ij1} + y_{ij2} + y_{ij3})$$

$$= \sum_{i=1}^{3}[(y_{i11} + y_{i12} + y_{i13}) + (y_{i21} + y_{i22} + y_{i23}) + (y_{i31} + y_{i32} + y_{i33})]$$

$$= [(y_{111} + y_{112} + y_{113}) + (y_{121} + y_{122} + y_{123}) + (y_{131} + y_{132} + y_{133})]$$
$$+ [(y_{211} + y_{212} + y_{213}) + (y_{221} + y_{222} + y_{223}) + (y_{231} + y_{232} + y_{233})]$$
$$+ [(y_{311} + y_{312} + y_{313}) + (y_{321} + y_{322} + y_{323}) + (y_{331} + y_{332} + y_{333})]$$

$$= [(9 + 10 + 12) + (10 + 12 + 14) + (16 + 12 + 13)]$$
$$+ [(14 + 16 + 12) + (12 + 10 + 16) + (16 + 18 + 20)]$$
$$+ [(12 + 14 + 13) + (13 + 10 + 11) + (15 + 16 + 20)]$$

$$= (31 + 36 + 41) + (42 + 38 + 54) + (39 + 34 + 51)$$

$$= 108 + 134 + 124$$

$$= 366$$

2.7 MEASURES OF CENTRAL TENDENCY

A measure of central tendency can be defined as a single score that describes the aggregate of the dataset. In other words, it can be considered as an average score around which all the scores lie. Such a measure is also known as a *measure of central location*. There are three measures of central tendency, namely, the *mean*, *median*, and *mode*. They are useful in different situations. These measures are discussed in detail in the following sections.

2.7.1 The Mean

The mean is the best measure of central tendency when data are measured on interval or ratio scale, and their distribution is symmetrical or nearly symmetrical. It is the most stable and widely used measure of central tendency. In other words, its sampling fluctuation is the least in comparison to that of the median and mode. The mean is also termed as *average*. It gives the most representative value of the scores in the dataset. It is an indicative of what an average score looks like. For instance, suppose the runs scored by a batsman in five matches are 30, 45, 49, 40, and 46. The batting average of this player becomes 42. This simply indicates that it is likely that this player would score somewhere near this score in the next match. It may be noticed that the mean is often not one of the actual values that are observed in the dataset. In this case, the mean value 42 is not present in the dataset. The mean is actually a model value of the dataset. It is the value that is most common. Since the mean depends on all the scores, it is considered to be the most accurate measure of central tendency. The mean can be computed for both discrete and continuous data. The mean is obtained by dividing the sum of all the scores by the number of scores in the dataset. However, the mean is not an appropriate measure of central tendency in case of a skewed distribution.

If $x_1, x_2, \ldots, x_n$ are the n scores in the sample, then the sample mean $(\bar{x})$ is computed as

$$\bar{x} = \frac{\sum x}{n} = \frac{x_1 + x_2 + \ldots . x_n}{n} \tag{2.1}$$

In statistics, different scripts are used to denote the sample and population means, although the formulas for their computations are the same. The sample mean is denoted by $\bar{x}$, whereas the population mean is denoted by the lower case Greek letter "mu," denoted as μ. Thus, the population mean is given by

$$\mu = \frac{1}{N}\sum x \tag{2.2}$$

where N is the number of scores in the population.

Mean for Raw Data

The mean is obtained by dividing the sum of all the scores by the number of scores. For raw data, it can be computed by using formula (2.1). If the heights of five athletes are 66, 68, 67, 70, and 69 in., then the mean would be computed as

> **FACTS TO KNOW**
>
> A measure of central tendency is a score that represents the dataset

$$\bar{x} = \frac{\sum x}{n} = \frac{66+68+67+70+69}{5} = \frac{340}{5} = 68 \text{ in.}$$

Mean for Grouped Data If the scores $x_1, x_2, \ldots, x_n$ occur with frequencies $f_1, f_2, \ldots, f_n$, respectively, then the mean of n scores is given by

$$\bar{x} = \frac{\sum f_i x_i}{n} \tag{2.3}$$

where f_i is the frequency of x_i. In case the scores are arranged in class interval form, then the x_i's are obtained by computing the midpoint of the class intervals. The procedure of computing the mean in case of grouped data is discussed in the following example. Consider the data on push-ups obtained on 24 subjects, arranged in the form of class intervals as shown in Table 2.6.

The procedure for computing the mean is summarized as follows.

Steps for computing the mean

1. Write the class intervals in column 1 and the corresponding frequencies in column 2.
2. Compute the midpoint of the class intervals in column 3. The midpoint of the class interval is computed by taking the average of both the limits of the class

TABLE 2.6 Data on Push-Ups

Push-Ups Class Interval (1)	Frequency f (2)	Midpoint x (3)	fx (4)
21–25	2	23	46
26–30	3	28	84
31–35	1	33	33
36–40	5	38	190
41–45	4	43	172
46–50	6	48	288
51–55	3	53	159
	$\sum f = n = 24$		$\sum fx = 972$

interval. For example, the midpoint of the class interval 41–45 is obtained as (41 + 45)/2, that is, 43.

3. Multiply the frequency of each class interval by its corresponding midpoint in column 4.
4. Find the value of $\sum f$ and $\sum fx$ by adding the scores in columns 2 and 4, respectively.
5. Compute the mean by substituting the values of $\sum f$ and $\sum fx$ in formula (2.3). Thus,

$$\bar{x} = \frac{\sum f_i x_i}{n} = \frac{972}{24} = 40.5 \approx 41$$

Remark

1. The symbols x_i and f_i can also be represented by x and f, respectively. Similarly, $\sum f_i x_i$ can also be written as $\sum fx$.
2. In case of ungrouped data, n represents the total number of scores, whereas in grouped data n signifies the total of all the frequencies. Hence, $\sum f_i = n$.

Mean for Grouped Data using the Deviation Method The mean can also be computed by using the deviation method. This method is used especially when the frequencies in different class intervals are large. In the deviation method, the midpoints (x) of the class intervals are transformed into deviations (d) by changing the origin and scale. The formula for computing the mean by the deviation method is given by

$$\bar{x} = \text{AM} + \frac{\sum fd}{n} \times i \qquad (2.4)$$

where

AM = assumed mean
i = size of the class interval
n = total number of scores

To compute the mean using the deviation method, let us consider the data of Table 2.6 once again. After computing the midpoint (x) of the class intervals, it is transformed into the deviation (d) by using the origin as 38 and scale as 5. Usually, the origin (AM) is taken as the midpoint of the middlemost class interval and the scale (i) is taken as the width of the class interval. The following steps explain the computation of the mean.

Steps for computing the mean

1. Write the class intervals and their respective frequencies in columns 1 and 2, respectively, as shown in Table 2.7.

TABLE 2.7 Computation of the Mean by Deviation Method

Push-Ups Class Interval (1)	Frequency (f) (2)	Midpoint (x) (3)	$d = \frac{X - 38}{5}$ (4)	fd (5)
21–25	2	23	−3	−6
26–30	3	28	−2	−6
31–35	1	33	−1	−1
36–40	5	38	0	0
41–45	4	43	1	4
46–50	6	48	2	12
51–55	3	53	3	9
	$\sum f = n = 24$			$\sum fd = 12$

2. Find the midpoint of each class interval by taking the average of the two limits. For example, the midpoint of the class interval 51–55 is (51 + 55)/2, that is, 53.
3. Take the assumed mean (AM) as the midpoint of the middlemost class interval. Here, the middlemost class interval is 36–40, hence the AM is 38. In case the number of class intervals is even, select the AM from either of the two middle classes.
4. Find the width i of the class interval by taking the difference of any two consecutive LLs or upper limits of the class intervals.
5. In column 4, subtract the AM from each of the scores of column 3 and divide this difference by the width of the class interval i to get the value of the deviation d.
6. Compute fd in column 5 by multiplying the value of f by the corresponding value of d.
7. Add all the entries in columns 2 and 5 to obtain the values of $\sum f$ and $\sum fd$, respectively.
8. Substitute the values in formula (2.4) to calculate the mean.
   Here, AM = 38, $i = 5$, $\sum f = n = 24$, and $\sum fd = 12$.
   Substituting these values in formula (2.4),

$$\bar{x} = \text{AM} + \frac{\sum fd}{n} \times i$$

$$= 38 + \frac{12}{24} \times 5 = 40.5$$

Remark In the earlier example, the class intervals are discrete as there is a gap between the upper limit of a class interval and the LL of the next higher class. What happens if a score is 30.4? It can be placed neither in 26–30 nor in 31–35. But if the score 30.4 is rounded off, it becomes 30. Similarly, rounding off the score

30.5, it becomes 31. The same result is obtained when the actual limit of any class interval is obtained by subtracting 0.5 from its LL. However, this problem does not arise in case of continuous class intervals in which the LL of any class interval is the actual LL of that class.

Properties of the Mean The mean is the most efficient measure of central tendency. It has the following characteristics:

1. The mean is the most reliable measure of central tendency as it is calculated on the basis of all the scores.
2. The sum of the deviations of a set of scores from their arithmetic mean is always 0. In other words,

$$\sum(x-\bar{x})=0$$

   To prove this, expand the left-hand side of this expression

$$\sum(x-\bar{x})=\sum x-\sum\bar{x}$$
$$=n\bar{x}-n\bar{x}=0$$

3. The sum of the squared deviations of the scores from the mean is least in comparison to the deviation taken about any other measures of central tendency. Owing to this property, the mean is the most stable measure in comparison to the median or mode. Its fluctuation is least from sample to sample drawn from the same population.
4. In most distributions, the sample mean is the most efficient estimate of the population mean.

Effect of Change of Origin and Scale on the Mean Let us see how the transformations of scores affect the computation of the mean value. In using the transformation, any value that is subtracted from all the scores is known as the *origin*, and the score by which all the scores are divided is known as the *scale*. Thus, if all the scores x are transformed to d by using the following transformation, then A is known as the *origin* and i as the *scale*.

$$d=\frac{x-A}{i}$$

The choice of origin and scale is up to the researcher, but one should use these values so as to simplify the data and computation.

To see the effect of change of origin and scale on the computation of the mean, let us take the summation on both sides of the earlier equation

$$\sum d = \sum \left(\frac{x-A}{i}\right)$$

$$\Rightarrow \quad \sum (x-A) = i \times \sum d$$

$$\Rightarrow \quad \frac{\sum (x-A)}{n} = \frac{i \times \sum d}{n}$$

$$\Rightarrow \quad \frac{1}{n}\sum x - \frac{n \times A}{n} = i \times \frac{1}{n}\sum d$$

$$\Rightarrow \quad \bar{x} = A + i \times \bar{d}$$

From this result, it may be concluded that if the original scores x are transformed into d by changing origin and scale (by subtracting A from all the scores and dividing them by i), then the mean of x is equal to the sum of the origin and the product of the mean of d and scale value i.

Example 2.3 Compute the mean by transforming the following scores using 55 as the origin and 10 as the scale and check its relationship with the mean of the actual data.

x:	15	25	35	45	55	65	75	85

Solution: Here, the scores x are transformed to d by subtracting 55 and dividing by 10. In this problem, the origin (A) and scale (i) are 55 and 10, respectively. The transformed scores d are shown in Table 2.8.

Here, $n = 8$, $A = 55$, and $i = 10$

In column 3, the scores x have been transformed to d by subtracting 55 from each of the x scores first and then dividing it by 10 later. Let us see what is the difference between the mean of x and d.

$$\text{Mean of } x = \bar{x} = \frac{\sum x}{n} = \frac{400}{8} = 50$$

$$\text{Mean of } d = \bar{d} = \frac{\sum d}{n} = \frac{-4}{8} = -0.5$$

TABLE 2.8 Computation of the Mean by Changing the Origin and Scale

x (1)	x − AM (2)	$d = \frac{x-A}{i}$ (3)
15	−40	−4
25	−30	−3
35	−20	−2
45	−10	−1
55	0	0
65	10	1
75	20	2
85	30	3
$\sum x = 400$		$\sum d = -4$

Now let us see the relationship between the mean of x and that of d. We see that

$$\begin{aligned}\bar{x} &= A + i \times \bar{d} \\ &= 55 + 10 \times (-0.5) \\ &= 50\end{aligned}$$

Thus, it can be concluded that if the scores are transformed by changing the origin (A) and scale (i) then the original mean ($\bar{x}$) can be obtained by multiplying the new mean ($\bar{d}$) by the scale value i and adding it to the origin A. It is therefore inferred that the mean is not independent of change of origin and scale.

2.7.2 The Median

The median can be defined as the middlemost score of a distribution. The median is also known as the *positional average*. The median is computed for ordinal data. However, it can be computed for ratio or interval data when the dataset is highly skewed. Further, the median is the most useful measure if the effect of extreme scores needs to be avoided. Consider a situation where a student's playing ability in hockey needs to be evaluated by a panel of three judges. Since there is no objective criterion for assessing the playing ability, it is quite likely that the marks given by the judges may fluctuate to a great extent. In that case, to do away with the influence of lenient and strict marking, the median score may be used as the measure of central tendency.

Median for Ungrouped Data If $x_1, x_2, \ldots, x_n$ are the n scores arranged in the ascending or descending order, then the median score is computed as

$$M_{\mathrm{d}} = \left(\frac{N+1}{2}\right)\text{th score} \qquad (2.5)$$

To compute the median, the scores are arranged in ascending or descending order first and then $(n + 1)/2$ is computed. The score lying at this position is the median. Consider the scores representing the runs scored by the players in a cricket match as 38, 23, 28, 6, 21, 33, 15, and 39.

After arranging the scores,

Sr. No.	1	2	3	4	5	6	7	8
No. of Runs:	6	15	21	23	28	33	38	39

Here, $n = 8$,

Thus, $$M_d = \left(\frac{8+1}{2}\right)\text{th} = 4.5\text{th score} = \frac{(23+28)}{2} = 25.5$$

If the number of scores is odd, then only one middle score exists, which becomes the median; but in case the number of scores is even, there exist two middle scores and in that case their average becomes the median.

Median for Grouped Data While computing the median for grouped data, it is assumed that the frequencies are evenly distributed in the class intervals. In calculating the median, the middlemost value of the distribution, which lies in the median class, is interpolated. The median is computed from the grouped data by using the following formula:

$$M_d = \text{LL} + \frac{\frac{n}{2} - F}{f_m} \times i \qquad (2.6)$$

where

LL = lower limit of the median class
n = frequency total
F = cumulative frequency of the class just lower than the median class
f_m = frequency of the median class
i = width of the class interval

The computation of the median is discussed by using the data of Table 2.9, which indicates the scores on a fitness test. The following steps are involved.

Steps for computing the median

1. Write the class intervals and their corresponding frequencies in columns 1 and 2, respectively, and find the total in column 2 to get the frequency total as shown in Table 2.9.

TABLE 2.9 Frequency Distribution of Fitness Scores

	Class Interval (Fitness Scores) (1)	Frequency (f) (2)	Cumulative Frequency (F) (3)	
	10–14	6	6	
	15–19	7	13	
	20–24	3	16	← F
Median class →	25–29	5	21	← f_m (points to 5)
	30–34	2	23	
	35–39	4	27	
	40–44	6	33	
	45 and more	3	36	
		$\Sigma f = n = 36$		

2. In column 3, find the cumulative frequencies starting from the lowest class interval onward. The value of the cumulative frequency for the last class interval is the total of all the scores. This value and the total of column 2 should be the same.
3. Determine the median class by computing $n/2$. The median class is the class interval in which the median lies. To find the median class, look for the value $n/2$ in the column of cumulative frequency. The class interval for which the cumulative frequency includes the value $n/2$ is the median class.
4. After identifying the median class, substitute the values in formula (2.6) to get the median score.
   Here, $n = 36$ and therefore $\frac{n}{2} = \frac{36}{2} = 18$.

To determine the median class, we look for 18 in the column for cumulative frequency. The class interval 25–29 has the cumulative frequency 21, which includes the value $n/2 = 18$. Thus, 25–29 is the median class. Once the median class is decided, the median is computed by substituting the values in formula (2.6).

In this example,

LL = lower limit of the median class 24.5
f_m = frequency of the median class 5
F = cumulative frequency of the class just lower than the median class 16
i = width of the class interval 5

Substituting these values in formula (2.6),

$$M_d = \text{LL} + \frac{\frac{n}{2} - F}{f_m} \times i$$

$$= 24.5 + \frac{18 - 16}{5} \times 5$$
$$= 24.5 + 2 = 26.5$$

The LL of the median class is computed by subtracting 0.5 from the LL because the class interval is discrete. Since any value that is equal to or greater than 24.5 falls in the class interval 25–29, the actual LL of this class interval is therefore taken as 24.5 instead of 25. On the other hand, if the class interval is continuous, we do not subtract 0.5 from the LL as it is the actual LL of the class interval. In case of continuous class intervals, it is assumed that the upper limit is excluded from the class interval. This is done so as to make the class intervals mutually exclusive.

In Table 2.9, the last class interval is truncated as a result of which its midpoint cannot be calculated; hence, the mean may not be computed in this situation. Thus, if the class intervals are truncated at one or both the ends, the median is the best measure of central tendency.

Properties of the Median

1. The sum of the absolute deviations of all the scores in a set from their median, that is, $|x - M_d|$ is the least. The two vertical lines | | indicate absolute difference, that is, the difference is always positive.
2. The median is a positional average and is calculated if the scores are in the form of ranks.
3. The median is not affected by the extreme scores. Hence, if the effect of extreme scores needs to be avoided, the median is the best measure of central tendency.
4. When the class interval is cut off or open at any one end or both the ends, the median is the only choice as a measure of central tendency. Let us see why this is so. Consider the frequency table shown in Table 2.10 where the upper class interval is open. Sometimes, this is also called a *truncated distribution*. Since the class interval 30 or more is an open class, its midpoint (X) and the deviation (d) cannot be calculated. Thus, it is not possible to calculate the mean. The only choice therefore is to work out the median value as it does not depend on the extreme scores.

TABLE 2.10 Truncated Frequency Distribution

Class Interval	f	X	d
30 or more	3	Not possible	Not possible
25–29	4	27	0
20–24	6	22	−1

2.7.3 The Mode

Most of the time, we are interested in phenomena such as which sport is popular in a college, which brand of tennis racket is in demand, or which type of food is liked the most in a population. In these situations, the mode is the best measure of central tendency. In other words, when a phenomenon of maximum occurrence is required, the mode is the best measure of central tendency. Thus, the mode can be defined as the score that occurs most frequently in the dataset. It is represented by M_0. The mode is least affected by extreme scores. It is usually computed when the data are categorical in nature. However, it may be computed for intervals as well as ratio data. At times, there may be two scores in the dataset that appear more frequently, and in that case the distribution will have two modes. Thus, if the distribution has one mode it is said to be unimodal and if it has two modal values it is known as bimodal. A distribution having more than two modes is said to be multimodal.

Mode for Ungrouped Data According to its definition, the mode is the score that appears most frequently. and therefore one should identify the score that appears the maximum number of times in the dataset as the mode. Consider a series of scores obtained by a set of students in an examination, X: 2, 5, 4, 7, 6, 4, 7, 4, 8, 1, 9, 4, 10, 4, 2, 4, and 7. Here, the score 4 is repeated a maximum number of six times, and therefore the mode for this dataset would be 4. The following steps are involved in the computation of the mode in ungrouped data.

Steps for computing the mode

1. Select the score x that is repeated the maximum number of times in the dataset. The score x so identified is the mode.
2. If two adjacent values of x are repeated equal number of times and are greater than the frequency of occurrence of the remaining values, then the mode is the average of two such adjacent scores.
3. If two nonadjacent values of x are such that their frequencies are either equal or nearly equal and are greater than the frequencies of all other values, then each value of x may be taken as a mode and the distribution is said to be *bimodal*.
4. In case of a symmetrical or nearly symmetrical distribution, the mode can also be computed by an empirical formula:

$$\text{Mode} = 3\ \text{Median} - 2\ \text{Mean}$$

Mode for Grouped Data The mode can be computed if the data are grouped into a frequency distribution. However, if a large dataset is given, it may be converted first into a frequency distribution before computing the mode. The formula for computing the mode is given by

$$M_0 = \text{LL} + \frac{f_\text{m} - f_1}{2f_\text{m} - f_1 - f_2} \times i \tag{2.7}$$

where

LL = lower limit of the modal class
f_m = frequency of the modal class
f_1 = frequency of the class just before the modal class
f_2 = frequency of the class just after the modal class
i = width of the class interval

The procedure for computing the mode is explained by means of the dataset obtained in a cricket match as shown in Table 2.11. The following steps make the process clear.

Steps for computing the mode

1. Arrange the scores in class intervals along with their frequencies in the table.
2. Find the class interval whose frequency is the maximum. The class so identified is the modal class. In this case, the class interval 39–43 has the largest frequency, and hence this is the modal class.
3. The frequency of the class before the modal class is identified as f_1 and that of the class following the modal class is identified as f_2. Here, $f_1 = 2$ and $f_2 = 3$.
4. The LL of the modal class is obtained by subtracting 0.5 from its lower limit if the class interval is discrete. Since, here, the class interval is discrete, the value of LL would be $39 - 0.5 = 38.5$. However, in case of continuous class intervals, the LL will be the value of the lower limit of the modal class.
5. Substituting the values in formula (2.7) will give the value of the mode.

   Here, the modal class is 39–43, $\text{LL} = 38.5$, $f_\text{m} = 6$, $f_1 = 2$, $f_2 = 3$, and $i = 5$.

TABLE 2.11 Runs Scored by the Players in a Cricket Match

	Class Interval (CI)	Frequency (f)
	24-28	4
	29-33	2
	34-38	2
Modal class →	39-43	6
	44-48	3

Substituting these values in the formula

$$M_0 = \text{LL} + \frac{f_m - f_1}{2f_m - f_1 - f_2} \times i$$
$$= 38.5 + \frac{6 - 2}{2 \times 6 - 2 - 3} \times 5$$
$$= 38.5 + 2.86 = 41.36$$

Properties of the Mode

1. The mode is the most desirable measure of central tendency when the phenomenon of frequent occurrence is required. For example, if it is required to find out which tactic is used by the majority of hockey teams in a tournament or which sport is more popular in a country, the mode is the appropriate measure of central tendency.
2. It is very easy to compute.
3. The mode is least affected by outliers.

Limitations of the Mode

1. Although the mode is a measure of central tendency, it does not actually represent the group of scores.
2. It is considered to be the crudest measure of central tendency.
3. The mode may not be unique in a dataset. There may be more than one mode in a distribution.
4. If no value is repeated twice in the dataset, then every score is the mode, which is useless.
5. The mode cannot be used for any algebraic manipulation.

2.8 COMPARISON OF THE MEAN, MEDIAN, AND MODE

Of the three measures of central tendency, the mean is most frequently used for data measured on an interval or ratio scale, provided the data are symmetrical or nearly symmetrical. The standard error of the mean is least compared to that of the median and mode, and therefore it is the most reliable measure of central tendency. It is very frequently used in advanced statistics.

The median is a positional value and its calculation is based on the ordinal properties of the data. However, even if the data are measured on interval or ratio scale, and if the distribution is highly skewed (positive or negative) or truncated, the median is the better choice in comparison to the mean. Further, the median is usually limited to descriptive use in statistical work.

The mode is seldom used. It is very easy to compute, but at the same time it is very unstable. However, if the data are measured on a nominal scale, the mode is

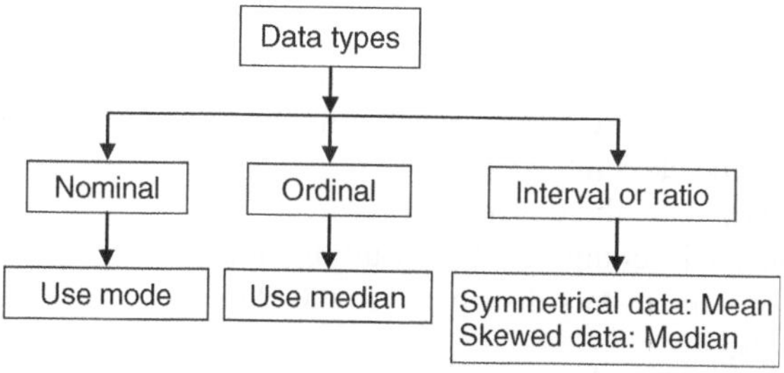

Figure 2.1 Use of different measures of central tendency according to the data types.

the best measure of central tendency. Suitability of different measures of central tendency under different data types has been shown in Figure 2.1.

Check Your Progress

Note: Tick the correct answer by using the sign ($\surd$).

	True	False
1. Raw scores are compiled scores.	-	-
2. A variable may be quantitative or qualitative.	-	-
3. An independent variable is the one that an experimenter cannot manipulate.	-	-
4. The mean is a positional average.	-	-
5. A single score refers to a whole number or integer score.	-	-
6. A dependent variable is the one that is affected by the changes in the independent variable.	-	-
7. The mean can be computed for data measured on a nominal scale.	-	-
8. A continuous variable can take values within a certain range.	-	-
9. Attributes refer to qualitative characteristics.	-	-
10. A discrete variable can assume fractional values also.	-	-
11. If data are presented in the form of a frequency distribution, the identity of individual scores is lost.	-	-
12. Nominal data refer to ranked data.	-	-
13. Ordinal data are also known as metric data.	-	-
14. The mean is a parametric statistic.	-	-
15. Nominal data are also known as categorical data.	-	-

16.	The median is a parametric statistic.	-	-
17.	The median is based on the assumption that the frequencies are concentrated at the mid-point of the class intervals.	-	-
18.	In interval data, there is no real zero.	-	-
19.	The mean is computed by assuming that the scores are evenly distributed in the class intervals.	-	-
20.	If a constant number b is added to all the scores, the new mean will be b plus the old mean.	-	-
21.	The median is a weighted average.	-	-
22.	In ratio data, the doubling principle holds.	-	-
23.	If the class intervals are continuous, the lowest limit of the class 15.5–20.5 is 15.5.	-	-
24.	The mean can be computed for ordinal data.	-	-
25.	Ratio data are obtained by measuring any phenomenon in an objective manner.	-	-
26.	In continuous class intervals, the lowest limit of the class 20–25 is 19.5.	-	-
27.	The mode can be computed for ratio data.	-	-
28.	The sum of the deviations of all the scores from their mean is a positive number.	-	-
29.	The mean is affected by the change of origin but is independent of the scale.	-	-
30.	The standard error of the mean is least compared to that of the other measures of central tendency.	-	-
31.	The mean may be computed even if the class interval is truncated at one end.	-	-
32.	To find the brand popularity of sports shoes among athletes, the median should be computed.	-	-
33.	The median can be computed for interval data.	-	-
34.	In discrete class intervals, the lowest limit of the class 21–25 is 20.5.	-	-
35.	If the ratio data are skewed, the median is the best measure of central tendency.	-	-
36.	In a symmetrical distribution, the values of the mean, median, and mode are the same.	-	-
37.	The median class indicates that the median lies immediately after this class.	-	-

38. If the data are symmetrical and measured on an interval scale, then the mean is the best measure of central tendency.	-	-
39. The standard error of the median is less than that of the mean.	-	-
40. Outliers affect the mode.	-	-
41. The median is the best measure of central tendency in case of ordinal data.	-	-
42. In skewed data, the mean is the best measure of central location.	-	-
43. The mode is appropriate for categorical data.	-	-
44. The mode is difficult to compute for ordinal, interval, or ratio datasets.	-	-
45. The mean should be calculated if outliers are present in the dataset.	-	-
46. The modal class is the one in which the frequency is least.	-	-

PRACTICE EXERCISE

1. Compute the mean and median for the following data:

12	16	15	18	20	19	8	22	7

2. Find the mode for the following data:

23	26	25	28	27	27	32	34	27

3. Compute the mean, median, and mode for the following data:

25	65	68	72	29	45	34	38	43
44	56	29	47	55	51	48	29	45

4. Find the mean of the following scores and also compute it by changing the origin by subtracting 50 from each score. Test whether these two means are the same.

10	20	30	40	50	60	70	80	90

5. Find the mean of the following data and compute it by changing their scale by dividing each score by 10. Check whether the two means are the same.

5	10	15	20	25	30	35	40	45

6. The chin-up scores of eight athletes are 13, 9, 16, 8, 12, 11, 14, and 20. Compute the median.
7. If the mean is 34 and the median is 40, what would be the value of the mode?
8. The mean of 10 scores is computed as 38. Later it was found that two scores were wrongly read as 45 and 40 instead of 35 and 30. What would be the corrected mean if these wrong values are replaced by the corrected values?
9. Which measure of central tendency is the most appropriate for the data shown in each of the following frequency distributions?

a		b		c	
Scores	Frequency	Scores	Frequency	Scores	Frequency
1	25	1	11	1	0
2	4	2	10	2	5
3	12	3	9	3	4
4	9	4	8	4	3
5	7	5	5	5	5
6	5	6	8	6	1
7	0	7	9	7	2
8	3	8	10	8	2
9	14	9	11	9	17

Example 2.4 Given the set of data x: 4, 8, 6, 12, 8, 11, and 7. Calculate the mean, median, and mode.

Solution:

x:	4	8	6	12	8	11	7

Calculation of the Mean: Here, $n = 7$ and $\sum x = 56$

$$\text{Mean} = \bar{x} = \frac{\sum x}{n} = \frac{56}{7} = 8$$

Calculation of the Median:

After Arranging the Scores x:	4	6	7	8	8	11	12

$$\text{Median} = M_d = \left(\frac{N+1}{2}\right)\text{th score}$$

$$= \left(\frac{7+1}{2}\right)\text{th score}$$

$$= \text{4th score} = 8$$

Calculation of Mode:

$$\because \text{Mode} = 3\ \text{Median} - 2\ \text{Mean}$$

After substituting the values of the mean and median,

$$\text{Mode} = 3 \times 8 - 2 \times 8 = 8$$

Example 2.5 The following table shows the distribution of scores on the shooting accuracy of 51 basketball players. Compute the mean, median, and mode of the distribution.

Distribution of Scores on Shooting Accuracy

Shooting Accuracy	Frequency
0–3	8
3–6	6
6–9	7
9–12	9
12–15	11
15–18	5
18–21	3
21–24	2

Solution: Since the data are given in the class interval form, the deviation method is used to compute the value of the mean. In computing the mean, median, and mode, it is required to find the values $\sum f$ and $\sum fd$. These computations are shown in the following table.

Computation Table for the Mean, Median, and Mode for the Data on Shooting Accuracy

	Class Interval (Shooting Score) (1)	Frequency (f) (2)	CF (F) (3)	Midpoint (X) (4)	$d = \frac{X-10.5}{3}$ (5)	fd (6)
	0 – 3	8	8	1.5	−3	−24
	3 – 6	6	14	4.5	−2	−12
	6 – 9	7	21	7.5	−1	−7
Median class →	9 – 12	9	30	10.5	0	0
Modal class →	12 – 15	11	41	13.5	1	11
	15 – 18	5	46	16.5	2	10
	18 – 21	3	49	19.5	3	9
	21 – 24	2	51	22.5	4	8
		$n = 51$				$\Sigma fd = -5$

Computation of the mean Here, there are eight class intervals and therefore either of the two middle class intervals can be selected for finding the AM. The class interval 9–12 is selected to find the AM. The midpoint of this class interval is 10.5, hence the assumed mean, AM = 10.5 and the width of the class interval $i = 3$. Further, summing the values in columns 2 and 6 gives the values of n and $\sum fd$.

Substituting the values of AM, $\sum fd$, n, and i in the formula, the mean becomes

$$\text{Mean} = \overline{X} = \text{AM} + \frac{\sum fd}{n} \times i$$

$$= 10.5 + \frac{(-5)}{51} \times 3$$

$$= 10.21 \approx 10$$

Computation of the median The median class needs to be identified before computing the value of median. To do so, the cumulative frequencies have been calculated in column 3 as shown in the above table. Since $n = 51$,

$$\frac{n}{2} = \frac{51}{2} = 25.5$$

Since the cumulative frequency of the class interval 9–12 includes the value 25.5, this is the median class. After locating the median class, the different values are as follows:

Lower limit of the median class, LL = 9
Frequency of the median class, $f_m = 9$
Cumulative frequency of the class just before the median class, $F = 21$
Width of the class interval, $i = 3$

Substituting these values in the formula

$$M_d = \text{LL} + \frac{\frac{N}{2} - F}{f_m} \times i$$

$$= 9 + \frac{25.5 - 21}{9} \times 3 = 9 + 1.5 = 10.5 \approx 11$$

Computation of the mode The modal class needs to be identified first before computing the mode. Here, the class interval 12–15, which has the maximum frequency, is the modal class.

For the modal class 12–15,

Lower limit of the modal class, LL = 12
Frequency of the modal class, $f_m = 11$
Frequency of the class just before the modal class, $f_1 = 9$
Frequency of the class just after the modal class, $f_2 = 5$
Width of the class interval, $i = 3$

Substituting these values in the formula, we get

$$M_0 = \text{LL} + \frac{f_m - f_1}{2f_m - f_1 - f_2} \times i$$

$$= 12 + \frac{11 - 9}{2 \times 11 - 9 - 5} \times 2$$

$$= 12 + 0.5$$

$$= 12.5 \approx 13$$

2.9 MEASURES OF VARIABILITY

A measure of variability can be defined as an index that measures the variability of scores. In the previous section, a detailed discussion was made about the measures of central tendency but that

> **FACTS TO KNOW**
>
> A measure of variability refers to the variation of scores around their average value

alone does not explain the characteristics of a distribution correctly. This is because an average index gives only an idea about the central location of the distribution of scores but does not tell us anything as to how the scores are distributed around the average value of the scores. Consider the following two sets of measurement on x and y:

x:	5	7	9	11	13
y:	1	5	9	13	17

In both x and y series, the mean values are same, that is, 9. But the series y seems to vary more than x around the mean value 9. In other words, series x is more consistent than y. Thus, the two series may have same mean but may differ in their variations about the central value. In order to measure the magnitude of variation among scores in a series about any central value, an index, which is known as measure of variability, is required.

Thus, to have a better idea about the nature of the distribution, one requires both a measure of central tendency and a measure of variability. In general, there are four measures of variability, which are discussed in this section.

2.9.1 The Range

The range is the crudest measure of variability. It provides the maximum variation in the dataset and does not provide the information about the internal variation of the scores. It is therefore computed when the information about the maximum variation of scores within the dataset is required. For example, one may be interested in knowing the maximum variation of height among the players in a tournament or one may want to know the maximum variation of marks obtained by the students in a class. Since range measures the maximum variation among the scores in the distribution, it is used in constructing class intervals from the raw scores. Since it depends on two scores only, it is the most unstable measure of variability. The range is obtained by the following formula:

$$\text{Range} = \text{Maximum score} - \text{Minimum score}$$

Consider the following scores x : 7, 16, 47, 19, 12, 36, 42, and 51. For this dataset, the minimum score is 7 and maximum score is 51; therefore, the range would be

$$\text{Range} = 51 - 7 = 44$$

The range is very sensitive toward the outliers. For instance, if in the above set of scores, 51 is replaced by 121, then the range will become $121 - 7 = 114$. Thus, you can see by changing one score only, the range has changed from 44 to 114. Since the range depends only on the two extreme scores, it is the most unstable measure of variability.

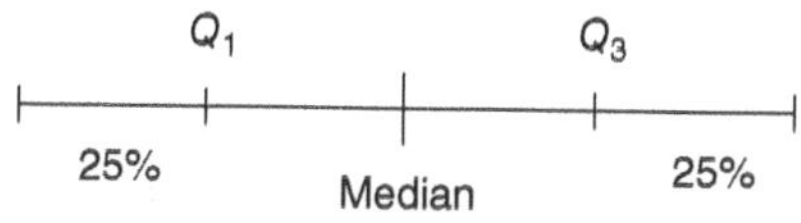

Figure 2.2 The graphical positions of Q_1 and Q_3.

2.9.2 The Quartile Deviation (QD)

The QD is a measure of variability that measures the variation of the middle 50% of the scores around median value. The QD is a nonparametric statistic and is computed in a situation where the scores are measured on an ordinal scale. However, it can be computed for the interval as well as ratio data. For any dataset, if the median is the best measure of central tendency, then the QD is the best measure of variability. Since QD is calculated on the basis of the first and third quartiles, it is not affected by the change in the first 25% and the last 25% of the data in the distribution. For this reason, it is least affected by the outliers. Thus, if the effect of the extreme scores is to be avoided, the QD is the better measure of variability. Since QD measures the variation of the middle 50% of the scores around the median value, it is considered to be the better measure of variability in comparison to the range. The QD is computed by the following formula:

$$\text{QD} = \frac{Q_3 - Q_1}{2} \tag{2.8}$$

where Q_1 and Q_3 are the first and third quartiles. By definition, if the scores are arranged in ascending order, Q_1 is the point in the distribution that has 25% of the scores below it and similarly Q_3 is the point that has 75% of the scores below it. These are illustrated in Figure 2.2.

Quartile Deviation for Ungrouped Data The QD is calculated on the basis of Q_1 and Q_3; hence, the procedure for computing these quartiles is discussed first. Since Q_1 is the score below which 25% of the scores in the distribution lies, it is computed by the formula

$$Q_1 = \left(\frac{N+1}{4}\right) \text{th score} \tag{2.9}$$

On the other hand, Q_3 is the score below which 75% of the scores in the distribution lies, hence it is computed as

$$Q_3 = \left(\frac{3\,(N+1)}{4}\right) \text{th score} \tag{2.10}$$

Consider the following series of scores x : 3, 6, 2, 12, 16, 18, 9, and 20. To compute Q_1 and Q_3, let us first arrange the scores in ascending order:

x:	2	3	6	9	12	16	18	20

Here, $N = 8$.

Q_1 is computed as

$$
\begin{aligned}
Q_1 &= \left(\frac{8+1}{4}\right)\text{th score} \\
&= 2.25\text{th score} \\
&= \text{2nd score} + \frac{1}{4}\,(\text{3rd score} - \text{2nd score}) \\
&= 3 + \frac{1}{4}(6-3) \\
&= 3.75
\end{aligned}
$$

Q_3 is computed as

$$
\begin{aligned}
Q_3 &= \left(\frac{3\,(N+1)}{4}\right)\text{th score} \\
&= \left(\frac{3\,(8+1)}{4}\right)\text{th} = 6.75\text{th score} \\
&= \text{6th score} + \frac{3}{4}(\text{7th score} - \text{6th score}) \\
&= 16 + \frac{3}{4}(18-16) \\
&= 17.5
\end{aligned}
$$

Thus, the QD is

$$
\begin{aligned}
\text{QD} &= \frac{Q_3 - Q_1}{2} \\
&= \frac{17.5 - 3.75}{2} \\
&= 6.875
\end{aligned}
$$

Quartile Deviation for Grouped Data QD can also be computed for grouped data. Since the QD depends on the values of Q_1 and Q_3, these quartiles need to be computed first. To obtain the values of Q_1 and Q_3, the class intervals need to be identified first and then by using formulas (2.11) and (2.12), respectively, these values can be calculated.

The first quartile Q_1 is obtained by the formula

$$
Q_1 = \text{LL} + \frac{\frac{N}{4} - F}{f_1} \times i \qquad (2.11)
$$

where

LL = lower limit of the Q_1 class
N = frequency total
F = cumulative frequency of the class interval just lower than the Q_1 class
f_1 = frequency of the Q_1 class
i = width of the class interval

Similarly, the third quartile is computed as

$$Q_3 = \text{LL} + \frac{\frac{3N}{4} - F}{f_3} \times i \qquad (2.12)$$

where

LL = lower limit of the Q_3 class
N = frequency total
F = cumulative frequency of the class interval just lower than the Q_3 class
f_3 = frequency of the Q_3 class
i = width of the class interval

The procedure for the computation of the QD in case of grouped data is discussed with the help of the following example.

Consider the distribution of runs scored by the players in a cricket tournament as shown in Table 2.12. The QD can be computed by going through the following steps described:

Steps for calculating the quartile deviation

1. Arrange the class intervals and their corresponding frequencies in columns 1 and 2, respectively, as shown in Table 2.12.

TABLE 2.12 Calculation of the QD for the Distribution of Scores in a Cricket Tournament

	Class Interval (1)	f_i (2)	Cum. Frequency (F) (3)
	1 – 10	2	2
	11 – 20	4	6
Q_1 class →	21 – 30	6	12
	31 – 40	8	20
	41 – 50	5	25
Q_3 class →	51 – 60	6	31
	61 – 70	2	33
	71 – 80	4	37
	81 – 90	3	40
	91 – 100	1	41
		$N = 41$	

2. In column 3, find the cumulative frequencies. Total the frequencies in column 2 to get the value of N.
3. For Q_1, find the value of $N/4$. In this case, it is $41/4 = 10.25$. Look for the value 10.25 in column 3. The class interval for which the cumulative frequency includes 10.25 is the Q_1 class. Here, the cumulative frequency of the class interval 21–30 is 12, which includes 10.25; hence, this is the Q_1 class.
4. Once the Q_1 class is identified, substitute the values of LL, f_1, F, and i in formula (2.11) to calculate the value of Q_1.
5. Similarly, for Q_3, find the value of $3\,N/4$. In this case, it is $123/4 = 30.75$. Look for this value 30.75 in column 3. The class interval for which the cumulative frequency includes 30.75 is the Q_3 class. Here, the cumulative frequency of the class interval 51–60 is 31, which includes 30.75; hence, this is the Q_3 class.
6. Once the Q_3 class is identified, substitute the values of LL, f_3, F, and i in formula (2.12) to calculate the value of Q_3.
7. After computing the values of Q_1 and Q_3, compute the QD by using formula (2.8).

Computation of Q_1: Here, the class interval 21–30 is the Q_1 class; hence, $\text{LL} = 20.5, f_1 = 6, F = 6$, and $i = 10$.

Substituting these values in formula (2.11)

$$Q_1 = \text{LL} + \frac{\frac{N}{4} - F}{f_1} \times i$$

$$= 20.5 + \frac{\frac{41}{4} - 6}{6} \times 10$$

$$= 20.5 + 7.08$$

$$= 27.58$$

Computation of Q_3: Here, the class interval 51–60 is the Q_3 class; hence, $\text{LL} = 50.5, f_3 = 6, F = 25$, and $i = 10$

Substituting these values in formula (2.12)

$$Q_3 = \text{LL} + \frac{\frac{3N}{4} - F}{f_3} \times i$$

$$= 50.5 + \frac{\frac{3 \times 41}{4} - 25}{6} \times 10$$

$$= 50.5 + 9.58$$

$$= 60.08$$

Computation of the QD

Therefore, $$\text{QD} = \frac{Q_3 - Q_1}{2}$$

Substituting the values of Q_1 and Q_3

$$\text{QD} = \frac{60.08 - 27.58}{2} = 16.25$$

Properties of Quartile Deviation

1. It is easy to calculate.
2. Since QD measures the variation of the middle 50% of the scores around the median value of the distribution, it is a better measure of variability compared to the range.
3. If the data are obtained on the ordinal scale, QD is the best measure of variability.

Drawback of the Quartile Deviation

1. The QD is not a stable measure of variability as it is significantly affected by sampling fluctuation.
2. It does not tell us anything about 50% of the distribution.
3. It is not suitable for algebraic manipulation.

2.9.3 The Mean Deviation

The mean deviation (MD) is another measure of variability that depends on the absolute deviation of scores from any average value. It is a better measure of variability compared to the range as it depends on all the scores. The MD about the mean is computed by the following formula:

$$[\text{MD}]_{\text{mean}} = \frac{1}{n}\sum |x - M| \tag{2.13}$$

where n is the sample size and M is the sample mean. Here, the absolute deviation is taken to compute the MD because of the fact that $\sum(x - M)$ is always zero.

Similarly, the MD about the median and mode are given by formulas (2.14) and (2.15), respectively.

$$[\text{MD}]_{\text{median}} = \frac{1}{n}\sum |x - M_{\text{d}}| \tag{2.14}$$

$$[\text{MD}]_{\text{mode}} = \frac{1}{n}\sum |x - M_{\text{o}}| \tag{2.15}$$

TABLE 2.13 Calculation of the Mean Deviation about the Mean

x	$x-M$	$\lvert x-M\rvert$
36	15	15
28	7	7
32	11	11
22	1	1
16	−5	5
24	3	3
21	0	0
10	−11	11
12	−9	9
9	−12	12
$\sum x = 210$		$\sum \lvert x-M\rvert = 74$

Mean Deviation for Ungrouped Data The MD of ungrouped data can be computed by first computing the average around which the MD is required to be computed. The procedure is illustrated by means of the dataset shown in Table 2.13.

Steps for computing the mean deviation

1. Arrange the scores in the first column.
2. Calculate the mean (M) by dividing the total $\sum x$ by the number of scores n.
3. Calculate the deviation of scores from its calculated mean M in column 2.
4. In column 3, convert the difference into absolute difference $\lvert x-M\rvert$. In doing so, all the negative scores in column 2 are converted into positive scores in column 3.
5. Calculate the total of absolute deviation, that is, $\Sigma\lvert x-M\rvert = 74$.
6. Use formula (2.13) to compute the MD about the mean.
   Here, the number of scores $n = 10$

$$M = \frac{\sum x}{n} = \frac{210}{10} = 21$$

$$[\mathrm{MD}]_{\mathrm{mean}} = \frac{1}{n}\sum \lvert x-M\rvert$$

$$= \frac{74}{10} = 7.4$$

Mean Deviation for Grouped Data If the scores $x_1, x_2, \ldots, x_n$ occur with frequencies $f_1, f_2, \ldots, f_n$, then the MD around the mean can be computed by formula (2.16)

$$[\text{MD}]_{\text{mean}} = \frac{1}{n}\sum f|x - M| \tag{2.16}$$

where n is the total number of scores in the dataset and M is the mean.

Similarly, the MD about the median and mode can be computed from grouped data by using formulas (2.17) and (2.18), respectively,

$$[\text{MD}]_{\text{median}} = \frac{1}{n}\sum f|x - M_{\text{d}}| \tag{2.17}$$

$$[\text{MD}]_{\text{mode}} = \frac{1}{n}\sum f|x - M_{\text{o}}| \tag{2.18}$$

where M_{d} and M_{o} represent the median and mode, respectively. The procedure for computing the MD about the mean has been shown by using the following data:

Sit-Ups Score:	1–5	6–10	11–15	16–20	21–25	26–30	31–35	36–40	41–45	46–50
Frequencies (f):	1	4	2	6	3	9	4	6	2	3

Steps for computing

1. Write the class intervals and their frequencies in columns 1 and 2, respectively, as shown in Table 2.14.
2. In column 3, find the midpoint (x) of the class intervals.

TABLE 2.14 Calculation of Mean Deviation for the Distribution of Sit-Ups Scores

CI (1)	f (2)	x (3)	d (4)	fd (5)	$x - M$ (6)	$\|x - M\|$ (7)	$f\|x - M\|$ (8)
1–5	1	3	−5	−5	−24	24	24
6–10	4	8	−4	−16	−19	19	76
11–15	2	13	−3	−6	−14	14	28
16–20	6	18	−2	−12	−9	9	54
21–25	3	23	−1	−3	−4	4	12
26–30	9	28	0	0	1	1	9
31–35	4	33	1	4	6	6	24
36–40	6	38	2	12	11	11	66
41–45	2	43	3	6	16	16	32
46–50	3	48	4	12	21	21	63
	$n = 40$			$\sum fd = -8$			$f\|x - M\| = 388$

3. In column 4, find the deviation by taking the AM as the midpoint of the middlemost class interval. In case of even number of class intervals, AM can be taken from any of the two middlemost class intervals. Here, the AM is taken as 28. For detail discussion in computing d values, refer to the computation of the mean with grouped data.
4. In column 5, find the value of fd by multiplying the entries of columns 2 and 4.
5. Compute the mean (M) by using the formula for grouped data.
6. In column 6, find the deviation of scores x from the mean value M.
7. In column 7, find the absolute deviation by converting all the negative scores of column 6 into positive scores. The positive scores will remain as they are.
8. In column 8, find $f|x - M|$ for all the class intervals by multiplying the entries of columns 2 and 7.
9. Substitute the values of n and $\sum f|x - M|$ in formula (2.16) to compute the MD about the mean.

For computing the MD about the mean, it is required to compute the mean value first.

Here, $n = 40$, AM $= 28$, $i = 5$, and $\sum fd = -8$.

Thus,

$$M = \text{AM} + \frac{\sum fd}{n} \times i$$

$$= 28 + \frac{-8}{40} \times 5 = 27$$

After substituting the value of $\sum f|x - M|$ and n in formula (2.16), we get

$$[\text{MD}]_{\text{mean}} = \frac{1}{n}\sum f|x - M| = \frac{1}{40} \times 388$$

$$= 9.7$$

Remark The MD around median and mode can also be computed by using the above procedure. The only difference is that instead of the mean, the median or mode may be used for calculating the deviation.

Properties of the Mean Deviation

1. The MD is a better measure of absolute variability as it is computed from all the scores.
2. The MD is more efficient in assessing the variability compared to the range and QD.

Drawbacks of the Mean Deviation Since MD is computed by taking the absolute deviation of the scores from any of the measures of central tendency, it creates artificiality and so it is not used in statistical inference.

The MD is thus rarely used. It is not readily amenable to algebraic manipulation because no logical reason is assigned to convert the deviation of scores from their mean into absolute deviation. In order to overcome this problem, a better measure of variability is defined by taking the square of the deviations. This measure is known as the *standard deviation*. In general, in statistical work, the use of absolute values should be avoided as far as possible.

2.9.4 The Standard Deviation

The standard deviation is the positive square root of the average deviations of all scores in the dataset around their mean value. It measures the variability of scores around the mean value of the distribution. The standard deviation is calculated for the data measured on the interval or ratio scale. The standard deviation is used as a measure of variability in a situation where the mean is the best measure of central tendency. It is the most efficient and widely used measure of variability because it takes into account every score in the dataset. Among all the measures of variability, the standard deviation is the most stable measure, and thus it is widely used in statistical inference. The standard deviation is small if scores in the dataset are tightly bunched together and relatively large if they are wide apart. The square of the standard deviation is known as the *variance*. Instead of the standard deviation, the variance is normally used in defining different distributions. The standard deviation is represented by the Greek letter σ (termed *sigma*) and is computed by the following formula:

$$\sigma = \sqrt{\frac{1}{N}\sum (X-\mu)^2}$$

where N is the number of scores in the dataset and μ is the mean of the dataset. This formula can be simplified by expanding the expression.

Thus,

$$\sigma = \sqrt{\frac{1}{N}\sum (X^2+\mu^2-2\mu X)}$$

$$= \sqrt{\frac{1}{N}\sum X^2 + \frac{\sum \mu^2}{N} - 2\mu\frac{\sum X}{N}}$$

$$= \sqrt{\frac{1}{N}\sum X^2 + \mu^2 - 2\mu^2}$$

$$= \sqrt{\frac{1}{N}\sum X^2 - \mu^2}$$

$$\Rightarrow \quad \sigma = \sqrt{\frac{1}{N}\sum X^2 - \left(\frac{\sum X}{N}\right)^2} \tag{2.19}$$

The term σ is used for population standard deviation, whereas S is used for the sample standard deviation.

The sample standard deviation S can be estimated from the sample data by the following formula:

$$S = \sqrt{\frac{1}{n-1}\sum (X - \overline{X})^2}$$

After simplifying,

$$S = \sqrt{\frac{1}{n-1}\sum X^2 - \frac{\left(\sum X\right)^2}{n(n-1)}} \tag{2.20}$$

If $X_1, X_2, X_3, \ldots, X_n$ are the n scores with $f_1, f_2, f_3, \ldots, f_n$ frequencies, respectively, then the standard deviation is given by

$$\sigma = \sqrt{\frac{1}{N}\sum f(X - \mu)^2}$$

After simplification,

$$\sigma = \sqrt{\frac{1}{N}\sum fX^2 - \left(\frac{\sum fX}{N}\right)^2} \tag{2.21}$$

Standard Deviation for Ungrouped Data The standard deviation for ungrouped data can be computed by using formula (2.20). The computation is shown by means of the data in Table 2.15, which represent the number of goals made by eight soccer teams in a tournament. The following steps are used to compute the standard deviation.

Steps for computing

1. Arrange the scores in column 1 as show in Table 2.15.
2. Calculate the square of each score in column 2.
3. Find the totals in columns 1 and 2 to get the sums $\sum x$ and $\sum x^2$, respectively.
4. Substitute the values in formula (2.20) to get the value of the standard deviation σ.
5. If the scores are given along with their frequencies, then find the sums $\sum fx$ and $\sum fx^2$ and substitute these values in formula (2.21) to compute the standard deviation.

TABLE 2.15 Number of Goals by the Soccer Teams

x	x^2
19	361
17	289
16	256
12	144
5	25
3	9
6	36
2	4
$\sum x = 80$	$\sum x^2 = 1124$

Here, $N = 8$, $\sum x = 80$, $\sum x^2 = 1124$.
Substituting these values in formula (2.18),

$$\sigma = \sqrt{\frac{1}{N}\sum X^2 - \left(\frac{\sum X}{N}\right)^2}$$

$$= \sqrt{\frac{1124}{8} - \left(\frac{80}{8}\right)^2}$$

$$= \sqrt{140.5 - 100}$$

$$= 6.36$$

Remark The above standard deviation has been computed by taking the number of scores as N. However, the sample standard deviation can be computed by taking the sample size $n-1$ and using formula (2.20).

Standard Deviation for Grouped Data The computation of the standard deviation can be done for grouped data by using the deviation method. In this method, the scores x are transformed into d by changing the origin and scale. Usually, the origin is taken as the midpoint of the middlemost class interval and the scale as the width of the class interval. Thus, the formula for computing the standard deviation by using the deviation method is given by

$$\sigma = i \times \sqrt{\frac{1}{N}\sum fd^2 - \left(\frac{\sum fd}{N}\right)^2} \tag{2.22}$$

where

d = deviation of score from the AM divided by the width of the class interval (i)
f = frequency of the class interval

N = sample size
i = width of the class interval

The procedure for computing the standard deviation is discussed by considering the data in Table 2.16, which represent the scores on modified push-ups. The following steps are used to compute the standard deviation by using the deviation method.

Steps for computing

1. Arrange the class intervals and their corresponding frequencies in columns 1 and 2, respectively.
2. Find the midpoint of the class intervals in column 3.
3. Take the value of the AM as the midpoint of the middlemost class interval and i as the width of the class intervals. Here, the value of AM is 53 and the value of i is 5. If the number of class intervals are even, there will be two middlemost class intervals. In that case, AM may be the midpoint of either of the two class intervals.
4. Find the value of d in column 4 by subtracting the value of AM from x and divide by the value of i.
5. In column 5, find the value of fd by multiplying the entries of columns 2 and 4.
6. Find the value of fd^2 by multiplying the entries of columns 4 and 5.
7. Add up the entries in columns 2, 5, and 6 to get the values of N, $\sum fd$, and $\sum fd^2$, respectively.
8. Substitute the values of N, $\sum fd$, and $\sum fd^2$ in formula (2.22) to compute the value of the standard deviation.

TABLE 2.16 Computation of the Standard Deviation for the Scores on Modified Push-Ups

Class Interval (1)	f (2)	x (3)	$d = \frac{x-AM}{i}$ (4)	fd (5)	fd^2 (6)
26–30	1	28	−5	−5	25
31–35	2	33	−4	−8	32
36–40	3	38	−3	−9	27
41–45	5	43	−2	−10	20
46–50	4	48	−1	−4	4
51–55	5	53	0	0	0
56–60	2	58	1	2	2
61–65	5	63	2	10	20
66–70	4	68	3	12	36
71–75	6	73	4	24	96
76–80	3	78	5	15	75
	$N = 40$			$\sum fd = 27$	$\sum fd^2 = 337$

Here, $N = 40$, $\sum fd = 27$, and $\sum fd^2 = 337$. Substituting these values in formula (2.22),

$$\sigma = i \times \sqrt{\frac{1}{N}\sum fd^2 - \left(\frac{\sum fd}{N}\right)^2}$$

$$= 5 \times \sqrt{\frac{337}{40} - \left(\frac{27}{40}\right)^2}$$

$$= 5 \times \sqrt{8.425 - 0.456}$$

$$= 14.11$$

Effect of Change of Origin and Scale on Standard Deviation Let us see what happens to the value of the standard deviation if a number A is subtracted from all the scores x and simultaneously divided by the number i. In other words, what would be the impact on the standard deviation if the scores x are transformed to d by changing its origin and scale. Let the scores x be transformed to d by using the following transformation:

$$d = \frac{x - A}{i}$$

$$\Rightarrow \quad x = A + i \times d$$

where A is the origin and i is the scale. By taking summation on both sides and dividing by N, we get

$$\frac{1}{N}\sum x = \frac{1}{N}\sum A + i \times \frac{1}{N}\sum d$$

$$\Rightarrow \quad \bar{x} = A + i \times \bar{d}$$

Since

$$\sigma_x = \sqrt{\frac{1}{N}\sum f(x - \bar{x})^2}$$

let us compute

$$x - \bar{x} = A + i \times d - (A + i \times \bar{d}) = i \times (d - \bar{d})$$

Substituting the value of $(x - \bar{x})$, we get

$$\sigma_x = \sqrt{\frac{1}{N}\sum i^2 f(d - \bar{d})^2} = i \times \sqrt{\frac{1}{N}\sum f(d - \bar{d})^2}$$

$$\Rightarrow \quad \sigma_x = i \times \sigma_d \tag{2.23}$$

From equation (2.23), it may be concluded that the standard deviation is free from change of origin but is affected by the change of scale. The original standard deviation can be obtained by multiplying the new standard deviation by the scale value.

Example 2.6 What would be the impact of subtracting number 10 from the following series of scores on the standard deviation?

X:	4	6	8	10	12	15	20

Solution: Let us transform the scores x into u by using the transformation $u = x - 10$.

Computation of the Standard Deviation

x	x^2	$u = x - 10$	u^2
4	16	−6	36
6	36	−4	16
8	64	−2	4
10	100	0	0
12	144	2	4
15	225	5	25
20	400	10	100
$\sum x = 75$	$\sum x^2 = 985$	$\sum u = 5$	$\sum u^2 = 185$

In order to see the impact of change of origin on the standard deviation, the standard deviation of x and u is computed. Here, $N = 7$.

The standard deviation of x is equal to

$$\sigma_x = \sqrt{\frac{1}{N}\sum x^2 - \left(\frac{\sum x}{N}\right)^2}$$

$$= \sqrt{\frac{985}{7} - \left(\frac{75}{7}\right)^2}$$

$$= \sqrt{140.71 - 114.70}$$

$$= 5.1$$

The standard deviation of u is equal to

$$\sigma_u = \sqrt{\frac{1}{N}\sum u^2 - \left(\frac{\sum u}{N}\right)^2}$$

$$= \sqrt{\frac{185}{7} - \left(\frac{5}{7}\right)^2}$$

$$= \sqrt{26.43 - 0.51}$$

$$= 5.1$$

Thus,

$$\sigma_x = \sigma_u$$

Since the standard deviation of x and u are same, it may be concluded that there is no change in the standard deviation if 10 is subtracted from all the scores. In other words, change of origin has no impact on the standard deviation.

Example 2.7 What would be the impact on standard deviation if the following series of scores is divided by a constant number 10?

X:	10	20	30	40	50	60

Solution: The scores x after transforming into v obtained by dividing 10 are shown in the following table.

Computation of the Standard Deviation

x	x^2	$v = x/10$	v^2
10	100	1	1
20	400	2	4
30	900	3	9
40	1600	4	16
50	2500	5	25
60	3600	6	36
$\sum x = 210$	$\sum x^2 = 9100$	$\sum v = 21$	$\sum v^2 = 91$

The effect of dividing the scores by 10 on the standard deviation can be studied after computing the standard deviation of both the variables x and v.

The standard deviation of x is equal to

$$\sigma_x = \sqrt{\frac{1}{N}\sum x^2 - \left(\frac{\sum x}{N}\right)^2}$$

$$= \sqrt{\frac{9100}{6} - \left(\frac{210}{6}\right)^2}$$

$$= \sqrt{1516.67 - 1225}$$

$$= 17.08$$

The standard deviation of v is equal to

$$\sigma_v = \sqrt{\frac{1}{N}\sum v^2 - \left(\frac{\sum v}{N}\right)^2}$$

$$= \sqrt{\frac{91}{6} - \left(\frac{21}{6}\right)^2}$$

$$= \sqrt{15.17 - 12.25}$$

$$= 1.708$$

Thus,

$$\sigma_x = 10 \times \sigma_v$$

It is therefore concluded that if all the scores are divided by a constant number 10, then the new standard deviation is also reduced to one-tenth of the original standard deviation. In other words, the standard deviation is affected by the change of scale.

Properties of Standard Deviation

1. The standard deviation is the most suitable measure of variability if the scores are measured on the interval or ratio scale.
2. The standard deviation is the most reliable measure of variability because it is computed on the basis of all the scores.
3. It is the most stable measure of variability because it fluctuates less from sample to sample in a sampling distribution compared to other measures of variability.
4. Since no algebraic manipulation is done as in the case of MD, it does not create any artificiality in its calculation.
5. It is not affected by the change of origin but is affected by the change of scale.

Grouping Error While computing statistics from grouped data, we assume that the frequencies are concentrated at the midpoint of the class intervals. Owing to this, an error is committed in calculating the standard deviation of grouped data. This error is known as the *grouping error*. Owing to this error, the calculated standard deviation from grouped data is somewhat greater than what it actually should be. To correct this error, a formula was given by Sheppard, commonly known as *Sheppard's correction*.

$$\sigma_c = \sqrt{\sigma^2 - \frac{i^2}{12}} \tag{2.24}$$

where

σ_c = corrected standard deviation
σ = standard deviation obtained from the grouped data
i = width of the class interval.

2.9.5 Variance

The square of the standard deviation is known as the *variance*. It can be defined as the average deviation of scores around the mean value. Similar to standard deviation, it is also used as a measure of variability among the scores around the mean value. It measures the lack of consistency in the data. Higher variance indicates more heterogeneity, whereas lower variance indicates more homogeneity in the data. As with standard deviation, variance is also computed when the scores are measured on the interval or ratio scale. In fact, in all statistical distributions and statistical inferences, the mean and variance are widely used as the measures of central tendency and of variability. The variance is denoted by σ^2 and is computed as follows:

FACTS TO KNOW

Variation refers to the spread of scores around their mean value, whereas variance is the index used to measure it

$$\sigma^2 = \frac{1}{N}\sum(x-\mu)^2 \tag{2.25}$$

The population variance σ^2 can be estimated efficiently by the sample variance S^2, which is computed as follows:

$$S^2 = \frac{1}{n-1}\sum(x-\bar{x})^2$$

$$= \frac{1}{n-1}\sum x^2 - \frac{\left(\sum x\right)^2}{n(n-1)} \tag{2.26}$$

2.10 STANDARD ERROR

The standard error of any statistic can be defined as the standard deviation of that statistic in the sampling distribution. Standard error is a measure of sampling fluctuation of the statistic and is widely used in statistical inference. It measures how well a sample is a true representative of the population. The standard error is small in a homogeneous population and large in a heterogeneous population.

The standard error of any statistic is affected by the population standard deviation and the sample size. In general, the standard error decreases with an increase in sample size and a decrease in the population standard deviation. It is denoted by σ with a subscript of the statistic for which it is computed.

Let $\overline{x}_1, \overline{x}_2, \overline{x}_3, \ldots, \overline{x}_n$ be the means of n samples drawn from the same population. Then, the standard error of the sample mean can be computed by

$$\sigma_{\overline{x}} = \frac{\sigma}{\sqrt{n}} \tag{2.27}$$

where σ is the population standard deviation and n is the sample size. However, if the population standard deviation is not known, it may be estimated by computing S (sample standard deviation). In this case, the standard error of the sample mean is

$$\sigma_{\overline{x}} = \frac{S}{\sqrt{n}}$$

Similarly, the standard error of the sample standard deviation is given by the following formula:

$$\sigma_{s} = \frac{\sigma}{\sqrt{2n}} \tag{2.28}$$

Similar to the standard error of the mean, the standard error of the standard deviation also measures the fluctuation of standard deviations among the samples. In this case also, the estimate of σ, that is, S, can be used if the population standard deviation is unknown.

2.11 COEFFICIENT OF VARIATION

The coefficient of variation can be defined as an index that measures the variability of a dataset in relation to its mean value. The standard deviation is a measure of absolute variability, whereas the coefficient of variation measures relative variability. The coefficient of variation is free from units, and therefore it can be used to compare the variability of two groups of data having

FACTS TO KNOW

The mean and standard deviation are appropriate if the data are measured on at least the interval scale and are symmetric or nearly symmetric in nature

different units. Consider a situation in which we are interested in knowing whether the performance of college athletes is more consistent in a 100 m event or in long jump. In this case, units of the two events are different and therefore the coefficient of variation can be used to compare the variability of athletes in their performance in the 100 m event as well as in long jump. In this case, the standard deviation cannot be used to compare the variability of these two groups of data because their units are different. The coefficient of variation can also be used to compare the variability of two groups of data whose means are not equal. However, if the group means are equal, the standard deviation can be used to compare the variability, provided the data in both the groups have the same units.

Since the coefficient of variation is a relative measure of variability and it is measured in terms of percentage, it can be used to assess the variability of a single group as well. On the other hand, no conclusion can be drawn about the variability of a group on the basis of its standard deviation because it indicates the absolute variability.

The coefficient of variation, denoted by CV, is computed as

$$CV = \frac{S}{\bar{x}} \times 100 \tag{2.29}$$

where S is the sample standard deviation and $\bar{x}$ is the sample mean of the dataset.

Consider the mean and standard deviation of the two groups as shown in Table 2.17. Let us see how to compute the coefficient of variation of these two groups and interpret the findings.

$$\text{CV of group A} = \frac{S}{\bar{x}} \times 100 = \frac{4}{50} \times 100 = 8\%$$

$$\text{CV of group B} = \frac{S}{\bar{x}} \times 100 = \frac{5}{80} \times 100 = 6.25\%$$

Since the coefficient of variation for group A is greater than that of group B, it may be concluded that group A is more heterogeneous than group B. You may note that the standard deviation of group A is smaller than that of group B but the variability of group A is greater

> **FACTS TO KNOW**
>
> Median and QD are appropriate if the data are measured on an ordinal scale. They are also appropriate for metric data if the distribution is skewed

TABLE 2.17 Mean and Standard Deviation of the Groups

	Group A	Group B
$\bar{x}$	50	80
S	4	5

than that of group B. This situation has arisen because of the difference between the means of the groups A and B. Had the means of these two groups been equal, the variability could have been compared by using the values of the standard deviations.

2.12 ABSOLUTE AND RELATIVE VARIABILITY

The standard deviation measures absolute variability, whereas the coefficient of variation measures relative variability. The standard deviation alone does not provide any information about the magnitude of the variability in a dataset. However, standard deviation can be used to compare the variability of two groups provided the data in both the groups have the same units and their means are equal. On the other hand, the coefficient of variation measures relative variability as it is computed with reference to the mean value. Because of this, the coefficient of variation is used to assess the amount of variation present in a dataset. This can be understood by the following example: suppose a student has secured 60 marks in a particular test. The score of 60 has no meaning because it is an absolute number. To make it meaningful, we have to specify the maximum marks out of which 60 marks have been obtained. If the maximum marks are 150, then the percentage of marks obtained in the test would be $(60/150)\times 100 = 40\%$, which is meaningful.

Example 2.8 Compute the range and QD for the following dataset.

x:	2	4	6	8	7	5	9	8	1

Solution:

Computation of the Range In the dataset, Maximum score = 9 and Minimum score = 1.

Thus, the value of range would be

$$\text{Range} = \text{Maximum score} - \text{Minimum score}$$
$$= 9 - 1 = 8$$

Computation of the Quartile Deviation Since the QD is computed on the basis of Q_1 and Q_3, these quartiles are computed first. Here, $N = 9$. After arranging the scores in ascending order, they can be written as follows:

x:	1	2	4	5	6	7	8	8	9

Q_1 is computed as

$$\begin{aligned} Q_1 &= \left(\frac{9+1}{4}\right) \text{th score} \\ &= 2.5\text{th score} \\ &= 2\text{nd score} + \tfrac{1}{2}(3\text{rd score} - 2\text{nd score}) \\ &= 2 + \frac{1}{2}(4-2) \\ &= 3 \end{aligned}$$

Q_3 is computed as

$$\begin{aligned} Q_3 &= \left(\frac{3(N+1)}{4}\right) \text{th score} \\ &= \left(\frac{3(9+1)}{4}\right) \text{th} = 7.5\text{th score} \\ &= 7\text{th score} + \tfrac{1}{2}(8\text{th score} - 7\text{th score}) \\ &= 8 + \frac{1}{2}(8-8) \\ &= 8 \end{aligned}$$

Thus, the QD is

$$\begin{aligned} \text{QD} &= \frac{Q_3 - Q_1}{2} \\ &= \frac{8-3}{2} \\ &= 2.5 \end{aligned}$$

Example 2.9 The hits of a baseball player during his last 45 games are shown in the following table. The number of games in which the player had 0, 1, 2, 3, and 4 hits are recorded in the table.

Distribution of Hits in Baseball Games

Number of Hits	Frequency
0	12
1	18
2	11
3	3
4	1

Determine the average number of hits per game and the standard deviation of the distribution.

Solution: It is required to compute the mean and the standard deviation of the distribution. To compute these, it is required to compute $\sum fx$ and $\sum fx^2$. These computations have been done in the following table.

Steps in Computing the Mean and Standard Deviation for the Number of Hits

Number of Hits (x)	Frequency (f)	fx	fx^2
0	12	0	0
1	18	18	18
2	11	22	44
3	3	9	27
4	1	4	16
	$n = 45$	$\sum fx = 53$	$\sum fx^2 = 105$

$$\text{Mean} = \bar{x} = \frac{\sum fx}{n} = \frac{53}{45} = 1.18$$

$$\text{Standard deviation} = \sigma = \sqrt{\frac{1}{N}\sum fx^2 - \left(\frac{\sum fx}{N}\right)^2}$$

$$= \sqrt{\frac{105}{45} - \left(\frac{53}{45}\right)^2}$$

$$= \sqrt{2.33 - 1.39}$$

$$= 0.97$$

Example 2.10 The following is the frequency distribution of heights of 49 college athletes. Assuming these as population data, compute the QD and population standard deviation.

Frequency Distribution of Heights

Height (ft.)	Frequency
5.0–5.2	3
5.2–5.4	4
5.4–5.6	8
5.6–5.8	16
5.8–6.0	12
6.0–6.2	5
6.2–6.4	1

Solution: To compute the QD, Q_1 and Q_3 need to be computed first. In order to locate the Q_1 and Q_3 classes, the cumulative frequencies need to be worked out. Since the scores are given in the class interval form, the deviation method is used to compute the standard deviation. To compute Q_1, Q_3, and the standard deviation, the necessary computations have been done in the following table

Computation Table for the Quartile Deviation and Standard Deviation for the Data on Height

	Class Interval (Height in ft.) (1)	Frequency (f) (2)	CF (F) (3)	Midpoint (X) (4)	$d = \frac{X-5.7}{0.2}$ (5)	fd (6)	fd^2 (7)
	5.0 – 5.2	3	3	5.1	−3	−9	27
	5.2 – 5.4	4	7	5.3	−2	−8	16
Q_1 class	5.4 – 5.6	8	15	5.5	−1	−8	8
	5.6 – 5.8	16	31	5.7	0	0	0
Q_3 class	5.8 – 6.0	12	43	5.9	1	12	12
	6.0 – 6.2	5	48	6.1	2	10	20
	6.2 – 6.4	1	49	6.3	3	3	9
		N = 49				$\Sigma fd = 0$	$\Sigma fd^2 = 92$

Calculation of quartile deviation

To compute Q_1 and Q_3, it is required to locate the Q_1 and Q_3 class intervals.

Computation of Q_1 $\frac{N}{4} = \frac{49}{4} = 12.25.$

Since the cumulative frequency of the class interval 5.4–5.6 includes 12.25, this is the Q_1 class. For this class interval, the different values are as follows:

Lower limit of the Q_1 class, LL = 5.4

Frequency of the Q_1 class, $f_1 = 8$

Cumulative frequency of the class just before the Q_1 class, $F = 7$
Width of the class interval, $i = .2$

On substituting these values,

$$Q_1 = \text{LL} + \frac{\frac{N}{4} - F}{f_1} \times i$$

$$= 5.4 + \frac{\frac{49}{4} - 7}{8} \times 0.2$$

$$= 5.4 + 0.13 = 5.53$$

Computation of Q_3 $\frac{3N}{4} = \frac{3\times49}{4} = 36.75.$

Since the cumulative frequency of the class interval 5.8–6.0 includes 36.75, this is the Q_3 class. For this class interval, different values are as follows:

Lower limit of the Q_3 class, LL = 5.8
Frequency of the Q_3 class, $f_3 = 12$
Cumulative frequency of the class just before the Q_3 class, $F = 31$
Width of the class interval, $i = .2$

On substituting these values,

$$Q_3 = \text{LL} + \frac{\frac{3N}{4} - F}{f_3} \times i$$

$$= 5.8 + \frac{\frac{3\times49}{4} - 31}{12} \times 0.2$$

$$= 5.8 + 0.096 = 5.896$$

$$\text{The quartile deviation} = \text{QD} = \frac{Q_3 - Q_1}{2}$$

$$= \frac{5.896 - 5.53}{2}$$

$$= 0.183$$

Computation of the standard deviation: To compute the standard deviation, the values d, fd, and fd^2 have been computed in the 5th, 6th, and 7th columns respectively, in the previous table. From this table, $N = 49$, $\sum fd = 0$, and $\sum fd^2 = 92$.

Substituting these values in the formula, we get

$$\sigma = i \times \sqrt{\frac{1}{N}\sum fd^2 - \left(\frac{\sum fd}{N}\right)^2}$$

$$= 0.2 \times \sqrt{\frac{1}{49} \times 92 - \left(\frac{0}{49}\right)^2}$$

$$= 0.2 \times 1.37$$

$$= 0.274$$

2.13 BOX-AND-WHISKER PLOT

The box-and-whisker plot is a graphic way of showing the distribution of scores. The "box" in the box-and-whisker plot highlights the middle half of the data points in the distribution. In creating the box-and-whisker plot, the first step is to arrange the data in ascending order. After arranging the scores, the values of the median, Q_1, and Q_3 are computed to construct the box in the box-and-whisker plot. The lowest and highest scores in the dataset are used to draw the whisker on both the sides of the box.

The procedure for drawing the box-and-whisker plot is discussed by means of the following data, which represent the runs scored by a batsman in a tournament.

X:	20	27	12	42	65	8	29	55	26	47

The box-and-whisker plot can be created by using the following steps:

Steps in constructing box-and-whisker plot

1. Arrange the scores in ascending order and find the number of scores N.
2. Find the median by identifying the scores at the $[(N+1)/2]$th position.
3. Find the value of Q_1 by identifying the score at the $[(N+1)/4]$th position.
4. Find the value of Q_3 by identifying the score at the $[3(N+1)/4]$th position.
5. Find the lowest and highest score in the dataset.
6. Plot the value of the lowest scores, Q_1, median, Q_3, and highest score on a linear scale as shown in Figure 2.3.
7. Draw a box around the median by taking the endpoints at Q_1 and Q_3.
8. Extend the line from the Q_1 point at the box to the lowest score and from Q_3 point to the highest score for creating the whiskers.

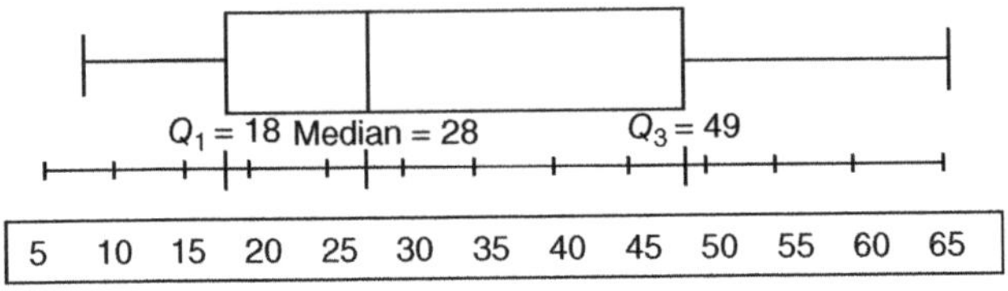

Figure 2.3 Box-and-whisker plot for the data on runs scored.

After arranging the scores in ascending order, we get

X:	8	12	20	26	27	29	42	47	55	65

Before creating the box-and-whisker plot, the values of the median, Q_1, and Q_3 are computed. Here, $N = 10$, lowest score = 8, and highest score = 65.

Computation of the Median:

$$\begin{aligned}\text{Median} &= \left(\frac{N+1}{2}\right)\text{th score}\\ &= \left(\frac{10+1}{2}\right)\text{th}\\ &= 5.5\text{th score} = (27+29)/2\\ &= 28\end{aligned}$$

Computation of Q_1:

$$Q_1 = \left(\frac{N+1}{4}\right)\text{th score} = \left(\frac{10+1}{4}\right)\text{th score} = 2.75\text{th score}$$

$$= \text{2nd score} + {}^3\!/_4(\text{3rd score} - \text{2nd score}) - 12 + \frac{3}{4}(20 - 12)$$

$$= 18$$

Computation of Q_3:

$$Q_3 = \left(\frac{3\,(N+1)}{4}\right)\text{th score} = \left(\frac{3\,(10+1)}{4}\right)\text{th score} = 8.25\text{th score}$$

$$= \text{8th score} + {}^1\!/_4(\text{9th score} - \text{8th score}) = 47 + \frac{1}{4}(55 - 47)$$

$$= 49$$

2.13.1 Creating the Box-and-Whisker Plot

A scale is drawn so that it includes lowest and highest scores. Q_1, the median, and Q_3 are marked on the scale. A box is made with lower and upper boundaries as Q_1 and Q_3. A line is extended from the Q_1 point to the lowest score, which becomes the lower whisker. Another line is drawn from the Q_3 point to the highest score on the scale, which shows the upper whisker. The graph so obtained is known as the *box-and-whisker plot* and is shown in Figure 2.3.

Can you find out from Figure 2.3, what is the value below which three quarters of the data lies? It is possible to answer this question from the plot. One can see that 49 is the score below which three quarters of the data lies.

2.14 SKEWNESS

> **FACTS TO KNOW**
>
> If a distribution is positively skewed, most of the data lie below the mean, whereas in case of a negatively skewed distribution, most of the data lie above the mean

Skewness measures the symmetricity of data. If the curve is not symmetrical, it is said to be *skewed*. The curve can be skewed toward the positive or negative side. The curve is said to be positively skewed if its tail in the positive side is stretched more than the negative side. Similarly, the curve is said to be negatively skewed if its tail is stretched more in the negative side than the positive side. For a positively skewed curve, the mean is higher than the mode and most of the scores are less than the mean value. On the other hand, for a negatively skewed curve, the mean is less than the mode and most of the scores are more than the mean value. Figure 2.4(a and b) illustrates positively and negatively skewed curves.

The skewness is denoted by β_1 and is computed by the following formula:

$$\beta_1 = \frac{\mu_3^2}{\mu_2^3} \tag{2.30}$$

where μ_2 and μ_3 are the second and third central moments around the mean value. In general, the rth central moment μ_r is computed as

$$\mu_r = \frac{1}{n}\sum (X - \overline{X})^r \tag{2.31}$$

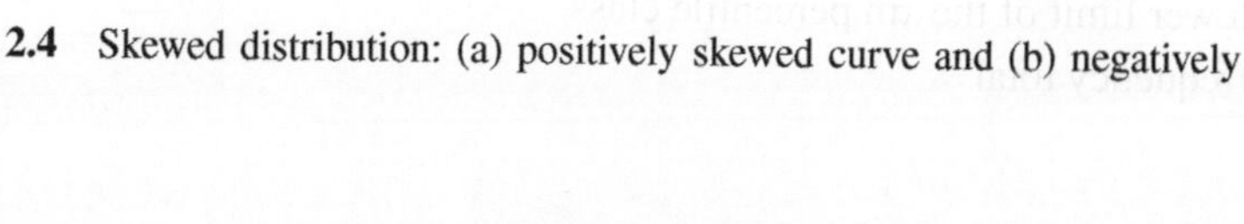

Figure 2.4 Skewed distribution: (a) positively skewed curve and (b) negatively skewed curve.

If the distribution is symmetrical, the value of β_1 is zero. For a positively skewed distribution, the value of $\beta_1 > 0$, whereas for a negatively skewed distribution, $\beta_1 < 0$. Skewness can also be computed by using other formulas as shown later.

2.14.1 Pearson's Skewness Coefficients

If the mean, median, mode, and standard deviation are known for a given dataset, then the Pearson's first or second skewness coefficients may be used. These can be computed as

$$\text{Pearson's first skewness coefficient} = \frac{3(\text{Mean} - \text{Mode})}{\sigma} \tag{2.32}$$

and

$$\text{Pearson's second skewness coefficient} = \frac{3(\text{Mean} - \text{Median})}{\sigma} \tag{2.33}$$

2.14.2 Bowley's Skewness Coefficient

Another index for computing the skewness is known as *Bowley's skewness coefficient*. It is also known as the *quartile skewness coefficient* and is defined by

$$\text{Bowley's skewness coefficient} = \frac{(Q_3 - Q_2) - (Q_2 - Q_1)}{Q_3 - Q_1} = \frac{Q_3 + Q_1}{Q_3 - Q_1} \tag{2.34}$$

2.15 PERCENTILES

A given percentile P_x is a point below which $x\%$ of the scores lies. For instance, the 40th percentile is a score below which 40% of the scores in the distribution lies. The percentile is denoted by P along with a subscript. Thus, 40th percentile is denoted by P_{40}. The percentile is used to find the relative position of an individual in the group on a particular parameter. The procedure for computing any given percentile is similar to that for computing quartiles because Q_1 and Q_3 are equivalent to P_{25} and P_{75}, respectively.

Percentiles are used in developing the norms for any parameter. They can be computed to know the position of an individual in the group on any parameter. For instance, one can develop the norms for events such as 100 m or long jump, or for parameters such as fat percentage, sit-ups, push-ups, and so on. These norms can be used to assess the performance level of an individual in a particular population.

The generalized formula for computing the xth percentile is given by

$$P_x = \text{LL} + \frac{\frac{xn}{100} - F}{f} \times i \tag{2.35}$$

where

LL = lower limit of the xth percentile class
n = frequency total

$F =$ cumulative frequency of the class interval just before the xth percentile class

$f =$ frequency of the xth percentile class

$i =$ width of the class interval

The computation procedure of the percentile P_{45} is shown by means of the data on the 1-min sit-ups performance obtained on college athletes shown in the form of the frequency distribution as in Table 2.18.

The value of P_{45} is computed by first locating the class interval in which P_{45} lies. To find this class, one should look for the class interval whose cumulative frequency includes the value $45 \times n/100$.

Here, $n = 72$ and therefore $\dfrac{45 \times n}{100} = \dfrac{45 \times 72}{100} = 32.4$

To determine the P_{45} class, look for 32.4 in the cumulative frequency column. The class interval 31–35 has a cumulative frequency 42, which includes the value $45 \times n/100 = 32.4$. Thus, 31–35 is the class in which P_{45} lies. Once this class is decided, the value of P_{45} can be obtained by substituting the following values in formula (2.35).

Here,

LL = lower limit of the P_{45} class 30.5

$f_m =$ frequency of the P_{45} class 15

$F =$ cumulative frequency of the class just below the P_{45} class 27

$i =$ width of the class interval 5

Substituting these values in formula (2.35),

$$P_{45} = 30.5 + \frac{\frac{45 \times 72}{100} - 27}{15} \times 5$$

$$= 30.5 + \frac{32.4 - 27}{15} \times 5 = 30.5 + 1.8 = 32.3$$

TABLE 2.18 Frequency Distribution of the Sit-Ups Scores

	Class Interval (Sit-Ups Scores) (1)	Frequency (f) (2)	Cumulative Frequency (F) (3)	
	6–10	2	2	
	11–15	5	7	
	16–20	8	15	F
P_{45} class	21–25	4	19	
	26–30	8	27	
	31–35	15	42	
	36–40	18	60	
	41–45	12	72	f_m
		$n = 72$		

Check Your Progress

Note: Tick the correct answer by using the sign (√).

	True	False
47. The range is affected by outliers.	-	-
48. The standard deviation measures the variability of scores around the mean value.	-	-
49. The QD is the best measure of variability in case of ordinal data.	-	-
50. The standard deviation is the most appropriate measure of variability for all types of data.	-	-
51. The Q_1 class is the class interval in which the value of P_{25} lies.	-	-
52. Since the range is the crudest measure of variability, it cannot be used in any situation.	-	-
53. If a constant number K is added to all the scores, the new standard deviation will be unaffected.	-	-
54. The QD is affected by the extreme scores.	-	-
55. Sampling fluctuation of the QD is more than that of the standard deviation.	-	-
56. In identifying the Q_3 class one needs to compute the value of $3N/4$.	-	-
57. The standard deviation is not affected much by outliers.	-	-
58. The value of Q_1 can be obtained by computing $(N+1)/4$.	-	-
59. The standard error of mean is σ/n.	-	-
60. The QD measures the variability of the middle 50% of the scores around mean value.	-	-
61. MD is the average of the absolute deviation of scores from the mean.	-	-
62. The sampling fluctuation of the standard deviation is the least among all measures of variability.	-	-
63. The QD is a parametric statistic.	-	-
64. Q_3 is also known as P_{75}.	-	-
65. The standard deviation is affected by the change of origin.	-	-
66. The QD is a better measure of variability compared to the range.	-	-
67. The coefficient of variation is used to compare the variability of two groups when their means are not equal.	-	-

68.	The value of standard deviation cannot be negative.	-	-
69.	Variance is the square of standard deviation.	-	-
70.	The standard error of any statistic is its standard deviation.	-	-
71.	The coefficient of variation is not free from units.	-	-
72.	In a positively skewed curve, the mode is greater than the mean.	-	-
73.	The box-and-whisker plot is used to show the distribution of scores.	-	-
74.	If the standard deviation is 105, it indicates that the variability among the scores is very high.	-	-
75.	The standard deviation is not affected by a change of scale.	-	-
76.	In a box-and-whisker plot, the box is plotted with the boundaries at Q_1 and Q_3.	-	-
77.	The coefficient of variation is an index of relative variability.	-	-
78.	The standard deviation is an appropriate measure of variability for ratio data.	-	-
79.	In a negatively skewed curve, the mode is smaller than the mean.	-	-
80.	P_{63} is a score above which 63% scores lies in the distribution.	-	-
81.	The values of median and P_{50} are same in the distribution.	-	-

PRACTICE EXERCISE

10. Find Q_1 and Q_3 for the following dataset and prepare the box-and-whisker plot.

2	26	30	16	18	8	22	60

11. Compute the MD about the mean and the standard deviation for the following population data.

7	8	9	4	5	7	6	9

12. Find the population standard deviation for the following data and also compute it by changing the origin of the scores by subtracting 50 from each score. Are these two standard deviations the same or not?

20	30	40	50	60	70	80	90

13. Find the standard deviation for the following population data and also compute it by changing the scale of the scores by dividing each score by 10. Check whether the two standard deviations are same.

5	10	15	20	25	30	35	40	45

14. Compute P_{35} and P_{70} for the following data.

35	12	67	80	45	56	78	34

2.16 COMPUTING WITH EXCEL

2.16.1 Computing Descriptive Statistics with Excel

Most of the descriptive statistics can be computed by using the Excel Analysis ToolPak. These descriptive statistics may be used for understanding the nature of the data. The computation of various descriptive statistics such as the mean, standard error, median, mode, standard deviation, sample variance, kurtosis, skewness, range, minimum, maximum, sum, count, largest score, and smallest score of variable(s) with Excel has been discussed by means of the following example.

Remark The descriptive statistics discussed below can only be computed if the Add-Ins “Analysis ToolPak” is already installed in your Excel. The readers can install this Add-Ins “Analysis ToolPak” in their Excel by following the procedure described in Chapter 1.

Example 2.11 Following are the data on standing long-jump performance and flexibility obtained on college women. Compute various descriptive statistics by using Excel.

Standing Long Jump (in.):	59	65	68	65	64	63	68	70	62	61
Flexibility (cm):	32	40	41	35	32	37	39	36	35	34

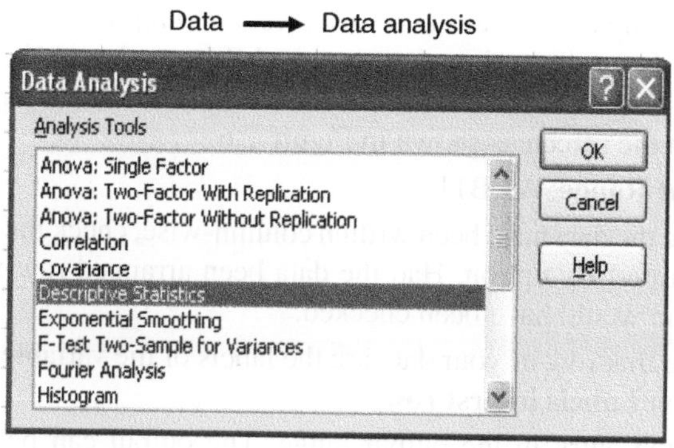

Figure 2.5 Command for descriptive statistics.

Solution:

1. To compute various descriptive statistics, click the following commands in Excel and you will get the screen as shown in Figure 2.5.
2. Bring the cursor on the option **Descriptive Statistics** and then click OK on the screen as shown in Figure 2.5. This will take you to the screen as shown in Figure 2.6. You can now define the range of data that you would like to use for computing various descriptive statistics.

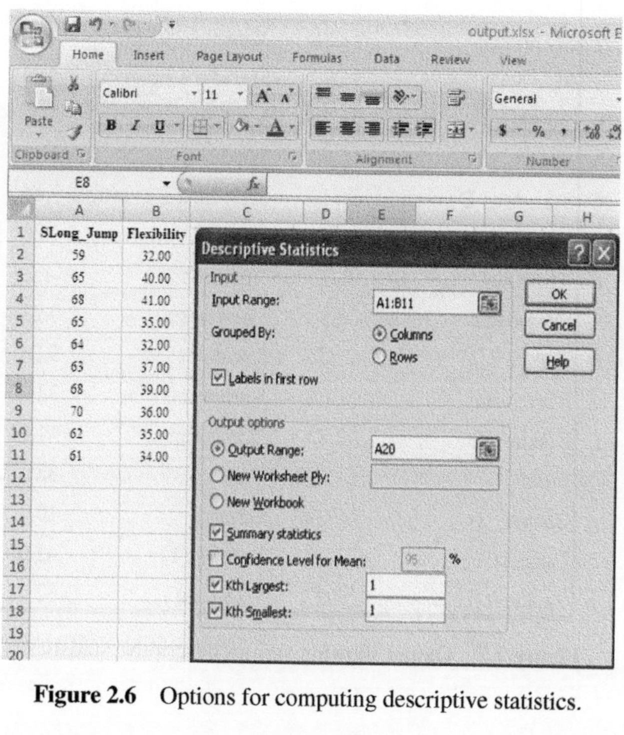

Figure 2.6 Options for computing descriptive statistics.

3. In this example, there are two variables *Standing long jump* and *Flexibility* that have been shown in columns A and B in the Excel sheet in Figure 2.6. The data range therefore would be A1:B11. Do the following steps to fill the entries in the screen as shown in Figure 2.6.
   i. **Input Range**: A1:B11
   ii. Since the data have been written column-wise, check the "Column" in the **Grouped By** option. Had the data been arranged row-wise, the "Row" option would have been checked.
   iii. If the first row of your data are the labels of the variables, then check the option **Labels in first row**.
   iv. Fill the entry in the output range. The output can be obtained on the same Excel sheet, new worksheet, or new workbook. Here, the output is obtained on the same sheet, starting from location A20 onward and therefore the following entry should be filled.
   Output Range: A20
   v. Check the relevant entries if you want the **Summary statistics, Largest, and Smallest** score for each variable.
   vi. Click **OK** to get the output as shown in Figure 2.7.

20	**Long_Jump**		**Flexibility**	
21				
22	Mean	64.50	Mean	36.10
23	Standard Error	1.09	Standard Error	0.99
24	Median	64.50	Median	35.50
25	Mode	65.00	Mode	32.00
26	Standard Deviation	3.44	Standard Deviation	3.14
27	Sample Variance	11.83	Sample Variance	9.88
28	Kurtosis	-0.72	Kurtosis	-1.06
29	Skewness	0.08	Skewness	0.23
30	Range	11.00	Range	9.00
31	Minimum	59.00	Minimum	32.00
32	Maximum	70.00	Maximum	41.00
33	Sum	645.00	Sum	361.00
34	Count	10.00	Count	10.00
35	Largest(1)	70.00	Largest(1)	41.00
36	Smallest(1)	59.00	Smallest(1)	32.00

Figure 2.7 Output showing various descriptive statistics.

IMPORTANT DEFINITIONS

Raw scores are the scores obtained in any experiment on which no statistical treatment has been done so far.

A ***single score*** is the score represented in the form of a whole number or integer.

A ***variable*** is a phenomenon that keeps changing from time to time, person to person, and place to place.

An ***attribute*** refers to a qualitative characteristic.

A variable is said to be an ***independent variable*** if it can be manipulated by the researcher.

A variable is a ***dependent variable*** if it is affected by changes in the independent variable.

A variable that can assume any real number value is known as a ***continuous variable***.

A variable is said to be ***discrete*** if it can assume only whole number values.

A ***frequency distribution*** is the representation of scores and their frequency in a tabular format.

A ***measure of central tendency*** is a single score that represents the aggregate of the whole dataset.

The mean is a weighted average of the scores in a dataset and is obtained by dividing the sum of all the scores by the total number of scores.

The median is the middlemost score in a distribution such that half the observations fall above and half below.

The mode is a score that is repeated maximum number of times in the dataset.

A ***measure of variability*** is an index that measures the variability of scores in the dataset around the mean, median, or mode.

The range is the maximum variation in the dataset and is obtained by subtracting the minimum score from the maximum score.

The quartile deviation is an index that measures the variability of the middle 50% of the scores around the median of the distribution.

The mean deviation is the measure of variability obtained by taking the average of absolute deviations of scores around the mean, median, or mode.

The standard deviation is the measure of variability of scores in a dataset from its mean.

The variance is the average of the squared deviations of the scores from the mean.

The standard error of any statistic is the standard deviation of that statistic.

The coefficient of variation is an index that measures the variability of the dataset in relation to its mean value.

Skewness measures the symmetricity of the distribution.

A ***percentile*** P_x is a score below which x percentage of scores lies.

IMPORTANT FORMULAS

Population mean for ungrouped data

$$\mu = \frac{1}{N}\sum x$$

Sample mean for grouped data

$$\bar{x} = \frac{\sum f_i x_i}{n}$$

Sample mean for grouped data (deviation method)

$$\bar{x} = \text{AM} + \frac{\sum fd}{n} \times i$$

Median for ungrouped data

$$M_\text{d} = \left(\frac{N+1}{2}\right)\text{th score}$$

Median for grouped data

$$M_\text{d} = \text{LL} + \frac{\frac{n}{2} - F}{f_\text{m}} \times i$$

Mode for symmetrical data

$$\text{Mode} = 3\ \text{Median} - 2\ \text{Mean}$$

Mode for grouped data

$$M_\text{o} = \text{LL} + \frac{f_\text{m} - f_1}{2f_\text{m} - f_1 - f_2} \times i$$

Range for ungrouped data

$$\text{Range} = \text{Maximum score} - \text{Minimum score}$$

Quartile deviation

$$\text{QD} = \frac{Q_3 - Q_1}{2}$$

First quartile for ungrouped data

$$Q_1 = \left(\frac{N+1}{4}\right)\text{th score}$$

Third quartile for ungrouped data

$$Q_3 = \left(\frac{3(N+1)}{4}\right)\text{th score}$$

First quartile for grouped data

$$Q_1 = \text{LL} + \frac{\frac{N}{4} - F}{f_1} \times i$$

Third quartile for grouped data

$$Q_3 = \text{LL} + \frac{\frac{3N}{4} - F}{f_3} \times i$$

MD about the mean

$$[\text{MD}]_{\text{mean}} = \frac{1}{n}\sum |x - M|$$

MD about the median

$$[\text{MD}]_{\text{median}} = \frac{1}{n}\sum |x - M_{\text{d}}|$$

MD about the mode

$$[\text{MD}]_{\text{mode}} = \frac{1}{n}\sum |x - M_{\text{o}}|$$

Population standard deviation for ungrouped data

$$\sigma = \sqrt{\frac{1}{N}\sum (X - \mu)^2}$$

$$\sigma = \sqrt{\frac{1}{N}\sum X^2 - \left(\frac{\sum X}{N}\right)^2}$$

Sample standard deviation for ungrouped data

$$S = \sqrt{\frac{1}{n-1}\sum X^2 - \frac{\left(\sum X\right)^2}{n(n-1)}}$$

Population standard deviation for grouped data

$$\sigma = \sqrt{\frac{1}{N}\sum fX^2 - \left(\frac{\sum fX}{N}\right)^2}$$

$$\sigma = i \times \sqrt{\frac{1}{N}\sum fd^2 - \left(\frac{\sum fd}{N}\right)^2}$$

Grouping error

$$\sigma_c = \sqrt{\sigma^2 - \frac{i^2}{12}}$$

Population variance

$$\sigma^2 = \frac{1}{N}\sum (x - \mu)^2$$

Standard error of mean

$$\sigma_{\overline{x}} = \frac{\sigma}{\sqrt{n}}$$

Standard error of standard deviation

$$\sigma_s = \frac{\sigma}{\sqrt{2n}}$$

Coefficient of variation

$$\text{CV} = \frac{s}{\overline{x}} \times 100$$

Skewness

$$\beta_1 = \frac{\mu_3^2}{\mu_2^3}$$

*r*th central moment

$$\mu_r = \frac{1}{n}\sum (X - \overline{X})^r$$

Pearson's first skewness coefficient

$$\frac{3(\text{Mean} - \text{Mode})}{\sigma}$$

Pearson's second skewness coefficient

$$\frac{3(\text{Mean} - \text{Median})}{\sigma}$$

Bowley's skewness coefficient

$$\frac{(Q_3 - Q_2) - (Q_2 - Q_1)}{Q_3 - Q_1} = \frac{Q_3 + Q_1}{Q_3 - Q_1}$$

*x*th percentile

$$P_x = \text{LL} + \frac{\frac{xn}{100} - F}{f} \times i$$

KEY TERMS

absolute and relative variability	measures of central tendency	skewness
box-and-whisker plot	measures of variability	

CHAPTER EXERCISE

1. Write short notes on the following:
   a. Variables and attributes
   b. Independent and dependent variables
   c. Continuous and discrete variables
2. Discuss four different levels of measurements that are used to record research data. Explain with suitable examples.
3. What are the two assumptions used while computing various statistics from grouped data? Discuss with examples.
4. Why are the mean and standard deviation frequently used as the measure of central tendency and measure of variability, respectively, in parametric data?
5. Can the mean be used always as a measure of central tendency in the case of ratio data? Explain your answer with an example.
6. Discuss the properties of the mean.
7. Show how the mean is affected both by change of origin and change of scale.
8. Discuss the situations where the median is the appropriate measure of central tendency.
9. What are the limitations of the mode?
10. "The measure of central tendency alone is sufficient to describe the nature of data." Comment on this statement with your arguments.
11. Discuss the situations where the QD may be used.
12. Discuss the properties of the standard deviation.
13. Show that the standard deviation is unaffected by change of origin but affected by change of scale.

14. Write short notes on the following:
    a. Grouping error
    b. Standard error
    c. Coefficient of variation
    d. Skewness
    e. Percentiles
15. What do box-and-whisker plots reveal? Take a dataset and construct the box-and-whisker plot by showing the steps involved in it.
16. Following are the weights of 54 college athletes measured in lbs.

126	132	135	145	153	142	158	162	167
174	136	144	135	127	167	155	145	176
168	162	151	149	132	138	156	174	173
168	165	163	151	157	142	139	144	131
129	128	167	145	167	135	143	149	158
167	136	129	166	155	145	128	156	169

   i. Construct the frequency distribution by taking approximately 10 class intervals.
   ii. Compute the mean and standard deviation with the data arranged in class intervals.
   iii. Find the number of scores that fall between the intervals of the sample mean ±2 standard deviation.

17. The following data represent the sit-ups performance of 60 athletes arranged in class intervals. Compute the mean value.

Sit-Ups Performance of Athletes

Sit-Ups	Frequency
1–5	4
6–10	8
11–15	6
16–20	8
21–25	15
26–30	10
31–35	5
36–40	4

18. The distribution of IQ scores for a group of students is shown below. Compute the mean, median, and mode.

IQ Scores	
Class Interval	Frequency
71–75	6
76–80	12
81–85	10
86–90	8
91–95	25
96–100	20
101–105	9

19. In a university soccer tournament, the distribution of the goals scored by different teams in a single match is given in the following table. Find the mean, median, and mode.

Distribution of Goals Scored in Soccer by Different Teams	
Goals Scored	Number of Teams
0	3
2	6
3	4
4	5
5	8
6	4
8	3
10	1

20. Following are the 400 m timings (in s) for a sample of 50 athletes in a tournament. Arrange these scores in class interval form by constructing 8 to 12 class intervals.

50.5	51.9	50.2	51.5	51.7	50.5	51.2	50.7	51.1
50.9	50.7	50.1	50.5	50.4	50.9	50.1	50.2	50.3
50.8	50.7	51.6	51.9	51.8	51.4	51.3	51.2	50.4
51.3	51.4	51.6	51.8	51.7	50.1	50.2	50.4	50.6
50.8	50.9	50.7	50.3	50.2	51.2	51.4	51.8	51.0
50.1	50.8	50.6	50.4	51.8				

Compute the sample mean and sample standard deviation from the raw scores as well as from the data arranged in class interval form.

21. The mean and standard deviation of the marks obtained by the students in sections A and B in the subject, test, and measurement are shown in the following table.

Mean and Standard Deviation for the Marks in the Test and Measurement

	Section A	Section B
Mean	75	65
SD	9	9

Compute the coefficient of variation for both the sections and explain your findings.

22. The mean and standard deviation of the sit-ups score obtained for rowing and badminton players are shown below. Compute the coefficient of variation to explain which group is more consistent in their sit-ups performance.

Mean and Standard Deviation of the Sit-Ups Score

	Rowing	Badminton
Mean	68	52
SD	12	8

23. If the distribution of heights for the students of a college is shown in the following class interval form, what would be the MD about the mean and the standard deviation?

Heights of the Students in cm

Class Interval	Frequency
150–155	12
155–160	10
160–165	20
165–170	25
170–175	15

24. The weights of 55 men were obtained and are shown in the following frequency table. Find the values of P_3, P_{15}, P_{70}, and P_{80}.

Weight in kg	
Class Interval	Frequency
51–55	5
56–60	25
61–65	10
66–70	12
71–75	3

25. The following are the 100 m timings of 73 athletes arranged in different class intervals. Find Q_1, Q_3, and the QD.

Distribution of 100 m Timings of Athletes

100 m Timings (s)	Number of Athletes
11.5–11.7	2
11.7–11.9	4
11.9–12.1	6
12.1–12.3	4
12.3–12.5	15
12.5–12.7	11
12.7–12.9	18
12.9–13.1	7
13.1–13.3	2
13.3–13.5	4

26. A random sample of 85 students is classified by age groups, as shown by the following data. Calculate the sample standard deviation.

Students Classified by Age Group

Age Group	Frequency
18–21	25
21–24	18
24–27	16
27–30	10
30–33	9
33–36	5
36–39	2

27. The following table shows the systolic blood pressures of 85 chess players. Considering these as the population data, do the following:
    i. Determine the QD.
    ii. Determine the MD about the mean.
    iii. Determine the population standard deviation.
    iv. Determine the coefficient of variation.

Systolic Blood Pressure (in mm of Mercury)

Class Interval	Frequency
90–94	4
95–99	8
100–104	6
105–109	14
110–114	16
115–119	3
120–124	8
125–129	4
130–134	3
135–139	4

28. Prepare box-and-whisker plots for the following two datasets.

a.	17	18	20	31	34	39	40	51	53	54	56		
b.	62	62	63	65	66	69	70	74	75	75	77	78	79

ANSWERS

Check Your Progress

1. F	10. F	19. F	28. F	37. F	46. F	55. T	64. T	73. T
2. T	11. T	20. T	29. F	38. T	47. T	56. T	65. F	74. F
3. F	12. F	21. F	30. T	39. F	48. T	57. F	66. T	75. F
4. F	13. F	22. T	31. F	40. F	49. T	58. F	67. T	76. T
5. T	14. T	23. T	32. F	41. T	50. F	59. F	68. T	77. T
6. T	15. T	24. F	33. T	42. F	51. T	60. F	69. T	78. T
7. F	16. F	25. T	34. T	43. T	52. F	61. T	70. T	79. F
8. T	17. F	26. F	35. T	44. T	53. T	62. T	71. F	80. F
9. T	18. T	27. T	36. T	45. F	54. F	63. F	72. F	81. T

Practice Exercise

1. Mean = 15.22, $[MD]_M = 16$
2. Mode = 27
3. Mean = 45.72, $[MD]_M = 45$, Mode = 29
4. Mean = 50, By changing the origin, Mean = 0
5. Mean = 25, By changing the scale, Mean = 2.5
6. $[MD]_M = 12.5$
7. Mode = 52
8. 36
9. a. Median, b. Mean, and c. Mode
10. $Q_1 = 10$, $Q_3 = 29$
11. $[MD]_M = 1.406$, SD = 1.69
12. SD = 22.91 and after changing origin, SD = 22.91
13. SD = 12.91 and after changing scale SD = 1.291
14. $P_{35} = 34.8$, $P_{70} = 62.6$

Chapter Exercise

17. ii. Mean = 148.24, SD = 14.64, iii. All scores fall in between $M \pm 2\sigma$
18. Mean = 29.28
19. Mean = 90.22, Median = 92.3 and Mode = 91.27
20. Mean = 4.18, Median = 4, and Mode = 5
21. Raw scores: Mean = 50.91, SD = 0.57;
    From class intervals: Mean = 50.81, SD = 0.57
22. CV for A = 12% and CV for B = 13.85%
23. CV for Rowing = 17.65% and CV for Badminton = 15.38%
24. $[MD]_M = 6.22$, SD = 6.47
25. $P_3 = 52.15$, $P_{15} = 56.15$, $P_{70} = 64.75$, $P_{80} = 67.17$
26. $Q_1 = 12.33$, $Q_3 = 12.84$, and QD = 0.255
27. SD = 5.05
28. i. QD = 8.18, ii. $[MD]_M = 1.86$, iii. $\sigma = 11.84$, iv. CV = 10.83%

FURTHER READING

1. Babbie E. The Practice of Social Research. 10th ed. Wadsworth: Thomson Learning Inc.; 2004. ISBN 0-534-62029-9.
2. Benjamini Y. Opening the box of a boxplot. The American Statistician 1988; 42(4):257–262. DOI: 10.2307/2685133. JSTOR 2685133.
3. Cliff N, Keats JA. Ordinal Measurement in the Behavioral Sciences. Mahwah, NJ: Erlbaum; 2003. ISBN 0-8058-2093-0.

4. Hector G. Excel data analysis: modeling and simulation. 1st ed. Germany: Springer 2010. ISBN 978-3-642-10834-1 Publication year(s): 2010
5. Lord FM. On the statistical treatment of football numbers. American Psychologist, USA 1953;8(12):750–751. DOI: 10.1037/h0063675.
6. Luce RD, Tukey JW. Simultaneous conjoint measurement: a new scale type of fundamental measurement. Journal of Mathematical Psychology 1964;1:1–27.
7. Maranell GM, editor. Chapter 31. In: Scaling: A Sourcebook for Behavioral Scientists. New Brunswick, New Jersey & London, UK: Aldine Transaction; 2007. p 402–405. ISBN 978-0-202-36175-8. Accessed 2012 Sep 16.
8. McGill R, Tukey JW, Larsen WA. Variations of box plots. The American Statistician 1978;32(1):12–16. DOI: 10.2307/2683468. JSTOR 2683468.
9. Michell J. Measurement scales and statistics: a clash of paradigms. Psychological Bulletin 1986;3:398–407.
10. Michell J. Quantitative science and the definition of measurement in psychology. British Journal of Psychology 1997;88:355–383.
11. Michell J. Measurement in Psychology – A Critical History of a Methodological Concept. Cambridge University Press: Cambridge; 1999.
12. Reed JF, Lynn F, Meade BD. Use of coefficient of variation in assessing variability of quantitative assays. Clinical and Diagnostic Laboratory Immunology 2002;9(6):1235–1239. DOI: 10.1128/CDLI.9.6.1235-1239.
13. Roy FB, Robert AG. Exploratory data analysis using Fisher information. UK: Springer 2007. ISBN 978-1-84628-506-6
14. Rozeboom WW. Scaling theory and the nature of measurement. Synthese 1966;16:170–233.
15. Sokal RR, Rohlf FJ. Biometry. 3rd ed. New York: Freeman; 1995. p 58ISBN 0-7167-2411-1.
16. Stevens SS. On the theory of scales of measurement. Science 1946;103(2684):677–680 Bibcode 1946;Sci.103.677S. DOI: 10.1126/science.103.2684.677. PMID 17750512. Accessed 2010 Sep 16.
17. von Eye A. Review of Cliff and Keats, ordinal measurement in the behavioral sciences. Applied Psychological Measurement 2005;29:401–403.

3

WORKING WITH GRAPHS

3.1 INTRODUCTION

A graphical picture conveys a lot more than numerical data. It is often of great help in understanding facts at a glance. It also provides a comparison between two or more frequency distributions. A graph can be said to be a mathematical picture. It provides a way of analyzing a problem in visual terms. Many problems can be reduced to visual form and such reductions often facilitate the understanding and solving of problems. It is difficult to draw any conclusion about a player's performance by just looking at a cricket score sheet. However, if the score sheet contents are shown in terms of graphics, it conveys a lot more information in a simple format and grabs the attention of a large audience. During a live cricket match, you must have seen the vertical bars showing the runs scored per over or the hawk-eyed analysis that shows ball movement graphically. These graphics enhance the interest of the audience in the game as they convey a lot about match analysis in a simple format.

Although graphic representation has many forms, only those forms that are useful in visualizing the important properties of frequency distribution and that facilitate comparison of two or more frequency distributions are discussed in this chapter. The latest software packages have helped students in creating different types of graphs with varied options, and therefore, it is recommended that students understand the concepts discussed in this chapter, which explains various graphical designs. Before discussing the construction of different types of graphs, the general guidelines common to most of the graphical presentation are discussed first.

Statistics for Exercise Science and Health with Microsoft® Office Excel®, First Edition. J. P. Verma.

3.2 GUIDELINES FOR CONSTRUCTING A GRAPH

There are varieties of graphs that can be used to show the results of research data. The selection of a graph depends on the nature of the data. Irrespective of the graphic option that one may choose, there are some guidelines that are common in constructing most graphic display.

3.2.1 Defining the $x-y$ Axis

There are two elements of measurement in a two-dimensional graphic display. The independent variable is measured along the horizontal axis and is known as abscissa or the x-axis. The dependent variable is measured along the vertical axis and is called the ordinate or the y-axis. In the case of grouped data, class interval is taken along the x-axis and frequencies along the y-axis.

3.2.2 Taking Origin as Zero

The scale of y must begin with zero as the origin. In case the frequency starts from 25 and ends at 35, then a cut is marked on the y-axis near zero in order to accommodate the frequency from 0 to 25 and then frequencies are marked from 25 onwards. Similarly, if some values of x need to be accomodated, then a similar cut should be made along the x-axis near the origin (Figure 3.1).

3.2.3 Using a Single Vertical Scale

If two curves are to be compared in a single graph, one should use only one vertical scale. This provides a real comparison of the data. If two different vertical scales are used on the left and right sides of the graph, then a valid visual comparison of the two curves cannot be made.

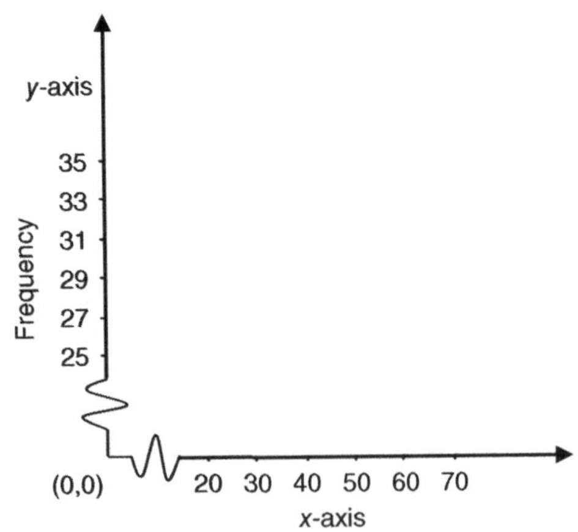

Figure 3.1 Marking scales on the x- and y-axis.

3.2.4 Deciding the Scale Unit

The scale unit is decided based on the nature of the data and their fluctuations. For example, stretching the *x*-axis will tend to de-emphasize fluctuations while stretching the *y*-axis will tend to overemphasize them. As a convention, the proportion of *y* and *x* scales must be in the ratio of 3:4.

3.2.5 Plotting the Data

If the scores given in a class interval (CI) form are to be plotted, the midpoints of the CIs are taken along the *x*-axis and frequencies along the *y*-axis. In a two-dimensional *x*–*y* plane, the cross-section points are located by taking the midpoints of the CIs along the *x*-axis and their corresponding frequencies along the *y*-axis. All such points in the *x*–*y* plane are encircled or marked with a cross. The picture so obtained is known as scatter plotting. Consider the grouped data shown in Table 3.1.

Here, the midpoints of the CIs are plotted along the *x*-axis and frequencies along the *y*-axis. The scatter plot has been obtained by identifying the cross-section points where the midpoints of the CIs on the *x*-axis and their corresponding frequencies on the *y*-axis meet each other. The scatter plot so obtained is shown in Figure 3.2.

TABLE 3.1 Frequency Distribution of the Sit-Ups Score

Class Interval	Midpoint	*f*
26–30	28	13
31–35	33	16
36–40	38	15
41–45	43	14
46–50	48	12

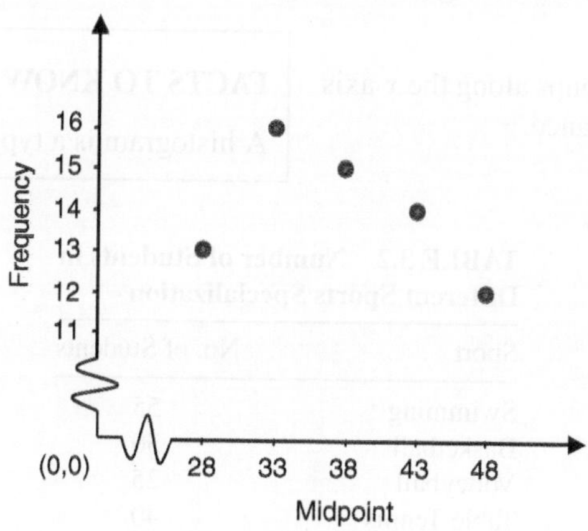

Figure 3.2 Scatter diagram of the sit-ups score.

In the case of the histogram discussed in the following section, CIs are marked differently along the x-axis.

3.2.6 Labeling the Graph

The title of the graph must indicate the objective for which it has been prepared. The heading should be brief and the legends must be self-explanatory. Variable names and their levels if any must be defined at the bottom of the graph. The scale of measurement of x and y may be written on the extreme right corner of the graph.

3.2.7 Highlighting the Lines

Usually, the curve and the axis lines are thicker than the rest of the graph. If more than one curve is plotted on the same graph, then different types of formatting must be used for each curve. The curve may be shown in the bold, dotted, dot–dash, or dashed format. Each line should be labeled at the bottom of the graph.

3.3 BAR DIAGRAM

A bar diagram is a graphic display of the data shown in discrete groups. It can be either vertical or horizontal. In this diagram, separate bars showing different groups are erected with the size proportionate to their frequencies. The distances between all the bars are fixed. This type of graphic display facilitates an instant comparison of the groups. The procedure for constructing the bar diagram is explained by means of the data shown in Table 3.2.

In this table, five discrete sports specialization groups along with their frequencies are shown; hence, five bars shall be erected. The following are the steps involved in the construction of the bar diagram.

3.3.1 Steps in Constructing a Bar Diagram

1. Mark the groups along the x-axis at equal distance.

> **FACTS TO KNOW**
>
> A histogram is a type of bar diagram

TABLE 3.2 Number of Students in Different Sports Specialization

Sport	No. of Students
Swimming	55
Basketball	30
Volleyball	25
Table Tennis	40
Athletics	20

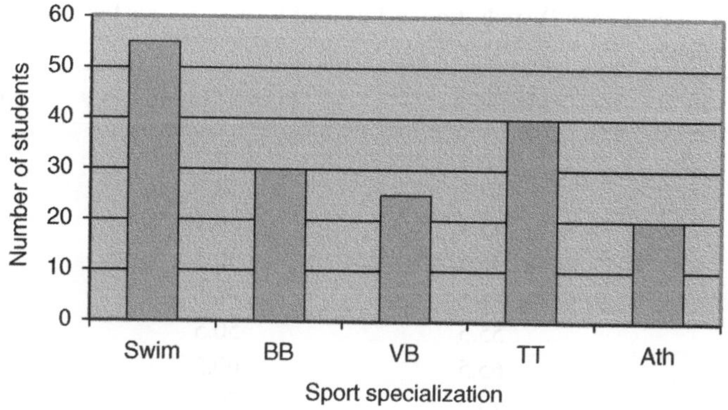

Figure 3.3 Bar diagram showing the number of students in different sports specialization groups.

2. Take the frequencies along the *y*-axis.
3. For each of the group on the *x*-axis, erect a rectangle with the height equal to their frequencies. The width of each bar should be equal.
4. Write an appropriate title for the graph.

After following the above-mentioned steps, the bar diagram so obtained is shown in Figure 3.3.

3.4 HISTOGRAM

A histogram is a diagrammatic representation of the frequency distribution of scores when CIs are continuous in nature. It is constructed by erecting rectangles for each of the CIs where the heights of these rectangles are equivalent to the frequencies of the respective CIs. In plotting the histogram, frequencies are marked along the *y*-axis while the CIs are taken along the *x*-axis. A histogram is a kind of bar diagram where all the bars are adjacent to each other. A histogram can also be constructed for the discrete data, but in this case, it is assumed that the upper limit of the CI is equivalent to the lower limit of the next higher CI. Besides showing the frequency distribution of the scores, the histogram also helps understand the trend of the data. The values of frequency distribution of the physical fitness scores of college students for the construction of histogram are provided in Table 3.3.

The procedure for constructing the histogram can be summarized in the following steps.

3.4.1 Steps in Constructing a Histogram

1. Find the lower limit of each of the CIs and mark it on the *x*-axis.
2. Mark the frequencies on the *y*-axis.

TABLE 3.3 Frequency Distribution of Physical Fitness Scores for a Sample of 50 College Students

Class Intervals	Midpoint (*x*)	Lower Limit	Frequency (*f*)
1–10	5.5	0.5	2
11–20	15.5	10.5	7
21–30	25.5	20.5	5
31–40	35.5	30.5	5
41–50	45.5	40.5	9
51–60	55.5	50.5	8
61–70	65.5	60.5	6
71–80	75.5	70.5	5
81–90	85.5	80.5	2
91–100	95.5	90.5	1

3. Erect the bars on each of the CIs with the height equal to their frequencies. While drawing the vertical bars, one must ensure that the higher limit of the CI must coincide with the lower limit of the next CI.
4. Write an appropriate title for the graph.

By following the above-mentioned steps, the lower limits of the CIs have been plotted along the *x*-axis and the frequencies have been plotted along the *y*-axis. After erecting the bars on each of the CI, the histogram will appear as shown in Figure 3.4.

Remark In the case of continuous CIs, the upper limit of the CI is equal to the lower limit of the next higher CI. However, in this example, CIs are discrete in nature; hence, it is assumed that the higher limit of the CI is equal to the lower limit of the next higher CI.

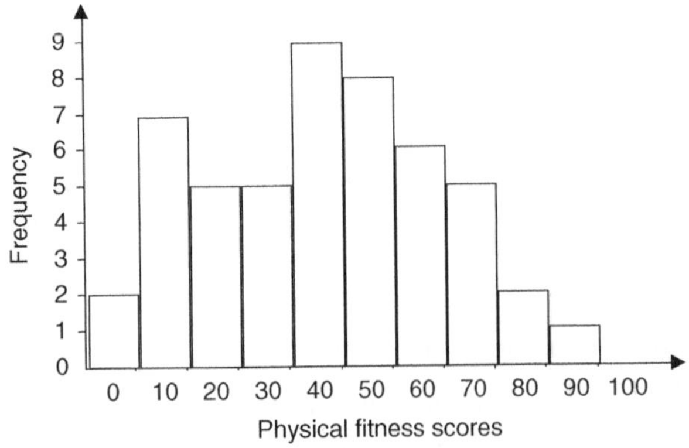

Figure 3.4 Histogram for the data on physical fitness.

3.5 FREQUENCY POLYGON

A frequency polygon is a graphic representation for showing the trend of the data. In constructing the frequency polygon, it is assumed that the frequency is uniformly distributed in the CI. It is also assumed that the frequencies are concentrated at the midpoint of the CIs. In constructing the frequency polygon, the midpoints of the CIs along the x-axis are plotted against their frequencies on the y-axis. The graph obtained by joining these points by a straight line is known as a frequency polygon. The frequency polygon may also be obtained by joining the midpoints of the bars at the top in the histogram by straight lines. By using the frequency polygon, one can interpolate or extrapolate the values. The procedure for drawing the frequency polygon is explained by considering the data provided in Table 3.3. The following are the steps involved in the construction of a frequency polygon.

3.5.1 Steps in Constructing a Frequency Polygon

1. Mark the midpoints of the CIs along the x-axis and frequencies along the y-axis.
2. Mark the points obtained by plotting the midpoints of the CIs on the x-axis against their frequencies on the y-axis.
3. Join the points obtained in step 2 by straight lines to get the frequency polygon.
4. Write an appropriate title for the frequency polygon.

By following the above steps, the points have been marked in Figure 3.5 by using the data provided in Table 3.3. These points have been joined by straight lines to get the frequency polygon.

3.6 FREQUENCY CURVE

The procedure for drawing a frequency curve is similar to that of a frequency polygon, except that in a frequency curve the points are joined by freehand instead of

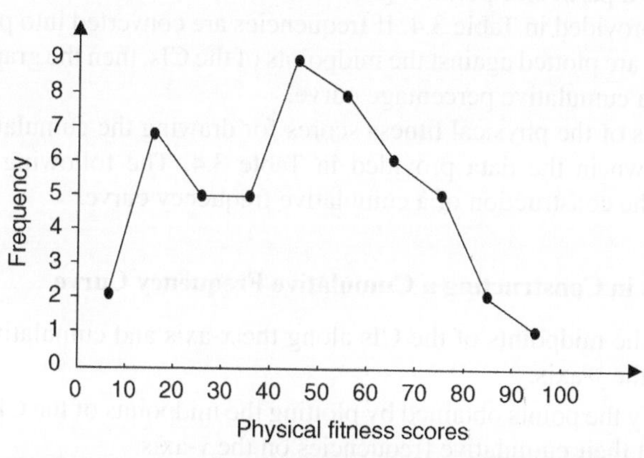

Figure 3.5 Frequency polygon of physical fitness score.

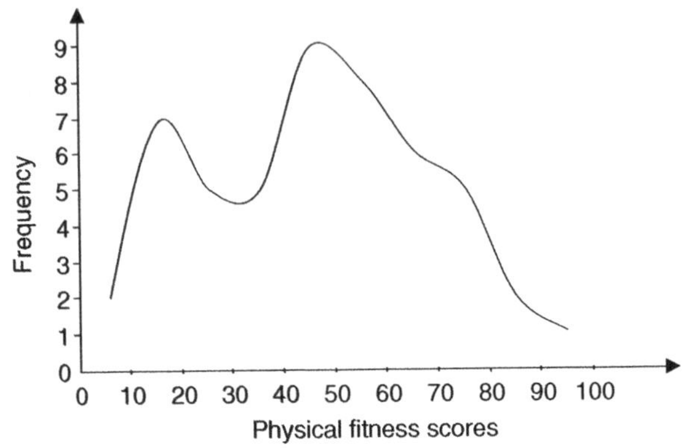

Figure 3.6 Frequency curve of physical fitness scores.

straight lines as in the frequency polygon. Thus, if the points obtained by plotting the midpoints of the CIs along the x-axis and frequencies along the y-axis are joined by freehand, the curve so obtained is known as a frequency curve. At times when the distribution of scores is such that the frequency polygon appears in a zigzag manner, it is preferred to show the distribution of scores by a frequency curve instead of a frequency polygon. However, frequency polygons give more accurate information in comparison with the frequency curves. The frequency curve for the same set of data provided in Table 3.3 is shown in Figure 3.6.

3.7 CUMULATIVE FREQUENCY CURVE

In cumulative frequency curves, instead of frequencies the cumulative frequencies are plotted against the midpoints of the CIs. The curve obtained by joining these points by freehand is known as a cumulative frequency curve. The cumulative frequency curve is used to find the percentiles of the scores. It provides the number of scores below a particular point. Figure 3.7 shows the cumulative frequency curve for the data provided in Table 3.4. If frequencies are converted into percentage frequencies and are plotted against the midpoints of the CIs, then the graph so obtained is known as a cumulative percentage curve.

The values of the physical fitness scores for drawing the cumulative frequency curve is shown in the data provided in Table 3.4. The following are the steps involved in the construction of a cumulative frequency curve.

3.7.1 Steps in Constructing a Cumulative Frequency Curve

1. Mark the midpoints of the CIs along the x-axis and cumulative frequencies along the y-axis.
2. Identify the points obtained by plotting the midpoints of the CIs on the x-axis against their cumulative frequencies on the y-axis.

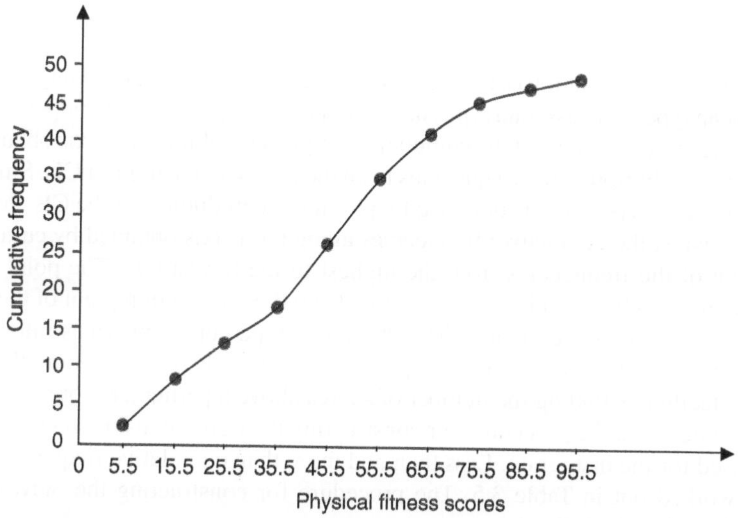

Figure 3.7 Cumulative frequency curve of physical fitness scores.

TABLE 3.4 Frequency Distribution of Physical Fitness Scores

Class Intervals	Midpoint (x)	Frequency (f)	Cumulative frequency
1–10	5.5	2	2
11–20	15.5	7	9
21–30	25.5	5	14
31–40	35.5	5	19
41–50	45.5	9	28
51–60	55.5	8	36
61–70	65.5	6	42
71–80	75.5	5	47
81–90	85.5	2	49
91–100	95.5	1	50

3. Join the points obtained in step 2 by freehand to get the cumulative frequency curve.
4. Write an appropriate title for the graph.

By following the above-mentioned steps, the midpoints of the CIs shown in Table 3.4 have been marked along the x-axis and cumulative frequencies along the y-axis. The points obtained by plotting the midpoints along the x-axis and cumulative frequencies along the y-axis are marked. After joining these marked points by freehand, the curve so obtained is the cumulative frequency curve as shown in Figure 3.7.

3.8 OGIVE

An ogive is a combination of two curves that are known as the less than type and the more than type. The less than type curve is obtained by plotting the midpoints of the CIs along the x-axis against the cumulative frequencies along the y-axis obtained by cumulative addition of the frequencies from the lowest to the highest CIs. Similarly, the more than type curve is obtained by plotting the midpoints of the CIs along the x-axis against the cumulative frequencies along the y-axis obtained by cumulative addition of the frequencies from the highest to the lowest CIs. The point on the x-axis obtained by dropping a vertical line from the intersection point of these two curves is known as the median. The "less than type curve" provides information about the number of scores below a particular score, whereas the "more than type curve" facilitates finding the number of scores above a particular score.

To understand the procedure for constructing the ogive, consider once again the data used for the histogram. Less than and more than cumulative frequencies have been worked out in Table 3.5. The procedure for constructing the ogive can be summarized in the following steps.

3.8.1 Steps in Constructing an Ogive

1. Find the midpoints of the CIs and mark them along the x-axis.
2. Find the "less than" frequencies by cumulatively adding the frequencies from the lowest to the highest CIs as shown in Table 3.5.
3. Similarly, find the "more than" frequencies by cumulatively adding the frequencies from the highest to the lowest CIs as shown in Table 3.5.
4. Mark these cumulative frequencies along the y-axis by choosing the scale appropriately.
5. Identify the points by plotting the midpoints of the CIs on the x-axis against the less than type frequencies on the y-axis. Joining these points by freehand will provide the "less than type curve."

TABLE 3.5 Ogive Curve Comprising Less Than Type and More Than Type Frequencies

Class Interval	Midpoint	Frequency	Less than c.f.	More than c.f.
1–10	5.5	2	2	50
11–12	15.5	7	9	48
21–30	25.5	5	14	41
31–40	35.5	5	19	36
41–50	45.5	9	28	31
51–60	55.5	8	36	22
61–70	65.5	6	42	14
71–80	75.5	5	47	8
81–90	85.5	2	49	3
91–100	95.5	1	50	1

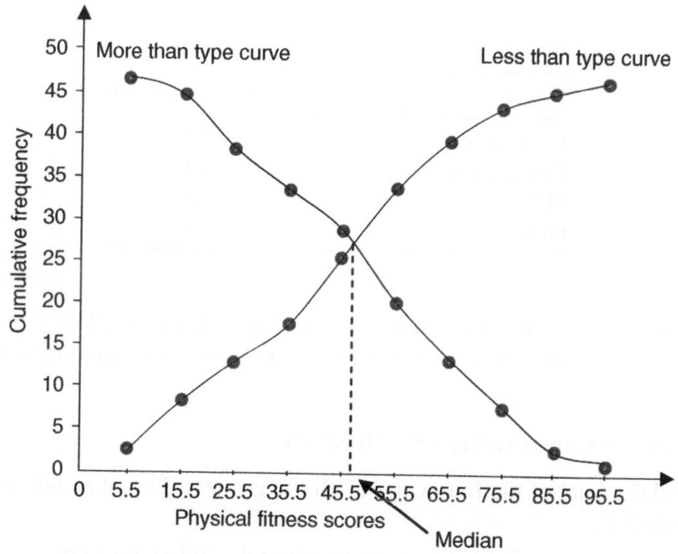

Figure 3.8 Ogive for the data on physical fitness test.

6. Similarly, identify the points by plotting the midpoints of the CIs on the x-axis against the more than type frequencies on the y-axis. Joining these points by freehand will provide the "more than type curve."
7. The graph obtained by drawing the curves in steps 5 and 6 will provide you the ogive curve as shown in Figure 3.8. Draw a perpendicular line on the x-axis from the intersection point of the curves to get the value of the median.
8. Write an appropriate title for the graph.

After following the above-mentioned steps, the curve so obtained has been shown in Figure 3.8.

3.9 PIE DIAGRAM

A pie diagram is a circular diagram in which the circle is divided into triangular areas proportionate to the percentages of the whole chart. Here, the scores for the various groups are represented by means of different pokes or triangular sections of a circle. The angles of these triangular sections are obtained by dividing the whole 360° angle into different angles proportionate to the magnitude of the frequencies represented by the different groups. Once the angles are calculated, the different sections of the circle can be constructed by using the protractor. Different patterns could be used to distinguish different groups. Sometimes, if a particular group is to be highlighted, it is cut and removed slightly outside the circle. To illustrate the procedure for constructing the pie diagram, consider the number of students enrolled in a college for different courses as shown in Table 3.6.

TABLE 3.6 Number of Students in Different Courses

Courses	Number of Students
Undergraduate	90
Postgraduate	80
M.Phil.	40
Ph.D.	30

The procedure shall be explained by using the data provided in Table 3.6. The following steps explain the procedure for constructing a pie diagram more clearly.

3.9.1 Steps in Constructing a Pie Diagram

1. Find the total of the frequency of all the groups. Here, it is 240 as shown in Table 3.7.
2. Calculate the angles for each group using the following formula:

$$\text{Angle for the group} = \frac{360}{\text{Total of all the frequencies}} \times \text{frequency of the group} \quad (3.1)$$

3. Divide the circle into different segments by using the protractor and write the angles and labels of these segments. The diagram so obtained is the pie diagram.
4. Write an appropriate title for the graph.

Using the above-mentioned steps, the angles for different groups shall be as follows:

$$\text{Angle for the undergraduate group} = \frac{360}{240} \times 90 = 135°$$

$$\text{Angle for the postgraduate group} = \frac{360}{240} \times 80 = 120°$$

$$\text{Angle for the M.Phil. group} = \frac{360}{240} \times 40 = 60°$$

TABLE 3.7 Pie Diagram for the Data on Different Courses

Courses	No. of Students	Angle
Undergraduate	90	135°
Postgraduate	80	120°
M.Phil.	40	60°
Ph.D.	30	45°
Total	240	

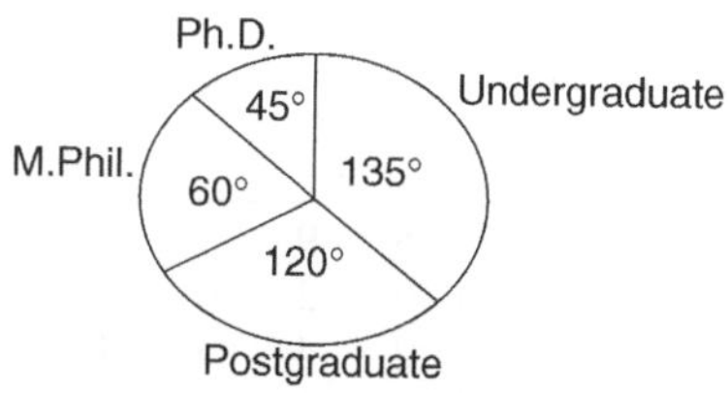

Figure 3.9 Pie diagram showing the number of students in different courses.

$$\text{Angle for the Ph.D. group} = \frac{360}{240} \times 30 = 45°$$

The frequencies of different groups along with their computed angles are shown in Table 3.7. The pie diagram so obtained is shown in Figure 3.9.

3.10 STEM AND LEAF PLOT

> **FACTS TO KNOW**
>
> If the number of categories is less, bar diagrams and pie diagrams are more appropriate than line diagrams

A stem and leaf plot is a method of showing the frequency distribution of data in terms of the stem and leaf. The stem represents the tens digit and the leaf represents the ones digit. The stem and leaf plot is an alternate solution to showing the frequency distribution of data in the form of either CIs or histograms. In representing the distribution either by CIs or by histogram, the identity of individual scores is lost. For instance, if the frequency of a CI 20–29 is 4, one may not be able to say what the four scores are. On the other hand, the stem and leaf plot can show the distribution of scores and can also tell us what the individual scores are in each CI. To show the procedure for constructing a stem and leaf plot, consider the distribution of scores obtained by the students on a sit-ups test as shown below.

Sit-Ups Score:	56	76	79	86	80	81	29	45	30	44	65	72	36	71	32	48	25	42	51

3.10.1 Steps in Constructing a Stem and Leaf Plot

1. Construct a table with two columns. Write the heading of the first and second columns as Stem and Leaf, respectively, as shown in Table 3.8.
2. Look at the minimum and maximum scores in the dataset. Here, the lowest and highest scores are 25 and 86. Write the stem value from 2 to 8 in the first column of the table. If the lowest and the highest scores would have been 45 and 135, then stem values would have been from 4 to 13.

TABLE 3.8 Stem and Leaf Plot for the English Scores

Stem	Leaf			
2	5	9		
3	0	2	6	
4	2	4	5	8
5	1	6		
6	5			
7	1	2	6	9
8	0	1	6	

3. Look at the scores that start with 2. Here, such scores are 29 and 25; hence, write the rightmost digits of these numbers, that is, 5 and 9 in the leaf column against the stem value 2.
4. Similarly, scores starting with 3 are 30, 32, and 36; hence, their last digits, that is, 0, 2, and 6 are written in front of the stem value 3. Keep placing all the scores in the stem and leaf plot table against their respective stem scores.
5. The plot so obtained is known as the stem and leaf plot.
6. Write an appropriate title for the plot.

The stem and leaf plot obtained by following the above-mentioned steps is shown in Table 3.8. The plot is similar to the distribution of scores shown in the CI form. One can see from this plot that there are two scores 25 and 29 in the CI 20–29 and three scores 30, 32, and 36 in the CI 30–39. This plot is also similar to the histogram. It can be seen from Table 3.8 that the frequencies of the CIs 20–29 and that of 50–59 are the same and are equal to 2. Thus, the stem and leaf plot can be considered to be the graphical display of the distribution of scores; it also reveals the identity of each and every score.

Check Your Progress

Note: Tick the correct answer by using the sign (√).

	True	False
1. Hawk-eyed analysis is used for showing graphics during the basketball match.	–	–
2. The *y*-axis is known as the ordinate.	–	–
3. If the coordinates of the point *A* are (0,3), then it lies on the *x*-axis.	–	–
4. Usually, a dependent variable is marked along the *y*-axis.	–	–
5. In a bar diagram, the distance between the bars may not necessarily be the same.	–	–
6. In a histogram, the bars are adjacent to each other.	–	–

7.	The x-axis is known as the ordinate.	–	–
8.	In a bar diagram, the bars can be erected vertically as well as horizontally.	–	–
9.	A frequency curve is obtained by adding the points with straight lines.	–	–
10.	In a frequency polygon, the points are joined by freehand.	–	–
11.	Stretching the x-axis more than the y tends to de-emphasize fluctuations.	–	–
12.	If the coordinates of the point B are (6, 0), then it lies on the x-axis.	–	–
13.	In drawing a histogram, the CIs are marked along the x-axis.	–	–
14.	If the stem and leaf plot is moved vertically, then it looks like a pie diagram.	–	–
15.	In a stem and leaf plot, the identity of scores is not lost.	–	–
16.	A frequency polygon is used to find the trend of the dataset.	–	–
17.	A cumulative frequency curve can be used for finding the percentile.	–	–
18.	In ogive, more than cumulative frequency is obtained by cumulative addition of frequencies starting from lower to higher CIs.	–	–
19.	In a pie diagram, the 360° angle is divided into different groups proportionate to their frequencies.	–	–
20.	The x-axis is known as the abscissa.	–	–
21.	In a stem and leaf plot, the stem represents the ones digit.	–	–
22.	The y-axis is known as the abscissa.	–	–
23.	The range can be computed from the stem and leaf plot.	–	–
24.	The intersection point of both the curves in the ogive facilitates computing the median value.	–	–

PRACTICE EXERCISE

1. Construct a bar diagram for the preference of sports by students.

Groups:	Basketball	Tennis	Wrestling	Swimming	Cricket
Frequency:	50	35	15	25	60

2. Construct a histogram and frequency polygon for the following data on shooting score in basketball.

CI:	1–4	5–8	9–12	13–16	17–20	21–24	25–28
Frequency:	3	5	8	5	12	4	6

3. The following table shows how Jacob spends each working day in the college. Construct a pie diagram to show this data.

Activity:	Class	Sports	Extra-curricular	Sleep	Routine Activity
Percentage Time Spent:	25	10	15	30	20

4. Write the stems that would be required to plot each set of the following data.

   a. 23, 45, 56, 12, 27, 58, 37
   b. 8, 11, 23, 37, 31, 42, 59

5. Complete a stem and leaf plot for the following set of runs scored by the players in a cricket match.

   Runs: 51 70 40 56 61 72 28 32 97 88 44 96 84 69
   77 21 20 92 72 29 34 48 55 78 52 65 79

   Answer the following questions.

   i. If the stem and leaf plot is turned vertically what kind of graph will it look like?
   ii. What is the lowest score of the players?
   iii. What is the highest score of the players?
   iv. In which interval did most of the players score the runs?

6. A survey was conducted to know how students spend their after-college time. The following table shows the findings of the survey. Construct a bar diagram and answer the below-mentioned questions.

Activities That Are Favored by the Students During After-College Hours

Activity	Number of Students
Friendship	35
Sports	25
Talking on phone	65
Part-time job	24
Computer	80
Club	32
TV watching	70

i. What is the range of values on the (vertical) scale?
ii. How many groups are there in the graph?
iii. Which after-college activity do students like the most?
iv. Which after-college activity do students like the least?

3.11 COMPUTING WITH EXCEL

3.11.1 Constructing Histograms to Understand the Distribution of Data

Excel can be used to create different types of graphs. However, the Analysis ToolPak can create the histogram only. This facility can be used to understand the distribution of data. The procedure for creating histograms using Excel has been discussed using the following example.

Remark The histogram discussed below can only be constructed if the Add-Ins "Analysis ToolPak" is already installed in your Excel. The readers can install this Add-Ins "Analysis ToolPak" in their Excel by following the procedure mentioned in Chapter 1.

Example 3.1 A basketball coach wanted to assess the performance of athletes in basketball shooting. Each of the 15 subjects was given 20 attempts to try shooting from a specific distance. The number of successful attempts was counted for each athlete, which is shown below. Construct a histogram to see the distribution of shooting performance of athletes.

Shooting Performance of Athletes														
2	3	8	6	10	12	15	17	9	11	14	12	7	6	13

Solution:

1. To construct a histogram, click the following commands in Excel and you will get the screen as shown in Figure 3.10.

   Data ⟶ Data analysis

2. Bring the scroll on the option **Histogram**, and then click OK in the screen as shown in Figure 3.10. This will take you to the screen as shown in Figure 3.11. You can now define the range of data that you would like to use for constructing the histogram.
3. In this example, the scores on shooting performance are in the first column and CI in the second column of the Excel sheet, as shown in Figure 3.11. The data range therefore would be *A*1:*A*16 for the shooting variable and *B*1:*B*6 for the CI. Do the following steps to fill the entries in the screen shown in Figure 3.11.

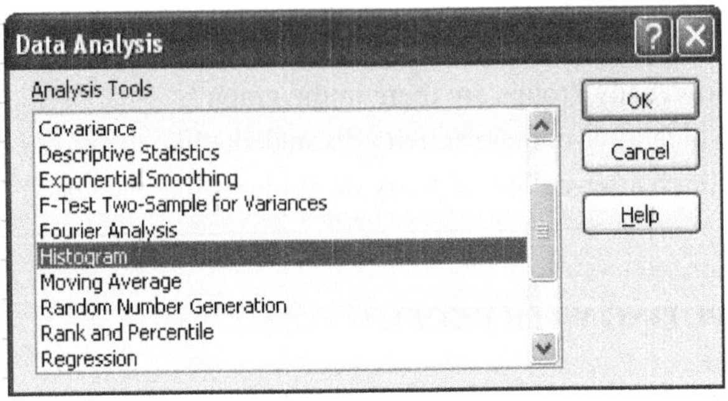

Figure 3.10 Command for histogram.

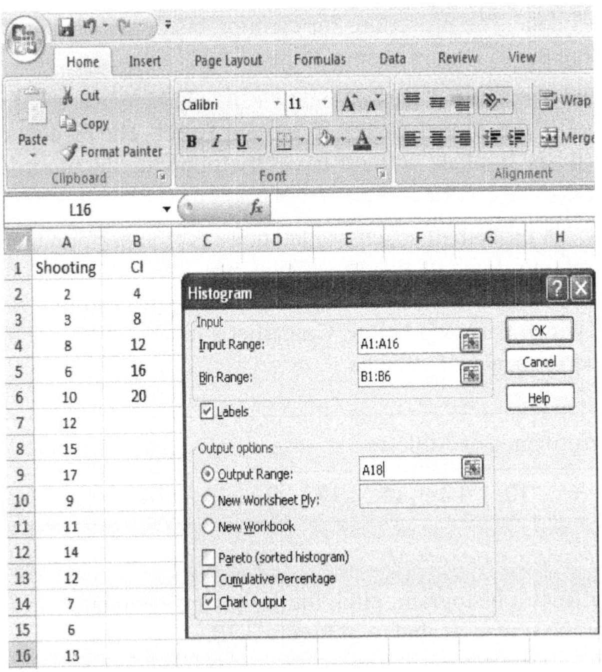

Figure 3.11 Options for computing the histogram.

Input Range: $A1{:}A16$

i. Bin Range: $B1{:}B6$

(Bin denotes the CI. Users can define it to suit the data. Since, in this example, the minimum and maximum performances of the shooting scores can be 0 and 20, respectively, a CI of width 4 has been chosen.)

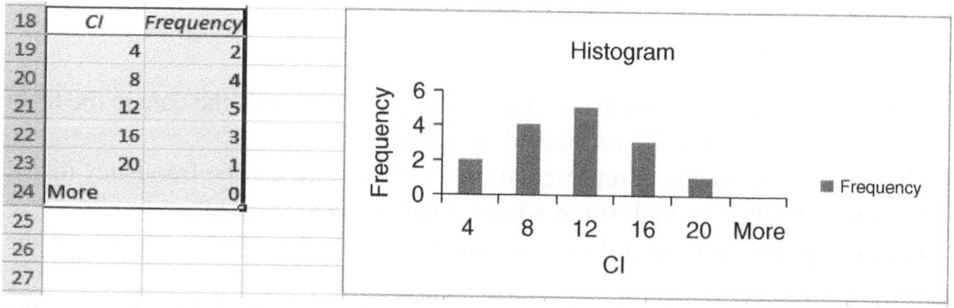

Figure 3.12 Output showing the histogram along with the data.

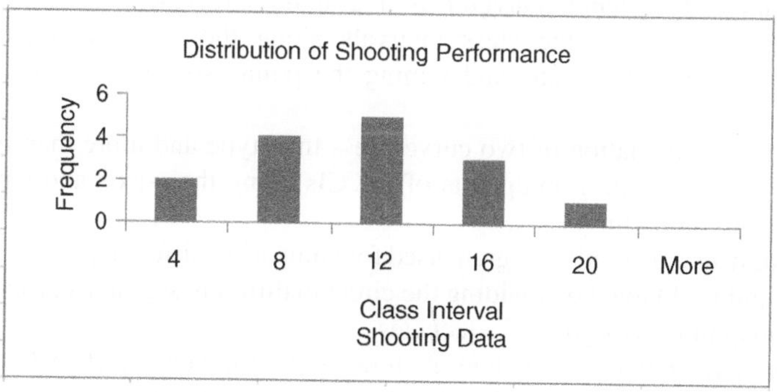

Figure 3.13 Histogram showing the distribution of shooting performance.

ii. If the first row of your data contains the variable name, then check the option **Labels** in the first row.

iii. Fill the entry in the output range. The output can be obtained on the same Excel sheet, new worksheet, or new workbook. Here, the output is obtained on the same sheet starting from A18, and therefore the following entry should be filled.

Output Range: A18

iv. Check the option **Chart Output**. Other entries are optional; readers can check them if so required.

v. Click **OK** to get the output as shown Figure 3.12.

4. The output obtained in Figure 3.12 can be customized by changing the labels. To change the label, double click "CI" and retype the required label. Similarly, the heading "Histogram" can also be changed. To do away with the "Frequency" on the right of the figure, double click on it and delete. The customized figure of the histogram is shown in Figure 3.13.

IMPORTANT DEFINITIONS

Bar diagram can be defined as a graphical representation of the data in the form of horizontal or vertical bars erected at equal distance.
Histogram is a graphical representation used for showing the frequency distribution of the data in the form of adjacent bars erected vertically.
Frequency Polygon is a line diagram used for showing the trend of the dataset.
Frequency Curve is a diagrammatic representation used for showing the trend of the dataset and is obtained by joining the plotted points by a smooth curve.
Cumulative Frequency Polygon is a graphical representation of the data obtained by plotting the class intervals along the x-axis and cumulative frequency along the y-axis and joining the points so obtained by a smooth curve.
Ogive is a combination of two curves, less than type and more than type, and is obtained by plotting midpoints of the CIs along the x-axis and cumulative frequencies along the y-axis.
Pie Diagram is a circular diagram used for comparing different parts of the same whole and is obtained by dividing the circle in different segments proportionate to the magnitudes of group frequencies.
Stem and Leaf Plot is a method of showing the frequency distribution of data in terms of stem and leaf so that the identity of scores is not lost.

IMPORTANT FORMULAS

Angle in the pie diagram

$$\text{Angle for the group} = \frac{360}{\text{Total of all the frequencies}} \times \text{frequency of the group}$$

KEY TERMS

cumulative frequency curve

histogram

ogive

stem and leaf plot

CHAPTER EXERCISE

1. Construct a frequency curve and cumulative frequency polygon for the following data on weight reduction in a 1-week health awareness program.

CI (Weight in lbs)	Frequency
0–0.5	5
0.5–1.0	8
1.0–1.5	12
1.5–2.0	11
2.0–2.5	9
2.5–3.0	3
3.0–3.5	2

2. Construct ogive for the following data on push-ups.

CI (Push-Ups)	Frequency
5–10	3
10–15	6
15–20	8
20–25	10
25–30	15
30–35	12
35–40	4

3. Construct a stem and leaf plot for the following data on age of the coaches in an organization.

23	26	24	25	28	31	33
31	27	25	27	34	36	37
38	54	45	44	34	43	23
26	42	45	44	47	53	52
44	46	23	27	45	43	28

4. Students were tested for their abdominal strength by means of 1-min sit-ups test and the data so obtained are shown below.

Sit-Ups:	45 32 23 18 26 34 41 54 46 48 62 30 68 22 21 12 40 56 58

Prepare a stem and leaf plot and answer the following questions.

i. What was the highest number of sit-ups performed by the student?
ii. Find the difference between the highest and lowest sit-ups performed by the students.
iii. How many students performed more than 48 sit-ups?

5. The following are the number of injuries reported in the health center of a sports college during the last 1 year. How will you find the trend of the injuries occurring in the college by preparing a suitable graph?

Month-Wise Distribution of Injuries

Month	No. of Injuries
Jan	30
Feb	35
Mar	51
Apr	39
May	32
Jun	48
Jul	85
Aug	94
Sep	62
Oct	73
Nov	64
Dec	52

6. The following are the scores of 10 athletes on their physical fitness index and shot-put performance.

Performance of Athletes

Physical Fitness Index	Shot-Put Performance (in ft.)
65	34
76	37
86	40
59	33
90	42
87	44
95	48
81	41
72	36
61	30

Plot these data along with the trend line and answer the following.

i. Do you observe any correlation between the physical fitness index and shot-put performance?

ii. On the basis of the trend line what would be the estimate of shot-put performance of an athlete if his physical fitness index is 71?

7. Construct a bar diagram to show the number of students who opted for different sports in the match practice.

Data on Preferences of Sports

Sport	No. of Subjects
Basketball	20
Gymnastics	12
Volleyball	18
Tennis	25
Judo	12

8. Following is the break-up of the hours spent per month by the students of exercise science on different activities.

Frequency Distribution of the Number of Hours Spent on Different Activities

Activities	Hours Spent
Classroom learning	60
Field activities	80
Lesson plan	10
Match practice	25
Extracurricular	15

Construct a bar diagram to represent this data.

9. The following are the number of push-ups performed by the subjects. Find the midpoint, relative frequency, and cumulative frequency and construct a histogram.

Push-Up Performance

Push-Ups	No. of Subjects
1–5	8
6–10	14
11–15	20
16–20	10
21–25	16
26–30	9
31–35	4

10. The following data indicate the scores on the arm length of 50 tennis players.

Frequency Distribution of the Arm Length (in cm)

CI (Arm Length)	Frequency
65–69	12
70–74	11
75–79	20
80–84	8
85–89	10
90–94	6

i. Draw a histogram of the data.
ii. Draw a frequency polygon and frequency curve.

11. In a cricket tournament, the runs made by the batsman were recorded, which is shown in the following table. Draw the histogram and frequency polygon.

Runs Scored in the Cricket Tournament

CI (Runs)	No. of Players
0–15	5
16–30	24
31–45	12
46–60	6
61–75	4
76–90	4
91–105	3
106–120	1
121–135	2

12. In an undergraduate program, the number of students who opted for different specialization papers are as follows:

Students Opting for Different Papers

Subject	Frequency
Exercise physiology	12
Sports biomechanics	25
Sports psychology	40
Sports pedagogy	5
Health education	18

i. Draw a pie diagram to show the data.
ii. Draw a bar diagram for the above-mentioned data.

13. The following IQ scores of the students have been shown in the form of frequency distribution. Construct an ogive and find the median IQ of the students graphically.

Data on IQ

CI	No. of Students
81–83	2
84–86	12
87–89	11
90–92	25
93–95	4
96–98	6
99–101	8

14. The following are the marks of the students in health education. Prepare an ogive and find its median. Check whether the median obtained by the ogive is equal to the median obtained by computing its value.

Marks of the Students in Health Education

CI	Frequency
11–15	3
16–20	5
21–25	10
26–30	6
31–35	12
36–40	7
41–45	5
46–50	1

15. In an experiment the pulse rate of 80 gymnasts were recorded. These data are shown in the following table.

Frequency Distribution of the Pulse Rate (in Numbers) of Gymnasts

CI	Frequency
65–69	12
70–74	11
75–79	20
80–84	5
85–89	2

i. Construct "less than" and "more than" cumulative frequency distribution.
ii. Draw an ogive and hence compute the value of the median.

16. The following are the grip strength scores obtained on some undergraduate students. Prepare a stem and leaf plot and interpret the findings.

35	30	31	37	70	67	45	54	34	75	74	67
68	56	64	63	32	35	43	45	34	37	41	42
43	51	53	65	57	58	63	65	68	69	73	74

17. The following statistics show the number of male and female students participating in the different sports teams of a university. The authorities want to make a presentation of this fact. What kind of graph would you suggest?

Details of Students Participating in Different Sports

Sport	Male	Female
Baseball	14	12
Soccer	22	16
Hockey	21	18
Tennis	14	6
Basketball	16	11

18. The following is the line diagram indicating the number of students at different times of a day in the college canteen.

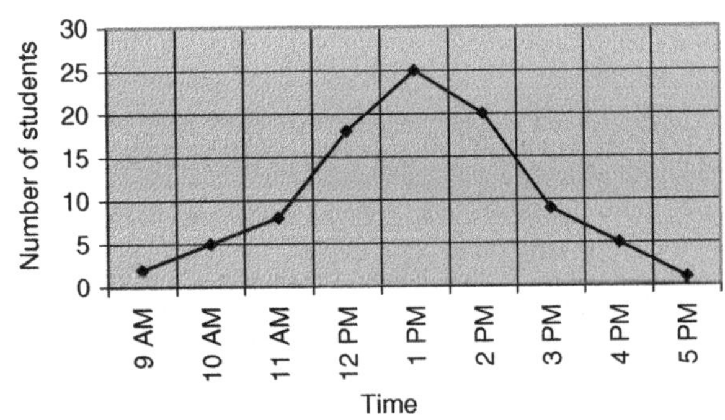

By reading the graph answer the following questions:

i. What does the graph tell you?

ii. What is the busiest time of day in the canteen?

iii. From what time onward do the students start coming in less than 10 numbers?

iv. When the canteen opens, how many students are there?

19. The following pie chart shows the preferences of a sample of students in a university for different leisure activities.

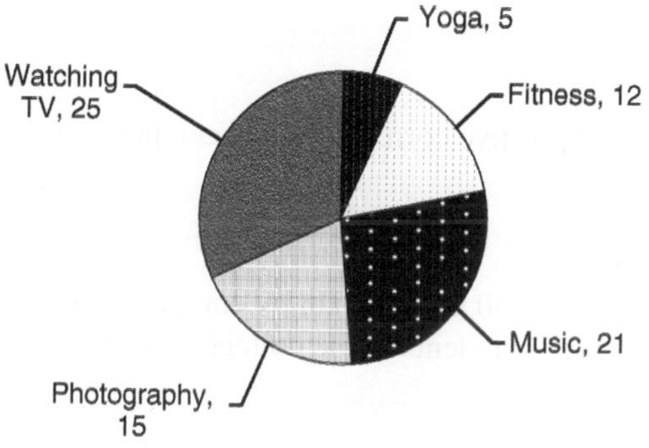

Find the following:

i. Which is the most popular leisure activity in the university?
ii. What is the percentage of students that prefer photography?
iii. Following the same pattern, if 40 students prefer watching TV, how many students in total were surveyed?
iv. Assuming that the same pattern holds for the students of the entire university, if 25 students prefer photography, how many students would have chosen yoga as a leisure activity?

ANSWERS

Check Your Progress

1. F	4. T	7. F	10. F	13. T	16. T	19. T	22. F
2. T	5. F	8. T	11. T	14. F	17. T	20. T	23. T
3. F	6. T	9. F	12. T	15. T	18. F	21. F	24. T

Practice Exercise

5. i. Histogram
   ii. 20
   iii. 97
   iv. 70–79
6. i. 24–80
   ii. 7
   iii. Computer
   iv. Part-time job
   v. Club and friendship

Chapter Exercise

4. i. 68
   ii. 56
   iii. 5
6. i. Yes, there is a positive correlation between physical fitness index and shot-put.
   ii. 35
13. Median = 90.5
14. Median from ogive = 30 and Median by computation = 30.71
18. i. Arrival pattern of students in the college canteen
    ii. 1 PM
    iii. 3 PM
    iv. 2
19. i. Watching TV
    ii. 19.23
    iii. 125
    iv. 8

FURTHER READING

1. C. Jeff. "Neoformix". Multi-level Pie Charts [2]; 2006.
2. Cleveland WS. The Elements of Graphing Data. Pacific Grove, CA: Wadsworth & Advanced Book Program; 1985. ISBN 0-534-03730-5.
3. Dean, S., & Illowsky, B. Descriptive Statistics: Histogram. Retrieved from the Connexions Web site. Available at http://cnx.org/content/m16298/1.11/ Accessed 2013 Nov 19; 2009.
4. Everitt BS. The Cambridge Dictionary of Statistics. 2nd ed. Cambridge: Cambridge University Press; 2002.
5. Good PI, Hardin JW. Common Errors in Statistics (and How to Avoid Them). Wiley; 2003. ISBN 0-471-46068-0.
6. Harris RL. Information Graphics: A comprehensive Illustrated Reference. Oxford University Press; 1999. ISBN 0-19-513532-6.
7. Howitt D, Cramer D. Statistics in Psychology. Prentice Hall; 2008.
8. Nancy RT. Seven Basic Quality Tools. The Quality Toolbox. Milwaukee, WI: American Society for Quality; 2004. p 15. Retrieved 2010-02-05.
9. Phillip IG, James WH. Common Errors in Statistics (and How to Avoid Them). Wiley; 2003. ISBN 0-471-46068-0.
10. Scott DW. On optimal and data-based histograms. Biometrika 1979;66(3):605–610. DOI: 10.1093/biomet/66.3.605.
11. Shimazaki H, Shinomoto S. A method for selecting the bin size of a time histogram. Neural Computation 2007;19(6):1503–1527. DOI: 10.1162/neco.2007.19.6.1503. PMID 17444758.

12. Spence I. No humble pie: the origins and usage of a statistical chart. Journal of Educational and Behavioral Statistics 2005;30(4):353–368.
13. Tufte E. The Visual Display of Quantitative Information. Graphics Press; 2001. ISBN 0-9613921-4-2.
14. van Belle G. Statistical Rules of Thumb. Wiley; 2002. ISBN 0-471-40227-3.
15. Wilkinson L. The Grammar of Graphics. 2nd ed. Springer; 2005. ISBN 0-387-24544-8.

4

PROBABILITY AND ITS APPLICATION

4.1 INTRODUCTION

Probability is a chance of an event happening in the future. In our day-to-day decisions, we use the concept of probability. While driving the car we assume that the probability of accidents is very low, or we would not drive the car. During a cricket match, we often assume a low probability of being hit by another player. During a tennis match, a player needs to take a call on whether the ball will cross the side-line, and if he feels that it is highly probable that the ball would fall outside the line, he leaves it. If the player does not make that assumption, he would probably not leave the ball for fear of losing a point. In assuming many probabilities, we constantly live in fear of the horrible things that might happen to us. Decisions based on probability and statistics provide us with the ability to cope with uncertainty. It has tremendous power in improving the accuracy in our decision-making capacity and in testing new ideas. Within probability and statistics, there are many applications with profound or unexpected results. Let us see how the concept of probability came into existence.

Probability theory grew out of attempts to understand gambling. Gambling was popular before the theory of probability was formed. Gamblers used to identify simple laws of probability by witnessing the events firsthand. The notion of probability has been around for thousands of years, but probability theory as a branch of mathematics did not come into existence until the mid-seventeenth century. Several works on probability were noticed during the fifteenth century. Computing probabilities

Statistics for Exercise Science and Health with Microsoft® Office Excel®, First Edition. J. P. Verma.

became more noticeable during this period even though mathematicians in Italy and France remained unfamiliar with these calculation methods.

During the mid-seventeenth century, a simple question posed to Blaise Pascal by his friend led to the birth of probability theory as we know it today. Chevalier de Méré used to gamble frequently to increase his wealth. He bet on the throw of a dice that at least one 6 would appear during a total of four throws. From his past experience, he knew that he was more successful than not with this game of chance. He was tired of this approach and wanted to do something different. He bet that he would get a total of 12 in throwing two dice 24 times.

> **FACTS TO KNOW**
>
> The use of probability provides confidence in decision-making about population characteristics on the basis of a sample

Quickly, he realized that his earlier approach to the game resulted in more money. He asked his friend Blaise Pascal why his new approach was not as profitable. Pascal worked thoroughly on this problem and came to the conclusion that the probability of winning using the new approach was only 49.1% compared to 51.8% using the old approach (Smith, 1996).

This problem raised by Chevalier de Méré is said to be the start of the famous correspondence between Pascal and Pierre de Fermat. They started exchanging their thoughts on mathematical principles and problems through a series of letters. Historians believe that the first letter written was associated with the above problem and other issues dealing with probability theory. Thus, Pascal and Fermat are the mathematicians credited with the founding of probability theory.

In the seventeenth century, Galileo wrote down some ideas about dice games. This led to discussions and papers that formed the earlier parts of probability theory. There were and have been a variety of contributors to probability theory since then, but it is still one of the least understood areas of mathematics.

4.2 APPLICATION OF PROBABILITY

Probability is the basis of all statistical decision-making processes. In statistical inference, we are concerned with estimating population parameters on the basis of sample data. The big question is how accurate the estimate is. This question can be answered by using the concept of probability. For instance, if the IQ of college students is estimated on the basis of a sample, where the sample mean is 80 and standard deviation is 10, then using statistical theory one can make a probabilistic statement such as "there is a 95.44% chance that the limits 60 to 100 would include the population mean." In other words, one can be 95.44% confident that the average IQ of the college students would be between the limits. As the width of the limits increases, the probability of its containing the population mean keeps increasing.

The application of probability can be seen in different situations. In comparing the effectiveness of two different training programs, the researcher may be interested in knowing which program is better in improving the skill of subjects. This can be answered by conducting an experiment on two random samples of subjects. Since the conclusion is based on the sample data, the inference is bound to have some errors. Here, the concept of probability is used in explaining the accuracy of the findings. By using statistical theory, one can conclude that the first training program is better than the second program in improving the skill with a p value 0.05. This means that the researcher is 95% confident in saying that the first training program is superior than the second program. This fact can be understood as follows. If such an experiment is conducted 100 times, the second training program may prove to be better than the first one for a maximum of 5 occurrences. Similarly, in assessing the relationship between 100 m performance and leg strength, one may infer that the relationship is significant at the 5% level. In other words, it may be concluded that the probability of this statement being true is 0.95. Thus, by using the concept of probability, the validity of findings can be ensured.

Since statistical tests used in hypothesis testing use the concept of probability, the decision of whether to reject or not reject the null hypothesis is always accompanied by some probability. In fact, the entire estimation theory is based on the concept of probability.

4.3 SET THEORY

The concept of set theory is essential to understand various phenomena in probability theory. Let us first understand what a set is, the different operations carried out on it, and the rules involved in set theory.

4.3.1 Set

A *set* is a collection of all possible objects having given properties and specified according to a well-defined rule. The objects of the set are called *elements*. Sets are usually denoted by capital letters, namely, A, B, C, and so on.

If an element of the set A is x, it is denoted as $x \in A$; if x does not belong to A, we write $x \notin A$. Usually, sets are defined by describing the properties of their elements. Thus,

$$A = \{x : x \text{ is even}, \quad x > 0\}$$

It means that all positive even numbers are the elements of the set A. Similarly, one may define the sets of odd numbers, prime numbers, whole numbers, and so on.

4.3.2 Null Set

A set that has no element is known as a *null set*. The null set is also known as an empty set. It is denoted by ϕ or { }. There is only one null set. This is because there is logically only one way that a set can contain nothing.

Remarks

1. Every set is a subset of itself.
2. An empty set is a subset of every set.
3. In probability theory, we shall have one universal set S all the time and we would be interested in the elements of this set S, which changes from situation to situation.

4.3.3 Complement

The complement of any set A consists of those elements of the universal set S that do not belong to A. It is denoted by $\overline{A}$ and given by

$$\overline{A} = S - A$$

Let the sets S and A be defined as

$$S = \{1, 7, 4, 5, 8, 9, 3, 15, 12, 10\} \text{ and } A = \{3, 4, 12\}$$

Then, the complement of A will be the set consisting all the elements of S minus the elements of A and is given by

$$\overline{A} = \{1, 5, 7, 8, 9, 10, 15\}$$

Graphically, the complement of A can be shown as in Figure 4.1.

4.3.4 Subset

If A and B are two sets, then set A is said to be the subset of B if all the elements of A belong to B. It is represented as follows:

$$A \subseteq B$$

By definition, the empty set { } and the universal set S are subsets of every set. Set A is said to be a proper subset of B if all the elements of A belong to set B and there is at least one element in set B that does not belong to set A.

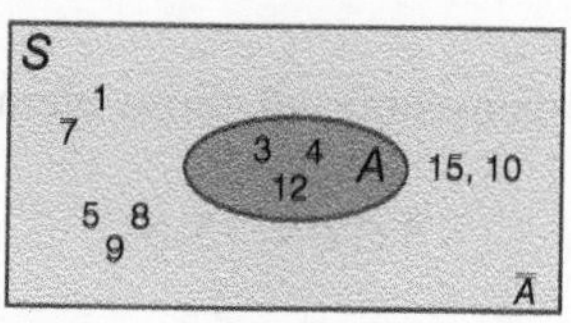

Figure 4.1 Venn diagram showing $\overline{A}$.

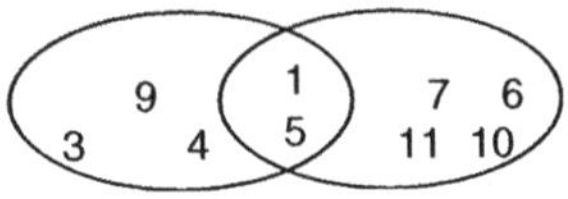

Figure 4.2 Venn diagram showing $A \cup B$.

4.3.5 Operations on Sets

Let us see how different operations are performed on the sets. Learning the concepts of complementary event, union, intersection, and the difference of two sets is important in solving problems on probability.

Union The union of the two given sets A and B is defined as a set consisting of elements that belong to either A or B or both and is denoted by

$$A \cup B = \{x : x \in A \text{ or } x \in B\}$$

For instance, if the sets A and B are defined as

$$A = \{1, 5, 9, 3, 4\} \text{ and } B = \{7, 6, 11, 5, 10, 1\}$$

then $A \cup B$ shall be the set consisting of all those elements that belong to A or B. One should take care that the common elements in both the sets occur once in $A \cup B$ as shown below.

$$A \cup B = \{1,\ 3,\ 4,\ 5,\ 6,\ 7,\ 9,\ 10,\ 11\}$$

Graphically, it can be represented as in Figure 4.2.

Intersection The intersection of the two sets A and B is defined as a set consisting of those elements that belong to both A and B and is denoted by

$$A \cap B = \{x : x \in A \text{ and } x \in B\}$$

If the sets A and B are defined as

$$A = \{3, 8, 5, 9\} \text{ and } B = \{6, 8, 10, 5, 15\}$$

then $A \cap B$ shall be the set consisting all those elements that belong to both A and B.

$$A \cap B = \{5, 8\}$$

Graphically, the intersection of A and B can be shown by Figure 4.3.

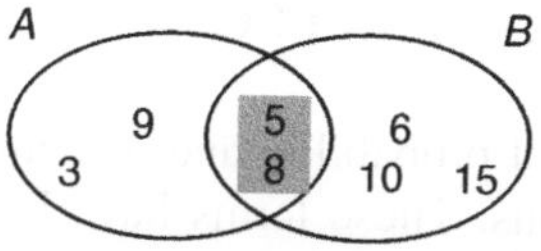

Figure 4.3 Venn diagram showing $A \cap B$.

Difference The difference of the two sets A and B is a set consisting those elements of A that do not belong to B. The difference of A and B is denoted by

$$A - B = \{x : x \in A \text{ and } x \notin B\}$$

If $A = \{1, 6, 9, 3, 5, 4\}$ and $B = \{6, 3, 4\}$, then $A - B = \{1, 5, 9\}$.

4.3.6 Algebra of Sets

The following are some important properties of the operations of sets. If A, B, and C are three subsets of the universal set S, then the following laws hold.

Commutative law:
$$A \cup B = B \cup A$$
$$A \cap B = B \cap A$$

Associative law:
$$(A \cup B) \cup C = A \cup (B \cup C)$$
$$(A \cap B) \cap C = A \cap (B \cap C)$$

Distributive law:
$$A \cap (B \cup C) = (A \cap B) \cup (A \cap C)$$
$$A \cup (B \cap C) = (A \cup B) \cap (A \cup C)$$

Complementary law:
$$A \cap \overline{A} = \phi$$
$$A \cup \overline{A} = S$$
$$A \cup S = S$$
$$A \cap S = A \because (A \subseteq S)$$

Law of difference:
$$A - B = A \cap \overline{B}$$

Law of involution:
$$\overline{\overline{A}} = A$$

Law of idempotent:
$$A \cup A = A$$
$$A \cap A = A$$

4.4 TERMINOLOGIES USED IN PROBABILITY

To understand the concept of probability and its computation procedure, it is necessary to know certain terms. These terms have been discussed in detail in the following sections.

4.4.1 Experiment

An experiment is a systematic procedure of manipulating one or more variables while holding the other variables constant to get the answer to a particular question. Tossing a coin is an experiment. Here, the coin is tossed to know the outcome while all other conditions are kept constant. Similarly, other examples of experiments are rolling a dice, drawing a card from a deck of playing cards, tossing a coin, and so on.

4.4.2 Sample Space

Sample space is the collection of all possible outcomes of an experiment. It is represented by S. Consider an experiment of tossing a single coin. In this experiment, only two outcomes H and T are possible, and therefore the sample space S would be given by

$$S = \{H, T\}$$

If a coin is tossed twice, then the sample space S consists of the following four elements.

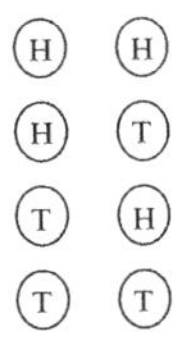

$$S = \{HH, HT, TH, TT\}$$

In general, if a coin is tossed n times, there would be 2^n exhaustive cases.

In rolling a dice, any of the six faces, that is, 1, 2, 3, 4, 5, or 6 may turn up, and therefore the sample space in this case would be

$$S = \{1,\ 2,\ 3,\ 4,\ 5,\ 6\}$$

4.4.3 Event

Any single outcome or a combination of outcomes in an experiment may be called an *event*. The sample space itself may be an event. In tossing a coin, getting H or T is an event. An event may be denoted by E. In rolling a dice, getting an odd number or getting a number that is a multiple of 2 and 3 is an example of an event.

4.4.4 Elementary Events

An elementary event can be defined as any single outcome or element of a sample space in the experiment. In tossing a coin twice, any of the following elements such as *HH* or *TH* in the sample space *S* is known as an elementary event.

$$S = \{HH, HT, TH, TT\}$$

4.4.5 Exhaustive Cases

The total number of all possible outcomes of an experiment is known as an *exhaustive case*. One must note that the sample space is the collection of all such outcomes, whereas exhaustive cases are the number of such outcomes in the sample space. Thus, in tossing a coin twice, the sample space would contain four elements, that is, *HH*, *HT*, *TH*, and *TT*, and the exhaustive number of cases would be $n = 4$.

4.4.6 Trial

The number of times an experiment is repeated is known as a *trial*. To find the probability of getting heads once if a coin is tossed n times, the experiment is said to have n trials.

4.4.7 Equally Likely Events

Events are said to be equally likely if the chances of their occurrences are same. In tossing a coin, the chances of getting heads or tails are the same; hence, heads and tails are equally likely events. Similarly, in rolling a dice, getting all the numbers from 1 to 6 is equally probable; hence, the events of getting 2 or 4 are equally likely.

Let us consider an experiment in which a card is drawn from a deck of playing cards and the events E_1, E_2, and E_3 are defined as follows:

E_1: The card is a black card
E_2: The card is a red card
E_3: The card is an ace card

Then, the events E_1 and E_2 are equally likely because there are equal numbers of black and red cards, and both these types of cards have equal probability of occurring. On the other hand, the events E_1 and E_3 are not equally likely as the chances of getting a black card is more than that of getting an ace card.

4.4.8 Mutually Exclusive Events

Events are said to be mutually exclusive if the occurrence of one event precludes the occurrence of other events. In other words, if one event occurs, the other cannot occur simultaneously. In tossing a coin, either heads or tails can occur; hence, both these events are mutually exclusive. Let us see in what situation events are not mutually exclusive. Consider an experiment in which a dice is rolled and the events defined are as follows:

E_1: Getting an even number
E_2: Getting an odd number
E_3: Getting a multiple of 2 and 3

Here, E_1 and E_2 are mutually exclusive events because any number that is even cannot be odd. On the other hand, the events E_1 and E_3 are not mutually exclusive because the number 6 is even as well as a multiple of 2 and 3.

4.4.9 Independent Events

Events are said to be mutually independent if the happening of an event is not affected by supplementary knowledge concerning the occurrence of other events. If a coin is tossed 2 times, the outcome of the second tossing does not depend on the occurrence in the first tossing, and therefore the events of getting heads or tails are independent events. Here, getting *H* or *T* in the first trial does not affect getting *H* or *T* in the second trial.

4.4.10 Factorial

The factorial of any number n is denoted by $n!$ and is obtained by cumulative multiplication of all the terms from 1 to n.

That is,

$$n! = n(n-1)(n-2)\ldots 1 \tag{4.1}$$

If $n = 5$, then $5! = 5 \times 4 \times 3 \times 2 \times 1 = 120$
Similarly, $6! = 6 \times 5 \times 4 \times 3 \times 2 \times 1 = 720$

4.4.11 Combination

The number of combinations of r elements out of n elements is denoted by ${}^nC_r$ and is obtained by the following formula:

$${}^nC_r = \frac{n!}{r!(n-r)!} \tag{4.2}$$

The following are the universal results of the combination:

i. ${}^nC_0 = 0$
ii. ${}^nC_n = 1$
iii. ${}^nC_r = {}^nC_{n-r}$

Thus, if three teams *A*, *B*, and *C* participate in a tournament where all the teams play with each other, then the number of such matches can be obtained by calculating

$$^{3}C_{2} = \frac{3!}{2!(3-2)!} = \frac{3 \times 2 \times 1}{2 \times 1 \times 1} = 3$$

Here, n is 3 because the total number of teams is 3, and r is 2 because we need to find the combination of two teams at a time.

Shortcut Method Computing of combinations can be done by a shortcut, which is explained below. The procedure shall be explained by computing $^{7}C_{3}$.

1. Write the lower digit of the combination (here, it is 3 in $^{7}C_{3}$) in the denominator and multiply it with all its preceding terms till 1, that is, $3 \times 2 \times 1$.
2. Write the upper digit of the combination (here, it is 7 in $^{7}C_{3}$) in the numerator and multiply it with its preceding numbers till the total number of scores in the numerator is equal to the number of scores in the denominator. Since there are three scores in the denominator, there will be three scores in the numerator also, that is, $7 \times 6 \times 5$.

Following the above-mentioned method,

$$^{7}C_{3} = \frac{7 \times 6 \times 5}{3 \times 2 \times 1} = 35$$

Similarly,

$$^{6}C_{4} = \frac{6 \times 5 \times 4 \times 3}{4 \times 3 \times 2 \times 1} = 15$$

Since $^{n}C_{r} = {}^{n}C_{n-r}$, $^{6}C_{4}$ can be solved as

$$^{6}C_{6-4} = {}^{6}C_{2} = \frac{6 \times 5}{2 \times 1} = 15$$

Example 4.1 If a bag contains two white and three red balls, write all the elements of the sample space.

Solution: Let W_1 and W_2 be two white balls and R_1, R_2, and R_3 be three red balls. The sample space points would be

$$S = \{W_1, W_2, R_1, R_2, R_3\}$$

Since there are five elements in the sample space, the exhaustive cases (n) would be 5.

Example 4.2 If 5 persons are randomly selected from a group of 3 girls and 4 boys, what will be the number of favorable cases that 2 girls and 3 boys are selected?

Solution:

$$\text{Sample space} = S = \{3G,\ 4B\}$$
$$\text{Exhaustive cases } n = 7$$

Number of ways 2 girls can be selected out of 3 = ${}^3C_2 = 3$
Number of ways 3 boys can be selected from 4 boys = ${}^4C_3 = 4$

Thus, the number of favorable cases for selecting 2 girls and 3 boys is ${}^3C_2 \times {}^4C_3 = 12$.

Example 4.3 Compute the following combinations: ${}^6C_2, {}^8C_3, {}^9C_4, {}^{10}C_5$.

Solution: Since

$${}^nC_r = \frac{n!}{r!(n-r)!}$$

In evaluating ${}^6C_2$, $n = 6$ and $r = 2$

$${}^6C_2 = \frac{6!}{2!(6-2)!} = \frac{6 \times 5 \times 4 \times 3 \times 2 \times 1}{2 \times 1 \times 4 \times 3 \times 2 \times 1} = 15$$

The value of the combination can be calculated by using the shortcut as well.

$${}^8C_3 = \frac{8 \times 7 \times 6}{3 \times 2 \times 1} = 56$$

$${}^9C_4 = \frac{9 \times 8 \times 7 \times 6}{4 \times 3 \times 2 \times 1} = 126$$

$${}^{10}C_5 = \frac{10 \times 9 \times 8 \times 7 \times 6}{5 \times 4 \times 3 \times 2 \times 1} = 252$$

Check Your Progress

Note: Tick the correct answer by using the sign (√).

	True	False
1. Probability is used in decision-making processes.	-	-
2. The concept of hypothesis is used in testing the significance of relationships.	-	-

3. The null element is a subset of every set. - -
4. The null set consists of zero elements. - -
5. The set A is a proper subset of B if there is at least one element in B that does not belong to A. - -
6. $A-B$ consists of those elements that belong to A but do not belong to B. - -
7. In defining a set, it is not necessary to define the rules for its elements. - -
8. In conducting an experiment, a sample space may have infinite outcomes. - -
9. In tossing a coin, the event E (getting a heads or tails) is an elementary event. - -
10. In rolling a dice, the events E_1 (getting a multiple of 2) and E_2 (getting a multiple of 3) are mutually exclusive events. - -
11. $A \cup B$ means that the elements belong to both the groups. - -
12. If a coin is tossed 4 times, then the exhaustive cases would be 32. - -
13. The value of ${}^6C_2$ is 15. - -
14. In tossing a coin 3 times, there can be more than 8 events. - -
15. $A \cap B$ consists of those elements that belong to either A and B. - -
16. In tossing a coin twice, getting a heads in the first toss and getting a tails in the second toss are the independent events. - -
17. A set is a subset of itself. - -
18. The factorials ($n!$) and $(n-1)!$ are the same. - -
19. If 3 men are to be selected from a group of 6 men and 4 women, the number of favorable cases for the event would be 20. - -
20. A trial is nothing but the outcome of an experiment. - -
21. In drawing a card from a deck of playing cards, the events E_1 (getting an ace card) and E_2 (getting a ten) are equally likely events. - -
22. The value of ${}^1C_4$ is 1. - -
23. Two cards are drawn without replacement. Getting a queen in the first draw and getting an ace in the second draw are independent events. - -

24. If two balls are drawn from a bag that contains 6 red and 5 white balls, the number of exhaustive cases would be 110.	-	-
25. The values of the factorial ${}^{10}C_4$ and ${}^{10}C_6$ are the same.	-	-

PRACTICE EXERCISE

1. If a coin is tossed 3 times, how many sample space points will it have? Write all the cases.
2. If a coin is tossed 2 times, what would be the probability of getting one heads and one tails?
3. Compute ${}^{10}C_4$ and ${}^{10}C_6$ and check whether these two are the same.
4. If two dice are rolled and you are required to find the probability of getting the number on the second dice larger than first, enumerate the number of cases favorable for the event.
5. In finding the probability of getting the odd number on the first dice and even number on the second dice while rolling the dice twice, write all the favorable cases for this event.
6. A coin is tossed continuously until tails occurs for the first time. Enumerate the sample space.
7. A coach examines two athletes for fitness. Each person may be fit (F) or unfit (U). What is the sample space?

4.5 BASIC DEFINITIONS OF PROBABILITY

There are different approaches in computing probabilities. These approaches have been evolved from the earliest era to modern times. In chronological order, these approaches can be sequenced as classical probability, empirical probability, subjective probability, and axiomatic probability. In fact, this is a unifying perspective. The logic needed for subjective probability can be proved to hold for the classical and empirical definitions. Similarly, the logic that is used in axiomatic definition can be used with any of the above three perspectives.

4.5.1 Classical Definition of Probability

The earliest definition of computing probability is known as classical probability. This can be stated as follows. If an experiment results in N mutually exclusive and equally likely cases out of which m are favorable to the event E, then the probability of the event E is given by

$$P(E) = \frac{\text{Number of times the event } E \text{ occurs}}{\text{Total number of outcomes}} = \frac{m}{N} \tag{4.3}$$

For example, in computing the probability of drawing a queen of diamonds from a randomly shuffled single deck of cards, we would divide the number of favorable cases by the total number of all possible outcomes. As there are 52 possible outcomes, only one of which is favorable to the event, the probability of drawing a queen of diamonds from a single deck is 1/52.

The classical definition of probability can be applied in a situation in which all possible outcomes and favorable cases for the event A can be counted. This definition is due to Laplace (1749–1827). The classical definition is also known as an *a priori definition of probability*. The word *priori* is used because the definition is based on previous knowledge that the outcomes are equally likely. One should note that classical probabilities can be deduced from knowledge of the sample space and its assumptions. Nothing has to be observed in terms of outcomes to deduce the probabilities.

In tossing a coin, the probability of getting heads is ½ . This probability is computed by using the classical definition of probability. Before computing the probability, it is assumed that the occurrence of the events H and T are equally likely. The probability of any event is a number that lies between 0 and 1. If the event is impossible, its probability is 0 because there is no case favorable to the event. If the event is a sure event, its probability is 1 because all the cases of the sample space are favorable to the event. For instance, in tossing a coin, getting both heads and tails is an impossible event, whereas getting heads or tails is a sure event.

The classical definition is applicable only when the events are equally likely and countable. This definition is not applicable when it is difficult to count the total number of outcomes or the cases favorable to the event. It is difficult to count the number of people who play cricket in the country. Thus, it is difficult to find the probability of selecting a batsman of some age, say, more than 21 years old. The classical definition of probability fails if any of these conditions are not satisfied.

4.5.2 Empirical Definition of Probability

The empirical approach of probability is also known as the method of relative frequency of occurrence. Empirical probability does not assume all simple events to be equally likely. This approach of computing probability depends on the observed data only, and no conditions are imposed on the characteristics of the events. Here, the probability that event E will happen is figured out empirically by looking at the relative frequency with which E occurs in the observed data. Thus, empirical probabilities are based on our observation or experimentation, rather than on theoretical reasoning or an assumed knowledge of a process. The empirical definition of probability can be stated as follows.

If a random sample of size n is drawn from the population of interest and if there are m cases favoring the attribute E in the sample, then the relative frequency of E in the sample is given by

$$\text{Relative frequency of } E = \frac{\text{Number of sample observations possessing attribute } E}{\text{Number of observations in the sample}} = \frac{m}{n} \qquad (4.4)$$

This relative frequency of E in the sample is an estimate of $P(E)$. The basis of this approach is that there is some $P(E)$ that cannot be deduced as in the case of the classical approach but one can estimate it. This is because this definition is applicable in a situation where events are not finite and equally likely.

For example, if one tosses a coin (which may or may not be fair) 80 times and observes heads 48 times, then one's estimate of the probability of heads is 0.60. Frequency probability allows the estimation of probabilities when classical probability fails.

4.5.3 Subjective Definition of Probability

The subjective approach of finding the probability of any event is based on one's experience, intuition, or a hunch about the event. In a situation where one can neither determine the number of events nor collect the data, both classical and relative frequency methods of assigning probability fail. In such a situation, the subjective approach is used to find the probability of an event. Here, one comes up with a subjective opinion about the probability of an event. Of course, the probability value estimated in this way is subjective, and different people can be expected to assign different values to the same event. For instance, based on experience, one can find the probability of a female candidate qualifying in a junior research fellowship examination in a college.

4.5.4 Axiomatic Definition of Probability

The modern definition of probability is known as *axiomatic probability*. This approach of computing probability is used when the classical approach fails. That is, in a situation where events are infinite or/and not equally likely, the axiomatic approach of probability is used to compute the probabilities. The axiomatic definition of probability is stated as follows:

Any real-valued function P is said to be the probability of an event E if the following three axioms are satisfied:

1. $0 \leq P(E) \leq 1$ for every allowable event E.
2. $P(S) = 1$, S is the sample space. In other words, the probability of a sure event is 1.

3. If $E_1, E_2, \ldots, E_n$ are the n mutually exclusive events, then

$$P(E_1 \cup E_2 \cup \ldots \cup E_n) = P(E_1) + P(E_2) + \ldots P(E_n)$$

4.6 SOME RESULTS ON PROBABILITY

By using the axiomatic definition of probability, the following properties of probability can be deduced.

1. For any null event ϕ, $P(\phi) = 1$.
2. For any event A, $P(\overline{A}) = 1 - P(A)$.
3. If $A, B \in S$ and $A \subseteq B$, then $P(A) \leq P(B)$.
4. For any $A_1, A_2, \ldots, A_n \in S$, $P(A_1 \cup A_2 \cup \ldots \cup A_n) \leq P(A_1) + P(A_2) + \ldots P(A_n)$. This is called Boole's inequality.
5. If $A, B \in S$, then $P(A) = P(A \cap B) + P(A \cap \overline{B})$, that is, $P(A) = P(AB) + P(A\overline{B})$.
6. If $A, B \in S$, then $P(A \cap \overline{B}) = P(A) - P(A \cap B)$, that is, $P(A-B) = P(A) - P(AB)$.

4.7 COMPUTING PROBABILITY

To compute the probability of any event E, first the sample space S needs to be enumerated. The number of elements in the sample space is known as exhaustive cases. After writing all possible outcomes of an experiment in the sample space S, the number of favorable cases for the event E is counted. If the number of exhaustive cases is "N" and the number of favorable cases for the event E is "m," then the probability of the event E is obtained by

$$P(E) = \frac{\text{Number of favorable cases for the event } E}{\text{Exhaustive cases}} = \frac{m}{N}$$

Example 4.4 If a coin is tossed, what is the probability of getting the following events?

i. Getting heads
ii. Getting tails
iii. Getting heads or tails
iv. Getting heads and tails

Solution: To find the different probabilities, first list the sample space S. Since there are two possibilities in tossing a coin, that is, one may get heads (H) or tails (T), the sample space S would become

$$S = \{H, T\}$$

Thus,

$$\text{Exhaustive cases } = N = 2$$

i. *Getting Heads*

Let this event be denoted as E_1. Since the heads H can occur only in one way in the sample space S, the number of favorable cases for the event E_1 is $m = 1$.

Thus,

$$P(E_1) = P(\text{Getting a } H) = \frac{m}{N} = \frac{1}{2}$$

ii. *Getting Tails*

Let this event be denoted as E_2. Since the tails T can also occur only in one way in the sample space S, the number of favorable cases for the event E_2 is $m = 1$.

Thus,

$$P(E_2) = P(\text{Getting a } T) = \frac{m}{N} = \frac{1}{2}$$

iii. *Getting Heads or Tails*

Let this event be denoted as E_3. This event is said to occur if either heads or tails appears. Hence, both the outcomes in the sample space S are favorable to this event; therefore, $m = 2$.

Thus,

$$P(E_3) = P(\text{Getting } H \text{ or } T) = \frac{m}{N} = \frac{2}{2} = 1$$

iv. *Getting Heads and Tails*

Let this event be denoted as E_4. Since heads and tails cannot occur simultaneously, no case in the sample space S is favorable for this event; hence, $m =$ 0.

Thus,

$$P(E_4) = P(\text{Getting } H \text{ and } T) = \frac{m}{N} = \frac{0}{2} = 0$$

Example 4.5 In an experiment, three coins are tossed. Enumerate the sample space points and compute the following probabilities:

i. $P(3H)$
ii. $P(2H\ 1T)$
iii. $P(1H\ 2T)$

Solution: Since three coins have been tossed, the sample space S shall be

$$S = \{HHH, HHT, HTH, THH, TTT, TTH, THT, HTT\}$$

$$n = \text{ exhaustive cases} = \text{total number of outcomes in the sample space} = 8$$

i. $P(3H) = \dfrac{\text{Number of cases favorable for } 3H}{\text{Exhaustive cases}} = \dfrac{1}{8}$

ii. $P(2H\ 1T) = \dfrac{\text{Number of cases favorable for } 2H \text{ and } 1T}{\text{Exhaustive cases}} = \dfrac{3}{8}$

iii. $P(1H\ 2T) = \dfrac{\text{Number of cases favorable for } 1H \text{ and } 2T}{\text{Exhaustive cases}} = \dfrac{3}{8}$

Example 4.6 If two dice are rolled, what is the probability that the sum is (a) 9 and (b) greater than 10?

Solution: Let us first write the elements of the sample space S. Since two dice have been rolled, the sample space will be obtained by taking all possible combinations of the two dice.

		Dice 1					
		1	2	3	4	5	6
Dice 2	1	(1,1)	(1,2)	(1,3)	(1,4)	(1,5)	(1,6)
	2	(2,1)	(2,2)	(2,3)	(2,4)	(2,5)	(2,6)
	3	(3,1)	(3,2)	(3,3)	(3,4)	(3,5)	(3,6)
	4	(4,1)	(4,2)	(4,3)	(4,4)	(4,5)	(4,6)
	5	(5,1)	(5,2)	(5,3)	(5,4)	(5,5)	(5,6)
	6	(6,1)	(6,2)	(6,3)	(6,4)	(6,5)	(6,6)

i. Let the event A = sum of the two dice = 9. The event A can be obtained in the following manner:

Favorable Cases of A	
Dice 1	Dice 2
6	3
5	4
4	5
3	6

$$m = \text{Favorable number of cases for the event } A = 4$$

$$P(A) = \frac{\text{Number of cases favorable for the event } A}{\text{Exhaustive cases}} = \frac{4}{36} = \frac{1}{9}$$

ii. Let the event B denote that the sum on the two dice is greater than 10.
Event B can materialize in the following manner:

6	5
5	6
6	6

Here, $m = 3$. Thus,

$$P(B) = \frac{3}{36} = \frac{1}{12}$$

Example 4.7 An unbiased coin is tossed 3 times. Write the sample space and compute the probabilities of the following events:

i. getting exactly 1 tails
ii. more than 2 heads

Solution: If a coin is tossed n times, then there are 2^n exhaustive cases. Here, the coin is tossed 3 times; hence exhaustive cases are $n = 2^3 = 8$.

$$S = \{HHH, HHT, HTH, THH, TTH, THT, HTT, TTT\}$$

i. In tossing a coin 3 times, exactly 1 tail can materialize in the following manner:

$$HHT, HTH, \text{ and } THH$$

$$m = \text{favorable number of cases for getting exactly 1 tail} = 3$$

$$P\text{ (getting exactly 1 tail)} = \frac{m}{n} = \frac{3}{8}$$

ii. The outcome in the sample space that is favorable to the event of getting more than 2 heads is only HHH.

$$m = \text{favorable number of cases for getting more than 2 heads} = 1$$

$$P\text{ (getting more than 2 heads)} = \frac{m}{n} = \frac{1}{8}$$

Example 4.8 A coin is tossed 6 times. Assuming that the coin is fair, compute the following probabilities.

i. $P(6H)$
ii. $P(5H,\ 1T)$

iii. $P(4H, 2T)$
iv. $P(3H, 3T)$

Solution: If a coin is tossed n times, then the number of exhaustive cases are 2^n. Here, a coin is tossed 6 times; hence, the exhaustive cases n would be $2^6 = 64$.

i. In tossing a coin 6 times, the number of favorable cases for getting 6 heads is obtained by

$$m = {}^6C_6$$

$$P(6H) = \frac{\text{Number of favorable cases for } 6H}{\text{Exhaustive cases}} = \frac{{}^6C_6}{2^6} = \frac{1}{64} \qquad [\because {}^nC_n = 1]$$

ii. In tossing a coin 6 times, the number of favorable cases for getting $5H$ and $1T$ can be obtained by

$$m = {}^6C_5$$

Since ${}^nC_r = {}^nC_{n-r}$, ${}^6C_5$ is equivalent to ${}^6C_1$. Thus, the favorable cases for the event ($5H$, $1T$) can be obtained by solving either ${}^6C_1$ or ${}^6C_5$.

$$P(5H, 1T) = \frac{\text{Number of favorable cases for } 5H \text{ and } 1T}{\text{Exhaustive cases}} = \frac{{}^6C_1}{2^6} = \frac{6}{64} = \frac{3}{32}$$

iii. In tossing 6 coins, the number of favorable cases for getting $4H$ and $2T$ is obtained by

$$m = {}^6C_2 = \frac{6 \times 5}{2 \times 1} = 15$$

$$P(4H, 2T) = \frac{\text{Number of favorable cases for } 4H \text{ and } 2T}{\text{Exhaustive cases}} = \frac{{}^6C_2}{2^6} = \frac{15}{64}$$

iv. The favorable cases for getting $3H$ and $3T$ would be

$$m = {}^6C_3 = \frac{6 \times 5 \times 4}{3 \times 2 \times 1} = 20$$

$$P(3H, 3T) = \frac{\text{Number of favorable cases for } 3H \text{ and } 3T}{\text{Exhaustive cases}} = \frac{{}^6C_3}{2^6} = \frac{20}{64} = \frac{5}{16}$$

Example 4.9 Four cards are drawn from a pack of cards. What are the probabilities of getting

i. all cards of the same color
ii. all four cards of the same suit
iii. one card from each suit.

Solution:

i. Four cards can be drawn from 26 red cards in ${}^{26}C_4$ ways. Since these 4 cards should be either red or black, the number of favorable cases that all 4 cards are of the same color will be $2 \times {}^{26}C_4$. Further, 4 cards can be drawn from the pack of cards in ${}^{52}C_4$ ways.
Thus,

$$P(\text{All 4 cards are of the same color}) = \frac{2 \times {}^{26}C_4}{{}^{52}C_4}$$

ii. The number of favorable cases that all 4 cards are from one suit is ${}^{13}C_4$.
Since there are 4 suits, the number of favorable cases that all the 4 cards drawn are from any of the suits is $4 \times {}^{13}C_4$. Thus,

$$P(\text{All 4 cards are of the same suit}) = \frac{4 \times {}^{13}C_4}{{}^{52}C_4}$$

iii. The number of favorable cases that out of 4 cards drawn one belongs to each suit is ${}^{13}C_1 \times {}^{13}C_1 \times {}^{13}C_1 \times {}^{13}C_1$.

$$P(\text{1 card from each suit}) = \frac{{}^{13}C_1 \times {}^{13}C_1 \times {}^{13}C_1 \times {}^{13}C_1}{{}^{52}C_4}$$

Example 4.10 A bag contains 4 black, 3 red, and 5 white marbles. If 2 marbles are drawn at random, find the probability that

i. both marbles are white
ii. both marbles are of the same color
iii. one is black and the other is white.

Solution:

$$S = \{4B,\ 3R,\ 5W\}$$

i. Both marbles are white.
Since there are 12 marbles in the bag, 2 balls can be drawn in the following ways:

$${}^{12}C_2 = 66$$

The favorable cases for the event A are ${}^{5}C_2 = 10$:

$$P(A) = \frac{{}^{5}C_2}{{}^{12}C_2} = \frac{10}{66} = \frac{5}{33}$$

ii. Both marbles are of the same color.

Both marbles can be black, red, or white. Thus, the number of favorable cases for the event B is

$$^{4}C_2 + {}^{3}C_2 + {}^{5}C_2 = 6 + 3 + 10 = 19$$

$$P(B) = \frac{19}{^{12}C_2} = \frac{19}{66}$$

iii. One marble is black and the other is white.

$$\text{Favorable cases for the event } = {}^{4}C_1 \times {}^{5}C_1 = 20$$

$$P(C) = \frac{20}{^{12}C_2} = \frac{20}{66} = \frac{10}{33}$$

4.8 TYPES OF PROBABILITY

In this section, four specific types of probabilities, that is, marginal probability, union probability, joint probability, and conditional probability, have been discussed. Understanding these probabilities will help in solving different problems on probability.

4.8.1 Marginal Probability

Marginal probability is denoted by $P(E)$ and is obtained by dividing the number of cases favorable for the event E by the total number of cases. An example of marginal probability is the probability that a sports person plays tennis. This probability is computed by dividing the number of players who play tennis by the total number of players. The probability of a sports person using Nike shoes is also a marginal probability. This probability can be computed by dividing the number of sports persons using Nike shoes by the total number of sports persons.

4.8.2 Union Probability

Union probability is the probability of union of two events and is denoted by $P(A \cup B)$ where A and B are the two events. $P(A \cup B)$ is the probability that either A occurs or B occurs or both A and B occur. An example of union probability is the probability that a student plays basketball or volleyball. The union event shall occur if the student play at least any one of these two games. Another example is the probability of getting a red card or an ace card in drawing a card from a well-shuffled pack of playing cards. In a college, the probability that a person is a male or a lecturer is a union probability. A person qualifies for the union event by being male or by being a lecturer or by being both (a male lecturer).

4.8.3 Joint Probability

Joint probability is the probability of intersection of two events. If A and B are two events, then it is denoted by $P(A \cap B)$. The intersection event is said to occur if both events occur simultaneously. An example of joint probability is the probability of a student playing both sports: basketball and volleyball. Another example of joint probability is the probability of getting a number that is a multiple of 2 as well as a multiple of 3 in rolling a dice.

4.8.4 Conditional Probability

Conditional probability is denoted as $P(A/B)$. This indicates the probability that A will occur given that B is known to have occurred. In conditional probability, we are interested in those events of A where the event B has already occurred. An example of conditional probability is the probability that a student plays basketball given that he plays volleyball also. Here, our sample space consists of those students who play volleyball. Only those students who play basketball out of those who play volleyball also are the favorable cases of this conditional event. Another example of conditional probability is the probability of getting a king card given that it is red. Here, all those cards that are red belong to the sample space, and the king cards that are red also are the favorable cases of this conditional event.

4.9 THEOREMS OF PROBABILITY

There are two important theorems of probability known as *law of addition* and *law of multiplication*. These theorems, along with their applications, are discussed in this section.

4.9.1 Law of Addition of Probabilities

If A and B are any two events, then according to the law of addition, the probability of $A \cup B$ is given by

$$P(A \cup B) = P(A) + P(B) - P(A \cap B) \tag{4.5}$$

Case 1: Events A and B are mutually exclusive.

If the events A and B are mutually exclusive, then $A \cap B$ is a null event, and therefore, $P(A \cap B) = 0$. In this situation, the probability of $A \cup B$ becomes

$$P(A \cup B) = P(A) + P(B) \tag{4.6}$$

Case 2: Events A and B are mutually independent.

If the events A and B are mutually independent, then $P(A \cap B) = P(A)P(B)$. In this situation, the probability of $A \cup B$ becomes

$$P(A \cup B) = P(A) + P(B) - P(A)P(B) \tag{4.7}$$

Example 4.11 One card is drawn from a pack of 52 cards where drawing of all 52 cards is equally likely. Find the probability that the card drawn is

i. black
ii. a queen
iii. either a jack or red
iv. black and an ace

Solution: One card can be drawn from the pack in 52 ways; hence, n = exhaustive cases = 52.

i. Since there are 26 black cards, the number of favorable cases for drawing a black card (m) is 26

$$P(\text{drawing a black card}) = \frac{m}{n} = \frac{26}{52} = \frac{1}{2}$$

ii. There are 4 queen cards; hence, $m = 4$

$$P(\text{drawing a queen card}) = \frac{4}{52} = \frac{1}{13}$$

iii. Let the events be defined as
A: drawing a jack card
B: drawing a red card

$$P(A) = \frac{4}{52} = \frac{1}{13}$$

and

$$P(B) = \frac{26}{52} = \frac{1}{2}$$

Since there are 2 jack cards that are red also, the number of favorable cases for the event $A \cap B$ is $m = 2$.

$$P(A \cap B) = \frac{2}{52} = \frac{1}{26}$$

Here, both events A and B are not mutually exclusive; hence, by the law of addition,

$$P(A \cup B) = P(A) + P(B) - P(A \cap B)$$

Substituting the values,

$$P(A \cup B) = \frac{1}{13} + \frac{1}{2} - \frac{1}{26} = \frac{7}{13}$$

Example 4.12 If A and B are two events and $P(\overline{A}) = 2/3$, $P(\overline{B}) = 3/5$, and $P(A \cup B) = 1/2$, then find the values of (i) $P(A \cap B)$ and (ii) $P(\overline{A} \cap B)$.

Solution:

i. Given $P(\overline{A}) = 2/3$, $P(\overline{B}) = 3/5$, and $P(A \cup B) = 1/2$

$$P(A) = 1 - P(\overline{A}) = 1 - \frac{2}{3} = \frac{1}{3}$$

$$P(B) = 1 - P(\overline{B}) = 1 - \frac{3}{5} = \frac{2}{5}$$

Therefore, $P(A \cup B) = P(A) + P(B) - P(A \cap B)$

$$\Rightarrow P(A \cap B) = P(A) + P(B) - P(A \cup B) = \frac{1}{3} + \frac{2}{5} - \frac{1}{2} = \frac{7}{30}$$

ii. We know that $(\overline{A} \cap B) \cup (A \cap B) = B$

Since the events $(\overline{A} \cap B)$ and $A \cap B$ are disjoint events,

$$P((\overline{A} \cap B) \cup (A \cap B)) = P(\overline{A} \cap B) + P(A \cap B)$$

Thus,

$$P(\overline{A} \cap B) + P(A \cap B) = P(B)$$

$$\Rightarrow P(\overline{A} \cap B) = P(B) - P(A \cap B)$$

$$= \frac{2}{5} - \frac{7}{30} = \frac{1}{6}$$

Example 4.13 If the probability of occurrence of both events A and B is equal to 1/3 and that of occurrence of the event A or B is equal to 3/4, then compute $P(\overline{A}) + P(\overline{B})$.

Solution: Given that $P(A \cap B) = \frac{1}{3}$ and $P(A \cup B) = \frac{3}{4}$

$$P(A \cup B) = P(A) + P(B) - P(A \cap B)$$

$$\Rightarrow P(A) + P(B) = P(A \cup B) + P(A \cap B) = \frac{3}{4} + \frac{1}{3} = \frac{13}{12}$$

$$\Rightarrow 1 - P(\overline{A}) + 1 - P(\overline{B}) = \frac{13}{12}$$

$$\Rightarrow P(\overline{A}) + P(\overline{B}) = 2 - \frac{13}{12} = \frac{11}{12}$$

4.9.2 Law of Multiplication of Probability

If A and B are any two events, then according to the law of multiplication the probability of $A \cap B$ is given by

$$P(A \cap B) = P(B)P(A/B) \tag{4.8}$$

where the event $B \neq \phi$ and $P(A/B)$ is the probability of occurrence of event A where event B has already occurred.

Equation (4.8) can also be written as

$$P(A \cap B) = P(A)P(B/A) \tag{4.9}$$

where the event $A \neq \phi$ and $P(B/A)$ is the probability of occurrence of event B where event A has already occurred.

When Events A and B Are Independent If events A and B are independent, then the probability of occurrence of event A is not affected by the occurrence or nonoccurrence of event B; therefore,

$$P(A/B) = P(A)$$

Substituting the value of $P(A/B)$ in (4.8), we get

$$P(A \cap B) = P(A)P(B) \tag{4.10}$$

Remarks

1. Any two events A and B are independent if and only if $P(A \cap B) = P(A)\,P(B)$.
2. For any three independent events A, B, and C, $P(A \cap B \cap C) = P(A)\,P(B)\,P(C)$.

Example 4.14 A sports goods firm manufactures cricket bats. Two percent of all bats that are manufactured are defective. If 2 bats are chosen by the quality control manager one at a time, with replacement, what is the probability that the 2 bats selected are defective?

Solution: If the event E denotes a defective bat, then $P(E) = 0.02$. Here, it is determined that

$$P(E_1 \cap E_2)$$

Since the sampling is done with replacement, the two events are independent. Thus,

$$P(E_1 \cap E_2) = P(E_1)P(E_2) = (0.02)\ (0.02) = 0.0004$$

Example 4.15 In an organization, there are 1500 employees out of whom 800 are more than 55 years old and 900 are female. Given that 40% of the females are over 55 years of age, what is the probability that a randomly chosen employee from the organization is either female or over 55 years of age?

Solution:

A: Employee is more than 55 years of age

B: Employee is a female

Given that $P(A) = \frac{800}{1500} = \frac{8}{15}$, $P(B) = \frac{900}{1500} = \frac{3}{5}$, and $P(A/B) = \frac{2}{5}$

To find $P(A \cup B)$,

$$P(A \cap B) = P(A/B)P(B)$$
$$\Rightarrow P(A \cap B) = \frac{2}{5} \times \frac{3}{5} = \frac{6}{25}$$

Thus,

$$P(A \cup B) = P(A) + P(B) - P(A \cap B)$$
$$= \frac{8}{15} + \frac{3}{5} - \frac{6}{25} = \frac{67}{75}$$

4.9.3 Conditional Probability

If A and B are two events, then the conditional probability of an event A given that event B has already occurred is denoted as $P(A/B)$, and is given by

$$P(A/B) = \frac{P(A \cap B)}{P(B)} \tag{4.11}$$

where $P(A \cap B)$ is the probability of those cases where the events A and B occur simultaneously and $P(B)$ is the marginal probability of the event B. Conditional probability $P(A/B)$ refers to those cases where the event B has already occurred. To compute this probability, one should look for the favorable cases of A out of those cases where the event B has already occurred. Consider the following example to understand the concept of conditional probability.

In a study, 60% of athletes said that the quality of coaching (A) improves performance and 75% of athletes said that the Astroturf (B) improves performance. In addition, suppose 45% of the athletes believe that both the quality of coaching and Astroturf improve performance. An athlete is selected randomly and asked about performance. This athlete believes that quality of coaching improves performance. What is the probability that this athlete believes that the Astroturf would improve performance? In other words, what is the probability that a randomly selected athlete believes that the Astroturf would improve performance, given that he believes that the quality of coaching also improves performance? Symbolically, the question is

$$P(B/A) = ?$$

We know that

$$P(B/A) = \frac{P(A \cap B)}{P(A)}$$

Here,

$P(A)$ = Probability that the athlete believes the quality of coaching improves performance = 0.60

$P(B)$ = Probability that the athlete believes the Astroturf improves performance = 0.75

$P(A \cap B)$ = Probability that the athlete believes both the quality of coaching and Astroturf improve performance = 0.45

Substituting the three probabilities,

$$P(B/A) = \frac{0.45}{0.60} = 0.75$$

Example 4.16 The following are the response matrix and the corresponding probability matrix for the survey results of 100 postgraduate students who were asked to give their preference for a sport for match practice class and their choice of subject specialization. The students were allowed to select only one sport and one subject specialization.

Response Matrix

		Sport			
		Basket ball A	Badminton B	Swimming C	Total
Specialization	Sports Psychology D	19	13	8	40
	Exercise Physiology E	11	9	5	25
	Sports Biomechanics F	10	11	14	35
	Total	40	33	27	$N = 100$

Probability Matrix

		Sport			
		Basket ball A	Badminton B	Swimming C	Total
Specialization	Sports Psychology D	0.19	0.13	0.08	0.40
	Exercise Physiology E	0.11	0.09	0.05	0.25
	Sports Biomechanics F	0.10	0.11	0.14	0.35
	Total	0.40	0.33	0.27	1.00

Find the following probabilities:

i. $P(E)$
ii. $P(B \cap D)$
iii. $P(A \cup F)$
iv. $P(A/D)$
v. $P(C/E)$
vi. $P(C/B)$

Solution: The probability matrix can be prepared by dividing each frequency in the response matrix by the total (100).

i. $P(E)$ is the marginal probability and is obtained by adding the probabilities in the row E of the probability matrix. Thus,

$$P(E) = 0.25$$

ii. $P(B \cap D)$ refers to the probability of the students who prefer badminton (B) and opt for sports psychology (D). This probability is the value at the cross section of column B and row D in the probability matrix. Hence,

$$P(B \cap D) = 0.13$$

This indicates that 13% of the students prefer badminton and opt for sport psychology.

iii. Since A and F are not mutually exclusive events

$$P(A \cup F) = P(A) + P(F) - P(A \cap F)$$

$$P(A) = 0.40 \text{ (the sum of probabilities in column } A)$$

$$P(F) = 0.35 \text{ (the sum of the probabilities in row } F)$$

$$P(A \cap F) = 0.10 \text{ (value of the probability at the cross section of column } A \text{ and row } F)$$

Substituting these values in the equation,

$$P(A \cup F) = 0.40 + 0.35 - 0.10 = 0.65$$

This indicates that 65% of the students prefer either basketball (A) or sports biomechanics (F) or both basketball and sports biomechanics.

iv. We know that

$$P(A/D) = \frac{P(A \cap D)}{P(D)}$$

Here, the joint probability $P(A \cap D)$ appears in the cell of the matrix (0.19) and the marginal probability $P(D)$ is 0.40. Substituting these two probabilities in the formula, the required probability becomes 0.475.

$$P(A/D) = \frac{0.19}{0.40} = 0.475$$

This indicates that 47.5% of the students who take sports psychology as a specialization prefer basketball.

v.

$$P(C/E) = \frac{P(C \cap E)}{P(E)}$$

Here, the joint probability $P(C \cap E)$ in the probability matrix (cross-section point of column C and row E) is 0.05, and the marginal probability $P(E)$ that appears in row E is 0.25. Substituting these probabilities in the formula, the conditional probability becomes

$$P(C/E) = \frac{0.05}{0.25} = 0.2$$

One may conclude that 20% of the students specializing in exercise physiology prefer swimming.

vi.

$$P(C/B) = \frac{P(C \cap B)}{P(B)} = \frac{0.00}{0.33} = 0.00$$

Here, the events C and B are mutually exclusive; hence, $P(C \cap B)$ is 0 and therefore $P(C/B)$ is 0. This indicates that if a student has opted for badminton, he or she cannot opt for swimming.

4.9.4 Bayes' Theorem

Let $E_1, E_2, \ldots, E_n$ be the n exhaustive events of a random experiment such that the $P(E_i) > 0$, $\forall\, i = 1, 2, \ldots, n$. In other words, the events $E_1, E_2, \ldots, E_n$ constitute a partition of sample space S, that is, $\cup E_i = S$. If A is an arbitrary event of the sample space of the above experiment with $P(A) > 0$, then

$$P(E_i/A) = \frac{P(E_i)P(A/E_i)}{\sum_{j=1}^{n} P(E_j)P(A/E_j)};\ 1 \le i \le n \text{ and } 1 \le j \le n \qquad (4.12)$$

Example 4.17 In an undergraduate class there are 50 males and 30 females, and in the postgraduate class there are 40 males and 25 females. One student is randomly selected from one of the classes and is found to be male. Find the probability that he was selected from the postgraduate class.

Solution: Let us define the events as

E_1: the undergraduate class is chosen
E_2: the postgraduate class is chosen
A: the student selected is male

It is required to calculate $P(E_2/A) = P$(that the student is selected from the postgraduate class, given that the student is male).

Using Bayes' theorem (4.12)

$$P(E_2/A) = \frac{P(E_2)P(A/E_2)}{P(E_1)P(A/E_1) + P(E_2)P(A/E_2)}$$

Since the two classes are equally likely to be selected,

$$P(E_1) = P(E_2) = \frac{1}{2}$$

In addition,

$$P(A/E_1) = P(\text{male student is selected from the undergraduate class})$$
$$= \frac{50}{80} = \frac{5}{8}$$
$$P(A/E_2) = P(\text{male student is selected from the postgraduate class})$$
$$= \frac{40}{65} = \frac{8}{13}$$

$$\Rightarrow P(E_2/A) = \frac{\frac{1}{2} \times \frac{8}{13}}{\frac{1}{2} \times \frac{5}{8} + \frac{1}{2} \times \frac{8}{13}} = \frac{\frac{8}{13}}{\frac{5}{8} + \frac{8}{13}} = \frac{8}{13} \times \frac{104}{129} = \frac{832}{1677}$$

Example 4.18 In the match practice classes of badminton, gymnastics, and swimming, there are 60, 50, and 40 students, respectively, out of which 30, 40, and 10 students are women, respectively. The chances that the students leave the match practice in badminton, gymnastics, and swimming are 20%, 15%, and 10%, respectively, irrespective of the sexes. One student leaves the match practice and she is a female. What is the probability that she had swimming as the sport?

Solution: Let us define the events as

E_1: The student leaves the match practice in badminton.
E_2: The student leaves the match practice in gymnastics.
E_3: The student leaves the match practice in swimming.
A: The student is a female.

It is required to find $P(E_3/A) = P$(that the female student leaves, given that she is from the swimming group).

Using Bayes' theorem

$$P(E_3/A) = \frac{P(E_3)P(A/E_3)}{P(E_1)P(A/E_1) + P(E_2)P(A/E_2) + P(E_3)P(A/E_3)}$$

Given that $P(E_1) = 0.20$, $P(E_2) = 0.15$, $P(E_3) = 0.10$.

In addition,

$$P(A/E_1) = P(\text{female student leaves badminton}) = \frac{30}{60} = 0.5$$

$$P(A/E_2) = P(\text{female student leaves gymnastics}) = \frac{40}{50} = 0.8$$

$$P(A/E_3) = P(\text{female student leaves swimming}) = \frac{10}{40} = 0.25$$

$$\Rightarrow P(E_3/A) = \frac{0.10 \times 0.25}{0.2 \times 0.5 + 0.15 \times 0.8 + 0.10 \times 0.25}$$

$$= \frac{0.025}{0.100 + 0.120 + 0.025}$$

$$= \frac{0.025}{0.245} = 0.102$$

Check Your Progress

Note: Tick the correct answer by using the sign ($\surd$).

	True	False
26. In the classical definition of probability, the events need not be finite.	-	-
27. In classical probability, all the events are required to be equally likely.	-	-
28. Probability of the sample space need not necessarily be 1.	-	-
29. In rolling a dice, the event E, getting a odd or even number, is a sure event.	-	-
30. If the events A and B are not independent, then $P(B/A) = P(B)$.	-	-
31. If the events A and B are mutually exclusive, then $P(A \cup B) = P(A) + P(B)$.	-	-
32. If the events A and B are independent, then $P(A/B)$ and $P(B/A)$ are the same.	-	-
33. For mutually exclusive events, $P(A \cap B) = P(A)\ P(B)$.	-	-

34. In frequency probability, no condition is posed on the outcomes.	-	-
35. If the events A and B are independent, then $P(B)$ $P(A/B) = P(A)\ P(B/A)$.	-	-
36. If the events A and B are independent, then $P(A \cap B) = 0$.	-	-

PRACTICE EXERCISE

8. What is the probability that a leap year selected at random will have 53 Sundays?
9. In tossing two coins, find the following probabilities:
   i. Getting exactly one tails
   ii. Getting exactly two heads
   iii. No heads
10. If the events A and B are mutually exclusive and $P(\overline{A}) = 0.60$, $P(A \cup B) = 0.55$, find the value of $P(A)$.
11. If two dice are thrown, what is the probability that the sum of the numbers on the two dice is divisible by either 3 or 5.
12. An urn contains 6 red, 5 black, and 4 white balls. If three balls are drawn, what is the probability that it includes one red, one black, and one white?
13. The probabilities of occurrence for the events A and B are 0.35 and 0.55, respectively. The probability of their simultaneous occurrence is 0.12. Find the probability that neither A nor B occurs.
14. A class consists of 25 women and 40 men, out of which 6 women and 10 men are hockey players. If two students are selected at random from the class, what is the probability that either both are women or both are not hockey players.
15. In drawing 2 cards from a deck of 52 cards, what is the probability that both the cards are from the same suit?

4.10 COMPUTING WITH EXCEL

4.10.1 Finding the Probability

Excel can be used to find the probability of any event if the mean and standard deviation are given and the distribution of data is known. Here, a problem based on normal distribution has been discussed in the example.

Example 4.19 The lean body weight of boys in a college is supposed to be normally distributed with mean 150.5 lbs and standard deviation 4.5 lbs. Find the following:

a. What fraction of boys in the college will have less than 152.5 lbs of lean body weight?
b. What fraction of boys will have at least 142 lbs of lean body weight?

Solution:

1. To solve these two problems, NORMDIST function of Excel shall be used. Click the following commands in sequence in Excel and you get the screen as shown in Figure 4.4.

   Formulas ⟶ Insert Function ⟶ Statistical ⟶ NORMDIST

2. After clicking the OK button in Figure 4.4, you get the screen as shown in Figure 4.5, where you can write other parameters to get the required probability.
3. In this example, it is required to find the probability $P(X \leq 152.5)$. To find this probability, fill the entries in the screen in Figure 4.5 as shown below:
   i. $X = 152.5$
   ii. **Mean** = 150.5
   iii. **Standard_dev** = 4.5
   iv. **Cumulative** = True
   v. Click **OK** to get the output as shown in step 4.
4. $P(X \leq 152.5) = 0.671639357$. Thus, approximately 0.67 fraction of boys in the college will have less than 152.5 lbs of lean body weight.
5. To know the fraction of boys having at least 142 lbs of lean body weight, we need to know the probability $P(X \geq 142)$.

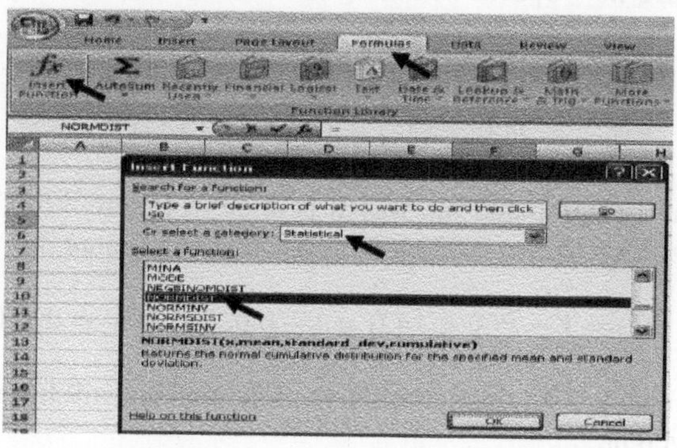

Figure 4.4 Command sequence for using the normal distribution function.

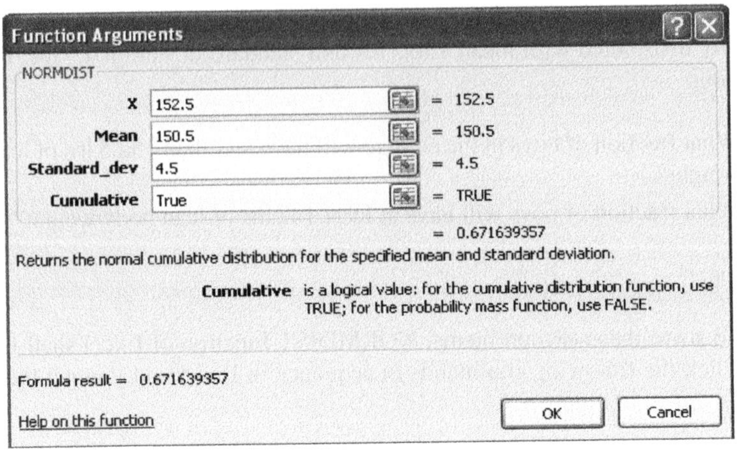

Figure 4.5 Options for finding cumulative distribution function.

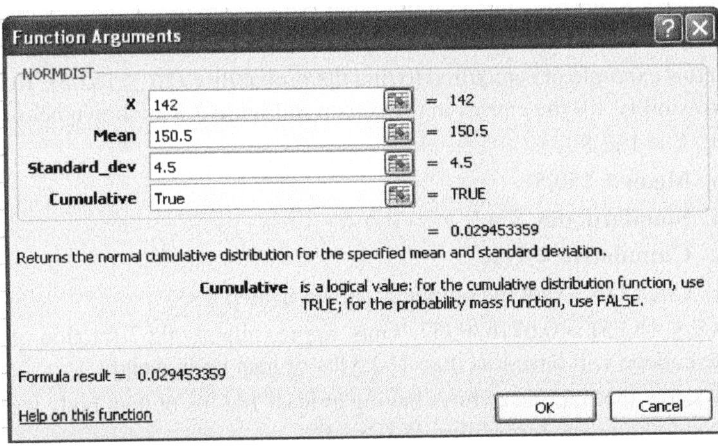

Figure 4.6 Options for finding cumulative distribution function.

Since

$$P(X \geq 142) = 1 - P(X < 142)$$

$P(X \leq 142)$ can be computed the way it is done in Figure 4.5. Taking $X = 142$, Excel will give $P(X \leq 142) = 0.029453359$ as shown in Figure 4.6. Thus,

$$P(X \geq 142) = 1 - P(X < 142) = 1 - 0.029453359 = 0.970546641$$

Thus, approximately 0.97 fraction of boys in the college will have at least 142 lbs of lean body weight.

IMPORTANT DEFINITIONS

A ***set*** can be defined as a collection of all elements having similar characteristics.
A ***null set*** is a set having no elements in it.
A set is said to be a ***complement*** of A if it contains the elements of S that do not belong to A.
Set A is said to be a ***subset*** of B if all the elements of set A belong to set B.
Set is said to be a ***proper subset*** of B if all elements of A belong to set B but there is at least one element of B that does not belong to set A.
The two sets A and B are said to be ***equal sets*** if all the elements of set A belongs to set B and all the elements of set B belongs to set A.
Union of the two sets A and B is a set whose elements belong to A or B or both.
Intersection of the two sets A and B is a set whose elements belong to both the sets A and B.
Difference of the two sets A and B, that is, $A - B$, is a set whose elements belong to A but do not belong to B.
An experiment is a means of getting the answer to a particular question.
A sample space is the collection of all possible outcomes of an experiment.
An event is a subset of a sample space.
An ***elementary event*** can be defined as any single outcome of a sample space in the experiment.
Exhaustive cases are the number of elements in the sample space.
Repeating an experiment a number of times is known as a ***trial***.
A ***factorial*** of any number n is a score obtained by multiplying n by all its preceding numbers.
A ***combination*** can be defined as all possible pairs of elements and is obtained by computing ${}^nC_r$, where n is the total number of elements and r is the number of elements whose combination is required to be obtained.
Events are said to be ***equally likely*** if their chances of occurrence are same.
Events are said to be ***mutually exclusive*** if the occurrence of one event discards the possibility of other events occurring.
Events are said to be ***independent*** if the occurrence of one event is not affected by the supplementary knowledge concerning the occurrence of other events.
As per the ***classical definition of probability*** if there are N mutually exclusive and equally likely cases out of which m are favorable to the event A, then the probability of the event A is given by m/N.
Empirical definition of the probability states that if a random sample of size n is drawn from the population of interest and if there are m cases favoring the attribute E in the sample, then the relative frequency of E in the sample is the estimated probability of the event E and is given by m/n. Events need not be equally likely.

As per the ***Axiomatic definition of probability***, any real-valued function P is said to be the probability of an event E if the following three axioms are satisfied.

1. $0 \leq P(E) \leq 1$ for all possible events E.
2. $P(S) = 1$, S is the sample space.
3. If $E_1, E_2, \ldots, E_n$ are n mutually exclusive events, then

$$P(E_1 \cup E_2 \cup \ldots \cup E_n) = P(E_1) + P(E_2) + \ldots P(E_n)$$

The ***marginal probability*** of any event is obtained by dividing the number of cases favorable for the event E by the total number of cases and is written as $P(E)$.
Union probability is the probability of union of two events and is denoted by $P(A \cup B)$.
Joint probability of any two events is the probability of the intersection of these two events. If A and B are two events, then it is denoted by $P(A \cap B)$.
The ***conditional probability*** of any event A is the probability of occurrence of the event A among those cases where the event B has already occurred and is written as $P(A/B)$.

IMPORTANT FORMULAS

The set is defined as

$$A = \{x : x \in A\}$$

Complement of the set

$$\overline{A} = S - A$$

A is the subset of B

$$A \subseteq B$$

Union of A and B

$$A \cup B = \{x : x \in A \text{ or } x \in B\}$$

Intersection of the sets A and B

$$A \cap B = \{x : x \in A \text{ and } x \in B\}$$

Difference of the set

$$A - B = \{x : x \in A \text{ and } x \notin B\}$$

Commutative law

$$A \cup B = B \cup A$$

$$A \cap B = B \cap A$$

Associative law

$$(A \cup B) \cup C = A \cup (B \cup C)$$

$$(A \cap B) \cap C = A \cap (B \cap C)$$

Distributive law

$$A \cap (B \cup C) = (A \cap B) \cup (A \cap C)$$

$$A \cup (B \cap C) = (A \cup B) \cap (A \cup C)$$

Law of complementary

$$A \cap \overline{A} = \phi$$

$$A \cup \overline{A} = S$$

$$A \cup S = S$$

$$A \cap S = A \quad (\because A \subseteq S)$$

Law of difference

$$A - B = A \cap \overline{B}$$

Law of involution

$$(\overline{\overline{A}}) = A$$

Law of idempotent

$$A \cup A = A$$

$$A \cap A = A$$

Factorial of n

$$n! = n(n-1)(n-2) \ldots 1$$

Combination

$$^{n}C_{r} = \frac{n!}{r!(n-r)!}$$

Results on the factorial

i. ${}^nC_0 = 0$
ii. ${}^nC_n = 1$
iii. ${}^nC_r = {}^nC_{n-r}$

Probability of any event E

$$P(E) = \frac{\text{Number of times event } E \text{ occurs}}{\text{Total number of outcomes}} = \frac{m}{N}$$

Frequency probability

Relative frequency of E

$$= \frac{\text{Number of sample observation possessing attribute } E}{\text{Number of observations in the sample}} = \frac{m}{n}$$

Law of addition of probability

$$P(A \cup B) = P(A) + P(B) - P(A \cap B)$$

Case 1: Events A and B are mutually exclusive

$$P(A \cup B) = P(A) + P(B)$$

Case 2: Events A and B are mutually independent

$$P(A \cup B) = P(A) + P(B) - P(A)P(B)$$

Multiplicative law of probability

$$P(A \cap B) = P(A)P(B/A)$$

When events A and B are independent

$$P(A \cap B) = P(A)P(B)$$

Conditional probability

$$P(A/B) = \frac{P(A \cap B)}{P(B)}$$

Bayes' theorem formula

$$P(E_i/A) = \frac{P(E_i)P(A/E_i)}{\sum_{j=1}^{n} P(E_j)P(A/E_j)}$$

KEY TERMS

Bayes' theorem	computing probability	probability
combination	factorial	set theory

CHAPTER EXERCISE

1. Explain the following with examples:
   i. Equally likely events
   ii. Mutually exclusive events
   iii. Independent events
2. Define classical and axiomatic definitions of probability.
3. Discuss the following terms with examples:
   i. Marginal probability
   ii. Union probability
   iii. Joint probability
   iv. Conditional probability
4. State the addition theorem of probability. What happens if the events are mutually exclusive and mutually independent?
5. What does the law of multiplication of probabilities mean? What happens when the events are independent?
6. State Bayes' theorem and explain a situation where it can be used.
7. Three pieces of papers bearing numbers 1, 2, and 3 are kept in a bowl. The bowl is mixed thoroughly. If a person is asked to draw two chits one by one without replacement, write the sample space points.
8. In a cricket tournament, three teams from the north and four teams from the south are participating. In drawing a fixture, write the favorable cases of the event of getting one team from the north and the other from the south.
9. An urn contains two black balls (B_1,B_2) and two white balls (W_1,W_2). Two balls are drawn from the urn, given that the first ball is replaced before the second ball is drawn. List all the outcomes in the sample space.
10. A coin is tossed. If it turns out to be heads we select a student from a group of 3 girls and 2 boys, and if turns out to be tails, we select a member from a group of 5 research scholars. What is the sample space associated with this experiment?
11. A coin is tossed twice. If the first toss results in tails, a dice is rolled. Describe the sample space associated with this experiment.
12. A coin is tossed repeatedly until a head comes up for the first time. Write the sample space for this experiment.

13. A dice is rolled repeatedly until a 5 comes up. What is the sample space for this experiment?
14. Let $A = \{1, 4, 3, 9\}$, $B = \{2, 3, 6, 8\}$, and $C = \{1, 5, 9, 11\}$ be the subsets of integers from 1 through 15. Find the events.
    i. $\overline{A}, \overline{B}, \overline{C}$
    ii. $A \cap B$
    iii. $A \cap B \cap C$
    iv. $A \cup B \cup C$
    v. $\overline{A} \cap \overline{B}$
15. If A, B, and C are three events, find the correct match for each of the following events:

i. At least one event occurs	a. $(A \cap B \cap \overline{C}) \cup (\overline{A} \cap B \cap C) \cup (A \cap \overline{B} \cap C)$
ii. Only C occurs	b. $A \cap B \cap C$
iii. At least two events occur	c. $\overline{A} \cap \overline{B} \cap \overline{C}$
iv. Two and no more events occur	d. $A \cup B \cup C$
v. All three events occur	e. $(A \cap B) \cup (A \cap C) \cup (B \cap C) \cup (A \cap B \cap C)$
vi. None occurs	f. $\overline{A} \cap \overline{B} \cap C$

16. A card is chosen from a deck of 52 cards. Given that the probability of drawing all the cards is equal, the events A, B, and C are defined as follows:
    A = Event of getting a red card
    B = Event of getting a face card
    C = Event of getting either a queen or a king
    Find the following probabilities.
    i. $P(A \cup B)$
    ii. $P(A \cup C)$
17. A six-sided dice is tossed twice. Given that the outcomes are equally likely, find the probability of the following events:
    i. A = Event that the total is 6
    ii. B = Event that the total is an even number
    iii. C = Event that both numbers are the same
    iv. D = Event that the first number is greater than the second
18. Expand $(H + T)^9$ and hence compute the probability of the following events:
    i. Getting $6H$ and $3T$
    ii. Getting $8T$ and $1H$
    iii. Getting $4H$ and $5T$
    iv. Getting $2T$ and $7H$
19. In rolling a pair of dice, what is the probability that
    i. the sum is greater than 7

ii. the sum is at least 6 and a multiple of 2

20. If three coins are tossed, what would be the probability of getting
    i. at the most two heads
    ii. exactly one heads
    iii. exactly two tails.
21. A dice is rolled. Find the following probability.
    i. Getting a prime number
    ii. Getting a number that is a multiple of 2 and 3
    iii. Getting a number greater than or equal to 3
22. Two dice are rolled. Find the probability of
    i. getting an even number on the first dice and odd number on the second dice
    ii. getting an odd number on both dice
    iii. getting the first number as a square of the second number
    iv. getting a total of at least 8
23. Three persons are to be selected at random from 4 men, 3 women, and 6 children. Find the probability of selecting
    i. 2 men and 1 woman
    ii. exactly two children
24. A box contains 12 tennis balls, of which just 4 are defective. If a random sample of 4 balls is drawn, find the probabilities that the sample contains
    i. exactly two defective balls
    ii. exactly three defective balls
    iii. no defective ball
25. A bowl contains 6 black and 5 red balls, out of which 4 balls are drawn. What is the probability that
    i. all will be black
    ii. 3 will be black and 1 red
26. What is the probability that an ordinary year has 53 Sundays?
27. Two persons *A* and *B* roll a pair of dice. If *A* throws 9, what are the chances of *B* throwing a higher number?
28. In rolling a pair of dice, what is the probability that the first number is the square of the second number?
29. Two unbiased dice are rolled. Find the probability that
    i. neither a doublet nor a total of 6 will appear
    ii. the sum of the numbers obtained on the two dice is neither a doublet nor a multiple of 2
30. If 4 cards are drawn from a pack of 52 playing cards, what is the probability of getting all the 4 cards of the same suit?

31. A number is selected at random from 1 to 30. What is the probability that the number is a multiple of 2 or 3?
32. In a tournament, the odds in favor of athletes Marshal, Tony, and Jacob are 1:2, 1:3, and 1:4, respectively. Find the probability that one of them wins the competition.
33. In rolling two dice, what is the probability that the sum of two numbers on the dice is divisible neither by 2 nor by 3?
34. The probability that Jane will be selected for the college basketball team is 3/5 and the probability that she will not be selected for the scholarship is 2/3. If the probability of getting at least one reward is 3/4, what is the probability that she will get both?
35. For the position of coach, three persons, Williams, Jackson, and Lewis, attended the interview. The probability of Williams being selected is thrice that of Jackson and the probability of Jackson being selected is twice that of Lewis. What are the respective probabilities of Williams, Jackson, and Lewis being selected?
36. An urn contains 5 red, 6 blue, and 3 black marbles. If 4 marbles are drawn randomly, then find the probability that it contains at least one marble for each color.
37. In an examination, Clark and Young appeared. The probability that Clark will qualify in the examination is 0.20 and that Young will qualify in the examination is 0.3. The probability that both will qualify in the examination is 0.15. Find the following probability.
    i. At least one of them will not qualify in the examination.
    ii. Only one of them will qualify in the examination.
38. In tossing two coins, what is the probability that both coins turn up as heads?
39. If you throw two dice, what is the probability that both dice show 5?
40. A bag contains 5 balls of each of 4 colors, that is, red, blue, white, and orange. If 2 balls are drawn, what is the probability that both balls are of the same color?
41. In throwing two dice, what is the probability that the sum of the numbers will be greater than 7 whereas the second dice shows 5?
42. If 2 cards are drawn randomly one by one without replacement from a deck of 52 cards, what is the probability of drawing two aces, given that the first card is an ace?
43. If A and B are two events such that $P(A) = 2/5$ and $P(A \cap B) = 1/5$, then find $P(B/A)$.
44. If $P(B) = 1/3$ and $P(A \cap B) = 1/4$, then find $P(A/B)$.
45. Three bags contain 4 red and 6 white; 5 red and 7 white; and 6 red and 4 white balls, respectively. One bag is randomly chosen and a ball is drawn from it. If the ball drawn is red, find the probability that it is drawn from the first bag.

ANSWERS

Check Your Progress

1. T	5. F	9. F	13. T	17. T	21. T	25. T	29. T	33. F
2. T	6. T	10. T	14. F	18. F	22. F	26. F	30. F	34. T
3. T	7. F	11. F	15. F	19. T	23. F	27. T	31. T	35. T
4. F	8. T	12. F	16. T	20. F	24. F	28. F	32. F	36. F

Practice Exercise

6. $S = \{T, HT, HHT, HHHT \ldots\}$
8. 2/7
10. $P(A) = 0.15$
13. 0.22
15. 12/51

Chapter Exercise

7. $S = \{12, 13, 23\}$
8. $N_1S_1, N_1S_2, N_1S_3, N_1S_4, N_2S_1, N_2S_2, N_2S_3, N_2S_4, N_3S_1, N_3S_2, N_3S_3, N_3S_4$
9. $B_1B_1, B_1B_2, B_1W_1, B_1W_2$
   $B_2B_2, B_2B_1, B_2W_1, B_2W_2$
   $W_1W_1, W_1W_2, W_1B_1, W_1B_2$
   $W_2W_2, W_2W_1, W_2B_1, W_2B_2$
10. $HG_1, HG_2, HG_3, HB_1, HB_2, TR_1, TR_2, TR_3, TR_4, TR_5$ (G: Girl, B: Boy, R: Research scholar)
11. $\{HH, HT, (TH,1), (TH,2), (TH,3), (TH,4), (TH,5), (TH,6), (TT,1), (TT,2), (TT,3), (TT,4), (TT,5), (TT,6)\}$
12. $\{H, TH, TTH, TTTH, \ldots\}$
13. {5, (1,5), (2,5), (3,5), (4,5), (6,5), (1,1,5), (1,2,5), (1,3,5), (1,4,5), (1,6,5), (2,1,5), (2,2,5), (2,3,5), (2,4,5), (2,6,5)}
14. i. $\overline{A} = \{2,5,6,7,8,10,11,12,13,14,15\}, \overline{B} = \{1,4,5,7,9,10,11,12,13,14,15\}, \overline{C} = \{2,3,4,6,7,8,10,12,13,14,15\}$
    ii. $A \cap B = \{3\}$
    iii. $A \cap B \cap C = \{\phi\}$
    iv. $A \cup B \cup C = \{1,2,3,4,5,6,8,9,11\}$
    v. $\{\overline{A} \cap \overline{B}\} = \{5,7,10,11,12,13,14,15\}$
15. i-d, ii-f, iii-e, iv-a, v-b, vi-c
16. i. 8/13, ii. 15/26
17. i. 5/36, ii. 1/2, iii. 1/6, iv. 5/12
18. i. 21/128, ii. 9/512, iii. 63/256, iv. 9/128
19. i. 5/12, ii. 7/18

20. i. 7/8, ii. 3/8, iii. 3/8
21. i. 1/2, ii. 1/6, iii. 2/3
22. i. 1/4, ii. 1/4, iii. 1/18, iv. 5/12
23. i. 9/143, ii. 105/286
24. i. 56/165, ii. 45/495, iii. 14/99
25. i. 1/22, ii. 10/33
26. 1/7
27. 1/6
28. 1/18
29. i. 13/18, ii. 1/2
30. 44/4165
31. 2/3
32. 47/60
33. 1/3
34. 11/60
35. P(William selected) = 2/3,
    P(Jackson selected) = 2/9, P(Lewis selected) = 1/9
36. 45/91
37. i. 0.95, ii. 0.38
38. 1/4
39. 1/36
40. 4/19
41. 1/9
42. 3/51
43. 1/2
44. 3/4
45. 24/85

FURTHER READING

1. Alan G. An Intermediate Course in Probability. 2nd ed. USA: Springer; 2009. ISBN 978-1-4419-0161-3.
2. Baclawski K. Introduction to probability with R. CRC Press; 2008. p 179. ISBN 978-1-4200-6521-3.
3. Bayes T, Price R. An Essay towards solving a Problem in the Doctrine of Chance. By the late Rev. Mr. Bayes, communicated by Mr. Price, in a letter to John Canton, MA and FRS. Philosophical Transactions of the Royal Society of London 1763; 53(0):370–418. DOI: doi:10.1098/rstl.1763.0053.
4. Daston L. Classical Probability in the Enlightenment. Princeton University Press; 1988. p 268. ISBN 0-691-08497-1.
5. Kallenberg O. Foundations of Modern Probability. Springer Series in Statistics. 2nd ed. USA: Springer; 2002. p 650. ISBN 0-387-95313-2.
6. Laplace P-S. A Philosophical Essay on Probabilities. English edition 1951 ed. New York: Dover Publications Inc.; 1814.

7. Laplace P-S. Memoir on the Probability of the Causes of Events. Statistical Science 1774/1986;1(3):364–378.
8. Mark JS. Theory of Statistics. USA: Springer; 1995. ISBN 978-0-387-94546-0
9. Mood AM, Graybill FA, Boes DC. Introduction to the Theory of Statistics. 3rd ed. McGraw-Hill; 1974. Section 2.3.
10. Olofsson P. Probability, Statistics, and Stochastic Processes, USA: Wiley-Interscience. 2005. p 504. ISBN 0-471-67969-0.
11. Pfeiffer PE. Concepts of Probability Theory. USA: Courier Dover Publications; 1978. p 47–48. ISBN 978-0-486-63677-1.
12. R D. Probability for Dummies. For Dummies. 2006. p 58. ISBN 978-0-471-75141-0.
13. Stigler SM. Who Discovered Bayes' Theorem? The American Statistician 1983; 37(4):290–296.
14. Tijms HC. A First Course in Stochastic Models. USA: John Wiley and Sons; 2003. p 431–432. ISBN 978-0-471-49880-3.
15. William M, Robert JB, Barbara MB. Introduction to Probability and Statistics. 13th ed. USA: Brooks/Cole; 2008. ISBN 978-0-87150-377-0.
16. Zwillinger D, Kokoska S. CRC Standard Probability and Statistics Tables and Formulae. USA: CRC Press; 2000. p 31. ISBN 1-58488-059-7.

5

STATISTICAL DISTRIBUTIONS AND THEIR APPLICATION

5.1 INTRODUCTION

Statistical methods are used to estimate a future event on the basis of the sampled data. For instance, by knowing the intensity of a training program, one may estimate the improvement in an athlete's performance. In other words, if the cause-and-effect relationship is known, estimation becomes more precise and one may be able to estimate the performance by manipulating the training component, provided other conditions are held constant. In statistical terms, if the probability distribution of the data is known, it helps in estimating a future event accurately on the basis of the known parameters. Probability distribution is a statistical model in which each outcome of a statistical experiment is provided with its probability of occurrence. Consider an experiment in which a coin is tossed twice. The outcomes of this experiment would be 0, 1, or 2 heads. The probability associated with these outcomes would be 1/4, 1/2, and 1/4, respectively. Thus, the probability distribution of the number of heads in tossing a coin twice can be represented as shown in the following table.

Probability Distribution of the Number of Heads

Number of Heads	0	1	2
Probability	1/4	1/2	1/4

If the events of an experiment are discrete in nature, then their probability distribution is known as *discrete probability distribution* as shown earlier.

Statistics for Exercise Science and Health with Microsoft® Office Excel®, First Edition. J. P. Verma.

However, if the events are continuous in nature, then their probability distribution is said to be a *continuous probability distribution.* In a continuous probability distribution, the probability that an event will assume a particular value is 0; therefore, it cannot be expressed in a tabular form similar to the discrete distribution. Instead, a formula is used to describe a continuous probability distribution, which is known as the probability density function. The probability density function can also be written as a density function, a PDF, or a pdf. In this chapter, only two of the important discrete distributions, namely, binomial and Poisson, and one continuous distribution, that is, normal, are discussed in detail.

5.2 TERMINOLOGIES USED IN STATISTICAL DISTRIBUTION

Before discussing discrete and continuous distributions and their applications, let us first understand the terms involved in this chapter.

5.2.1 Random Variable

A random variable can be defined as a variable whose possible values are the numerical outcomes of a random phenomenon. The random variable is usually represented by X and is of two types, discrete and continuous.

Discrete Random Variable A random variable is said to be discrete if it can assume only a countable number of distinct values such as 0, 1, 2, 3, and so on. In other words, if a random variable can assume only a finite number of distinct values, then it must be discrete. Examples of discrete random variables include the number of goals scored in a soccer match, the number of athletes selected in a team, and the number of medals an athlete has bagged in a tournament. Consider an experiment where the performance in push-ups is measured on 15 athletes to test their strength. This push-ups performance may be regarded as a discrete random variable, X, because it may assume any of the values such as 0, 1, 2, … , 25. Each of these values corresponds to a particular experimental outcome where the experiment consists of measuring the push-ups performance of athletes. This discrete variable X is said to be a discrete random variable because its values cannot be predicted with absolute certainty in advance.

Continuous Random Variable A random variable is said to be continuous if it can assume an infinite number of possible values within a given range. Usually, measurements obtained on any trait result in a continuous random variable. Examples of continuous random variables include height, weight, 100 m timings, long jump performance, and so on. The probability of a continuous random

FACTS TO KNOW

Knowledge of statistical distribution enables a researcher to estimate the performance parameter variable assuming any specific value is always 0. Thus, the probability of a continuous random variable is always computed over a range of values and is represented by the area under the curve. The probability is computed by using the concept of integral.

Remark If X_1 and X_2 are random variables and c, c_1, and c_2 are constants, then

1. $cX_1, X_1 + X_2$, and $X_1 \cdot X_2$ are also random variables,
2. $c_1X_1 + c_2X_2$ is a random variable. In particular, $X_1 - X_2$ is a random variable.

5.2.2 Probability Distribution Function

A probability distribution function is a real-valued function that provides the probability to each and every outcome of a random variable in an experiment. It is represented by $P(X=x)$, where X (capital letter) is a discrete random variable and x (small letter) is the value of the random variable. In short, the probability distribution function is written as $P(x)$, where $P(x) \geq 0$ for all values of X. The probability distribution function is a term used for discrete random variables; hence, it is also known as discrete probability distribution. It is also sometimes referred to as probability function or the probability mass function.

Properties of Probability Distribution Function

1. The probability associated with each value of the discrete random variable x in the sample space is greater than or equal to 0 and less than or equal to 1. In notation form, it can be represented as $0 \leq P(x) \leq 1$.
2. Probabilities of discrete random variables are additive.
3. The sum of the probabilities for all values of x in the sample space is 1.

5.2.3 Probability Density Function

Probability density function is a term used for a continuous random variable and is abbreviated as PDF. Probability density function can be defined as a function that can be integrated to obtain the probability that the random variable can have values in a given interval. For instance, if it is known that the random variable X follows a given probability distribution as shown in Figure 5.1, then the probability that X can take values between A and B, $P(A \leq X \leq B)$, can be defined as the area between A and B.

Properties of Probability Density Function The curve representing the function $p(x)$ must satisfy the following and is known as a density curve.

i. For all values of x, $p(x) \geq 0$.
ii. The area under the curve is equal to 1.

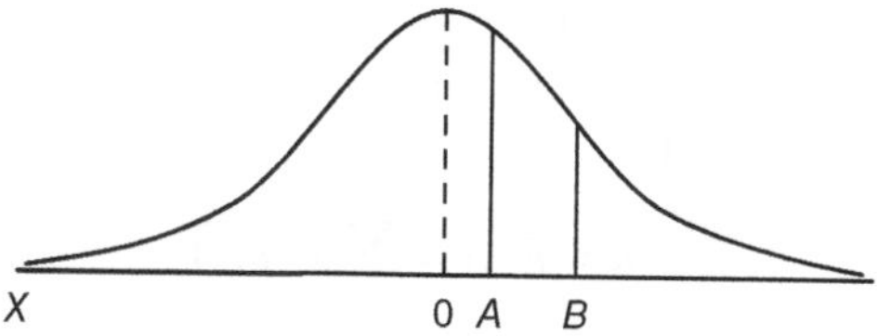

Figure 5.1 The variable X can take any value in between A and B.

5.2.4 Binomial Experiment

A binomial experiment is also known as a Bernoulli trial. Any statistical experiment is said to be a binomial experiment if it has the following properties:

1. The experiment consists of n repeated trials.
2. Each trial results in only two possible outcomes. One of the outcomes is known as success (p) and the other is failure (q) such that $q = 1 - p$.
3. The probability of success (p) is the same in each trial.
4. All the trials are independent of each other. In other words, the outcome in one trial does not affect the outcome of any other trial.

5.2.5 Expectation

The expectation of any random variable is its aggregate value. It is the same as the mean value. The mean of the random variable is referred to as the expected value and is not calculated by simply adding up the different variables. In computing the mean for grouped data, the frequency of each class interval is used as a weight to the class midpoint, whereas for discrete distribution, the probability of each occurrence is used as the weight in computing the expectation. The expected value of a random variable x is denoted by $E(x)$, and it is a value you expect if an experiment is conducted whose outcomes are represented by the random variable.

> **FACTS TO KNOW**
>
> The expected value of any variable is equal to its mean

$$\text{For discrete distribution } E(x) = \sum x \cdot p(x) \tag{5.1}$$

where x is a discrete random variable and $p(x)$ is the probability distribution function of the random variable x.

$$\text{For continuous distribution } E(x) = \int_{-\infty}^{\infty} x \cdot f(x)dx \tag{5.2}$$

where $f(x)$ is the probability density function of the continuous random variable.

Mean and Variance of Discrete Distributions If x is a discrete random variable with the probability distribution function $p(x)$, then the mean and variance of the discrete distribution are given by

$$\mu = E(x) = \sum x \cdot p(x) \tag{5.3}$$

$$\begin{aligned}\sigma^2 = E(x-\mu)^2 &= E(x-E(x))^2 = E(x^2) - (E(x))^2 \\ &= \sum (x-\mu)^2 \cdot p(x)\end{aligned} \tag{5.4}$$

Mean and Variance of Continuous Distributions If x is a continuous random variable with the probability density function $f(x)$, then the mean and variance of the continuous distribution are given by

$$\mu = E(x) = \int_{-\infty}^{\infty} x \cdot f(x)dx \tag{5.5}$$

$$\sigma^2 = E(x-\mu)^2 = \int_{-\infty}^{\infty} (x-\mu)^2 \cdot f(x)dx \tag{5.6}$$

Example 5.1 In rolling a dice if the probability of getting any number x is 1/6, then find the expected value and the variance for the random variable x.

Solution: Here, the probability distribution of the random variable shall be as follows.

Discrete Probability Distribution for Rolling a Dice

Outcome (x)	Probability (p)	xp	x^2	x^2p
1	1/6	1/6	1	1/6
2	1/6	2/6	4	4/6
3	1/6	3/6	9	9/6
4	1/6	4/6	16	16/6
5	1/6	5/6	25	25/6
6	1/6	6/6	36	36/6

$$\begin{aligned}\text{Mean} = E(x) &= \sum x \cdot p(x) \\ &= 1\cdot\frac{1}{6} + 2\cdot\frac{1}{6} + 3\cdot\frac{1}{6} + 4\cdot\frac{1}{6} + 5\cdot\frac{1}{6} + 6\cdot\frac{1}{6} \\ &= \frac{1}{6}(1+2+3+4+5+6) = \frac{21}{6} = 3.5\end{aligned}$$

To compute the variance of x, let us first find the value of $E(x^2)$:

$$E(x^2) = \sum x^2 \cdot p(x)$$
$$= 1 \cdot \frac{1}{6} + 4 \cdot \frac{1}{6} + 9 \cdot \frac{1}{6} + 16 \cdot \frac{1}{6} + 25 \cdot \frac{1}{6} + 36 \cdot \frac{1}{6}$$
$$= \frac{1}{6}(1 + 4 + 9 + 16 + 25 + 36) = \frac{91}{6} = 15.17$$

Therefore,

$$\sigma^2 = E(x^2) - (E(x))^2$$
$$= \frac{91}{6} - \left(\frac{21}{6}\right)^2 = \frac{546 - 441}{36} = \frac{35}{12}$$
$$= 2.92$$

Since the mean of the random variable is 3.5, it does not imply that if you roll a dice you will be likely to get 3.5. Rather, it simply means that if you average out the results of rolling a dice a large number of times, you will get 3.5.

Check Your Progress

Note: Tick the correct answer by using the sign (√).

	True	False
1. The weight of an individual is a discrete random variable.	-	-
2. In continuous probability distribution, $P(X = 2)$ is zero.	-	-
3. A continuous random variable may assume infinite number of values.	-	-
4. The purpose of statistics is to study a sample for drawing conclusions about sample characteristics.	-	-
5. Expectation is the mean of the distribution.	-	-
6. If x is a random variable, then cx is not a random variable where c is a constant.	-	-
7. The performance of an athlete in a 100 m event is a discrete variable.	-	-
8. Discrete probability distribution can also be referred to as probability density function.	-	-

9. If x and y are random variables, then $x+y$ will also be a random variable.	-	-
10. A continuous random variable can take a specific value.	-	-
11. In finding probability in discrete distributions, summation is used.	-	-
12. In discrete probability distribution, $P(x<2)$ can be obtained by adding $P(x=0)$ and $P(x=1)$.	-	-
13. Probability distribution is the characteristics of the data.	-	-
14. The probability in a continuous distribution is obtained by using integration.	-	-
15. Cumulative frequency curve can be used to show a discrete distribution graphically.	-	-
16. The number of goals in a soccer match is a random variable.	-	-
17. Continuous probability distribution is also known as probability mass function.	-	-
18. The sum of the probabilities, of all values of a random variable x in the sample space is 1.	-	-
19. In a discrete distribution, expectation is obtained by adding all the values of the random variable multiplied with their corresponding probabilities.	-	-

5.3 DISCRETE DISTRIBUTION

The distribution of probabilities associated with the outcomes of a discrete random variable in a statistical experiment is known as a *discrete distribution*. Usually, a histogram is used to show the discrete distribution graphically. Look at the discrete distribution shown in Table 5.1. Consider a situation where on every Saturday there is a 2-h intramural competition in the college, in which teams of different hostels take part. Injury is bound to happen during the tournament. In the past, the maximum number of injuries that have occurred is 5. The data on injuries were recorded for each Saturday in the whole season. Table 5.1 shows the distribution of injuries that occurred during the intramurals. For instance, there is a 0.36 probability that no injury will occur; 0.27 is the probability that 1 injury will occur; and similarly 0.06 is the probability that 4 injuries will occur. This probability distribution can be shown by constructing the histogram as shown in Figure 5.2. Here, the x-axis indicates the number of injuries that occurred, and the y-axis indicates the probabilities of these occurrences.

TABLE 5.1 Discrete Distribution of Occurrence of Injuries during Intramurals

Number of Injuries	Probability
0	0.36
1	0.27
2	0.16
3	0.11
4	0.06
5	0.04

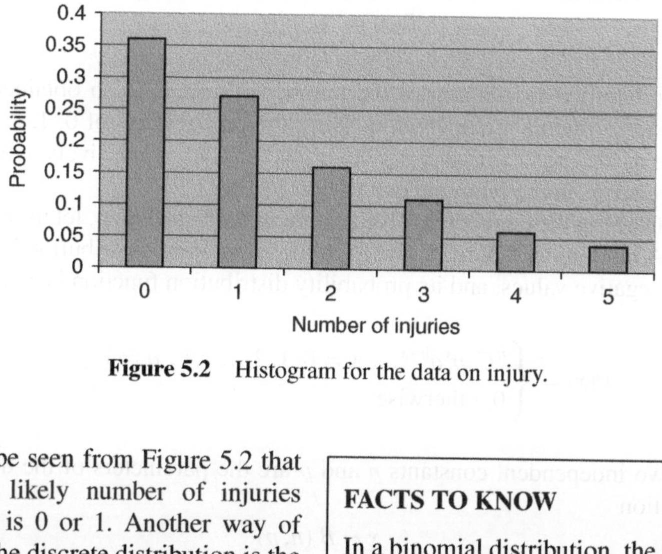

Figure 5.2 Histogram for the data on injury.

It can be seen from Figure 5.2 that the most likely number of injuries occurring is 0 or 1. Another way of showing the discrete distribution is the box-and-whisker plot as discussed in Chapter 2. In this chapter, only two important discrete distributions, *Binomial* and *Poisson*, are discussed.

> **FACTS TO KNOW**
>
> In a binomial distribution, the mean is always greater than the variance

5.4 BINOMIAL DISTRIBUTION

Binomial distribution is the most widely known distribution in the world. It was first proposed by James Bernoulli in the year 1700 and was first published posthumously in 1713. Let us understand the distribution by considering a binomial experiment in which a coin is tossed n times. Here, tossing a coin is a Bernoulli experiment. Let p be the probability of getting a head and q be the probability of getting a tail in a single trial so that $q = 1 - p$. The probability p is the same in all the trials, and all the trials are independent of each other. The probability of x successes and consequently $(n-x)$ failures in n trials in a specified order, say $SSFSF \ldots FSF$, is given by the multiplicative law of probability.

Thus,

$$P(SSFSF \ldots FSF) = P(S)\,P(S)\,P(F)\,P(S)\,P(F) \ldots P(F)\,P(S)\,P(F)$$

$$= \underbrace{p.p. \ldots\ldots\ldots p.p}_{x \text{ times}}.\underbrace{q.q.q.\ldots\ldots\ldots q}_{(n-x) \text{ times}}$$

$$= p^x q^{n-x}$$

However, x successes in n trials may occur in ${}^nC_x$ ways, and therefore, the probability for each of these ways is $p^x q^{n-x}$. Hence, the probability of x successes in n trials in any order is given by the additive law of probability by means of the following formula:

$$P(x) = {}^nC_x p^x q^{n-x} \tag{5.7}$$

The probability distribution of the number of successes so obtained is called the *binomial probability distribution*. Thus, the probabilities of 0, 1, 2, … , n successes are q^n, ${}^nC_1 pq^{n-1}$, ${}^nC_2 p^2 q^{n-2}$, ${}^nC_3 p^3 q^{n-3}$, … , p^n, respectively, which are the successive terms in the binomial expression $(q+p)^n$.

After learning the concept involved in binomial distribution, let us see how it is defined. A random variable x is said to follow a binomial distribution if it assumes only nonnegative values, and its probability distribution function is given by

$$P(x) = \begin{cases} {}^nC_x p^x q^{n-x}, & x = 0, 1, 2, \ldots, n, \; q = 1 - p \\ 0, \text{ otherwise} \end{cases}$$

The two independent constants n and p are the parameters of the distribution. The notation

$$x \sim B\,(n, p)$$

denotes that the random variable x follows the binomial distribution with parameters n and p, where n is the number of trials and p is the probability of success in a trial. The binomial distribution can be used to solve varieties of problems where an experiment consists of a Bernoulli trial. The following examples explain the utility of a binomial distribution.

5.4.1 Conditions for a Binomial Distribution

a. The number of trials must be a fixed number.
b. All the trials should be independent.
c. Each trial must have only two outcomes (success/failure, true/false, etc.).
d. The probability of success must be the same for each trial.

5.4.2 Mean and Standard Deviation of the Binomial Distribution

If x follows a binomial distribution with the parameters n (number of trials) and p (probability of success in a trial), then its mean and variance are given by the following formulas:

$$\text{Mean} = \mu = np$$

$$\text{Variance} = \sigma^2 = npq$$

Let us see what the relationship between the mean and variance of the binomial distribution is. Since p is the probability of success, which will always be greater than or equal to 0, that is, $p \geq 0$, q will always be less than or equal to 1, that is, $q \leq 1$. Thus,

$$npq < np$$

Hence, variance is always less than the mean in a binomial distribution.

Example 5.2 Compute the values of the mean and standard deviation of the binomial distribution having $n = 15$ and $p = 0.65$.

Solution:

$$\text{Mean} = \mu = np = 15 \times 0.65 = 9.75$$

$$\text{SD} = \sigma = \sqrt{npq} = \sqrt{15 \times 0.65 \times (1 - 0.65)} = 1.85$$

Example 5.3 If the variable x has a binomial distribution, find the following probabilities by using the binomial formula:

a. If $n = 5$ and $p = 0.3$, find $P(x = 2)$.
b. If $n = 5$ and $p = 0.5$, find $P(x \leq 3)$.

Solution:

a. For $n = 5, p = 0.3, P(x = 2) = {}^5C_2 \times 0.3^2 \times 0.7^3 = 0.3087$.
b. For $n = 5, p = 0.5$, it is required to find the probability of $P(x \leq 3)$.

Therefore,

$$P(x \leq 3) = 1 - P(x > 3) = 1 - [P(x = 4) + P(x = 5)]$$
$$= 1 - [{}^5C_4 \times 0.5^4 \times 0.5^1 + {}^5C_5 \times 0.5^5]$$
$$= 1 - 6 \times 0.5^5 = 0.8125$$

TABLE 5.2 Cross Section of the Binomial Table

$n = 5$

x \ p	0.1	0.2	0.3	0.4	0.5	0.6	0.7	0.8	0.9
0	0.59049	0.32768	0.16807	0.07776	0.03125	0.01024	0.00243	0.00032	0.00001
1	0.32805	0.40960	0.36015	0.25920	0.15625	0.07680	0.02835	0.00640	0.00045
2	0.07290	0.20480	0.30870	0.34560	0.31250	0.23040	0.13230	0.05120	0.00810
3	0.00810	0.05120	0.13230	0.23040	0.31250	0.34560	0.30870	0.20480	0.07290
4	0.00045	0.00640	0.02835	0.07680	0.15625	**0.25920**	0.36015	0.40960	0.32805
5	0.00001	0.00032	0.00243	0.01024	0.03125	0.07776	0.16807	0.32768	0.59049

5.4.3 Solving Problems Using Binomial Tables

Problems based on binomial distribution can also be solved by using the probabilities listed in the binomial table for each sample size n with varying values of p and x. These probabilities have been listed in Table A.2 in the appendix. A cross section of the binomial table for the sample size $n=5$ with different values of p and x is shown in Table 5.2. Let us see how the probability value can be seen from the table for a specific value of p and x.

If $n=5$, $p=0.6$, and $x=4$, the probability $P(x=4)$ can be located by first locating the table of the binomial distribution for $n=5$. Since Table 5.2 shows the probability distribution for $n=5$, it can be used to find the required probability. To find $P(x=4)$, locate the row for which $x=4$ and the column for which $p=0.6$. The value at the cross-section point of the identified row and column is the required probability 0.25920 as shown in the table.

Example 5.4 If the distribution of a variable x is binomial, find the following probabilities by using the binomial table.

a. If $n=15$ and $p=0.4$, find $P(x=10)$.
b. If $n=10$ and $p=0.6$, find $P(x>8)$.
c. If $n=12$ and $p=0.7$, find $P(x<10)$.

Solution:

a. From Table A.2, locate the binomial table for $n=15$. After locating the table, the value of probability at the cross-section point of $x=10$ and $p=0.4$ can be identified, which is 0.024.
b. Given that $n=10$, $p=0.6$, $P(x>8)$ can be computed as follows:

$$\begin{aligned}P(x>8) &= P(x=9)+P(x=10)\\ &= 0.04031+0.00605\\ &= 0.04636\end{aligned}$$

[From Table A.2 for $n=10$ and $p=0.6, P(x=9)=0.04031$ and $P(x=10)=0.00605$.]

c. Given that $n = 12$ and $p = 0.7$, $P(x < 10)$ can be computed as follows:

$$\begin{aligned} P(x < 10) &= 1 - [P(x = 10) + P(x = 11) + P(x = 12)] \\ &= 1 - [0.16779 + 0.07118 + 0.01384] \\ &= 0.74719 \end{aligned}$$

[From Table A.2 for $n = 12$ and $p = 0.7$, $P(x = 10) = 0.16779$, $P(x = 11) = 0.07118$, and $P(x = 12) = 0.01384$.]

Example 5.5 The past record of a college shows that 75% of the students were satisfied with the mess food. If a sample of 10 students is randomly selected and if the past record of the college still holds true as on date, what is the probability that exactly 9 students are satisfied with the mess food?

Solution: Let p denote the probability that the students are satisfied with the mess food and q denote the probability that the students are not satisfied. Here, $p = 3/4$, $q = 1/4$, and $n = 10$. It is required to find $P(x = 9)$.

Therefore,

$$P(x) = {}^{n}C_{x}p^{x}q^{n-x}$$

$$\Rightarrow P(x = 9) = {}^{10}C_{9}\left(\frac{3}{4}\right)^{9}\left(\frac{1}{4}\right)^{1}$$

The value of this probability can also be computed by using the binomial probability table.

Example 5.6 In a survey, it was found that 50% of the students were satisfied with the timings allotted to match practice classes. Suppose a random sample of 10 students was selected and if the survey result holds for them, what is the probability that exactly 4 students are satisfied with the timings of the class.

Solution: Given that $p =$ the probability that a student is satisfied with the timings $= 1/2$ and $n = 10$, it is required to compute the following probability.

$P(x = 4) =$ probability that exactly 4 students are satisfied in a random sample of 10 students.

Therefore,

$$P(x) = {}^{n}C_{x}p^{x}q^{n-x}$$

$$\Rightarrow P(x = 4) = {}^{10}C_{4}\left(\frac{1}{2}\right)^{4}\left(\frac{1}{2}\right)^{6}$$

$$= \frac{10 \times 9 \times 8 \times 7}{4 \times 3 \times 2 \times 1} \times \frac{1}{16} \times \frac{1}{64} = \frac{105}{512} = 0.205$$

The value of this probability $P(x=4)$ can also be seen from the binomial table in Table A.2. From this table, the value of $P(x=4)$ for $n=10$ and $p=0.50$ is 0.20508.

Example 5.7 The health center in a college reports that 10% of all the injuries reported in the center were of the knee. If 12 reported cases are selected randomly from the population, what is the probability that it includes 3 or less knee injuries?

Solution: Given that $p=$ the probability of knee injury reported $=1/10$, $q=9/10$, and $n=12$, it is required to find $P\ (x \le 3)$.

$$
\begin{aligned}
P(x \le 3) &= P(x=0) + P(x=1) + P(x=2) + P(x=3) \\
&= {}^{12}C_0\left(\frac{1}{10}\right)^0\left(\frac{9}{10}\right)^{12} + {}^{12}C_1\left(\frac{1}{10}\right)^1\left(\frac{9}{10}\right)^{11} + {}^{12}C_2\left(\frac{1}{10}\right)^2\left(\frac{9}{10}\right)^{10} \\
&\quad + {}^{12}C_3\left(\frac{1}{10}\right)^3\left(\frac{9}{10}\right)^9 \\
&= \frac{9^{12}}{10^{12}} + 12 \times \frac{9^{11}}{10^{12}} + 66 \times \frac{9^{10}}{10^{12}} + 220 \times \frac{9^9}{10^{12}} \\
&= 2515 \times \frac{9^9}{10^{12}} = 0.97
\end{aligned}
$$

$P(x \le 3)$ can also be solved by using the binomial table. From Table A.2, the probabilities for different values of x when $n=12$ and $p=0.10$ are as follows:

$$
\begin{aligned}
P(x=0) &= 0.28243 \\
P(x=1) &= 0.37657 \\
P(x=2) &= 0.23013 \\
P(x=3) &= 0.08523
\end{aligned}
$$

Thus,

$$
\begin{aligned}
P(x \le 3) &= P(x=0) + P(x=1) + P(x=2) + P(x=3) \\
&= 0.28243 + 0.37657 + 0.23013 + 0.08523 \\
&= 0.97436
\end{aligned}
$$

Example 5.8 As per past knowledge, 30% students of a college are girls. In conducting a random telephone survey on 10 students, what is the probability that 4 or less number of girl students were surveyed.

Solution: Given that p = probability that the student is a girl = 0.3 and n = 10, it is required to find $P(x \leq 4)$ where x is the number of girls surveyed.

$$P(x \leq 4) = P(x = 0) + P(x = 1) + P(x = 2) + P(x = 3) + P(x = 4)$$

For $n = 10$ and $p = 0.3$, the different probabilities from Table A.2 are as follows:

$$P(x = 0) = 0.02825$$
$$P(x = 1) = 0.12106$$
$$P(x = 2) = 0.23347$$
$$P(x = 3) = 0.26683$$
$$P(x = 4) = 0.20012$$

Thus,

$$P(x \leq 4) = 0.02825 + 0.12106 + 0.23347 + 0.26683 + 0.20012$$
$$= 0.84973$$

5.5 POISSON DISTRIBUTION

Poisson distribution is another important discrete distribution. This distribution was independently discovered by von Bortkiewicz, Rutherford, and Gosset. It is based on the happening of a rare event in a specific time period such as the number of injuries reported at the health center, the number of goals scored in a match, the number of double faults occurring in a tennis tournament, and so on. The Poisson distribution is determined by one parameter, which is known as lambda (λ). The distribution function for Poisson distribution is given by

> **FACTS TO KNOW**
>
> In Poisson distribution, the mean and variance are always the same

$$P(x) = \frac{e^{-\lambda} \lambda^x}{x!}, \quad x = 0, 1, 2, \ldots \tag{5.8}$$

Consider that the average goal scored per match by a team has been 4 in the past. One can determine the probability of scoring 0, 1, 2, 3, 4, or 5 goals in a particular match by using the Poisson distribution. Here, the mean λ is 4, and say, the probability of $P(x = 3)$ can be computed by using formula (5.8). Consider another example where in the student information center of a university, 4 cases of lost items are typically reported per day. This may be the authorities' expectation, but there will be a certain variation in this figure: sometimes a little more, sometimes a little less, and once in a while there may not be reporting of any case. Given only the average rate for a certain period of observation and assuming that the reporting of cases is essentially random in nature, the Poisson distribution can be used to find *how likely it is* that 0, 2, 4, or any other number of cases can be reported in the center during a day. In other words, it predicts the degree of variation around a known average rate of reporting.

5.5.1 Conditions for a Poisson Distribution

a. Occurrences of events are independent in nature.
b. The events can be counted in whole numbers.
c. Events must occur at a constant rate in a continuous time slot.
d. The average frequency of occurrence for the given time period is known.

5.5.2 Mean and Standard Deviation of the Poisson Distribution

If x follows Poisson distribution with the parameter λ, then its mean and variance are given as follows:

$$\text{Mean} = \mu = \lambda$$

$$\text{Variance} = \sigma^2 = \lambda$$

Thus, the mean and variance of the Poisson distribution are the same.

5.5.3 Solving Problems Using Poisson Tables

Computing probabilities in solving problems based on Poisson distribution may be a tough task because it requires solving the values of some power of exponential. In order to make this task easy, Poisson probabilities have been provided for each value of x associated with a given population mean (λ) in Table A.3. Table 5.3 gives the cross section of the Poisson table for different values of x and λ.

TABLE 5.3 Cross Section of the Poisson Table

x \ λ	0.1	0.2	0.3	0.4	0.5	0.6	0.7	0.8	0.9	1.0	1.2
0	0.9048	0.8187	0.7408	0.6703	0.6065	0.5488	0.4966	0.4493	0.4066	0.3679	0.3012
1	0.9953	0.9825	0.9631	0.9384	0.9098	0.8781	0.8442	0.8088	0.7725	0.7358	0.6626
2	0.9998	0.9989	0.9964	0.9921	0.9856	0.9769	0.9659	0.9526	0.9371	0.9197	0.8795
3	1.0000	0.9999	0.9997	0.9992	0.9982	0.9966	0.9942	0.9909	0.9865	0.9810	0.9662
4	1.0000	1.0000	1.0000	0.9999	0.9998	0.9996	0.9992	0.9986	0.9977	0.9963	0.9923
5	1.0000	1.0000	1.0000	1.0000	1.0000	1.0000	0.9999	0.9998	0.9997	0.9994	0.9985
6	1.0000	1.0000	1.0000	1.0000	1.0000	1.0000	1.0000	1.0000	1.0000	0.9999	0.9997

From this table, $P(x)$ can be located for different values of λ. For example, for $\lambda = 0.5$, the probability of $P(x = 3)$ can be located at the cross section of $x = 3$ and $\lambda = 0.5$. This value is 0.9982.

Example 5.9 During an intramural on every Saturday, one can expect 3 injuries. Find the probability that during intramural there will be at the most 1 injury during an intramural.

Solution: As the expected, the number of injuries that can happen in the intramural is 3, $\lambda = 3$. The variable x can be defined as the number of injuries that occur during an intramural.

Thus, it is required to compute $P(x \leq 1)$.

$$P(x \leq 1) = P(x = 0) + P(x = 1)$$
$$= \frac{e^{-3}3^0}{0!} + \frac{e^{-3}3^1}{1!}$$
$$= e^{-3} + 3e^{-3}$$
$$= 4e^{-3}$$

However, this problem can be solved by using the Poisson distribution table. From Table A.3, the probabilities of $P(x = 0)$ and $P(x = 1)$ can be seen for the mean $\lambda = 3$.

Thus,

$$P(x \leq 1) = P(x = 0) + P(x = 1)$$
$$= 0.0498 + 0.1494$$
$$= 0.1992$$

Example 5.10 A health center has determined that on an average 4 muscle injuries are reported per day. Find the probability that the health center receives at least 2 muscle injuries on a randomly selected day.

$$P(x \geq 2) = 1 - P(x < 2)$$
$$= 1-(p(x = 0) + P(x = 1))$$
$$= 1-(0.0183 + 0.0733)$$
$$= 1 - 0.0916$$
$$= 0.9084$$

Example 5.11 The number of goals scored in the interclass soccer games follows a Poisson distribution with a mean of 3 goals per game. Find the probability of scoring 2 goals in a randomly selected soccer match of the college.

Solution: Given that $\lambda = 3$, it is required to find $P(x = 2)$. Using the Poisson distribution formula given in equation (5.8) and substituting the values of x and λ,

$$P(x = 2) = \frac{e^{-3}3^2}{2!} = \frac{9}{2}e^{-3}$$

However, the above-mentioned probability can be computed by using Table A.3 for $\lambda = 3$ and $x = 2$.

$$P(x = 2) = 0.2240$$

Example 5.12 On an average, 4 ankle injuries per week are reported in a health center. Assuming that the occurrence of injury has a Poisson distribution, find the probability that in a given week

i. some ankle injuries are reported
ii. 2 or more but less than 4 ankle injuries are reported

Solution: Let x be the number of ankle injuries occurring per week. Since x is a Poisson variable, here the mean (λ) is 4.

1. The probability that some ankle injuries are reported can be obtained by

$$\begin{aligned} P(x > 0) &= 1 - P(x = 0) \\ &= 1 - \frac{e^{-4} \times 4^0}{0!} \\ &= 1 - e^{-4} \end{aligned}$$

   This probability can be obtained by using the Poisson table directly. From Table A.3, the value of $P(x = 0)$ for $\lambda = 4$ is equal to 0.0183. Hence, the required probability would be 1−0.0183, that is, 0.9817.

2. Probability that in a given week, 2 or more but less than 4 ankle injuries are reported can be obtained by

$$\begin{aligned} P(2 \le x < 4) &= P(x = 2) + P(x = 3) \\ &= \frac{e^{-4} \times 4^2}{2!} + \frac{e^{-4} \times 4^3}{3!} \\ &= 8e^{-4} + \frac{32\,e^{-4}}{3} \end{aligned}$$

   The above-mentioned probabilities can be obtained by using the Poisson table directly. From Table A.3, for $\lambda = 4$, $P(x = 2) = 0.14653$ and $P(x = 3) = 0.19537$.

   Thus,

$$P(2 \le x < 4) = 0.14653 + 0.19537 = 0.34190$$

Check Your Progress

Note: Tick the correct answer by using the sign (√).

		True	False
20.	A binomial distribution is a discrete distribution.	-	-
21.	In a binomial experiment, the probability of x successes in n trials in a specified order is given by ${}^nC_x p^x q^{n-x}$.	-	-
22.	The binomial distribution has two parameters n and p.	-	-
23.	In a binomial distribution if $n = 8$ and $p = 0.4$, then $P(x \geq 1)$ can be obtained by subtracting $P(x = 0)$ from 1.	-	-
24.	The standard deviation of the binomial distribution is npq.	-	-
25.	The number of accidents occurring during each intramural session is a binomial variable.	-	-
26.	The Poisson distribution has only parameter λ.	-	-
27.	In a binomial distribution, the probability of success (p) can be different in different trials.	-	-
28.	College athletes getting gold medals in the intervarsity tournament each year is a Poisson variable.	-	-
29.	In a binomial distribution, the variance can be more than the mean.	-	-
30.	The mean of a Poisson distribution is λ.	-	-
31.	In a binomial experiment, each trial should have only two outcomes.	-	-
32.	In a binomial experiment, the probability of x successes in n trials is given by $p^x q^{n-x}$.	-	-
33.	The mean of the binomial distribution is np.	-	-
34.	The standard deviation of the Poisson distribution is λ.	-	-
35.	The Poisson distribution is a continuous distribution.	-	-
36.	In a Poisson distribution, occurrences of events are independent of nature.	-	-

PRACTICE EXERCISE

1. Compute the mean and standard deviation for the following discrete distribution.

x	$p(x)$
1	0.15
2	0.30
3	0.20
4	0.35

2. Find the value of the mean and standard deviation of the binomial distribution having $n = 18$ and $p = 0.70$.
3. Find the following probabilities by using the binomial formula:
   a. $P(x = 5)$, if $n = 8$ and $p = 0.6$
   b. $P(3 \leq x \leq 5)$, if $n = 6$ and $p = 0.5$
4. Find the following probability by using the binomial table: $P(x < 4)$, if $n = 15$ and $p = 0.3$.
5. Find the following probabilities by using the Poisson distribution:
   a. $P(x = 2)$, given that $\lambda = 4.5$
   b. $P(x < 5)$, given that $\lambda = 5.2$
6. Find the following probabilities by using the Poisson distribution:
   a. $P(x \leq 3)$, given that $\lambda = 2.6$
   b. $P(x \geq 2)$, given that $\lambda = 4.1$

5.6 CONTINUOUS DISTRIBUTION

FACTS TO KNOW

Most of the behavioral parameters are normally distributed

Continuous distributions are the probability models that are used to describe variables that are continuous in nature. Continuous distributions deal with such a large sample size that its random variable values are treated on a continuum scale from $-\infty$ to $+\infty$, whereas discrete distributions deal with smaller populations and thus cannot be treated as if they are on a continuum scale. Because of this difference, different methods are used to analyze these two types of distributions. Continuous distributions are analyzed by using calculus, whereas discrete distributions are analyzed by using simple arithmetic. To be more specific, in continuous distribution, the probability that a random variable lies in between the two points is calculated by using integration, whereas in discrete distribution, the probability that a random variable takes a value within a range is computed by adding the different probabilities. There are many continuous distributions available, but the most important distribution is the normal distribution. In this chapter, only normal distribution is discussed in detail.

5.7 NORMAL DISTRIBUTION

Normal distribution is one of the most important continuous distributions. It plays a prominent role in both parametric and nonparametric inferential procedures because it provides a large sample approximation to the probability distributions for many estimators and test statistics. Normal distribution is defined by the following equation:

$$p(x) = \frac{1}{\sigma\sqrt{2\pi}} e^{-\frac{(x-\mu)^2}{2\sigma^2}}, \quad -\infty \leq x \leq \infty, \ -\infty \leq \mu \leq \infty, \text{ and } \sigma \geq 0 \qquad (5.9)$$

where x is the normal random variable, μ is the mean, σ is the standard deviation, π is approximately 3.14159, and e is approximately 2.71828. The function $f(x)$ is said to be the probability density function for the normal distribution. The statistics μ and σ are known as the parameters of the distribution. Thus, if x is normally distributed with mean μ and variance σ^2, then we can state that $x \sim N(\mu, \sigma^2)$. The curve so obtained by using the above-mentioned formula is known as a *normal curve*. The normal curve is also known as a Gaussian curve because it was invented by Carl Friedrich Gauss, a German mathematician. The normal curve is also referred to as an ideal curve because it can never be obtained in practice. This curve is used to test how far your data is close to the normal distribution. As the curve looks similar to a bell, it is also called a bell-shaped curve. In fact, a normal curve is not a single curve; it is rather an infinite number of possible curves, all described by the same algebraic expression (5.9). Different curves are obtained for different sets of parameters μ and σ, therefore, the normal curve is called a *family of distributions*. Each member of the family is determined by values of the parameters μ and σ of the model. Since μ can assume any value in the range $-\infty$ to $+\infty$ and σ can take any nonnegative value, the family of normal curves is quite large, consisting of an infinite number of members. This makes the normal curve a general-purpose model for describing a large number of happenings of natural phenomena. Although all the members of the family of normal curves are different, they have a number of properties in common. These properties include shape, symmetry, tails never touching the X-axis, and area under the curve. The area under the normal curve is always taken as 1. All members of the family of normal curves are bell shaped, provided the X-axis is scaled properly. The normal curve appears as shown in Figure 5.3. This curve is obtained by using formula (5.9) for a particular set of μ and σ.

5.7.1 Family of the Normal Curve

Let us see how the different curves of a normal curve family are obtained by changing the values of mean and standard deviation.

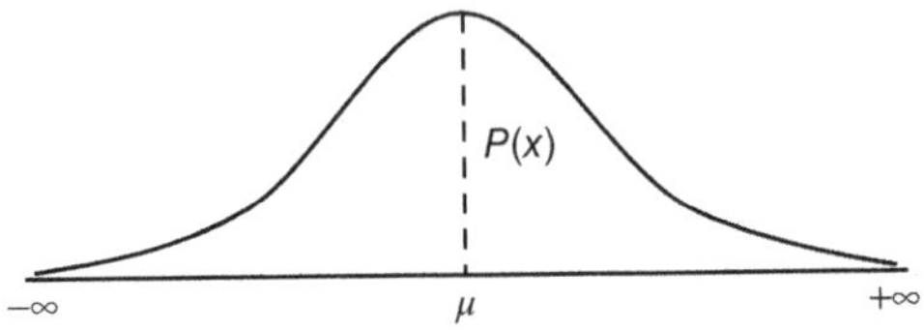

Figure 5.3 Normal curve with the mean (μ) and standard deviation (σ).

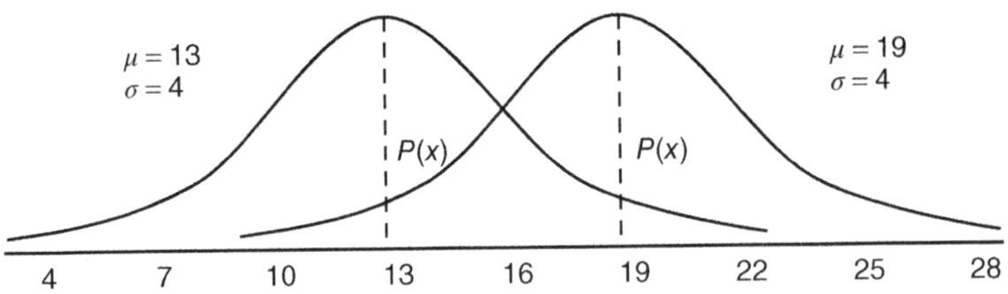

Figure 5.4 Two curves of the normal curve family having different means and same standard deviations.

The value of mean (μ) determines where the midpoint of the distribution falls. By changing the value of μ without changing the standard deviation, the distribution shall move to the right or left, depending on whether the new value of μ is greater or smaller than the first value.

Consider an example where the mean and standard deviation of the normally distributed variable x are 13 and 4, respectively. If the mean is changed to 19 while the standard deviation remains 4, then the shape of the two distributions remains the same except for the shifting of the distribution to the right because the new mean 19 is higher than the first mean 13. This has been shown in Figure 5.4.

On the other hand, let us see the effect of change in standard deviation without changing the mean value of the distribution of scores. Changes in the value of σ change the shape of the distribution without affecting the midpoint. It is so because σ affects the spread of the scores around its mean value. The larger the value of σ, the more is the spread of the score, whereas a smaller value of σ results in less spread of the scores. Let us understand this fact by means of the graphs shown in Figure 5.5. In this figure, the effect of increasing the value of σ is shown on the distribution of the scores. Let the score x be normally distributed with mean 16 and standard deviation 4. If the standard deviation of the scores is increased to 8 by changing the scale while the mean remains the same, 16, then drawing the two distributions on the same scale results in the graph as shown in Figure 5.5.

It can be noticed in the figure that the shape of the second distribution has changed dramatically, being much flatter than the original distribution. It must not be as high as the original distribution because the total area under the curve must be constant, that is, 1.00. The second curve is still a normal curve but looks different because it is drawn on a different scale on the X-axis. Since both these curves are from the family of the normal curve, the area among them would remain 1.

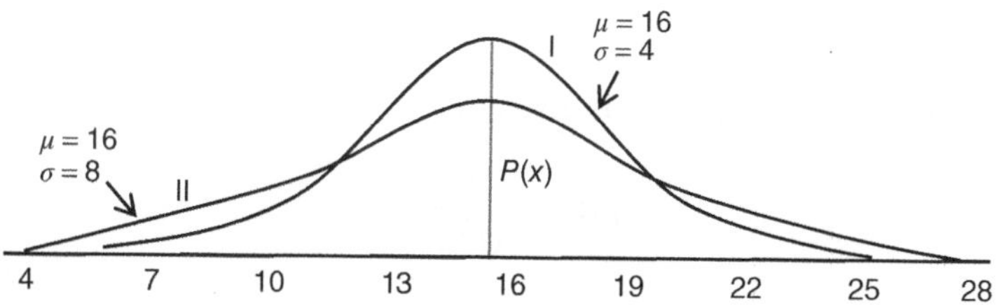

Figure 5.5 Two curves of the normal curve family having same means but different standard deviations.

5.7.2 Characteristics of the Normal Curve

A normal distribution is used to solve varieties of research problems; therefore, it is important to know its various characteristics. The following are the important properties of a normal distribution.

1. A normal distribution is a bilaterally symmetrical distribution; therefore, its mean, median, and mode coincide.
2. In a normal distribution, the curve does not touch the baseline. In other words, the curve is asymptotic toward the baseline.
3. The points of inflexion of the curve are given by $\mu \pm \sigma$. The point of inflexion is a point at which the curve changes its direction. Before $\mu + \sigma$ point the curve is concave, whereas after this point it becomes convex.
4. The quartile deviation of a normal distribution is 2/3.
5. In a normal distribution, 1σ limits cover the middle 68.26% of the area. In other words, 68.26% cases would fall within the range $\mu - \sigma$ to $\mu + \sigma$. Thus, the area under the normal curve is distributed as per the following limits:

Limits	Area (%)
$\mu-\sigma$ to $\mu+\sigma$	68.26
$\mu-2\sigma$ to $\mu+2\sigma$	95.44
$\mu-3\sigma$ to $\mu+3\sigma$	99.73

6. In a normal curve, the height of the mean ordinate is in a fixed proportion to the height of the ordinate at any given standard deviation distance from the mean.

5.7.3 Standard Normal Distribution

By changing the origin and scale of the data, the shape of the normal distribution gets changed. It is therefore difficult for the researcher to know as to which normal curve he or she should refer to. However, if the scores are converted into standard scores by using the transformation $z = (x - \mu)/\sigma$, then the distribution so obtained is known as a *standard normal distribution*. Thus, the probability density function of the standard normal distribution is given by

$$p(z) = \frac{1}{\sqrt{2\pi}} e^{-\frac{1}{2}z^2} \tag{5.10}$$

where z is the standard normal variate with mean 0 and variance 1 and usually the value of z lies between -3 and $+3$. Whatever is the unit of the scores, one can always convert it into its standard scores, and the distribution so obtained will always be the standard normal distribution. The standard normal distribution is unique with mean 0 and variance 1. Here onward, whenever a reference shall be made about the normal distribution it is actually a standard normal distribution, and the area shown in Table A.4 also refers to the area of the standard normal curve.

> **FACTS TO KNOW**
>
> Standard score facilitates comparison of athlete's performance in two different events having different units

5.8 STANDARD SCORE

The standard score indicates as to how many standard deviations a score is above or below the mean. It is also called z-score, z-value, or standardized variables. Each and every normal random variable x can be transformed into a z-score by using the following formula:

$$z = \frac{x - \mu}{\sigma} \tag{5.11}$$

where x is the normal random variable, and μ and σ are the mean and standard deviation of x, respectively. The following are the properties of the standard score (z):

1. Mean of z is 0.
2. Standard deviation of z is 1.
3. Standard score is free from units.
4. Limits of z are ± 3.

As the standard score z is free from units, it can be used to compare the performance of an individual on two different test items having different units. Consider an example in which it is desired to know whether an athlete's performance is better in high jump or in 100 m. Since high jump performance is measured in meters whereas 100 m performance is measured in seconds, comparison is not possible. But if the high jump and 100 m performances are converted into their respective standard scores, then these two performances can be compared as these two are pure numbers.

Example 5.13 If population mean and population standard deviation of the normal variable x are 15 and 3, respectively, find the standard score (z) of the scores x: 21, 18, 15, 12, and 8.

Solution: For each score x, the standard score z shall be computed by using the formula $z = \dfrac{x-\mu}{\sigma}$.

Computation of Standard Scores

x	$z=(x-\mu)/\sigma$
21	2
18	1
15	0
12	−1
8	−2.33

Remark As we refer to the standard normal distribution all the time, we take the liberty to call it a *normal distribution* here onward.

5.9 NORMAL APPROXIMATION TO THE BINOMIAL DISTRIBUTION

We know that if x is a binomial variate we write $x \sim b(n, p)$, where n and p are the parameters of the distribution. The parameter n represents the number of trials and p represents the probability of success in a single trial. If n, the number of trials, becomes infinite and p is equal to 1/2, then the binomial distribution approaches a normal distribution. Even if the number of trials is not very large, binomial distribution gives a better approximation to the normal distribution.

To demonstrate this fact, let us have a coin-tossing experiment. In tossing a coin 10 times, various probabilities of the events can be worked out by expanding the below-mentioned expression using binomial expansion. Each term represents the occurrence of some number of heads and some number of tails. For example, H^8T^2 represents the occurrence of 8 heads and 2 tails.

$$(H+T)^{10} = T^{10} + 10T^9H + 45T^8H^2 + 120T^7H^3 + 210T^6H^4 + 252T^5H^5 + 210T^4H^6 + 120T^3H^7 + 45T^2H^8 + 10T^1H^9 + H^{10}$$

The probability of occurrence of any event (term in the expression) is proportional to its coefficient. For example, the probability of getting $10H$ is least and that of getting $5H5T$ is maximum. It is so because the coefficient of H^{10} is 1, which is the least coefficient, and the coefficient of H^5T^5 is the maximum, which is 252.

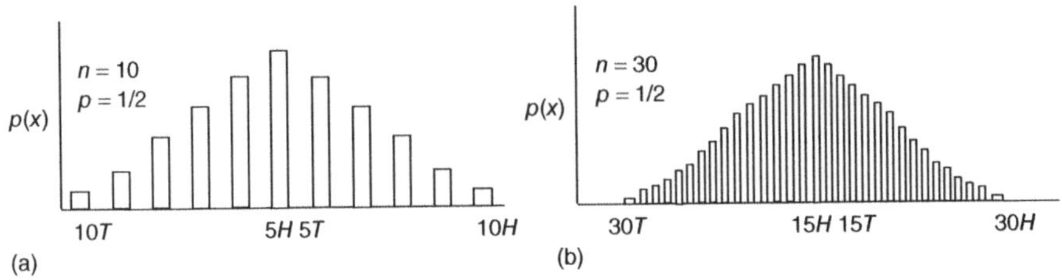

Figure 5.6 (a, b) Binomial distributions.

If each of the components in the above expansion is represented by a bar and the height of the bar by its corresponding probabilities, then the binomial distribution with $n = 10$ and $p = 1/2$ can be shown as in Figure 5.6a.

Similarly, at $n = 30$ with p equal to 1/2, the graph of binomial distribution can be shown as in Figure 5.6b.

The shape of the two graphs looks similar except that the width of the bars has decreased with an increase in the number of trials. If n, the number of trials, becomes infinite, the width of the bar will reduce to a point and all the bars will merge together, resulting in the normal distribution. If the probability p deviates more from 1/2, the curve will become more skewed, but if p is equal to 1/2 even for $n = 100$, the binomial distribution will closely resemble a normal distribution.

5.10 TESTING NORMALITY OF THE DATA

Normality of data can be tested by using skewness and kurtosis. Skewness measures the symmetricity of a curve, whereas kurtosis assesses whether the curve peakedness is comparable to the normal curve. For a curve to be normal, it should be symmetrical as well as mesokurtic in nature. In other words, both skewness and kurtosis should be 0 for a normal distribution; therefore, the farther away from 0 a distribution is, the more nonnormal it is. The details of these two characteristics are discussed below.

> **FACTS TO KNOW**
>
> Normality of data can be checked by using the Shapiro–Wilk test and Q–Q plot

5.10.1 Skewness

Skewness measures the lack of symmetry of a curve. If the curve is not symmetrical, it is said to skewed or asymmetrical. In a symmetrical curve, the mean, median, and mode coincide. A normal curve is a symmetrical curve; therefore, the mean, median, and mode are the same in the normal distribution. Skewness is represented by β_1 and is computed by the following formula:

$$\beta_1 = \frac{\mu_3^2}{\mu_2^3} \tag{5.12}$$

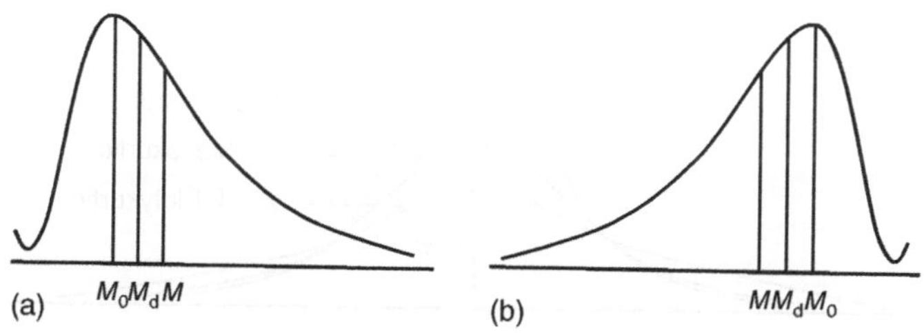

Figure 5.7 Curves with different skewness: (a) positively skewed curve $\beta_1 > 0$ and (b) negatively skewed curve $\beta_1 < 0$.

where μ_2 and μ_3 are the second and third central moments. A generalized formula for computing the rth central moment is

$$\mu_r = \frac{1}{n}\sum (X - \overline{X})^r$$

The skewness of the curve can be positive or negative. If the value of β_1 is 0, the curve is symmetrical. However, if β_1 is greater than 0 the curve is said to be positively skewed, and if it is less than 0 it is negatively skewed. In a positively skewed curve, the tail is more stretched on the right side in comparison to the left side and the mean is more than the mode. This means that in the positively skewed data, a large number of scores are less than the mean. Figure 5.7(a) shows the positively skewed curve.

On the other hand, in a negatively skewed curve, the tail is more stretched on the left side in comparison to the right side and the mean is less than the mode. This indicates that in the negatively skewed data, a large number of scores are more than the mean. Figure 5.7(b) shows the negatively skewed curve.

One must note that the normal curve is symmetrical, but all symmetrical curves need not necessarily be the normal curve. To find whether the distribution of scores is significantly skewed or not, it is required to compute the standard error (SE) of skewness. The SE error of skewness is given by

$$\text{SE}(\beta_1) = \sqrt{\frac{6n(n-1)}{(n-2)(n+1)(n+3)}} \tag{5.13}$$

where n is the sample size. In general, a skewness (absolute value) value more than twice its SE indicates a departure from symmetry.

5.10.2 Kurtosis

Kurtosis can be defined as a measure that describes the distribution of data around the mean. It can be used to find whether the distribution is more or less peaked than the normal distribution. The normal curve is known as a *mesokurtic curve*. A curve

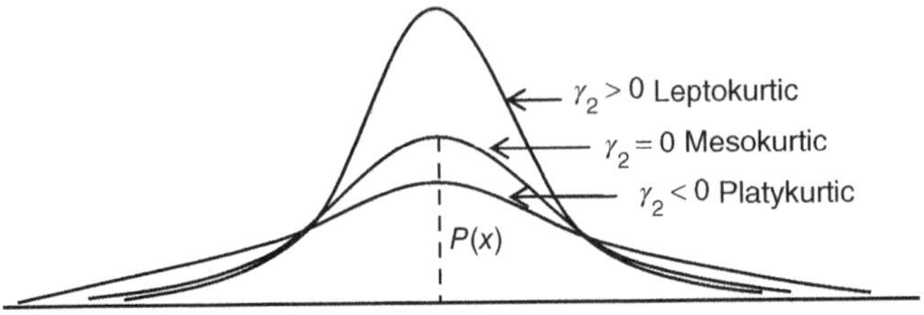

Figure 5.8 Curves with different kurtosis.

more peaked than the normal curve is known as a *leptokurtic curve*, whereas the curve that is less peaked than the normal curve is known as a *platykurtic curve*. Kurtosis is denoted by γ_2 and is computed by the following formula:

$$\gamma_2 = \beta_2 - 1 \tag{5.14}$$

where $\beta_2 = \frac{\mu_4}{\mu_2^2}$ and μ_2 and μ_4 are the second and fourth central moments, respectively.

For a mesokurtic curve γ_2 is 0 and for a leptokurtic curve it is greater than 0, whereas for a platykurtic curve it is less than 0. Here, it is worth mentioning that all the normal curves are mesokurtic, but all the mesokurtic curves need not necessarily be normal. It is because the mesokurtic curve may not be symmetrical at times. All three kinds of curves have been shown in Figure 5.8.

For a normal distribution, kurtosis (γ_2) is 0. To check whether kurtosis is significantly higher or lower than 0, it is required to compute the SE of the kurtosis. The SE of the kurtosis is given by

$$\text{SE}(\gamma_2) = 2 \times \text{SE}(\beta_1) \times \sqrt{\frac{n^2 - 1}{(n-3)(n+5)}} \tag{5.15}$$

where $\text{SE}(\beta_1)$ is the SE of skewness and n is the sample size. In general, a kurtosis (absolute value) value greater than twice its SE indicates that it is significant.

5.10.3 Test for Normality

The Kolmogorov–Smirnov test (K–S) and Shapiro–Wilk (S–W) test are the two established tests for testing the normality of data by taking into account the values of both skewness and kurtosis. These tests allow you to test the normality of data by comparing the distribution of sample data with the normal distribution. The data are normal if these tests are not significant. Thus, if the significance value (p-value) of these tests is more than 0.05, the data are considered to be normal, otherwise they are nonnormal. Consider the data on sit-ups

> **FACTS TO KNOW**
>
> Randomization facilitates data to be normally distributed

TABLE 5.4 Data on Sit-Ups and Height

Sit-Ups (in no.)	Height (in ft.)
24.00	5.40
30.00	5.50
22.00	5.50
42.00	5.60
38.00	5.60
21.00	5.60
24.00	5.70
30.00	5.70
22.00	5.70
24.00	5.70
23.00	5.80
23.00	5.80
28.00	5.80
24.00	5.90
21.00	5.90
45.00	6.00
24.00	5.80
23.00	5.50
28.00	5.60
30.00	5.60
22.00	5.70
28.00	5.70
24.00	5.70
45.00	5.80
42.00	5.90

TABLE 5.5 Tests of Normality

	Kolmogorov–Smirnov			Shapiro–Wilk		
	Statistics	df	Sig.	Statistic	df	Sig.
Sit-Ups	0.269	25	0.000	0.785	25	0.000
Height	0.140	25	0.200	0.963	25	0.484

performance and height obtained on 25 subjects in a random sample as shown in Table 5.4.

The results of K–S test and S–W test applied on these data are shown in Table 5.5. Looking at the values, it may be concluded that the data on sit-ups are nonnormal whereas those on height are normal because the S–W test for the sit-ups is significant whereas for height it is insignificant.

The S–W test is more appropriate for small sample sizes ($n < 50$) but can also be used for sample sizes as large as 2000. Because of this reason, this test is widely used for assessing the normality.

One of the limitations of these tests is that in the case of a large sample you are more likely to get significant results. In other words, these tests become significant even for slight deviation from normality in the case of a large sample.

5.10.4 Normal Q–Q Plot

Normality of the data can also be checked graphically. The "normal Q–Q plot" is a graphical way to check the level of normality of the data. The line indicates that the value of your sample should fall on it or close by if the data follow a normal distribution. The dots represent the data points in the sample. If these points deviate much from the line, it indicates that your data are nonnormal. The normal Q–Q plot obtained from the data mentioned in Table 5.4 is shown in Figure 5.9. In Figure 5.9a, the data deviate from the line indicating that the data on sit-ups are nonnormal, whereas in Figure 5.9b the data fall along the line indicating normality of the data on height.

Remark The K–S test and S–W test along with the normal Q–Q plot can be computed by any standard statistical software. However, in Statistical Package for the Social Sciences (SPSS), it can be obtained by using the following commands in the data file.

Analyze ⟶ Descriptive statistics ⟶ Explore

5.11 THE CENTRAL LIMIT THEOREM

The central limit theorem states that if a random sample is drawn from a population having mean μ and variance σ^2, which may or may not be normal, then the distribution of the sample mean tends to be normal with mean μ and variance σ^2/n, provided the sample is sufficiently large and is drawn randomly from the population. As the sample size keeps increasing, the distribution of the sample means becomes closer and closer to the normal distribution. A sample is said to be large if it is 30 or more, that is, $n \geq 30$. The concept of central limit theorem is used in testing many of the hypotheses related to population parameters.

5.12 SOLVING PROBLEMS BASED ON NORMAL DISTRIBUTION

Most of the behavioral parameters follow a normal (or near-normal) distribution. This encourages researchers to use the normal distribution as a model for finding probabilities associated with the happening of events of naturally occurring phenomena. Before solving varieties of problems based on normal distribution, let us first see how to use the normal distribution table. Solving any problem based on normal distribution involves the following steps.

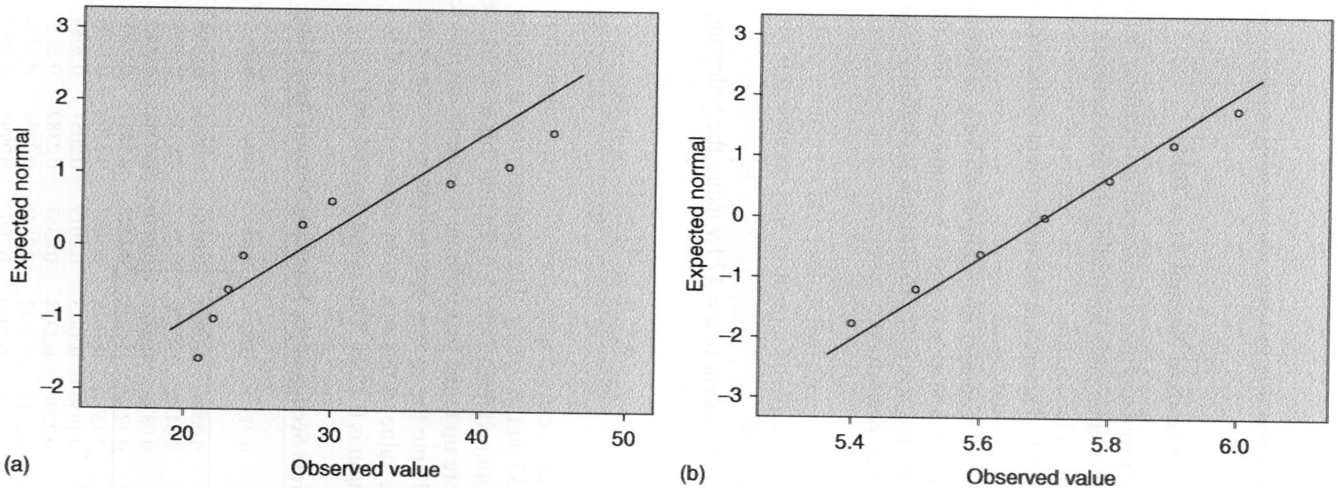

Figure 5.9 (a) Normal Q–Q plot for the data on sit-ups and (b) normal Q–Q plot for the data on height.

a. Convert the raw data into z-scores by using the transformation $z = (x - \mu)/\sigma$. The data need to be converted because the standard normal area table is based on z-scores.
b. Find the required probability by using the standard normal area table as shown in Table A.4.

5.12.1 How to Use the Standard Normal Area Table

Before starting to solve problems based on normal distribution, let us first see how to use the standard normal area table for finding the area between any two consecutive points. For ease of understanding, a cross section of the standard normal area table is shown in Table 5.6. The area in the table refers to the area in the standard normal curve between $z = 0$ and $z = z_1$.

For easy understanding, consider an example where x is normally distributed with mean 45 and standard deviation 6, and it is required to find the percentage of scores between mean 45 and score 47. To find this probability from the table, the following steps need to be performed.

1. Draw the normal curve with two scales z and x. On the x-scale, mark the value of mean 45 and score 47 (on a positive side because it is greater than 45) as shown in Figure 5.10.
2. Find the z-score equivalent to $x = 47$ by using the following transformation and locate it on the z-scale.

$$z = \frac{x - \mu}{\sigma} = \frac{47 - 45}{6} = 0.33$$

3. The area between mean 45 and score 47 is equivalent to the area between $z = 0$ and $z = 0.33$ on the z-scale. The required area is shaded in Figure 5.10, which can be obtained from Table 5.6. To find this area, locate $z = 0.33$ in the table. The z-score up to the first decimal is seen in the first leftmost column of the table and upto the second decimal place is seen in the first row of the table. Thus, the value of the area at the cross section of 0.3 in the row and 0.03 in the column is 0.1293. This is the desired area.

TABLE 5.6 Cross Section of the Standard Normal Area Table

z	0.00	0.01	0.02	0.03	0.04	0.05	0.06
0.0	0.0000	0.0040	0.0080	0.0120	0.0160	0.0199	0.0239
0.1	0.0398	0.0438	0.0478	0.0517	0.0557	0.0596	0.0636
0.2	0.0793	0.0832	0.0871	0.0910	0.0948	0.0987	0.1026
0.3	0.1179	0.1217	0.1255	**0.1293**	0.1331	0.1368	0.1406
0.4	0.1554	0.1591	0.1628	0.1664	0.1700	0.1736	0.1772
0.5	0.1915	0.1950	0.1985	0.2019	0.2054	0.2088	0.2123
0.6	0.2257	0.2291	0.2324	0.2357	0.2389	0.2422	0.2454
0.7	0.2580	0.2611	0.2642	0.2673	0.2704	0.2734	0.2764
0.8	0.2881	0.2910	0.2939	0.2967	0.2995	0.3023	0.3051

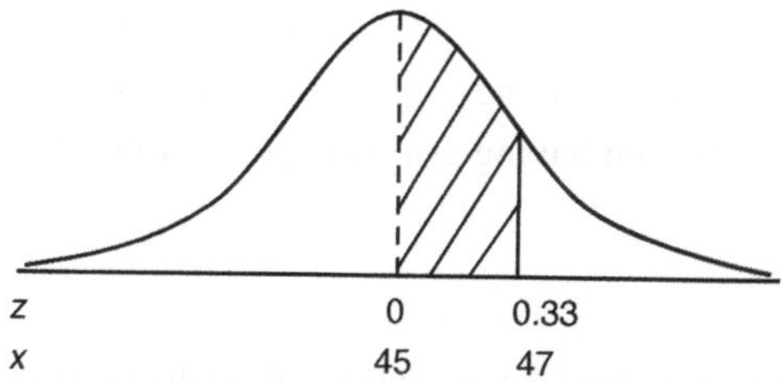

Figure 5.10 Marking the scores for computing the desired area.

Example 5.14 If the scores on sit-ups (x) obtained on athletes are normally distributed with mean 60 and standard deviation 12, find the percentage of athletes performing more than 78 sit-ups.

Solution: The required percentage of scores shall be the area in the normal curve above $x = 78$. Since the area in Table A.4 is tabulated in terms of the standard score, the value of x needs to be converted into z.

$$\text{For } x = 78, \ z = \frac{x - \mu}{\sigma} = \frac{78 - 60}{12} = 1.5$$

The area above $x = 78$ is required to be computed. Let this area be denoted by A_1.

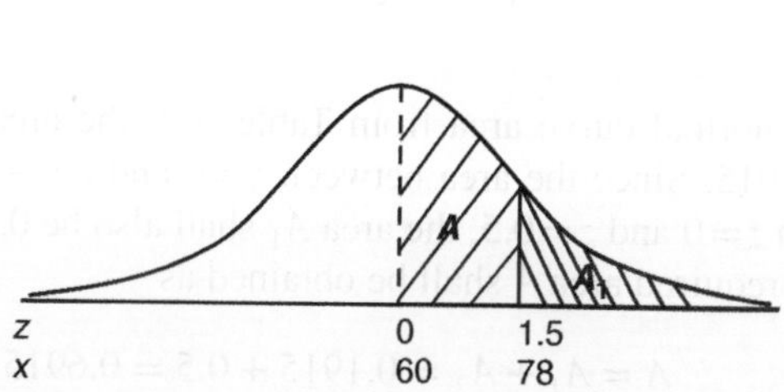

From the normal curve area from Table A.4, the area corresponding to $z = 1.5$ is 0.4332. This is the area between $z = 0$ and $z = 1.5$; hence, $A = 0.4332$.

Since the total area under the curve is 1, the area above the mean shall be 0.5 because of the symmetrical nature of the curve. The area A_1 can be obtained as

$$A_1 = 0.5 - A = 0.5 - 0.4332 = 0.0668$$

Since the normal curve covers 100% of the cases, 6.68% of the athletes' performance is more than 78.

Example 5.15 If the grip strength for the women in the category of 50–54 years of age is normally distributed with mean 54 lbs and standard deviation 10 lbs, calculate the following:

i. Percentage of women having grip strength more than 49 lbs
ii. Percentage of women having grip strength between 46 and 57 lbs
iii. Percentage of women having grip strength between 59 and 65 lbs

Solution:

i. Here, it is required to find the area above 49 in the normal curve shown below. Since 49 is less than the mean score 54, it lies on its left side. Let A be the required area, then

$$A = A_1 + A_2$$

A_1 can be obtained from the normal curve area table, whereas A_2 is 0.5 (as the area under the normal curve is 1).

$$\text{For } x = 49, \quad z = \frac{x-\mu}{\sigma} = \frac{54-49}{10} = -0.5$$

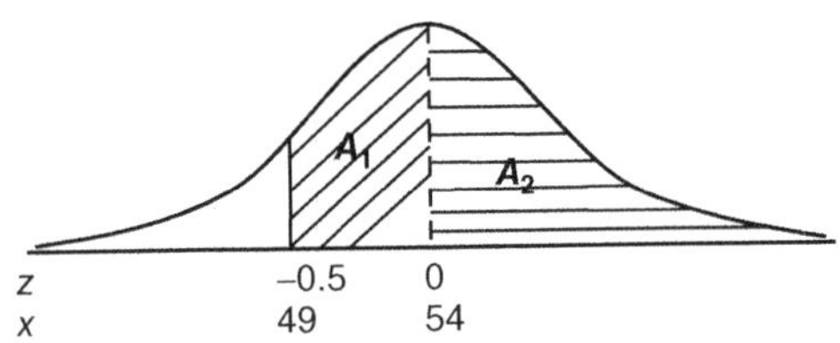

From the normal curve area from Table A.4, the area corresponding to $z=0.5$ is 0.1915. Since the area between $z=0$ and $z=-0.5$ is equal to the area between $z=0$ and $z=0.5$, the area A_1 shall also be 0.1915.

Thus, the required area A shall be obtained as

$$A = A_1 + A_2 = 0.1915 + 0.5 = 0.6915$$

Since the normal curve covers 100% of the cases, the grip strength of 69.15% women would be more than 49 lbs.

ii. The percentage of women having grip strength between 46 and 57 lbs can be calculated by finding the areas A_1 and A_2 as shown in the following figure. Thus, if A is the required area, then

$$A = A_1 + A_2$$

$$\text{For } x = 46, \quad z = \frac{x-\mu}{\sigma} = \frac{46-54}{10} = -0.8$$

$$\text{For } x = 57, \quad z = \frac{x-\mu}{\sigma} = \frac{57-54}{10} = 0.3$$

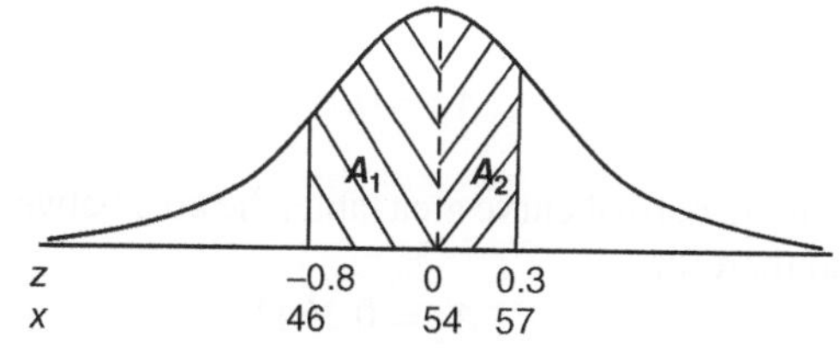

From Table A.4, the area between $z = 0$ and $z = 0.8$ is 0.281. Owing to the symmetrical nature of the curve, the area between $z = 0$ and $z = -0.8$ will also be 0.281, and therefore,

$$A_1 = 0.281$$

The area between $z = 0$ and $z = 0.3$ in the normal curve area table is 0.1179, and therefore,

$$A_2 = 0.1179$$

The required area shall be

$$A = 0.2810 + 0.1179 = 0.3989$$

Thus, the grip strength of 39.89% women would be between 46 and 57 lbs.

iii. It is required to find the percentage of women having grip strength between 59 and 65 lbs. Since both these scores are greater than the mean, they have been identified on the right side. If A_1 is the area between mean 54 and score 59 and A_2 is the area between mean 54 and score 65, then the required area A would be obtained as

$$A = A_2 - A_1$$

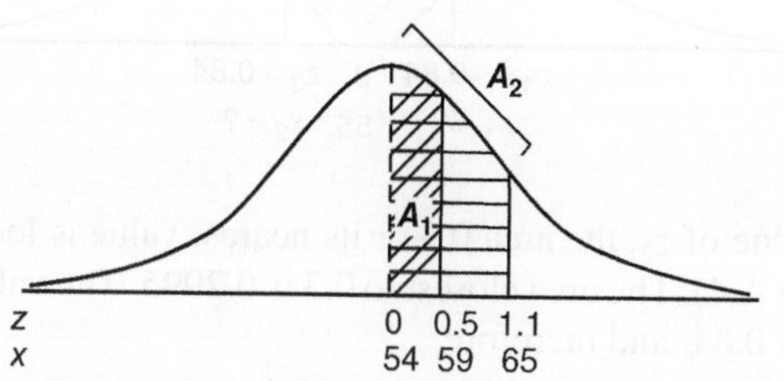

$$\text{For } x = 59, \quad z = \frac{x - \mu}{\sigma} = \frac{59 - 54}{10} = 0.50$$

$$\text{For } x = 65, \quad z = \frac{x - \mu}{\sigma} = \frac{65 - 54}{10} = 1.1$$

From Table A.4, the area between $z = 0$ and $z = 0.50$ is 0.1915, and therefore,

$$A_1 = 0.1915$$

Similarly, from the normal curve area table, the area between $z = 0$ and $z = 1.1$ is 0.3643, and therefore,

$$A_2 = 0.3643$$

The desired area A can be obtained by subtracting A_1 from A_2.

$$A = 0.3643 - 0.1915 = 0.1728$$

Thus, the grip strength of 17.28% women would be between 59 and 65 lbs.

Example 5.16 If weights of the women (x) are normally distributed with mean 55 kg and standard deviation 6 kg, what weight limits shall include the middle 60% of the women in the distribution?

Solution: In this problem, the area in the normal curve is known and it is required to find its corresponding limits.

Since the area of the normal curve is taken as 1, the middle 60% area would be divided on both the sides of the mean in the distribution. Thus, each of the area on both the sides would be 0.3. It is required to find the values of z_1 and z_2 as shown in the following figure. Converting z_1 and z_2 into their score values will give the score limits.

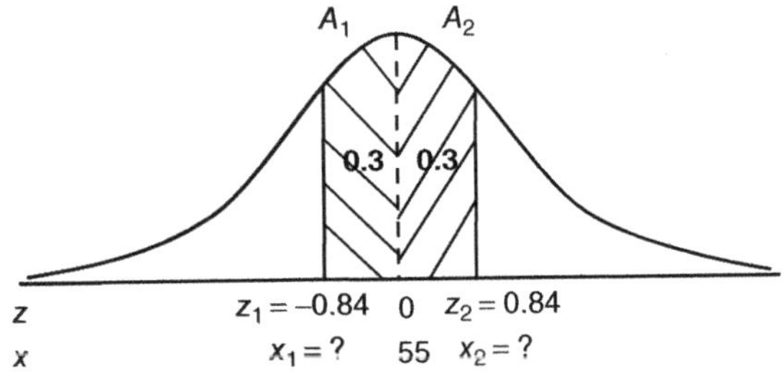

To find the value of z_2, the area 0.3 or its nearest value is located in the normal curve area (Table A.4). The area closest to 0.3 is 0.2995. The value of z corresponding to this area is 0.84, and therefore,

$$z_2 = 0.84$$

Because of the symmetrical nature of the curve, the corresponding z-value for the area on the left side would also be the same except for its sign.

Since the two scores on the z-scale have been located, their corresponding scores can be worked out as follows.

Since we know that

$$z = \frac{x - \mu}{\sigma}$$

for $z_1 = -0.84$,

$$-0.84 = \frac{x_1 - 55}{6}$$

$$\Rightarrow x_1 = 55 - 6 \times 0.84 = 49.96$$

Similarly, for $z_2 = 0.84$,

$$0.84 = \frac{x_2 - 55}{6}$$

$$\Rightarrow x_2 = 55 + 6 \times 0.84 = 60.04$$

Thus, the weight limits 49.96 and 60.04 kg will include 60% of the women in the distribution.

Example 5.17 In a statistics examination, students were graded in five categories: *A*, *B*, *C*, *D*, and *E*. If the grading was normally distributed, find the percentage of students securing each of the five grades.

Solution: Because of the symmetrical nature of the distribution, two of the grades *A* and *B* shall be on the left side, whereas two grades *D* and *E* shall be on the right side of the mean. The grade *C* will lie in the middle. Since 3σ limits cover 99.73% of the total cases, the width of the curve may be considered as 6 (the value of σ is 1).

$$\text{Width of each grade} = \frac{6}{5} = 1.2$$

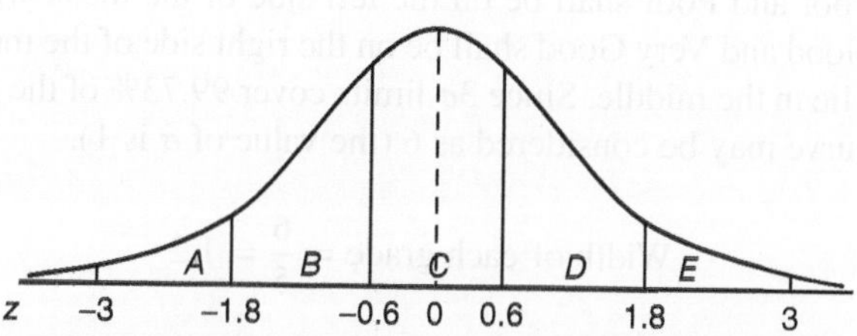

The normal curve can be divided into five grades as shown in the figure by taking the width of each grade as 1.2. As the mean of z is 0, boundary points of grade *C* would be −0.6 to 0.6. After adding 1.2, the boundary points of grade *D* will be 0.6 to 1.8 and that of grade *E* will be 1.8 to 3. Similarly, the boundary points of the grades *B* and *A* would be −0.6 to −1.8 and −1.8 to −3, respectively.

From Table A.4, the area between $z = 0$ and $z = 0.6$ is 0.2257. Owing to the symmetrical nature of the curve, the area between $z = 0$ and $z = -0.6$ would also be 0.2257. Thus,

$$\text{Area of grade } C = 2 \times 0.2257 = 0.4514$$

From Table A.4, the area between $z = 0$ and $z = 1.8$ is 0.4641. The area of the grade D would be obtained by subtracting the area 0.2257 from 0.4641. Thus,

$$\text{Area of grade } D = 0.4641 - 0.2257 = 0.2384.$$

Owing to the symmetrical nature of the curve, the area of grade B will also be 0.2384.

From Table A.4, the area between $z = 0$ and $z = 3$ is 0.4987. The area of grade E would be obtained by subtracting the area 0.4641 from 0.4987. Thus,

$$\text{Area of grade } E = 0.4987 - 0.4641 = 0.0346.$$

Owing to the symmetrical nature of the curve, the area of grade A will also be 0.0346.

Since 1 is taken as the area under the normal curve, 3.46% of the students would secure grades A and E, 23.84% of the students would secure grades B and D, whereas 45.14% of the students would secure grade C.

Example 5.18 In a psychological test, it is required to grade an individual on any one of the five categories, namely, Very Poor, Poor, Average, Good, and Very Good. If the scores are normally distributed with mean 32 and standard deviation 6, find the limits of each grade.

Solution: Owing to the symmetrical nature of the normal distribution, two of the grades Very Poor and Poor shall be on the left side of the mean whereas the two other grades Good and Very Good shall be on the right side of the mean. The grade Average shall lie in the middle. Since 3σ limits cover 99.73% of the total cases, the width of the curve may be considered as 6 (the value of σ is 1).

Thus,

$$\text{Width of each grade} = \frac{6}{5} = 1.2$$

By taking the width of each grade to be 1.2, the normal curve can be divided into five grades as shown in the figure. Since the mean of z is 0, boundary points of the grade Average would be from -0.6 to 0.6. After adding 1.2, the boundary points of grade Good shall be 0.6 to 1.8 and that of grade Very Good shall be 1.8 to 3. Similarly, the boundary points of the grades Poor and Very Poor would be -0.6 to -1.8 and -1.8 to -3, respectively.

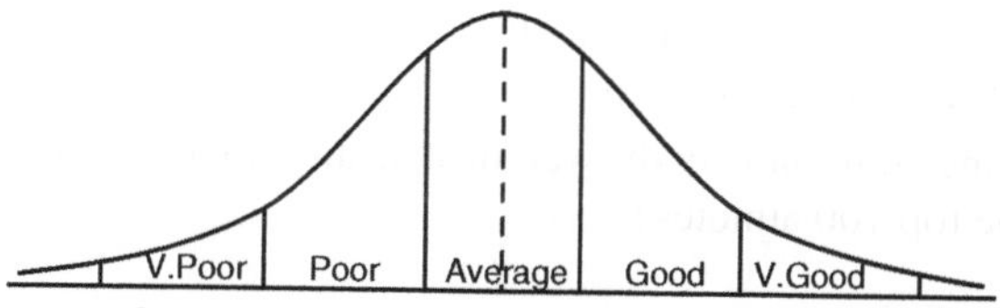

In order to find the limits of each grade, it is required to find the x-scores corresponding to each of the z-values. Computing the x-scores corresponding to z_1 and z_6 is optional if the researcher decides to keep the limits of the two extreme grades open. Therefore, the x-scores corresponding to z_1 and z_6 will not be computed in this problem.

Since

$$z = \frac{x - \mu}{\sigma}$$

$$\Rightarrow x = \mu + \sigma \times z$$

By using this formula, the x-scores corresponding to each of the z-values would be computed, given that the mean = 32 and SD = 6.

For $z_2 = -1.8$, $x_2 = 32 - 6 \times 1.8 = 32 - 10.8 = 21.2$
For $z_3 = -0.6$, $x_3 = 32 - 6 \times 0.6 = 32 - 3.6 = 28.4$
For $z_4 = 0.6$, $x_4 = 32 + 6 \times 0.6 = 32 + 3.6 = 35.6$
For $z_5 = 1.8$, $x_5 = 32 + 6 \times 1.8 = 32 + 10.8 = 42.8$

Thus, the limits of each grade for the marks in psychology would be as follows:

Grade	Score Limits
Very Poor	<21.2
Poor	21.2–28.4
Average	28.4–35.6
Good	35.6–42.8
Very Good	>42.8

Remark Since the score limits are continuous in nature, the upper limit is excluded from the class.

Example 5.19 The mean and standard deviation of the body weight obtained on 500 athletes are 122 and 8 lbs, respectively. Assuming that the distribution is normal, determine the following:

a. What is the minimum body weight that an athlete needs to be placed within the top 25% of the athletes in terms of the body weight?
b. What is the minimum body weight that an athlete needs to be positioned within the top 100 athletes?

Solution:

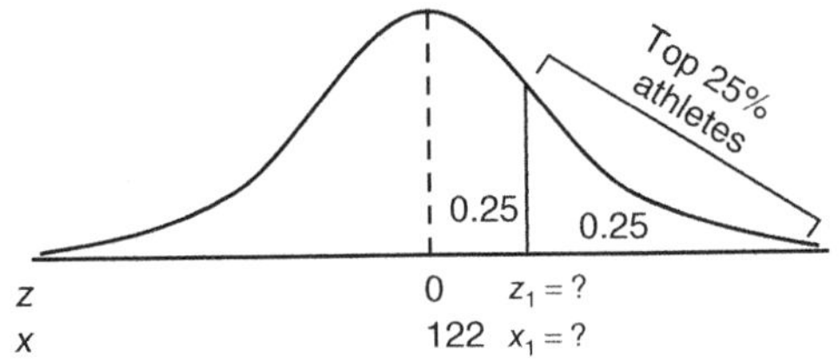

a. Since the area of the normal curve is 1, the top 25% of the athletes represents 0.25 area in the tail. The lower limit of this top 25% area is what is required to be computed. This lower limit is referred to as x_1. To find the value of x_1, first the value of z_1 corresponding to the area 0.25 needs to be located in the standard normal curve area table.

   From the normal curve area in Table A.4, the z-value corresponding to the area 0.2486 (closest value of 0.25 in the table) is 0.67.

$$\text{For } z_1 = 0.67, \qquad 0.67 = \frac{x_1 - \bar{x}}{s} = \frac{x_1 - 122}{8}$$

$$\Rightarrow x_1 = 122 + 8 \times 0.67 = 122 + 5.36 = 127.36$$

   Thus, an athlete needs more than 127.36 lb weight to be placed within the top 25% of the athletes in terms of body weight.

b. The top 100 athletes out of 500 refer to 0.2 area in the right tail of the normal curve. Thus, it is required to find the value of z_1 corresponding to the area 0.30 in the normal curve area table. The value of z_1 corresponding to 0.3 (0.2995 is the closest value in the table) in the table is equal to 0.84.

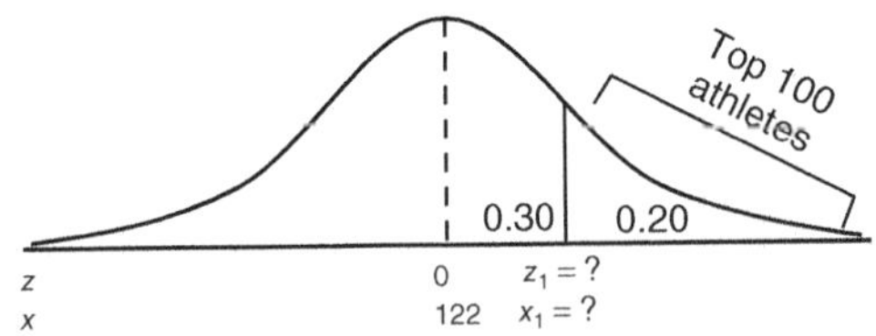

$$\text{For } z_1 = 0.84, \qquad 0.84 = \frac{x_1 - \bar{x}}{s} = \frac{x_1 - 122}{8}$$

$$\Rightarrow x_1 = 122 + 8 \times 0.84 = 122 + 6.72 = 128.72$$

   Thus, an athlete who has more than 128.72 lb body weight would be positioned within the top 100 athletes.

Check Your Progress

Note: Tick the correct answer by using the sign (√).

	True	False
37. A normal distribution is a discrete distribution.	-	-
38. The value of *e* is approximately 3.14159.	-	-
39. A normal distribution has parameters μ and σ^2.	-	-
40. For a symmetrical distribution, β_1 is 0.	-	-
41. In a standard normal distribution, the variance is 0 and mean is 1.	-	-
42. Two sigma limits in the normal distribution include 95% of the cases.	-	-
43. If *p* is 1/2 and the number of trials are infinite, then the binomial distribution approaches a normal distribution.	-	-
44. Points of inflexions are given by $\sigma \pm \mu$.	-	-
45. Skewness is considered to be significant if it is more than twice its SE.	-	-
46. In a leptokurtic curve, the dispersion of scores is more.	-	-
47. Standard score can be used in comparing the performance of an athlete in two different events having different units.	-	-
48. The value of π is approximately 3.14159.	-	-
49. A normal distribution is a single normal curve.	-	-
50. The quartile deviation of the normal distribution is 2/3.	-	-
51. Kurtosis (γ_2) for the normal distribution is 0.	-	-
52. The unit of standard score depends on the unit of data.	-	-
53. In a platykurtic curve, the scores are more dispersed than in the normal curve.	-	-
54. If significance value of the S–W test is more than 0.05, then the distribution of data is normal.	-	-
55. Whatever be the distribution of population, the distribution of sample mean in a large sample is always normally distributed.	-	-

PRACTICE EXERCISE

7. If x is normally distributed with the mean and standard deviation of 12 and 3, respectively, find the standard score of the following set of data.

x:	18	10	15	10	8	9	12

8. Find the probability for the area of the normal distribution described.
   a. $z \geq 2.58$
   b. $z < 0.53$
9. Let the shuttle run performance be denoted by X and have a normal distribution with mean 10.8 s and standard deviation 0.4 s. What is the value of k such that $P(X \geq k) = 0.95$?
10. If 50-yard dash performance of the volleyball players has a normal distribution with mean 7 s and standard deviation 0.3 s, find the probability that a randomly selected subject has a 50-yard dash performance between 6.5 and 7.4 s.
11. If the resting heart rate per minute is normally distributed with mean 62 and standard deviation 2, compute the heart rate limits that include the middle 50% cases.
12. Find the following probability where the variable x is normally distributed. $P(10 \leq x \leq 15)$, $\mu = 12$, $\sigma = 1.3$.

5.13 USES OF NORMAL DISTRIBUTION

Normal distribution is the basis of most of the statistical tests used in testing of hypotheses, especially when the sample is large. It has a wide range of applications in estimating the parameters of the population on the basis of sample information. In addition to this, many other applications in exercise science and health use the concepts of normal distribution. Some of them are listed below.

1. Most of the human traits such as height, weight, and blood pressure are normally distributed, and therefore to develop norms for these human traits various standard scales such as t, z and Stanine can be used. All these scales are based on the principle of normal distribution.
2. In developing standards and grading system for different fitness parameters such as speed, endurance, agility, and sit-ups, the principle of normal distribution is used.
3. Normal distribution can be used in estimating future events. For example, if the mean and standard deviation of the students appearing for an entrance examination are known, one can estimate what the probability would be that

the next year the number of students appearing for the test would be more than a specified number.

4. Normal distribution is used in testing various hypotheses concerning the mean, variance, and correlation coefficient of the population.
5. The test statistic based on normal distribution is used in comparing the means of the two populations when population variances are known.
6. Normal distribution is used in testing the significance of the difference between two population proportions.
7. In nonparametric data where the sample is large, the test statistic in most of the tests is normally distributed, which is used to test the null hypothesis.

5.14 COMPUTING WITH EXCEL

5.14.1 Finding the Probability

Excel can be used to compute the probability of any event if the mean and standard deviation are given and the distribution of the data is known. Here, problems based on binomial and Poisson distributions shall be discussed. Problems based on normal distribution have already been discussed in Chapter 4.

Remark The probabilities discussed below can only be computed if the Add-Ins "Analysis ToolPak" is already installed in your Excel. The readers can install this Add-Ins "Analysis ToolPak" in their Excel by following the procedure mentioned in Chapter 1.

Example 5.20 In a college, 15% students are smokers. Suppose 20 students have been randomly selected from the college. Find the following:

1. The probability that the sample includes 4 or fewer smokers
2. The probability that the sample includes 2 or more smokers

Solution: Given that $p =$ probability that the student is a smoker $= 0.15$ and $n = 20$.

1. To solve the two required probabilities, **BINOMDIST** function of Excel shall be used. Click the following commands in sequence in an Excel and you will get the screen as shown in Figure 5.11.

   Formulas → Insert Function → Statistical → BINOMDIST

2. After clicking the OK button as in Figure 5.11, you will get the screen as shown in Figure 5.12 where you can write other parameters to get the required probability.
3. In this example, it is required to find the probability $P(X \leq 4)$. To find this probability, fill the entries in the screen in Figure 5.12 as shown below:
   i. **Number_s** = 4 (This is the value of X.)

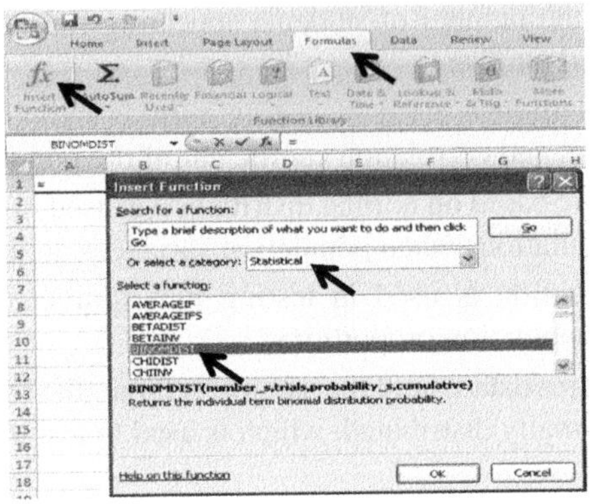

Figure 5.11 Command sequence for using the binomial distribution function.

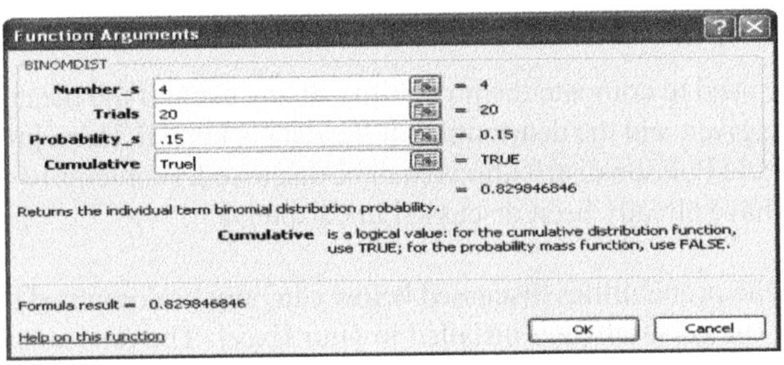

Figure 5.12 Options for finding cumulative distribution function $P(X \leq 4)$.

ii. **Trials** = 20 (This refers to the sample size, $n = 20$.)
iii. **Probability_s** = 0.15 (This refers to the probability of the event occurring in a single trial. Here, the probability (p) that the student is a smoker is 0.15.)
iv. **Cumulative** = True (This gives you the required probability.)
v. Click **OK** to get the output as shown in step 4.

4. $P(X \leq 4) = 0.829846846$. Thus, the probability that the sample includes 4 or fewer smokers is approximately 0.83.
5. To know the probability that the sample includes 2 or more smokers, it is required to calculate the probability $P(X \geq 2)$.

   Since $P(X \geq 2) = 1 - P(X \leq 1)$, $P(X \leq 1)$ can be computed similarly as shown in Figure 5.12. Taking $X = 1$, the Excel will give $P(X \leq 1) = 0.175557876$ as shown in Figure 5.13.

   Thus,

$$P(X \geq 2) = 1 - P(X < 1) = 1 - 0.175557876 = 0.824442124$$

Thus, the probability that the sample of 20 randomly selected students would include 2 or more smokers is approximately 0.82.

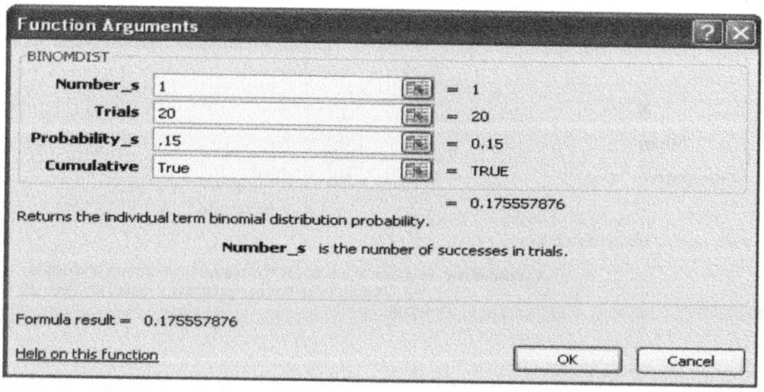

Figure 5.13 Options for finding the cumulative distribution function $P(X \leq 1)$.

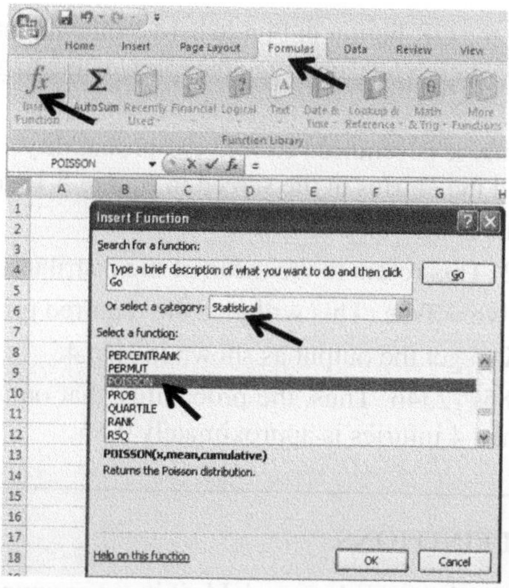

Figure 5.14 Command sequence for using the Poisson distribution function.

Example 5.21 The number of injuries in the interuniversity basketball championship follows a Poisson distribution with a mean of 2 injuries per day. Find the probability that on a particular day, there will be less than 4 injuries.

Solution: Given that mean $(\lambda) = 2$, it is required to find $P(x \leq 3)$.

1. To find the required probability, **POISSON** function of Excel shall be used. Click the following commands in sequence in Excel and you will get the screen as shown in Figure 5.14.

   Formulas → Insert Function → Statistical → POISSON

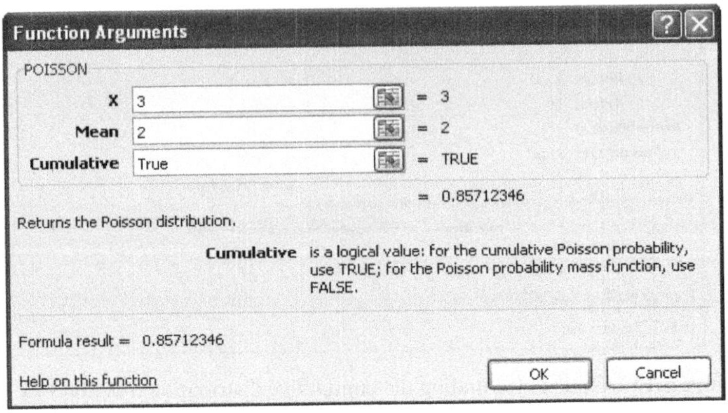

Figure 5.15 Options for finding the cumulative distribution function.

2. After clicking the OK button in Figure 5.14, you will get the screen as shown in Figure 5.15 where you can write other parameters to get the required probability.
3. In this example, it is required to find the probability $P(X \leq 3)$. To find this probability, fill the entries in the screen in Figure 5.15 as shown below:
   i. $\boldsymbol{X} = 3$ (This is the value of X.)
   ii. **Mean** = 2 (This refers to the mean of the distribution, $\lambda = 2$.)
   iii. **Cumulative** = True (This will give the required probability.)
   iv. Click **OK** to get the output as shown in step 4.
4. $P(X \leq 3) = 0.85712346$. Thus, the probability that on a particular day there will be less than 4 injuries is approximately 0.86.

IMPORTANT DEFINITIONS

A variable x is said to be a ***random variable*** if it can assume all possible numerical outcomes of a random phenomenon.
A random variable is said to be a ***discrete random variable*** if it can assume only a countable number of distinct values such as 0, 1, 2, 3, and so on.
A random variable is said to be a ***continuous random variable*** if it can assume an infinite number of possible values.
A ***probability distribution function*** is a real-valued function that provides the probability to each and every outcome of a random variable in an experiment.
The ***probability density function*** can be defined as a function that can be integrated to obtain the probability that the random variable can have values in a given interval.
An experiment of n repeated trials is said to be a ***binomial experiment*** if each trial results in only two outcomes and the probability of success is the same in each trial, whereas all the trials are independent of each other.

The ***expectation*** of any random variable is its aggregate value and is the same as the mean.
The distribution of probabilities associated with the outcomes of a discrete random variable in a statistical experiment is known as a ***discrete distribution***.
A ***continuous distribution*** can be defined as the probability model that is used to describe variables that are continuous in nature.
A ***normal curve*** is a bilaterally symmetrical curve with maximum concentration of scores at the center, following a particular probability law.
The ***standard score*** indicates by how many standard deviations a score is above or below the mean.
The ***expected value*** of a discrete random variable is the weighted mean of all possible outcomes in which the weights are the respective probabilities of those outcomes.
A ***binomial distribution*** can be defined as the probability function defined by $P(x) = {}^nC_x p^x q^{n-x}$, where x is the number of successes in a given set of independent Bernoulli trials.
A ***Poisson distribution*** can be defined as the probability function given by $P(x) = \frac{e^{-\lambda}\lambda^x}{x!}$, where x is the number of rare events in a specific time interval.
A ***normal distribution*** can be defined as the probability function given by $P(x) = \frac{1}{\sigma\sqrt{2\pi}} e^{\frac{(x-\mu)^2}{2\sigma^2}}$, where x is a continuous variable that lies between $-\infty$ and ∞ and μ and σ^2 are the mean and variance of the variable x.

IMPORTANT FORMULAS

For discrete distribution

$$\text{Mean} = E(x) = \sum x.p(x)$$

$$\text{Variance} = \sigma^2 = E(x-\mu)^2$$
$$= E(x^2) - (E(x))^2$$

For continuous distribution

$$\text{Mean} = E(x) = \int_{-\infty}^{\infty} x \cdot f(x)dx$$

$$\text{Variance} = \sigma^2 = E(x-\mu)^2$$

$$= \int_{-\infty}^{\infty} (x-\mu)^2 \cdot f(x)dx$$

For binomial distribution

$$P(x) = {}^{n}C_{x}p^{x}q^{n-x}, \quad x = 0, 1, 2, \ldots, n, \quad q = 1 - p$$

$$\text{Mean} = \mu = np$$

$$\text{Variance} = \sigma^2 = npq$$

$$\text{SD} = \sigma = \sqrt{npq}$$

For Poisson distribution

$$P(x) = \frac{e^{-\lambda}\lambda^x}{x!}$$

$$x = 0, 1, 2, \ldots$$

$$\text{Mean} = \mu = \lambda$$

$$\text{Variance} = \sigma^2 = \lambda$$

For normal distribution

$$p(x) = \frac{1}{\sigma\sqrt{2\pi}}e^{\frac{(x-\mu)^2}{2\sigma^2}}, \quad -\infty \leq x \leq \infty, \quad -\infty \leq \mu \leq \infty, \quad \sigma \geq 0$$

For standard normal distribution

$$p(z) = \frac{1}{\sqrt{2\pi}}e^{-\frac{1}{2}z^2}$$

Standard score

$$z = \frac{x - \mu}{\sigma}$$

Skewness

$$\beta_1 = \frac{\mu_3^2}{\mu_2^3}$$

rth central moment

$$\mu_r = \frac{1}{n}\sum (X - \overline{X})^r$$

Standard error (SE) of skewness

$$\text{SE}(\beta_1) = \sqrt{\frac{6n(n-1)}{(n-2)(n+1)(n+3)}}$$

Kurtosis

$$\gamma_2 = \beta_2 - 1$$

$$\beta_2 = \frac{\mu_4}{\mu_2^2}$$

Standard error (SE) of kurtosis

$$SE(\gamma_2) = 2 \times SE(\beta_1) \times \sqrt{\frac{n^2 - 1}{(n-3)(n+5)}}$$

KEY TERMS

binomial distribution function
central limit theorem
continuous distribution
discrete distribution
distribution function
expectation
normal distribution
poisson distribution
probability
probability density
random variable
testing normality

CHAPTER EXERCISE

1. Write short notes on the following:
   a. Random variable
   b. Probability distribution function
   c. Probability density function
   d. Expectation
2. Define a normal distribution and explain its properties.
3. Write a short note on standard score.
4. Write short notes on skewness and kurtosis.
5. How will you test the normality of data?
6. The following table shows the data of a study on the number of fouls committed by the teams in a basketball tournament. On the basis of the following data and its associated probabilities, compute the expected number of fouls and the standard deviation of the fouls.

Fouls (x)	Probability $p(x)$
0	0.05
1	0.22
2	0.15
3	0.25
4	0.33

7. Compute the mean, standard deviation, and variance of the following discrete distribution in a coin-tossing experiment.

Number of Heads $s(x)$	$p(x)$
0	0.05
1	0.10
2	0.20
3	0.30
4	0.20
5	0.10
6	0.05

8. Find the following probabilities by using the binomial table.
   i. $P(x \geq 16)$, if $n = 20$ and $p = 0.6$
   ii. $P(12 \leq x \leq 15)$, if $n = 17$ and $p = 0.8$
9. Solve the following problems, given that the variable x follows a binomial distribution.
   i. If $n = 4$, $p = 1/2$, find $P(x = 2)$
   ii. If $n = 6$, $p = 0.3$, find $P(x = 4)$
   iii. If $n = 7$, $p = 1/2$, find $P(2 < x < 5)$
10. Find the mean and variance of the binomial distribution in the following cases.
   i. $n = 25$ and $p = 0.8$
   ii. $n = 30$ and $q = 0.4$
   iii. $n = 200$ and $p = 0.65$
11. In a college 50% of the students are smokers. If a random sample of 8 students are selected, find the probabilities of the following cases.
   i. exactly 3 students are smokers
   ii. more than 5 students are smokers
12. Find the following probabilities by using the Poisson distribution.
   i. $P(x = 3/\lambda = 2)$
   ii. $P(x \leq 4/\lambda = 3)$
   iii. $P(3 \leq x < 5/\lambda = 2)$
13. In a match practice class of cricket, the probability that a cricketer will get injured and require physiotherapy treatment is 0.02. If a random sample of 100 cricketers playing in a match practice class is selected, what is the probability that exactly 2 of them will get an injury?
14. Find the following probabilities by using the Poisson distribution.
   i. $P(x = 4)$, given that $\lambda = 3$
   ii. $P(x > 3)$, given that $\lambda = 3.6$

15. Find the following probabilities by using the Poisson distribution.
    i. $P(x \leq 5)$, given that $\lambda = 6$
    ii. $P(X \geq 5)$, given that $\lambda = 4.8$
16. The placement cell of an institute shows that 5% of all the enrolled students remain unemployed in a year. If a random sample of 15 enrolled students is drawn, what is the probability that 2 or less would be unemployed?
17. The number of disciplinary cases reported to the proctorial committee in a college during a month follows a Poisson distribution with a mean of 5. Find the probability that less than 3 disciplinary cases will be reported during a randomly selected month.
18. The number of hits on a website occurs at the rate of 5 per day. What is the probability that there will be more than 6 hits on the website on a randomly selected day?
19. If the distribution of x is normal with the mean and standard deviation as 24 and 4, respectively, find the standard score of the following set of data.

x:	15	23	35	31	18	36	21	26

20. If the mean and standard deviation of a normally distributed variable are 5.8 and 0.2, respectively, then what would be the score values for the following standard scores?

z:	−2.1	1.6	1.8	−1.1	−2.9	1.7	0.8	−0.2

21. If the mean and standard deviation for the data on leg length of athletes in a college are 3.7 and 0.05 ft, respectively, then determine the z-scores for the following measurements obtained on leg length of the 5 athletes selected for the university team.

Leg length (in ft.):	3.62	3.75	3.68	3.71	3.69	3.77	3.74

22. The mean and standard deviation for the data on height of a group of athletes are 190 and 2 cm, respectively. Compute the raw scores of height if the data of the athletes are given in the form of the following z-scores:

Height (z-score):	2.2	1.75	−1.3	0.5	−1.8	−1.5	2.5

23. Find the probability for the area of the normal distribution described below.
    i. $-1.63 < z \leq 2.25$
    ii. $0.84 < z \leq 1.65$
    iii. $-2.5 < z \leq -1.1$

24. Find the following probabilities where the variable x is normally distributed.
    i. $x \leq 36$, $\mu = 32$, $\sigma = 4.5$
    ii. $x > 125$, $\mu = 110$, $\sigma = 25$
25. The average weight of a group of persons is 132 lb and the standard deviation is 8 lb. Given that the weight is normally distributed, determine the following.
    i. What percentage of persons would fall above 138 lb?
    ii. What percentage of persons would fall below 122 lb?
    iii. What percentage of persons would fall above 129 lb?
    iv. What percentage of persons would fall below 145 lb?
    v. What percentage of people would fall between 120 and 146 lb?
    vi. What percentage of people would fall between 122 and 130 lb?
    vii. What percentage of people would fall between 136 and 148 lb?
26. If push-ups is normally distributed with mean 25 and standard deviation 3, compute push-ups limits that include the middle 60% of the total score.
27. If grading developed for assessing an individual's health-related fitness is based on normally distributed data, what percentage of subjects would fall in each of the six grades: Very Poor, Poor, Satisfactory, Good, Very Good, and Excellent?
28. If the mean and standard deviation for the normally distributed IQ scores are 75 and 15, respectively, and it is desired to develop a grading criterion to grade an individual's IQ, what would be the limits for each of the five grades: Very Poor, Poor, Satisfactory, Good, and Very Good?
29. Vital capacity is normally distributed with mean 4.01 and standard deviation 0.31. If an individual is required to be graded in any of the five categories, Very Poor, Poor, Satisfactory, Good, and Very Good, what would be the limits of each grade?
30. If the mean body weight of the volleyball players is 175 lb and the median and standard deviation are 162 and 22 lb, respectively, what would you say about the skewness of the data? Interpret your findings.
31. If the lean body weights of a group of persons are normally distributed with the mean and standard deviation as 148 and 5 lbs, respectively, find the following.
    i. Percentage of persons having lean body weight above 150
    ii. Percentage of persons having lean body weight below 139
    iii. Percentage of persons having lean body weight above 141
    iv. Percentage of persons having lean body weight below 159
    v. Percentage of persons having lean body weight between 144 and 152
    vi. Percentage of persons having lean body weight between 135 and 142
    vii. Percentage of persons having lean body weight between 151 and 160

32. If the performance on a vertical jump measured on 100 subjects is considered to be normally distributed with mean 35 cm and standard deviation 3 cm, find the number of subjects whose performance is
    i. between 35 and 39 cm
    ii. between 30 and 35 cm
    iii. more than 36 cm
    iv. more than 38 cm
    v. less than 30 cm
    vi. less than 37 cm
    vii. between 29 and 42 cm
    viii. between 37 and 43 cm
33. Given that leg length of a group of people is normally distributed with mean 95 cm and standard deviation 3 cm, determine the following.
    i. limits of leg length that include the middle 60% of the scores
    ii. limits of leg length that include the middle 70% of the scores
34. Find the number k such that the standard random variable z has probability 0.99 that $z \leq k$.
35. If an individual is graded in one of the seven categories on the basis of 100 m performance, and if the grading is normally distributed, what percentage of subjects would be attached to each of the seven grades: Very Poor, Poor, Satisfactory, Average, Good, Very Good, and Excellent?
36. The push-ups performance measured on school students is normally distributed with $\mu = 22$ and $\sigma = 5$. Find the range of scores that can be used to determine the grades "Very Good," "Good," "Average," "Satisfactory," and "Poor," given that the grades are normally distributed. What are the grades corresponding to the actual scores 34, 12, 28, 19, and 23 obtained by the five students?
37. The mean and standard deviation for normally distributed body weight scores are 125 and 5 lb, respectively. What would be the limits for each of the five grades, Very Poor, Poor, Satisfactory, Good, and Very Good, if an individual needs to be graded in any of these five grades?
38. The mean and standard deviation of the marks obtained in mathematics by the students of class 12 are 75 and 10, respectively. Assuming normality of the distribution find the following
    i. percentage of students having marks more than 82
    ii. percentage of students having marks more than 70.
39. On the basis of scores obtained on a test, the students need to be divided into any of the three categories A, B, and C. If these categories are based on the assumption of normality, what percentage of students would be included in each of the three categories?

40. The mean and standard deviation of the scores obtained on leg length of soccer players are 98 and 3 cm, respectively. Assuming that the distribution of scores is normal, what limit will include the middle 65% of the area?
41. Given a distribution with mean 30 and standard deviation 5, assuming normality, what limits will include the highest 10% and lowest 20% of the distribution?
42. In an examination conducted for scholarships, 800 candidates participated, yielding a result that follows normal distribution with a mean of 65 marks and standard deviation of 10 marks. Calculate the following:
    i. What minimum score does a student need to be placed within the top 25% of the candidates in this test?
    ii. What minimum score does a student need to be positioned within the top 100 students?
43. The mean timing on 4×10 m shuttle run of the athletes is 10.5 s and the standard deviation is 0.3 s. The top 10% of the athletes needs to be selected for advanced training. Assuming that the timings are distributed normally, what is the minimum timing an athlete must get for inclusion in the advanced training program?
44. If the scores on statistics for a class is normally distributed with mean 62 and standard deviation 8, then what is the probability of obtaining a score greater than 74?
45. If the weight of a group of athletes is normally distributed with the mean and standard deviation as 135 and 10 lb, respectively, what is the probability of randomly choosing an athlete whose weight is between 131 and 142 lbs?

ANSWERS

Check Your Progress

1. F	7. F	13. F	19. T	25. F	31. T	37. F	43. T	49. F	55. T
2. T	8. F	14. T	20. T	26. T	32. F	38. F	44. F	50. T	
3. T	9. T	15. F	21. F	27. F	33. T	39. T	45. T	51. T	
4. F	10. F	16. T	22. T	28. T	34. F	40. T	46. F	52. F	
5. T	11. T	17. F	23. T	29. F	35. F	41. F	47. T	53. T	
6. F	12. T	18. T	24. F	30. T	36. T	42. F	48. T	54. T	

Practice Exercise

1. Mean = 2.75 and SD = 1.09
2. Mean = 12.6 and SD = 1.94
3. a. 0.279, b. 0.641
4. 0.298

5. a. 0.1125, b. 0.4062
6. a. 0.7360, b. 0.9155
7. z: 2, −0.67, 1, −0.67, −1.33, −1, 0
8. a. 0.0049, b. 0.7019
9. $k = 10.14$
10. 0.8607
11. 61–63
12. 0.9278

Chapter Exercise

6. $M(x) = 2.59$, $V(x) = 1.64$
7. $M(x) = 3$, $V(x) = 2.10$, $SD(x) = 1.45$
8. i. 0.051, ii. 0.7761
9. i. 0.375, ii. 0.06, iii. 0.546
10. i. $M(x) = 20$, $V(x) = 4$; ii. $M(x) = 18$, $V(x) = 7.2$; iii. $M(x) = 130$, $V(x) = 45.5$
11. i. 0.219, ii. 0.145
12. i. 0.1804, ii. 0.815, iii. 0.270
13. 0.2706
14. i. 0.168, ii. 0.485
15. i. 0.446, ii. 0.524
16. 0.02
17. 0.125
18. 0.238
19.

x:	15	23	35	31	18	36	21	26
z:	−2.25	−0.25	2.75	1.75	−1.5	3	−0.75	0.5

20.

z:	−2.1	1.6	1.8	−1.1	−2.9	1.7	0.8	−0.2
x:	5.38	6.12	6.16	5.58	5.22	6.14	5.96	5.76

21.

Leg length (x):	3.62	3.75	3.68	3.71	3.69	3.77	3.74
z:	−1.6	1	−0.4	0.2	−0.2	1.4	0.8

22.

Height (z-score):	2.2	1.75	−1.3	0.5	−1.8	−1.5	2.5
x:	194.4	193.5	187.4	191	186.4	187	195

23. i. 0.9362, ii. 0.1510, iii. 0.1295
24. i. 0.8130, ii. 0.2743

25. i. 22.66%, ii. 10.56%, iii. 64.62%, iv. 94.79%, v. 89.31%, vi. 29.57%, vii. 28.58%
26. 22.48 to 27.52
27. Very Poor and Excellent = 2.15%
    Poor and Very Good = 13.59%
    Satisfactory and Good = 34.13%
28.

Very Poor:	<48
Poor:	48–66
Satisfactory:	66–84
Good:	84–102
Very Good:	≥102

29.

Very Poor:	<3.46
Poor:	3.46–3.82
Satisfactory:	3.82–4.18
Good:	4.18–4.54
Very Good:	≥4.54

30. The curve is positively skewed and more number of scores are less than the mean scores.
31. i. 34.5%, ii. 3.59%, iii. 91.92%, iv. 98.61%, v. 57.62%, vi. 11.04%, vii. 26.61%
32. i. 41, ii. 45, iii. 37, iv. 34, v. 5, vi. 75, vii. 97, viii. 25
33. i. 92.48 to 97.52, ii. 91.88 to 98.12
34. $k = 2.35$
35. Very Poor and Excellent = 1.45%
    Poor and Very Good = 8.27%
    Satisfactory and Good = 23.51%
    Average = 33.28%
36.

Poor:	<13
Satisfactory:	13–19
Average:	19–25
Good:	25–31
Very Good:	≥31

37.

Very Poor:	<116
Poor:	116–122
Satisfactory:	122–128
Good:	128–134
Very Good:	≥134

38. i. 24.2%, ii. 69.15%
39. A: 15.8%, B: 68.26%, C: 15.8%
40. 95.21 cm to 100.79 cm
41. Limit of highest 10% score is 36.4
    Limit of lowest 20% score is 25.80
42. i. 71.75, ii. 76.5
43. 10.12
44. 0.0668
45. 0.4134

FURTHER READING

1. "Statistics | The Poisson Distribution". Umass.edu. Aug 24. Retrieved 2012 April 05; 2007.
2. Agresti A, Coull BA. Approximate is better than 'exact' for interval estimation of binomial proportions. The American Statistician 1998;52:119–126.
3. Shun-ichi A, Hiroshi N. Methods of Information Geometry. USA: American Mathematical Society 2000. ISBN: 978-0-8218-0531-2
4. Bernardo JM, Smith AFM. Bayesian Theory. UK: Wiley; 2000. ISBN 0-471-49464-X.
5. Box, George P, Hunter, William G, Hunter J, Stuart. Statistics for experimenters : an introduction to design, data analysis, and model building. USA: John Wiley & Sons; 1978. ISBN: 978-0-471-09315-2
6. Brown LD, Cai T, DasGupta A. Interval estimation for a binomial proportion (with discussion). Statistical Science, USA 2001;16:101–133.
7. Bryc W. The Normal Distribution: Characterizations with Applications. USA: Springer-Verlag; 1995. ISBN 0-387-97990-5.
8. Casella G, Berger RL. Statistical Inference. 2nd ed. Duxbury: BROOKS/COLE 2001. ISBN 0-534-24312-6.
9. David S. Elementary Probability. UK: Cambridge University Press 2003. ISBN: 0521534283
10. Gullberg J. Mathematics from the Birth of Numbers. New York: W. W. Norton; 1997. p 963–965ISBN 0-393-04002-X.
11. Halperin M, Hartley HO, Hoel PG. Recommended standards for statistical symbols and notation. COPSS Committee on Symbols and Notation. The American Statistician 1965;19(3):12–14. DOI: 10.2307/2681417. JSTOR 2681417.
12. Hamilton Institute. "The Binomial Distribution" October 20. 2010.
13. Hamza K. The smallest uniform upper bound on the distance between the mean and the median of the binomial and Poisson distributions. Statistics & Probability Letters 1995;23:21–25. DOI: 10.1016/0167-7152(94)00090-U. edit.
14. Hazewinkel M, editor. Normal Distribution. Encyclopedia of Mathematics: Springer; 2001. ISBN 978-1-55608-010-4.

15. Herrnstein RJ, Murray C. The Bell Curve: Intelligence and Class Structure in American Life. USA: Free Press; 1994. ISBN 0-02-914673-9.

16. Johnson NL, Kotz S, Kemp AW. Univariate Discrete distributions. 2nd ed. USA: Wiley. ISBN 0-471-54897-9; 1993. p 153.

17. Johnson NL, Kotz S, Balakrishnan N. Continuous Univariate DistributionsVolume 1. USA: Wiley; 1994. ISBN 0-471-58495-9.

18. Kaas R, Buhrman JM. Mean, median and mode in binomial distributions. Statistica Neerlandica 1980;34(1):13–18. DOI: 10.1111/j.1467-9574.1980.tb00681.x.

19. Kinderman AJ, Monahan JF. Computer generation of random variables using the ratio of uniform deviates. ACM Transactions on Mathematical Software 1977;3: 257–260.

20. Krishnamoorthy K. Handbook of Statistical Distributions with Applications. USA: Chapman & Hall/CRC; 2006. ISBN 1-58488-635-8.

21. Kruskal WH, Stigler SM. In: Spencer BD, editor. Normative Terminology: 'Normal' in Statistics and Elsewhere. Statistics and Public Policy. USA: Oxford University Press; 1997. ISBN 0-19-852341-6.

22. Laha RG, Rohatgi VK. Probability Theory. New York: John Wiley & Sons; 1989. p 233 ISBN 0-471-03262-X.

23. Le CL, Lo YG. Asymptotics in Statistics: Some Basic Concepts. 2nd ed. USA: Springer; 2000. ISBN 0-387-95036-2.

24. Lord N. Binomial averages when the mean is an integer. The Mathematical Gazette 2010;94:331–332.

25. Lukacs E, King EP. A Property of Normal Distribution. The Annals of Mathematical Statistics 1954;25(2):389–394. DOI: 10.1214/aoms/1177728796. JSTOR 2236741.

26. Marsaglia G. Evaluating the Normal Distribution. Journal of Statistical Software 2004;11(4).

27. McPherson G. Statistics in Scientific Investigation: Its Basis, Application and Interpretation. USA: Springer-Verlag; 1990. ISBN 0-387-97137-8.

28. Patel JK, Read CB. Handbook of the Normal Distribution. 2nd ed. USA: CRC Press; 1996. ISBN 0-8247-9342-0.

29. Rank AH. Handbook of the Poisson Distribution. New York: John Wiley & Sons, Ltd.; 1967.

30. Ross SM. Introduction to Probability Models. 9th ed. Boston: Academic Press. ISBN 978-0-12-598062-3; 2007. p 307–308.

31. Stigler SM. Mathematical Statistics in the Early States. The Annals of Statistics 1978;6(2):239–265. DOI: 10.1214/aos/1176344123. JSTOR 2958876.

32. Stigler SM. A modest proposal: a new standard for the normal. The American Statistician 1982;36(2):137–138. DOI: 10.2307/2684031. JSTOR 2684031.

33. Stigler SM. The History of Statistics: The Measurement of Uncertainty before 1900. USA: Harvard University Press; 1986. ISBN 0-674-40340-1.

34. Walker HM. De Moivre on the Law of Normal Probability. In: Smith DE, editor. A Source Book in Mathematics. New York: Dover; 1985. ISBN 0-486-64690-4.

35. Wilson EB. Probable inference, the law of succession, and statistical inference. Journal of the American Statistical Association 1927;22:209–212.

36. Zelen M, Severo NC. Probability Functions (chapter 26). Handbook of Mathematical Functions with Formulas, Graphs, and Mathematical Tables, by Abramowitz, M; and Stegun, IA.: National Bureau of Standards. New York: Dover; 1964. ISBN 0-486-61272-4.

6

SAMPLING AND SAMPLING DISTRIBUTION

6.1 INTRODUCTION

Decision-making is part and parcel of our daily life. We form an opinion about a person on the basis of a brief conversation, understand the popularity of a sport by interviewing a few persons, or buy a shuttlecock by inspecting a few pieces. In such situations, we try to assess the characteristics of the whole lot on the basis of a small section. Consider a study in which a researcher wishes to investigate whether most of the students in a college possess minimal muscular fitness. To address this issue, a random sample of students might be selected and tested for their muscular fitness. On the basis of the data obtained, one can draw a larger picture about the status of muscular fitness of the college students. In this study, there are two specific issues – firstly, whether the results would be more accurate if the entire lot of students in the college were tested; secondly, how far the conclusion drawn on a few randomly selected students would be valid. Let us investigate the first issue where the entire student body is tested. In this case, one might feel that the results would be more accurate because all the students are tested; but the scenario is just the reverse. In testing the whole lot it is possible that some students might not participate, and further it is difficult to have error-free measurements because of the large number of subjects. Thus, the results obtained would be far from accurate. In the second situation where a small number of randomly selected students are tested, there is greater likelihood that the conclusion drawn may not be accurate

Statistics for Exercise Science and Health with Microsoft® Office Excel®, First Edition. J. P. Verma.

because the result is based on a small number of students. This problem, however, can be tackled by drawing a representative sample of the students using a proper sampling technique. Further, because of the small number of subjects, it is easy to motivate them to perform the test. Thus, if we compare the trade-off, the findings drawn from the small representative set of students are much more accurate than the findings obtained from the whole lot of college students. In this chapter, a detailed discussion is given on how to draw a representative sample, issues in sampling and census, different types of sampling techniques, sampling distributions, strategies in choosing the sample, and other related issues of sampling.

6.2 POPULATION AND SAMPLE

In statistics, population refers to the collection of all the elements or entities under study. The elements could be the athletes participating at the national level, students opting for basketball, persons working as sports scientists in a country, and so on. The population can be defined as male or female teachers of exercise science in all the schools of a given state, all the high school children of a school, or the coaches in a particular discipline. All these examples consist of groups of individuals. Populations may also be defined as families, schools, colleges, and universities. Thus, the meaning of population changes from study to study. The first step in conducting any analytical study is to define the population correctly.

A sample is a subset of a population. Usually, a sample is drawn to investigate the population characteristics, and it is therefore essential that the sample should represent the population and possess similar characteristics as those of the population. If the sample drawn from the population is representative, only then can the findings drawn from it be generalized for the population. Random sampling is one of the main techniques of drawing a representative sample. There are many sampling techniques that can be used to draw a representative sample. Depending on the situation, a researcher may choose an appropriate sampling technique to draw a representative sample. Detailed discussions of all such techniques appear later in the chapter.

6.3 PARAMETER AND STATISTICS

Population characteristics can be assessed quantitatively or qualitatively. Quantitative characteristics of the population are measured by statistical constants that are known as parameters, whereas qualitative characteristics are measured by attributes.

> **FACTS TO KNOW**
>
> In general, a representative sample provides more accurate findings than a population

Quantitative characteristics shall be discussed in this chapter whereas the measurement of qualitative characteristics shall be discussed in Chapter 11, which deals with nonparametric techniques. A parameter can be defined as a statistical constant that is used to define the population characteristics in a quantitative manner. Some of the population parameters are μ, σ, and p, which refer to the mean, standard deviation, and proportion of the population, respectively.

Statistics is a function of sample observations that are used to define the characteristics of the sample. Some of the sample statistics are $\overline{\boldsymbol{x}}$, s, and $\widehat{\boldsymbol{p}}$, which are used to compute the mean, standard deviation, and proportion of the sample, respectively. Thus, *parameter* is a term used for a population characteristic, whereas *statistics* refers to the sample characteristics.

6.4 SAMPLING FRAME

Sampling frame is a list of all the population units from which the sample is drawn. The sampling frame may include individuals, teams, households, institutions, and so on. One needs to decide the sampling frame before starting the experiment. In fact, the population and the sampling frame are the same, but at times when the information regarding all the population units is not available, then the sampling frame is different from the population. If a survey about health status is conducted in the schools of Delhi, then the list of all the schools available with the administration will constitute the sampling frame. However, there may be some self-financing schools running in the suburbs whose information may not be available to the authorities; hence in this case, the sampling frame and the population may differ.

6.5 SAMPLING

Sampling is the procedure of drawing a sample from the population. The purpose of sampling is to draw inferences about the population characteristics on the basis of the sample. It is therefore important to draw a sample that is truly representative of the population. Different sampling techniques are used to draw a representative sample in different situations. Choosing a particular sampling technique depends on the nature of the population. Whatever the sampling technique chosen, the primary purpose is to obtain a representative sample. A researcher always resorts to sampling rather than studying the entire population. For instance, if the effect of circuit training on the improvement of basketball skills is to be studied on university basketball players, then the researcher will select a sample of those basketball players who have participated in university tournaments. The results obtained may be generalized for all the university basketball players. Whether studying the nutritional status of the women in a district, knowing the fitness status of school children, or the attitude of exercise scientists about competitive sports, in all such cases, a researcher always uses sampling to infer about population characteristics.

6.5.1 Advantages of Sampling

Studies conducted on a properly selected sample give more accurate findings than those conducted on the entire population. Researchers invariably use sampling because of its efficiency. There are several reasons why sampling is more advantageous than population studies.

Sampling is preferred because of its *low cost*. Since few population units are investigated in sampling, the cost involved in it is much lower than that of the population study. Fewer subjects means that lower number of field investigators and fewer resources are required for the study. This drastically reduces the cost of the sampling. Sampling is also preferred because it requires *less time*. Since fewer subjects are selected in sampling, the time involved in it is drastically reduced in comparison to a population study. As every research project needs to be completed in a limited time frame, time constraint is another reason for using sampling. Further, if a long time is taken to complete the study, it may lose its importance at times or the phenomenon under investigation may change during the course of the study. For instance, if a study is conducted to know the socioeconomic status of the people in a district and if many years are used on the pretext that the entire population will give the correct findings, the results may lose their purpose because of the delay; because of the long time involved in the study, the information obtained from the subjects at the beginning and end of the study may differ significantly, which may adversely affect the findings.

In sampling, *better control* can be achieved because the researcher can properly train the field investigators because of the smaller numbers. Because the number of subjects is small, the investigators can ensure reliability of data through cross-checks. One of the main problems in exercise science research is that the subjects need to be *properly motivated*; otherwise, it is difficult to get their optimum performance. In sampling, the subjects can be properly motivated to give their best performance by using extrinsic and intrinsic motivations. In fact, the investigator should keep a budget for motivating the respondents in their studies. As a goodwill gesture, the subjects may be offered a small gift, the cost of which may be included while planning the sample survey. The information obtained in sampling is much more *reliable* than that from the population study because the researcher can give personal attention during the data collection. Reliable data enhance accuracy in findings. Thus, if a proper sampling technique is used and a representative sample is drawn, then the conclusion drawn from the sample study is more efficient in comparison to the population study. In sampling, nonresponse error is less likely. *Nonresponse error* refers to the error due to nonparticipation of some of the subjects in the study. In sampling, it is easier to encourage maximum subject participation and there is, therefore, less dropout. To conclude, sampling is much more economical and less time consuming, and, at the same time, it gives more reliable information because of better control and better motivation of the subjects in the study.

Sampling provides reliable conclusions provided the sample obtained is truly representative of the population and no bias is involved in drawing the sample.

The results drawn from the sampling may not be accurate if the sampling frame is not properly defined or the population is not identified correctly.

6.6 CENSUS

> **FACTS TO KNOW**
>
> Probability sampling ensures external validity of findings, whereas nonprobability sampling lacks it

Census is the complete enumeration of a population. In census, the entire population units in the sampling frame are investigated. Because of the large size of the population, census studies take a long time to complete, and at the same time it is an expensive exercise. Census studies are also called population studies. The studies in which the entire population units are investigated require a large number of field investigators; therefore, it becomes difficult to control the functioning of these investigators resulting in loss of accuracy in collecting the information. In other words, population studies have less control, which affects the reliability of the findings. In population studies, nonresponse error is very high. It is because it is more likely that a particular section of the population may not cooperate with the field investigators.

Population studies seem to be more reliable because the information on all the population units is collected; the nonresponse error alone caused due to its reliability is drastically reduced. If a particular section of the population does not take part in the study, the results may be misleading.

However, in certain situations, census of the entire population is preferred provided there is sufficient time and finances available. In order to avoid a situation in which a sample does not truly represent the population, complete census may be preferred. For instance, in order to know the attitude of exercise scientists toward health and hygiene practices in a district, it is better to have the complete census of the population, provided there is no resource crunch. In such a situation, the sample may not truly represent the population because the subjects might have been selected as per the availability of teachers in the district. In addition to this, a census is also taken to protect the safety of an organization. For example, there are some products, such as sauna steam bath, whirlpool bath, blood analyzer, EMG machine, and so on, in which the functioning of these items is so critical to the organization that 100% of the articles are tested; and in such cases sampling is not a reasonable course of action.

6.7 PROBABILITY AND NONPROBABILITY SAMPLING

Samples can be drawn by using different sampling techniques. These techniques can be classified into probability and nonprobability sampling. The choice of probability and nonprobability sampling depends on the nature of the study. If used properly, probability sampling gives a representative sample. However, there are situations where probability sampling cannot be used for various reasons; therefore, in those conditions nonprobability sampling is the suitable option. There are a variety of probability and nonprobability sampling techniques available that are appropriate in different situations. A detailed discussion on these techniques is given in the following sections.

6.8 PROBABILITY SAMPLING

In probability sampling, every population unit has some known probability to be selected into the sample. In such sampling, a random selection method is used in drawing a sample from the sampling frame. In probability sampling, the procedure for drawing a sample is clearly defined, thus making it easy for the researcher to use it. Depending on the nature of the research problem, an appropriate probability sampling technique can be used to draw the representative sample. The results drawn by using probability sampling have more external validity. The following sampling techniques come under this category:

- Simple random sampling
- Stratified random sampling
- Systematic sampling
- Cluster sampling
- Multistage sampling

6.8.1 Simple Random Sampling

In simple random sampling, the sample is drawn from the population in such a way that every population unit has an equal chance of being included in the sample. This technique is suitable for a homogeneous population. For instance, in conducting a lifestyle study on college students belonging to higher socioeconomic status, the population may be considered to be homogeneous and simple random sampling can be used in drawing the sample. However, if the study is to be conducted on the entire group of male college students, then the population would be heterogeneous because in that situation the students belong to different socioeconomic statuses, resulting in heterogeneity in their lifestyle. In such a situation, simple random sampling may not be appropriate and the scholar may resort to some other techniques. A simple random sample can be drawn by using any of the three methods: lottery method, random number table method, and computer-generated method.

Lottery Method The lottery method is the most powerful and widely used method of drawing a simple random sample. In this method, all population units are numbered from 1 to N. This is known as a sampling frame. These numbers are written on small pieces of paper. These papers are placed in a bowl. All the pieces of paper must be of the same size; otherwise, the selected sample will not be truly random. After mixing thoroughly, a slip is drawn. After noting the number on the slip, it is replaced back into the bowl. The slips are again mixed in the bowl, and the next slip is selected. At some stage, if the slip drawn contains a previously selected number, then it is replaced into the bowl without any action. One keeps noting the slip numbers till the numbers noted are equal to the size of the sample. The population units bearing these numbers are selected as a sample for the study. The lottery method is useful in small population sizes.

Random Number Table Method A simple random sample can be drawn by using random number tables. These tables have been generated by many authors; however, the tables developed by the Tippet are mostly used by researchers. In Tippet's table, scores are arranged in rows and columns. To draw a simple random sample from a population, all the units of the population are numbered from 1 to N or 0 to $N-1$. Table 6.1 shows the cross section of the random number table. Let us see how this table can be used in drawing the sample. Let us suppose that the population consists of 80 subjects and it is required to draw a random sample of 12 subjects. The subjects in the population are numbered from 01 to 80.

The two-digit numbers are noted one after the other from Table 6.1. Any number above 80 is ignored because that number does not exist in the population. Further, if a number is repeated, then it is recorded only once. The population units bearing the selected numbers form the required sample. Twelve distinct numbers in pairs can be selected from the table starting from any row or column to draw a sample of size 12. Let us start from the first row in the table. The 12 random numbers would be 34, 66, 43, 44, 47, 74, 01, 54, 33, 70, 59, and 67. The two numbers 97 and 98 have not been recorded because the population does not contain these numbers. The numbers 33, 43, 47, and 74 have been observed more than once, and hence noted only once. The population units bearing these numbers will constitute the simple random sample.

TABLE 6.1 Cross-section View of the Random Number Table

3497	6643	4447	4798
7401	5433	3370	5974
4367	4574	3545	3346
9370	7483	3408	7767
5601	5946	3337	6907
7954	4943	3405	4075
7703	5956	3300	7643
3593	3084	6433	7943
6008	8376	4433	8776
7007	6933	8836	6446

In case the population consists of 100 units, they are numbered from 001 to 100, and one records the three-digit random numbers from the table. From the first row of the table, the random numbers are 349, 766, 434, 447, 479, 874, and 015 and so on. You can see that most of the numbers are above 100 except 015, and therefore much time is wasted in selecting the required sample. This problem can be overcome by numbering the population units from 00 to 99. In this way, only two-digit numbers will be recorded from the table and most of the numbers selected would form the required sample. Thus, if the population size N is 100, 1000, or 10,000, the population units should be numbered from 00 to 99, 000 to 999, or 0000 to 9999, respectively.

Computer-Generated Method A simple random sample can be drawn by generating the random numbers by a computer also. The random numbers can be generated by using different programs in the computer. For instance, the library function RND in BASIC language can be used to generate the random numbers. Similarly, in C language, the function RAND can be used to generate the random numbers. In generating random numbers by the computer, one faces a problem that on each run of the program, the numbers that are generated by the function are exactly the same, as it is dependent on the initial value called *seed*. Therefore, it is important to choose the initial value used by RAND function at program start-up in the C language, and this can be done by choosing another function called SRAND. Excel also provides the facility to draw a random sample. Toward the end of this chapter, a detailed procedure has been explained to draw a random sample using the Excel functionality.

Features of Simple Random Sampling In simple random sampling, prior knowledge of the population is not required, and the sample obtained is more representative provided the population is fairly homogeneous. A simple random sample is free from personal bias and sampling error can easily be calculated.

Simple random sampling is not suitable if the population is heterogeneous. In many situations, it is not possible to have a complete sampling frame. The selection of sample becomes difficult if the population units are widely dispersed.

6.8.2 Stratified Random Sampling

Stratified random sampling is suitable in a situation where the population is heterogeneous. In using this sampling, the whole population is divided into smaller homogeneous groups known as *strata*. A random sample is then drawn from each stratum in proportion to its size. The samples so drawn in each stratum are then pooled to form the stratified random sample. In using the stratified sampling, it is important to identify the criteria on which the population is divided into homogeneous strata. If proper stratification is not done or if the strata are not homogeneous within it, then the sample so obtained may not be a proper representative of the population.

Consider a situation in which the nutritional level of the girls in a school is to be studied. If the school has 1000 girls, one needs to divide the population into different homogeneous strata. Here, the stratification may be done on the basis of socioeconomic status because the nutritional level of the children depends on their family's socioeconomic status. On the other hand, if the stratification is done based on the age category or the locality from which they belong, then one may not get the representative sample. Therefore, it is essential to identify the correct stratification criterion for getting the representative sample.

Features of Stratified Random Sampling Stratified random sampling is preferred over simple random sampling if the population is heterogeneous. It provides greater precision than a simple random sample of the same size. Because of greater precision, stratified sampling requires a smaller sample, which becomes economical.

Stratified sampling is more complex in nature and requires greater effort than simple random sampling. At the same time, if the stratification criterion is faulty, the sample obtained may not be representative. In stratified random sampling, knowledge of the complete sampling frame is a must.

6.8.3 Systematic Sampling

Systematic sampling is used when the complete list of population units is available in a sequential or systematic order. In this type of sampling, every kth population unit in the list is selected from a randomly selected starting point. Systematic sampling can be considered to be a mixture of simple random sampling and stratified sampling. Here, the whole population can be considered to be divided into k strata, and the sample can be considered to be drawn randomly from each stratum because the first sample is drawn randomly from the first strata. This sampling plan is based on the concept of stratification as well as randomization. Thus, systematic sampling includes the characteristics of both simple random sampling and stratified sampling.

Let us see the procedure for drawing a systematic sample. Consider a population of size N, which is arranged in a systematic order out of which a sample of size n is to be drawn. A number k, which is known as *sample interval*, is obtained by dividing N by n. Out of the first k population units, the first unit is selected in a random manner, and thereafter every kth unit of the population is selected in the sample. This technique of drawing a sample is known as *systematic sampling*.

Consider a list of 500 faculties in a university, out of which a sample of 20 is to be selected. Then, the number k would be 25 (=500/20). Out of the first 25 faculties in the list, the first one is selected in a random manner. Suppose the first selected number is the 10th population unit, then this 10th faculty will constitute the first sample and thereafter every 25th faculty, that is, 35th, 60th, 85th, 110th faculty, would be included in the sample. In this way, a sample of 20 faculties can be obtained.

Features of Stratified Random Sampling Since systematic sampling possesses the characteristics of simple random sampling as well as stratified sampling whereby the sample is drawn from each section of the population, it is considered to be more representative.

The drawback of this sampling is that all the population units must be available in a systematic and sequential manner. Since only the first unit is drawn at random and thereafter every *k*th unit is selected, it may lead to systematic bias in the sample.

6.8.4 Cluster Sampling

At times, the population units are not a single unit but a cluster of units. In such situations, cluster sampling is done. In cluster sampling, each individual unit/member of the population is assigned to one, and only one, group. Each group is called a *cluster*. A school or a family can be considered to be a cluster because a school comprises many students and similarly a family may have several members in it. In conducting a study for assessing the expenditure incurred on health in different families in a city, the population unit would be a family, which is a cluster of family members. Similarly, in conducting a study on the basketball teams of various universities, each university would be a population unit, which is again a cluster of basketball players.

In cluster sampling, a sample is obtained by selecting clusters from the population by using any of the sampling plans. The sample consists of elements as randomly selected clusters. If a survey is to be conducted among the college students in a particular district, then all the colleges in that district are clusters. In drawing a sample of 30 colleges, one may use any of the sampling techniques, that is, simple random, stratified, or systematic. Thus, the sample elements obtained in a systematic sample are a group of clusters as each college is a cluster. If the purpose of the survey is to know the attitude of the faculty toward competitive sports in the colleges, then each faculty in the college must be interviewed because each college represents one cluster in the sample. Cluster sampling is very economical because in a single attempt all the units in a cluster are investigated. At the same time, it is very susceptible to sampling bias.

Cluster sampling is the most frequently used method. Cluster sampling is particularly useful in a situation where no list of the population is available. In this sampling, samples are selected by randomly selecting the subgroups of the population, possibly in several stages, and therefore it usually produces results equivalent to a simple random sample. Cluster sampling is used when well-defined clusters exist and a reasonable estimate of the number of elements in each level of clustering can be made. In using cluster sampling, the size of the sample must be fairly large for effective implementation of the sampling plan. Cluster sampling differs from stratified sampling. In stratified sampling, the sample includes elements from each stratum, whereas in cluster sampling, the sample includes elements only from sampled clusters.

Features of Cluster Sampling Cluster sampling is cost effective. A bigger sample can be obtained at limited cost. This sampling plan is specifically useful when the complete list of the population is difficult to obtain. This type of sampling plan is used if the researcher is interested in knowing the characteristics at the cluster level rather than at the individual level. For instance, in studying the fitness status of the children in schools of a district, cluster sampling would be more appropriate.

Clusters are required to be of the same level, but they may not have the same essential characteristics. For example, while studying the health status in the schools in urban areas, geographically the schools may belong to the urban areas but they may differ in terms of their status such as international schools, private schools, and government schools. Further, for the same sample size, cluster sampling usually provides less precision in comparison to simple random sampling and stratified sampling.

6.8.5 Multistage Sampling

Multistage sampling is a complex form of cluster sampling. In this sampling, the samples are selected in stages. In different stages, different sampling plans can be used to draw the clusters. The final sample is obtained by using simple random sampling in each of the clusters selected in the second last stage of the multistage sampling.

Multistage sampling is used when the population is large and can be organized in different clusters. For example, in investigating postural deformities among school children in a state, one may divide the state into districts where each district may further be divided into schools. Here, each district may be considered as a cluster of schools. In the first stage, few districts may be randomly selected in the sample by using simple random or stratified sampling. In the second stage, from each of these districts, a few schools may be selected by using simple random or stratified sampling. Finally, in the third stage, a few students may be randomly selected from each of the schools selected in the second stage. The pooled sample obtained in the third stage comprises the ultimate sample. Multistage sampling is easy to implement. It is used for its low cost. This technique is sometimes used when no general sample frame exists. Multistage sampling becomes two-stage or three-stage sampling if the ultimate samples are obtained in two or three stages, respectively.

Features of Multistage Sampling Multistage sampling is more accurate than cluster sampling for a same-size sample. The sample obtained in multistage sampling is more representative. This sampling plan is cost effective and can be performed speedily. Using multistage sampling is more convenient because it requires only a list of clusters and individuals in the selected clusters. Multistage sampling is more efficient than cluster sampling for same-size samples.

Multistage sampling is more complex in nature and combines limitations of cluster and stratified random sampling. It is less efficient than simple random sampling of the same size but more accurate for the same cost.

Check Your Progress

Note: Tick the correct answer by using the sign (√).

	True	False
1. If sample and population are the same, then the standard error of mean will be very low.	–	–
2. Population parameter μ depends on the sample value.	–	–
3. The term parameter can be used for the sample as well.	–	–
4. Census refers to population study.	–	–
5. In using stratified sampling, stratification can be done by using any criteria.	–	–
6. A sampling frame is a list of all the population units.	–	–
7. One should have complete knowledge of the sampling frame in stratified sampling.	–	–
8. In using systematic sampling, it is more essential that the population is homogeneous rather than that it is arranged in a sequential order.	–	–
9. Sampling is more efficient than population studies.	–	–
10. Nonresponse error refers to the wrong information from the respondent.	–	–
11. Population studies are usually less efficient on account of nonresponse errors.	–	–
12. μ, p, and S are parameters.	–	–
13. The value of a statistic changes with a change of sample values.	–	–
14. Sampling frame and population are always the same.	–	–
15. If there are 100 population units, then the units should be numbered from 1 to 100 in drawing the simple random sample.	–	–
16. Multistage sampling is more accurate than simple random sampling for the same cost.	–	–
17. In probability sampling, probability of all the population units for inclusion into the sample is same.	–	–
18. In stratified sampling, samples are drawn from each stratum proportionate to its size.	–	–
19. Simple random sampling can be used in heterogeneous population by dividing it into homogeneous groups.	–	–
20. In cluster sampling, one population unit may fall into two clusters simultaneously.	–	–
21. Cluster sampling is more prone to sampling bias.	–	–

22. Randomization reduces errors in sampling.	–	–
23. In using random number table, one always gets the same set of random sample irrespective of starting the selection from any row or column in the table.	–	–
24. In all the nonprobability sampling techniques, no systematic procedure is required to be followed in drawing the sample.	–	–
25. In random sampling, prior knowledge of the population is not required.	–	–
26. Sampling always results in a representative sample.	–	–
27. Generating random numbers in a computer always generates the same set of numbers.	–	–
28. Multistage sampling is more efficient than simple random sampling.	–	–
29. In stratified sampling, samples can be drawn from each stratum by using systematic sampling.	–	–
30. Systematic sampling inherits the characteristics from simple random sampling as well as from stratified sampling.	–	–
31. In cluster sampling, it is essential that all the clusters are mutually exclusive.	–	–
32. Sampling is used to draw the sample from the population.	–	–
33. Cluster sampling is not very economical.	–	–
34. Stratified random sampling provides more efficiency than simple random sampling for the same-size sample.	–	–
35. In using cluster sampling, sample size must be fairly large for effective implementation of the sampling plan.	–	–
36. Multistage sampling is a form of cluster sampling.	–	–
37. In using cluster sampling, stratified sampling can be used at some stage.	–	–

6.9 NONPROBABILITY SAMPLING

In nonprobability sampling, the probability of a population unit to be included in the sample is not known. Moreover, in using these techniques, all individuals in the population do not have an equal chance to be included in the sample. In some of the nonprobability sampling techniques, the procedure for selecting units from the population is clearly defined, just as in probability sampling techniques.

However, in other techniques such as purposive sampling, a researcher needs subjective judgment to select units from the population in drawing the sample. In using nonprobability sampling, a researcher needs to apply his theoretical knowledge and experience to select units from the population.

The conclusions drawn from the samples in nonprobability sampling cannot be generalized because they are not the true representative of the population, and hence they lack external validity. Validity of the sample can be enhanced by using random selection as much as possible and by making every possible attempt to avoid bias in sample selection. The following are the sampling techniques that come under the nonprobability sampling category.

- Sequential sampling
- Convenience sampling
- Consecutive sampling
- Quota sampling
- Purposive sampling
- Snowball sampling

6.9.1 Sequential Sampling

Sequential sampling is a nonprobability sampling because the probability for any population unit to be included in the sample is not known. In this technique, a sample of single subject or a group of subjects is drawn from the population, and the study is conducted to see whether some conclusion can be drawn. Unlike other sampling plans where a researcher has only two options, that is, either to reject or not to reject the null hypothesis on the basis of a sample, in sequential sampling if a researcher is in a position to neither reject the null hypothesis nor fail to reject the null hypothesis, he will have a third option wherein he can select an additional group of subjects and conduct the experiment once again for taking a decision. If the results are still inconclusive, additional groups of subjects are added to the sample. This means that the researcher can keep adding any number of subjects in the sample in a sequential manner till he decides either to reject the null hypothesis or not to reject it. This sampling technique gives the researcher unlimited chances of fine-tuning his research methods and gaining a vital insight into the study that he is currently pursuing.

Features of Sequential Sampling Sequential sampling provides a researcher an abundant opportunity in terms of sample size and sampling schedule. The sample size can be very small or excessively large depending on the decision made by the researcher. Sampling schedule is also completely dependent on the researcher since an extra sample can only be obtained after conducting the experiment on the initial group of samples. This technique enables the researcher to modify his research methods because the repetitive nature of this sampling method allows minor changes to be made in the methodology. Sequential sampling is neither costly nor time consuming. This sampling is usually used when the sampling is very costly or the sample obtained is destructive in nature.

The most disadvantageous feature of this sampling is that it is hardly representative of the population. The researcher may expect to get a near-representative sample only when the sample size is very large. The drawback of this sampling plan is that the conclusions drawn from the sample cannot be generalized for the entire population.

6.9.2 Convenience Sampling

Convenience sampling is the easiest and most commonly used sampling technique. In this sampling, the sample is selected on the basis of easy availability to the researcher; therefore, all population units do not have an equal chance to be selected in the sample. A convenience sample involves taking what you can get. This sampling technique is economical and least time consuming.

6.9.3 Consecutive Sampling

Consecutive sampling is very similar to convenience sampling except that it seeks to include all accessible subjects in the sample. Consecutive sampling is considered to be the best of all nonprobability sampling because it includes all subjects that are available in a single location. This makes the sample more representative of the entire population.

6.9.4 Quota Sampling

Quota sampling is based on the concept of selecting a fixed quota of samples from each segment of the population. The researcher draws either equal or proportionate quota of samples from different parts of the population. The segmentation of the population is based on different traits relevant to the study. In this sampling, the researcher deliberately sets the proportions of samples to be drawn from each stratum. This ensures inclusion of units from each segment of the population in the sample. Setting up of the quota for each stratum is independent of population characteristics. For example, if the quota is decided on the basis of a student's class and the researcher needs equal representation, then if the total sample size is 80, he might select 40 students from the undergraduate and another 40 from the postgraduate classes. Usually, the quota is decided on the basis of age, gender, class, race, religion, socioeconomic status, sport specialization, level of participation, and so on. Quota sampling ensures selection of adequate number of subjects with appropriate characteristics, but at the same time it lacks representativeness of the population.

6.9.5 Purposive Sampling

Purposive sampling is done for a specific purpose. In this sampling, the researcher is of the view that some subjects are more appropriate for the study in comparison to others, and that is why they are purposively chosen in the sample. A purposive sample is a nonrepresentative sample of the population. Thus, the findings may not be applicable to the population of interest. Purposive sample is selected because the study may be focused on some targeted group. For example, the sample may consist of those subjects who have basketball as a specialization or those subjects who have a sedentary lifestyle.

Sometimes, it may not be possible to specify the population, and therefore probability sampling cannot be used. In such situations, the researcher attempts to interview the target group wherever it is available. For instance, to know the attitude of studious students toward competitive sports, it is difficult to define or identify the population; hence, the researcher may select any group of studious students that is easily available for the study. In purposive sampling, the sample drawn is not easily defensible as being representative of the population because of the potential subjectivity of the researcher. Purposive sampling is also known as judgmental sampling.

6.9.6 Snowball Sampling

In snowball sampling, the sample is drawn by asking the initial subjects in the sample to identify another potential subject for the study who meet the criteria of the research. Here, the sample is drawn in a chain-like manner, and hence snowball sampling is also known as chain sampling. A snowball sample is obtained by asking a participant who is initially selected in the sample to suggest someone else who might be willing or appropriate for the study. This sampling is named as snowball because one picks up the samples along the way, analogous to a snowball accumulating snow. Snowball sampling is appropriate in a situation where it is difficult to track populations, such as absentees, dopers, criminals, and so on.

Snowball sampling is normally used in the case of small populations. This type of sampling involves utilizing well-informed people to identify the subjects who have a lot of information about a phenomenon. The researcher follows this chain of contacts in order to identify and accumulate critical cases. Such a sampling procedure is carried out by the investigators to identify dopers in the sports arena to reveal about the types of drugs and the way sports persons use them. In snowball sampling, it is possible to include members of the groups where no lists or identifiable clusters even exist. One of the drawbacks of this sampling is that the sample is not a true representative of the population.

6.10 WHEN TO USE PROBABILITY SAMPLING

In a survey research, drawing a representative sample is the key. Thus, it is essential to use the correct sampling plan so as to draw the most representative sample. The following are a few guidelines that can be used by the researchers to identify the correct sampling plan for their study.

Simple random sampling should be used in a situation where the entire population is nearly homogeneous on some criterion. Random sampling should also be used if the researcher is not aware of the more complex sampling techniques or if the population is completely unknown. If the sampling frame is known, one should use stratified sampling in which the population is divided into homogeneous strata. Stratified sampling gives a more representative sample than simple random sampling for a given sample size. If the population list is available in an arranged sequence, then systematic sampling should be used. Systematic sampling ensures representation of each portion of the population. Usually, this sampling plan is used when the population is not big and the entire population list is available. Cluster sampling is used when the population is structured in clusters and the information is obtained on the clusters rather than on the individual unit. Since multistage sampling is a complex form of cluster sampling, it should be used only when the population is very large and enough resources are available to the researcher.

6.11 WHEN TO USE NONPROBABILITY SAMPLING

Nonprobability sampling is used to investigate a specific phenomenon present in the population. If the researcher aims to do qualitative, pilot, or exploratory studies, nonprobability sampling is the best option. In a situation where the population is limitless, randomization cannot be done, and in that case the only option left to the researcher is to use nonprobability sampling. Sometimes, the researcher is not interested in generalizing the findings to the entire population outside his or her domain; in that case, nonprobability sampling is the best option. Nonprobability sampling is mostly used when the researcher has financial constraints and limited resources. Sometimes, these sampling plans are used by the researcher in an initial study after which the study is again carried out by using an appropriate probability sampling technique.

6.12 CHARACTERISTICS OF A GOOD SAMPLE

A small sample selected scientifically is much more reliable than a poorly selected large sample. One of the main characteristics of a good sample is that it should be representative in nature. In other words, it must possess the characteristics of the population under controlled experimental errors. The following are some of the important characteristics of a good sample.

a. It should be free from bias. No personal preferences should be used in drawing the sample.
b. It should possess the least sampling error.
c. It must be obtained by using some sampling plan.
d. It must have representation from all the sections in the population.

e. It must be optimum in size.
f. It must include only independent units.

6.13 SOURCES OF DATA

Data form one of the most integral parts of any research study. Research conducted in the field of exercise science and health may differ in methodology but is based on data that is analyzed and interpreted for concluding information. These data are either collected on the subjects by the researcher or obtained from other sources. Depending on whether the data have been collected by the researchers themselves or obtained from other sources, they can be classified as primary or secondary data, respectively. Both types of data are explained in detail in the following sections.

6.13.1 Primary Data

Data collected by the researcher himself or herself on the subjects during his study are known as *primary data*. Primary data are more reliable, authentic, and objective because the researcher himself or herself supervises the data collection. Since primary data have not been changed or altered by anyone, their validity is greater than that of secondary data. Secondary data are less reliable and may have biases because they have already been manipulated by their custodian. In experimental research or statistical surveys, it is necessary to derive information from primary data as the nature of data changes after some period of time. For example, an assessment of fitness level of the people in a district cannot be inferred from the data collected 5 years back. It is because the fitness status of people is dynamic in nature and keeps changing because of awareness on healthy habits in the society.

One of the main concerns in a research study is to obtain valid, reliable, and efficient findings. Therefore, using primary data improves the validity of the findings because they are more accurate and reliable. Primary data provide more reliable findings if the methods used for analysis are suitably chosen as per their data type. Reliability of the primary data can be questionable if the researcher uses personal biases or uses misleading information in the research. At the same time, primary data are expensive as well as time consuming.

6.13.2 Secondary Data

Secondary data are obtained from any source that has been published by other agencies. Without ensuring the authenticity of an organization if the data provided by it are used it may lead to unreliable findings. Nowadays, secondary data are often readily available but one has to see whether they suit their research requirements. With the explosion of the Internet facility, the availability of secondary data has become much easier. Secondary data may be less valid but still they are important. In a situation where getting primary data is difficult, one may consider getting it from secondary sources. At times, when it is not possible to collect the primary data, one has no option except to organize his or her research on the secondary data.

Secondary data can be obtained from a variety of sources. They may be obtained from the published literature. The data may be available in books, journals, or magazines. The main issue in using such data is their credibility, which depends on many factors such as the publisher, organization from where these publications are originated, and the credibility of such publishers and organizations. In using secondary data, one should prefer recent sources rather than old sources because new technology and research bring new findings and facts to light. Secondary data can be obtained from various sites on the Internet. Several researchers, companies, and organizations publish their data on the Internet, which can be used as a source of secondary data. Some of these organizations provide data free of cost to the researchers while others charge some amount of money for its use. Again, one needs to judge the reliability of the data source. Many government organizations such as National Sample Surveys Organization (NSSO), Central Statistical Organizations (CSO), National Information Centre (NIC), and different ministries publish their data on demography, census, population statistics, health statistics, and so on their websites. These data can be used free of cost by the researchers as secondary data. Further, many nongovernmental organizations (NGO) also provide their survey data on their website. These data can also be used by the researchers if they suit their requirements. Data from NGOs are often more comprehensive as they are obtained for some specific research purpose.

Secondary data are easy to obtain and are more economical but at the same time they lack originality. Most of the time, secondary data may not suit the objectives of the research study, which limits their use by the researchers. Secondary data are free from prejudice, but at the same time, great care and caution are required in using them.

6.14 METHODS OF DATA COLLECTION

In research studies, data are collected by using different methods. These methods have advantages as well as disadvantages. However, by carefully adopting these methods, reliable data can be obtained. Some of the important methods of data collection have been discussed in the following sections.

6.14.1 Observation Method

In the observation method, the data about the subjects are collected only by observing their activities. During data collection, the subjects may or may not know that they are being observed for their activities. Observations may be made in natural settings or in an artificially created environment. If the subjects are not aware that they are being observed by the experimenter, then they behave naturally, which improves the reliability of the data. The playing ability of sports persons during a game situation may be assessed by the observation method.

6.14.2 Interview Method

In interview method, face-to-face dialog is conducted with the respondents to get the response on different issues of the study. One of the advantages of interview method is that it provides an in-depth source of information. In this method, there is a fear that the respondent may deliberately hide the information on certain sensitive issues. It is therefore important that the interviewer must be trained enough to extract the correct information from the respondents by asking the questions without hurting their ego. The quality of data depends much on the skill set of the interviewer, who not only records the statements of the interviewee but also observes the body language, expressions, and other reactions to the questions too. This enables the interviewer to draw conclusions correctly. Parents' attitude toward their daughters participating in outdoor sports may be assessed by using the interview method.

6.14.3 Questionnaire Method

Data collection by using a questionnaire is the most widely used method in research. One must ensure the reliability and validity of a questionnaire before its use. A questionnaire meant for school children should not be used for college students. In the case of using a questionnaire developed by foreign experts, it must be standardized to the local environment before use; otherwise, it may not give valid findings. Usually, a questionnaire includes close-ended questions on which the responses are obtained. However, sometimes it may have open-ended questions as well. The data collected by using the questionnaire method are considered to be more reliable. While administering the questionnaire, the researcher must explain the purpose of the study and assure the respondents that the information given by them shall remain confidential. In addition, if the questionnaire is administered by mail, then an introductory statement must be made in the beginning of the questionnaire about its purpose and the confidentiality of the information. The questionnaire can be administered via personal contacts, telephone, mail, and electronic mail. One of the drawbacks of the mail method of conducting a questionnaire study is that the success rate of receiving the filled-in questionnaire is not more than 20–30%. Studies such as assessment of exercise infrastructure and its use or assessing the health status of the women in a village may be conducted by organizing the questionnaire study.

6.14.4 Experimental Method

In experimental method, the data are collected on subjects under controlled situations. It requires an artificial or natural setting in which the data are collected. Experimental methods are more suitable for studies in the area of exercise science, sports science, health sciences, and so on. In the experimental method, the researcher tries to control and minimize the effect of extraneous variables so as to see the real effect of the experimental treatments on certain dependent variables. For instance, one may be interested in comparing the effectiveness of three different circuit training programs on volleyball skills.

6.15 BIASES IN DATA COLLECTION

All sampling techniques are subjected to some or the other kind of bias. Bias refers to some kind of personal or procedural influences on the originality of data. Bias affects the real nature of data. Bias reduces the reliability of findings, and therefore researchers always try to reduce it to a minimum level. The following are the main types of biases in sample surveys.

6.15.1 Biases Due to Procedure

Bias in data collection may occur because of the procedure used. This type of bias is common to both complete enumeration and sampling. Bias may occur in the data set because of faulty responses of the respondents due to their ego. For example, one may furnish the wrong information if asked how much money he spends on fitness and health per month, or if a question about his salary is asked. Such bias is known as *prestige bias*. Because of this bias one may overstate one's fitness and health expenditure and monthly income. Further, one may furnish wrong information for the protection of self-interest; for example, the respondent may make an understatement of income sources and an overstatement of expenses. If the data are collected by observation method, it may create an *observational bias*. For example, assessing the playing ability of an athlete by the observation method may lead to either underestimation or overestimation in comparison to the assessment of the performance measured by any objective criteria.

In case some of the questions are not clear in the questionnaire and the respondent provides his response after listening to the suggestions from the interviewer, then such responses are likely to be influenced by the suggestion of the interviewer. This creates a bias in the data, which is known as *interviewer bias*.

Further, nonresponse may arise if the respondent is not willing to give the information for some or the other reason. Since nonresponse leads to a segment of the population with certain peculiar characteristics being excluded, it generally results in bias of some form. This kind of bias is known as the *nonresponse bias*. All the types of biases discussed in this section may occur because of the procedure, and therefore they are known as *procedural bias*.

6.15.2 Biases Due to Sampling

A *sampling bias* is caused by nonrandom sampling. Sampling bias is more in nonprobability sampling in comparison to that in probability sampling. The bias due to nonrandom sampling occurs because in such sampling a certain segment of the population having a specific attribute may not be represented in the sample. The exclusion of such segments of data can influence the conclusion and provide wrong information.

Biases due to sampling may occur in the absence of a complete sampling frame. For example, a survey of college athletes to assess the use of doping will be a biased sample because it does not include other athletes who are not studying in the college or who are dropouts. Biases may occur because of substitution on account of nonresponse from the respondent in the sample. The researcher generally replaces the subject by another subject if he or she finds that the subject is noncooperative. This may lead to an overrepresentation of the types of sample unit that already exists in the sample. Such biases that occur in the sample because of substitution are known as *biases due to substitution*.

6.16 SAMPLING ERROR

A *sampling error* can be defined as the error caused by the sampling procedure. If the sample is not a representative of the population, sampling error occurs and in that case sample and population characteristics differ. Usually, sampling error occurs if nonprobability sampling is used in drawing the sample because in that case the sample is not representative of the population. Sampling error is not an actual error but is the result of an unrepresentative sample. If the sample is drawn randomly, sampling error can be computed and analyzed. Can the sampling error be eliminated completely? This is only possible if the sample and the population are the same. Since a researcher always prefers sampling, one should try to minimize sampling error by using an appropriate probability sampling technique and by taking a large sample size.

6.17 NONSAMPLING ERRORS

Nonsampling errors refer to those errors that are due to human intervention. In fact, all errors other than sampling error are known as nonsampling errors. The errors due to missing data, tester error, instrumental error, respondent error, recording error, data feeding error, and processing error are all known as nonsampling errors. Other nonsampling errors include faulty definition of the sampling frame, unclear objectives, defective questionnaire, and faulty methodology in testing. There are no methods available to measure these nonsampling errors. All statistical techniques used for data analysis are based on the assumption that none of these nonsampling errors are committed during data collection. It is the responsibility of the researcher to minimize these nonsampling errors as far as possible for reliable conclusion.

6.18 SAMPLING DISTRIBUTION

Sampling distribution can be defined as the probability distribution of any statistic based on a random sample. Let us suppose that all possible samples of size n are drawn from a given population. Further, if we compute any statistic for each sample, then the probability distribution of this statistic is called the *sampling distribution*.

6.18.1 Central Limit Theorem

If samples of size n are randomly drawn from a population having mean μ and standard deviation σ, then the sample means, $\bar{x}$, are approximately normally distributed with mean μ and standard deviation $\sigma/\sqrt{n}$ for a sufficiently large sample ($n \geq 30$), irrespective of the shape of the population distribution. However, if the population is normally distributed, the sample means are normally distributed for any sample size.

6.18.2 Standard Error

The standard error is the standard deviation of the sampling distribution of a statistic. Standard error measures the accuracy with which a sample represents a population. When a random sample is drawn from a population, the sample mean deviates from the population mean; this deviation is explained by the standard error. In other words, standard error indicates how much sampling fluctuation a statistic will show. In the theory of estimation, the construction of confidence intervals and test of significance are based on standard error. The standard error of a statistic depends on the sample size: the larger the sample size, the smaller the standard error. The standard error is usually represented by the Greek letter sigma (σ) with a subscript indicating the statistic. For instance, the standard error of the mean is denoted by $\sigma_{\bar{x}}$.

6.18.3 Sampling Distribution of the Sample Mean

The sampling distribution of any statistic depends on the distribution of population, the sampling procedure used, and the size of the sample. Often, we are interested in testing whether the sampling distribution can be approximated to a normal distribution when $n \to \infty$. Consider a normal population having mean μ and variance σ^2. If all possible samples of a given size, say n, are drawn from this population and the mean is calculated for each sample, then the distribution of these sample means is known as the *sampling distribution of the sample mean.* The distribution of the sample mean (of any size) will be normal because the population from which these samples have been drawn is also normal. Thus, if random samples of size n are drawn from a normal population with mean μ and standard deviation σ, then the distribution of sample means $\bar{x}$ will also be normal with

$$\text{Mean} = \mu$$

and

$$\text{Standard deviation} = \sigma_{\bar{x}} = \frac{\sigma}{\sqrt{n}}$$

that is, $\bar{x} \sim N(\mu, \sigma^2/n)$, where σ^2/n is the variance of $\bar{x}$.

What happens if the distribution of population is not normal? This issue can be resolved by the central limit theorem. The sampling distribution of the sample mean will follow normal distribution if any of the following two conditions is satisfied:

a. The population is normally distributed and population standard deviation is known.
b. Sample size is sufficiently large ($n \geq 30$).

Illustration Let us see how the sample means are distributed if all possible samples are drawn from any population. Consider a finite population having the following eight scores.

x	12	15	17	21	22	26	27	28

If we draw the histogram for this population, the graph will appear as in Figure 6.1.

If we draw all possible samples of size 2 with replacement from this population, then the samples would be as follows.

12,12	12,15	12,17	12,21	12,22	12,26	12,27	12,28
15,12	15,15	15,17	15,21	15,22	15,26	15,27	15,28
17,12	17,15	17,17	17,21	17,22	17,26	17,27	17,28
21,12	21,15	21,17	21,21	21,22	21,26	21,27	21,28
22,12	22,15	22,17	22,21	22,22	22,26	22,27	22,28
26,12	26,15	26,17	26,21	26,22	26,26	26,27	26,28
27,12	27,15	27,17	27,21	27,22	27,26	27,27	27,28
28,12	28,15	28,17	28,21	28,22	28,26	28,27	28,28

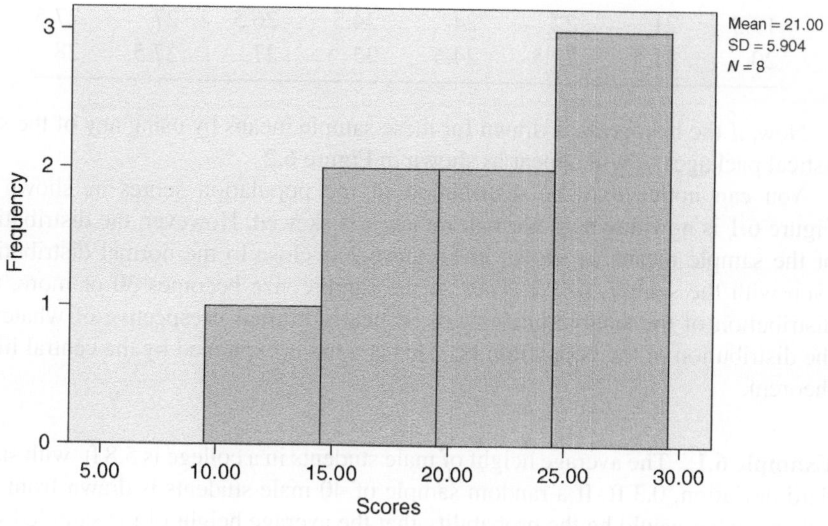

Figure 6.1 Histogram of the population scores.

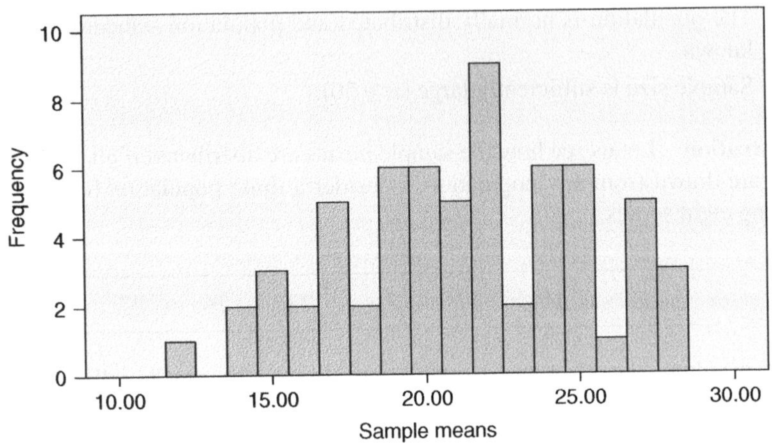

Figure 6.2 Histogram of the sample means.

The following are the means of these samples:

12	13.5	14.5	16.5	17	19	19.5	20
13.5	15	16	18	18.5	20.5	21	21.5
14.5	16	17	19	19.5	21.5	22	22.5
16.5	18	19	21	21.5	23.5	24	24.5
17	18.5	19.5	21.5	22	24	24.5	25
19	20.5	21.5	23.5	24	26	26.5	27
19.5	21	22	24	24.5	26.5	27	27.5
20	21.5	22.5	24.5	25	27	27.5	28

Now, if the histogram is drawn for these sample means by using any of the statistical packages, it will appear as shown in Figure 6.2.

You can notice that the distribution of the population scores as shown in Figure 6.1 is nowhere near normal; rather, it is skewed. However, the distribution of the sample means as shown in Figure 6.2 is close to the normal distribution even with the sample size 2. Thus, if the sample size becomes 30 or more, the distribution of the sample means will be nearly normal irrespective of whatever the distribution of the population be. This is what is explained by the central limit theorem.

Example 6.1 The average height of male students in a college is 5.8 ft. with standard deviation, 0.3 ft. If a random sample of 40 male students is drawn from the college, what would be the probability that the average height of the sampled students will be less than 5.7 ft.?

Solution: As per the central limit theorem, if the sample size is 30 or more the sample mean follows a normal distribution with the mean equal to the population mean μ and the standard deviation as given below:

$$\sigma_{\bar{x}} = \frac{\sigma}{\sqrt{n}}$$

Here, $n = 40$ and the population standard deviation is equal to 0.3 ft.; hence, the sample mean is normally distributed with mean 5.8 ft. and standard deviation $0.3/\sqrt{40} = 0.470$.

$$\sigma_{\bar{x}} = \frac{0.3}{\sqrt{40}} = 0.047$$

It is required to know the probability that the mean of the given sample is less than 5.7 ft. In other words, it is required to find the area A in the below-mentioned normal distribution.

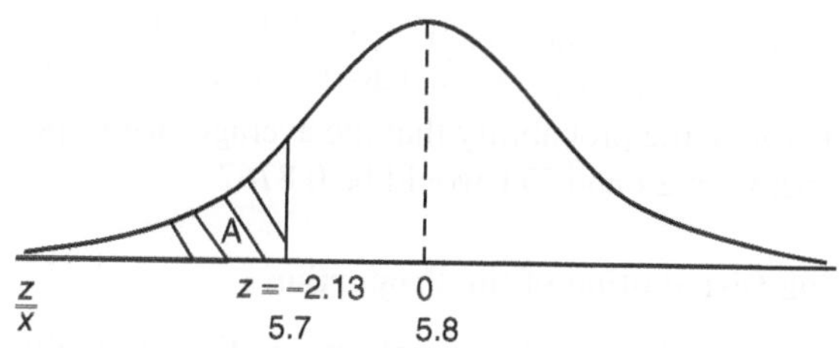

$$\text{For } \bar{x} = 5.7,\ z = \frac{\bar{x} - \mu}{\sigma/\sqrt{n}} = \frac{5.7 - 5.8}{0.047} = -2.13$$

From the normal curve area (Table A.4), the area between $z = 0$ and $z = -2.13$ is 0.4834. The required area A would be obtained by subtracting this value from 0.5.

$$\text{Area } A = 0.5 - 0.4834 = 0.0166$$

Thus, the probability that the average height of the sampled students is less than 5.7 ft. is equal to 0.0166.

Example 6.2 If the average sit-ups performance of the undergraduate students is 25 along with standard deviation 3, what would be the probability that a random sample of 36 undergraduate students will have their mean performance on sit-ups between 24 and 27?

Solution: Given that $\mu = 25$, $\sigma = 5$, and $n = 36$, it is required to find the probability that the mean sit-ups performance lies between 24 and 27. In other words, it is required to find $P(24 \leq \bar{x} \leq 27)$. Since the sample mean follows a normal distribution for a large sample size, in the below-mentioned normal distribution it is required to calculate the area $A_1 + A_2$.

$$\text{For } \bar{x} = 24, \ z = \frac{\bar{x} - \mu}{\sigma/\sqrt{n}} = \frac{24 - 25}{5/\sqrt{36}} = -1.2$$

$$\text{For } \bar{x} = 27, \ z = \frac{\bar{x} - \mu}{\sigma/\sqrt{n}} = \frac{27 - 25}{5/\sqrt{36}} = 2.4$$

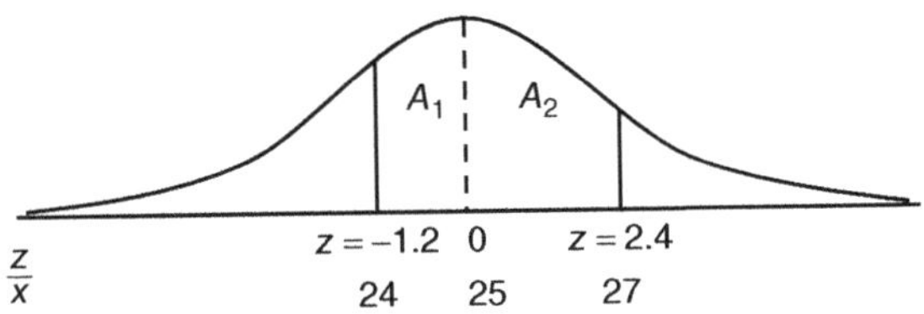

Corresponding to $z = -1.2$ the area A_1 from Table A.4 is 0.3849, and similarly corresponding to $z = 2.4$ the area A_2 is 0.4918. Thus, the required probability is 0.8767. In other words, the probability that the average sit-ups performance of the sample shall be between 24 and 271 would be 0.8767.

6.18.4 Sampling Distribution of the Proportion

At times, a researcher chooses the sample proportion to analyze the data. For instance, by looking at the sample of students, one may be interested to know whether the proportion of smokers in the college is 0.3. It is therefore important to know the sampling distribution of the sample proportion. Let us assume that p is the proportion of success of an event in the population and $\hat{p}$ represents the proportion of success of that event in the sample. If repeated samples of size n are drawn from the same population and the proportion of success $\hat{p}$ is determined for each sample, then the distribution of $\hat{p}$ (sample proportion) is known as the *sampling distribution of the sample proportion.*

As per the central limit theorem if the sample size n is sufficiently large so that $np > 5$ and $nq > 5$ (p is the population proportion and $q = 1 - p$), then the sample proportion $\hat{p}$ is approximately normally distributed with

$$\text{Mean } = p$$

and

$$\text{Standard deviation} = \sigma_{\hat{p}} = \sqrt{\frac{pq}{n}}$$

The standard deviation of the sample proportion is also referred to as the *standard error of proportion.*

Example 6.3 If 25% of the population are smokers, what is the probability that 15 or more persons would be smokers in a randomly selected sample of size 70?

Solution: Here, $p = 0.25$, $q = 0.75$, $\hat{p} = 15/70 = 0.21$, and $n = 70$. Since the sample is large, the sample proportion would be normally distributed.

$$z = \frac{\hat{p} - p}{\sqrt{\frac{pq}{n}}} = \frac{0.21 - 0.25}{\sqrt{\frac{0.25 \times 0.75}{70}}} = -\frac{0.04}{0.052} = -0.77$$

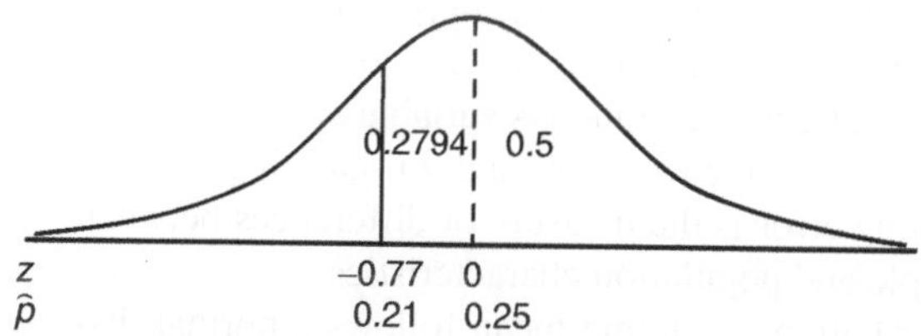

Table A.4 gives a probability of 0.2794 for a z value of −.77, which is the area between the sample proportion, 0.21, and the population proportion, 0.25. The answer to the problem is

$$P(\hat{p} \geq 0.21) = 0.2794 + 0.5 = 0.7794$$

Check Your Progress

Note: Tick the correct answer by using the sign (√)

	True	False
38. Nonprobability sampling lacks generalization.	_	_
39. Sequential sampling should be used when the samples are costly to evaluate.	_	_
40. In quota sampling, samples are selected proportionately from different parts of the population.	_	_
41. Sampling error may occur because of substitution.	_	_
42. In snowball sampling, each subject in the initial sample provides the knowledge about the other samples to be included in the sample.	_	_
43. Probability sampling is used in exploratory studies.	_	_
44. A good sample may have related units as well.	_	_
45. Primary data are more economical than secondary data.	_	_
46. In sequential sampling, a researcher has unlimited chances of fine-tuning his or her research methods.	_	_

47. The biases in sampling may occur because of the absence of the complete sampling frame.	–	–
48. In sequential sampling, one can either reject or not reject the null hypothesis on the basis of sample information.	–	–
49. The standard error of the sample proportion is $\sqrt{pq/n}$.	–	–
50. The success rate of receiving the response from the respondents in a questionnaire study is around 20–30%.	–	–
51. Standard error of the sample mean is $\sqrt{\sigma/n}$.	–	–
52. In an experimental method, data are collected by minimizing the effect of extraneous variables.	–	–
53. Sampling bias is the result of random sampling.	–	–
54. A sampling error is the measure of differences between the sample and population characteristics.	–	–
55. The distribution of sample mean follows a normal distribution in a large sample irrespective of whether the population standard deviation is known or not.	–	–
56. In the case of a large sample, the mean of the sample proportion is equal to that of the population proportion, p.	–	–

6.19 CRITERIA IN DECIDING SAMPLE SIZE

In general, increasing the size of the sample enhances the accuracy of the findings. This is so because with an increase in the sample size n, there is a decrease in the standard error of the sampling distribution of mean $\sigma/\sqrt{n}$. Since standard error is an indicator of sampling error, the lesser its value, the higher the accuracy of the findings based on the sample. However, as the sample size increases the cost of the study also increases. In addition, increasing the sample size beyond an optimum level reduces the accuracy of the findings because of operational factors. In fact, it is not the quantity but the quality of the sample that matters. At times, a sample of size 2000 may not be sufficient if the study is to develop the norms of certain test items of athletic fitness for different age categories in a district. On the other hand, a sample of size 15 would be good enough if the study is conducted on Olympic gold medalists. It is, therefore, important to decide an optimum sample size for the research study. The sample size is considered to be optimum if it can be managed within the available resources without sacrificing the accuracy of the findings. Finding the optimum size of the sample depends on two factors: cost and accuracy. Let us see the procedure for finding the sample size by considering these two criteria.

6.19.1 Cost Factor

Usually, every research study needs to be completed within the allotted budget unless it is a national project where there is no dearth of finances. It is, therefore, essential to decide the size of the sample within the allotted budget. In deciding the sample size, one needs to have a trade-off between the cost and accuracy factors. If the cost of the project is fixed, then the sample size can be worked out by deciding the various costs such as overhead cost, per unit evaluation cost, and motivation cost.

If C is the total cost of the study, then the required sample size can be determined by the following model:

$$C = a + nc_1 + \frac{C}{10} \tag{6.1}$$

where a is the overhead cost, c_1 is the cost of evaluating one unit, and n is the sample size. Here, $C/10$ is the contingency cost kept in reserve for coping with unforeseen expenditure or compensating for inflation during the conduct of the study.

Overhead cost refers to the expenditure that is incurred one time in conducting the research. This includes cost of the equipments, stationery, printing, computing, traveling, and so on. The value of c_1 is the cost of evaluating each subject. This includes the cost of the coordinator, the cost of the field investigator, and the cost of motivating the respondent. If the project is big, then the researcher needs to employ several field investigators to collect the data from specified subjects in the sample. These field investigators may be paid per unit evaluation. To monitor the field investigator's performance, a project coordinator may be appointed who can also be paid for per unit evaluation. The role of the project coordinator is to ensure the reliability of data collection by cross-checking. The project coordinator may visit some of the sampled cases to cross-check the responses. Finally, some money should be allotted for motivating the respondents as well. This is a gesture toward the respondents to encourage the correct response. This cost is a must in the studies conducted in exercise science because one needs to motivate the subject to extract his or her best performance on field. This cost should not be ignored as the entire findings depend on the correct responses of the respondents. The model in Equation (6.1) can also be used for submitting the proposal for funding a project because it provides justification for each of the costs in the study.

Example 6.4 It has been decided to invest \$50,000 on a project in which an investigator wants to study the attitude of exercise science teachers in a city toward smoking. The overhead expenditure is \$30,000. Per unit evaluation cost for the field investigator and supervisor are \$100 and \$25, respectively, whereas the motivation cost for each subject is \$20. What sample size would you recommend to the investigator for the project?

Solution: Given that $C = 50{,}000$, $a = 30{,}000$, $c_1 = 100 + 25 + 20 = 145$, and it is required to find the value of n.

$$C = a + nc_1 + \frac{C}{10}$$

Substituting these values

$$50000 = 30000 + 145n + \frac{50000}{10}$$
$$\Rightarrow 145n = 20000 - 5000 = 15000$$
$$\Rightarrow n = 15000/145 = 103.44$$

Thus, 103 samples may be selected for the project.

6.19.2 Accuracy Factor

In most of the studies, cost is the main consideration but if accuracy is of prime importance to the researcher, then the sample size is computed on the basis of the degree of accuracy required. Studies conducted by government organizations or private industries usually do not have financial constraints but accuracy of findings is of utmost importance. In that situation, an optimum size of the sample can be worked out for a specific degree of accuracy in findings.

Let us consider a study in which the researcher is interested in finding $(1-\alpha)$ level of confidence interval of the mean of a normal population where the variance is known in advance. Further, suppose that the mean is to be estimated within c units of the true mean. In that case, the desired length of the confidence interval is $2E$. Thus, we have

$$\left(\bar{x} + z_{1-\alpha/2}\frac{\sigma}{\sqrt{n}}\right) - \left(\bar{x} - z_{1-\alpha/2}\frac{\sigma}{\sqrt{n}}\right) = 2E$$

or

$$2z_{1-\alpha/2}\frac{\sigma}{\sqrt{n}} = 2E$$
$$\Rightarrow n = \frac{z^2_{1-\alpha/2}\sigma^2}{E^2} \tag{6.2}$$

Equation (6.2) provides the sample size "n" for $(1-\alpha)$ level of confidence in the findings. If n is a fraction, then the nearest whole number would be the sample size.

Example 6.5 Find the sample size required to estimate the population mean (μ) with 95% confidence that your estimate is within 3 units of μ, given that the population standard deviation (σ) is 25.

Solution: Here, $z_{1-\alpha/2} = 1.96$, $\sigma^2 = 125$, and $E = 3$.

Since

$$n = \frac{z^2_{1-\alpha/2}\sigma^2}{E^2}$$

substituting the values we get

$$n = \frac{1.96^2 \times 125}{3^2}$$
$$= 53.36 \approx 53$$

Thus, a sample of size 53 is required if the investigator desires to have the estimate of the mean within 3 units of the true mean.

Example 6.6 A researcher wants to obtain a 99% confidence interval for the mean modified sit-ups performance of the athletes and he desires that the estimate should be within 5 scores of the true value of the population mean modified sit-ups, where the standard deviation of the modified sit-ups is 22; then what should be the sample size?

Solution: Here, $z_{1-\alpha/2} = 2.58$, $\sigma^2 = 22^2 = 484$, and $E = 5$.
Since

$$n = \frac{z_{1-\alpha/2}^2 \sigma^2}{E^2}$$

substituting the values we get

$$n = \frac{2.58^2 \times 484}{5^2}$$
$$= 128.87 \approx 129$$

Thus, a sample of size 129 is required if the investigator desires to have the estimate of the mean modified sit-ups to be within 5 scores of the true population mean.

PRACTICE EXERCISE

1. A study is required to be conducted in a college to know the attitude of students toward smoking. The number of students in the college is as follows.

	Undergraduate	Postgraduate
Male	1000	400
Female	300	100

If a stratified sample of 90 students is to be selected, how many students in the sample would be selected from each category?

2. Determine the probability in each case.
   i. $P(\bar{x} < 26.7) =?$, given that n=55, $\mu = 29$, and $\sigma = 6$.
   ii. $P(\bar{x} \geq 101.5) =?$, given that $n = 49$, $\mu = 95$, and $\sigma = 20$.
   iii. $P(122 < \bar{x} < 124) =?$, given that $n = 81$, $\mu = 125$, and $\sigma = 15$.
3. If the population proportion p is 0.35, find the probability of getting each of the following sample proportions.
   i. $P(\hat{p} \leq 0.31)$, $n = 180$
   ii. $P(\hat{p} \leq 0.42)$, $n = 64$
   iii. $P(\hat{p} \geq 0.39)$, $n = 78$
   iv. $P(\hat{p} \geq 0.28)$, $n = 98$
   v. $P(0.32 \leq \hat{p} \leq 0.40)$, $n = 120$
4. It has been decided to invest \$42,000 on a project in which an investigator wants to study the attitude of exercise scientists toward smoking. The overhead expenditure is \$21,000 and per head evaluation cost of an experimental unit is \$100. What sample size would you recommend to the investigator for the project?
5. Find the sample size necessary to estimate the population proportion p for the following situation:

   $$E = 0.05,\ \hat{p} \text{ is } 0.40, \text{ and confidence level is } 98\%.$$

6. An experimenter wants to obtain a 95% confidence interval for the mean diastolic blood pressure of college athletes, and he wants the estimate to be within 3 counts of the true value. Assuming the variance to be 65, find the sample size.

6.20 COMPUTING WITH EXCEL

6.20.1 Finding a Random Sample Using Excel

Excel can be used to draw a random sample from a given population. Drawing a random sample is one of the most important assumptions for conducting research. It ensures external validity whereby the results can well be generalized for the population for interest. The procedure of drawing a random sample has been discussed by means of the below-mentioned example.

Remark The facility of drawing a random sample can only be used if the Add-ins "Analysis ToolPak" is already installed in your Excel. The readers can install this Add-ins "Analysis ToolPak" in their Excel by following the procedure mentioned in Chapter 1.

Example 6.7 In a survey study on old people about their attitude toward sports activities, a researcher wanted to draw a random sample from a population of 200 subjects. He allotted a distinct number to all the subjects in the population ranging from 1 to 200. Draw a random sample of size 25 by using Excel. The numbers allotted to the subjects are as follows:

Numbers allotted to the subjects in the population

65	186	113	143	23	183	181	108	150	35	115	61	14	125	17	76	105
22	98	44	114	104	47	100	190	75	107	52	53	154	165	56	57	116
145	62	138	26	85	144	19	40	89	90	147	178	194	157	140	160	121
45	103	66	110	184	59	80	129	20	187	46	163	134	135	197	180	200
161	162	12	13	7	179	167	168	169	60	171	172	10	37	175	176	9
117	101	149	148	102	30	156	28	106	185	32	34	155	112	77	38	39
153	118	120	141	189	188	142	70	196	68	146	21	72	74	195	152	78
79	193	158	96	51	84	48	43	122	93	15	86	41	92	54	97	50
87	16	11	198	2	136	91	124	88	83	130	133	55	126	81	132	94
137	127	1	42	18	99	8	131	164	128	123	170	173	95	166	174	49
6	177	4	5	3	82	58	139	111	119	182	27	29	31	109	33	191
192	36	151	159	24	67	69	71	73	63	199	64	25				

Solution: To find a random sample of size 25 from the population consisting 200 subjects, the following procedure shall be used:

1. Feed the population data in different columns of the Excel sheet.
2. To draw a random sample, click the following commands in sequence in Excel to get the screen as shown in Figure 6.3.

   Data ⟶ Data analysis

3. Bring the scroll on the option **Sampling**, and then click **OK** in the screen as shown in Figure 6.3. This will take you to the screen as shown in Figure 6.4. You can now define the range of population data from which a random sample needs to be drawn.
4. In this example, all scores allotted to the subjects in the population are written in A to L columns of the Excel sheet as shown in Figure 6.4. The data range would therefore be A1:L17. Do the following steps to fill the entries in the screen shown in Figure 6.4.

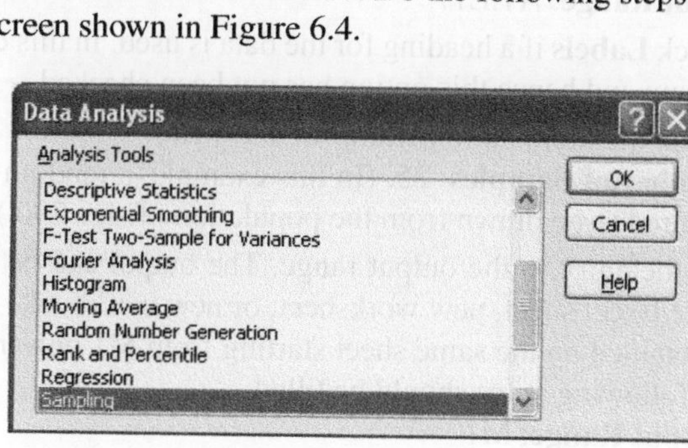

Figure 6.3 Command for drawing a random sample.

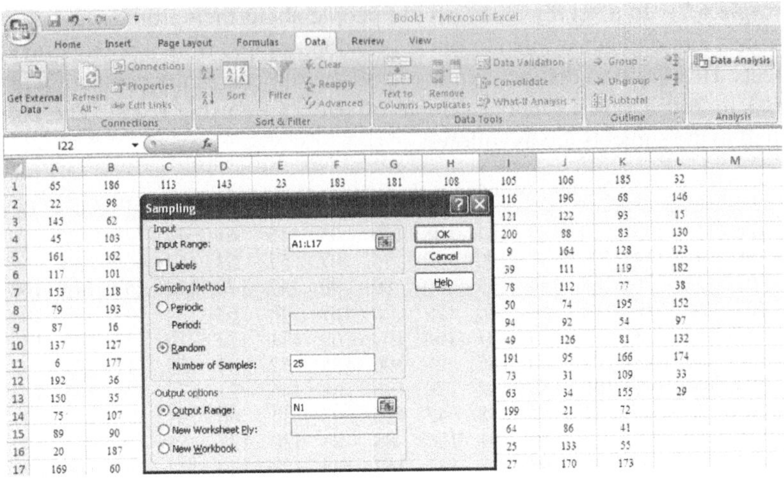

Figure 6.4 Options for drawing a random sample.

TABLE 6.2 Random Sample of Size 25

90	180
21	172
47	185
29	132
72	3
46	127
76	156
117	31
116	30
108	37
56	30
193	191
3	

i. **Input Range**: A1:L17

ii. Check **Labels** if a heading for the data is used. In this case, no heading is there and hence this option has not been checked.

iii. Check the radio button **Random** and write
Number of Samples: 25. (In this example, a random sample of 25 is required to be drawn from the population of size 200.)

iv. Fill the entry in the output range. The output can be obtained on the same Excel sheet, new worksheet, or new workbook. Here, the output is obtained on the same sheet starting from M1 onward, and therefore the following entry should be filled.
Output Range: M1

v. Click **OK** to get the output. The output obtained is shown in Table 6.2.

IMPORTANT DEFINITIONS

Population refers to a collection of all the elements or entities under study.
Parameter is a statistical constant that is used to define the population characteristics.
Statistic is a function of sample observations that are used to define the characteristics of a sample.
Sampling frame is a list of all those population units from which the sample is drawn.
Sampling is a procedure of drawing a sample from the population.
Census refers to the complete enumeration of a population.
Probability sampling is a group of sampling techniques in which population units have some known probability to be selected in the sample.
Simple random sampling is a technique of drawing a random sample from the population in such a way that every population unit has an equal chance to be included in the sample.
Stratified random sampling is a technique of drawing a random sample from the heterogeneous population after dividing it into homogeneous strata.
Systematic sampling is a technique of drawing a sample from the sequentially arranged population by first dividing it into *k* sample intervals and then choosing the first population unit from the first sample interval and every *k*th successive unit thereafter.
Cluster sampling is a technique of drawing a sample of clusters from the population by using any of the sampling techniques, that is, simple random sampling, stratified sampling, or systematic sampling.
Multistage sampling is a complex form of cluster sampling where the sample is selected in stages.
Nonprobability sampling is a group of sampling techniques in which the probability of population units to be included into the sample is not known.
Sequential sampling is a nonprobability sampling technique in which the decision about the hypothesis is taken first on the minimal number of sample and if a decision is not possible on this sample, the researcher keeps increasing the sample size in sequence till a decision about rejecting or not rejecting the null hypothesis is taken.
Convenience sampling is a nonprobability sampling technique in which the sample is selected on the basis of its availability.
Consecutive sampling is a technique of sample selection in which all subjects that are available in a single location are included in the sample.
Quota sampling is a technique of sample selection in which a fixed quota as decided by the researcher is selected from each segment of the population.
Purposive sampling is a technique of sample selection in which a researcher selects a specific sample as per his or her requirements for fulfilling a particular objective of the study.

Snowball sampling is a technique of selecting a sample on the basis of the feedback obtained from the subjects selected in the initial sample.
Primary data can be defined as the data that are collected by the researchers themselves and that have not been changed or altered by anyone.
Secondary data are those data that are obtained from any source and have already been published in some form.
Bias can be defined as the error due to preferential selection of subjects in the sample.
A ***sampling error*** can be defined as the error caused by the sampling procedure.
A ***nonsampling error*** refers to the error that results from human intervention.
Sampling distribution can be defined as the probability distribution of any statistic based on a random sample.
Standard error can be defined as the standard deviation of the sampling distribution of a statistic.

IMPORTANT FORMULAS

Standard error of sample mean

$$\sigma_{\overline{x}} = \frac{\sigma}{\sqrt{n}}$$

Standard error of sample proportion

$$\sigma_{\hat{p}} = \sqrt{\frac{pq}{n}}$$

z-Statistic for sample mean $\overline{x}$

$$z = \frac{\overline{x} - \mu}{\sigma/\sqrt{n}}$$

z-Statistic for sample proportion $\hat{p}$

$$z = \frac{\hat{p} - p}{\sqrt{\frac{pq}{n}}}$$

Model for computing sample size based on cost factor

$$C = a + nc_1 + \frac{C}{10}$$

Model for computing sample size based on accuracy factor

$$n = \frac{z_{1-\alpha/2}^2 \sigma^2}{E^2}$$

KEY TERMS

census	primary data	sampling frame
nonprobability sampling	probability sampling	sampling techniques
	sampling	secondary data

CHAPTER EXERCISE

1. Write short notes on the following:
   i. Population and sample
   ii. Parameter and statistics
   iii. Sampling frame
2. Discuss the advantage of sampling over complete census.
3. Differentiate between probability and nonprobability sampling.
4. Discuss the situations where simple random sampling, stratified sampling, and systematic sampling should be used.
5. Write short notes on the following:
   i. Cluster sampling
   ii. Multistage sampling
   iii. Sequential sampling
   iv. Snowball sampling
6. Explain different types of biases in data collection.
7. Define the following:
   i. Sampling error
   ii. Standard error
8. What are the considerations in deciding the sample size.
9. The following are the scores on vertical jump performance in centimeters obtained by 45 athletes.

36	40	32	45	46	36	32	36	50
32	45	31	40	40	38	35	40	49
37	46	30	35	32	36	31	46	48
42	32	50	46	33	40	35	32	31
36	33	48	40	45	46	45	33	38

   i. Draw a random sample of size 10 from this group (i) with replacement and (ii) without replacement.
   ii. In each case, give an estimate of the average vertical jump performance per student in the whole group.
   iii. Also, give in each case an estimate of the standard error.

10. Give an outline of a sample survey you would conduct if you need to study the attitude of college students toward physical activity in Delhi.
11. If the population consists of the scores x: 34, 35, 38, 40, 44, 45, 46, 47, graph the histogram and see its distribution. Draw all possible samples of size 2 from this population and find the mean for each sample. Graph the histogram for these sample means and compare it with the distribution of the population. Is the distribution of sample means near normal?
12. The average weight of college-going students is 180 lbs along with a standard deviation of 5.5 lbs. What is the probability that a random sample of size 45 will have an average weight of 177 lbs or more?
13. A random sample of size 49 is drawn from a population having a mean lean body weight of 150 lbs. If 69% of the time, the sample mean is less than 153 lb, what is the population standard deviation?
14. From a population whose standard deviation is 25, a random sample of size 110 is drawn. If 25% of the time, the sample mean greater than 150 is obtained, what is the mean of the population?
15. In a physical education university, authorities were interested in knowing the fitness status of their postgraduate students. A sample of 75 postgraduate students was selected at random and their fitness index was calculated. If the population mean and standard deviation of the fitness index were 67 and 20, respectively, what would be the probability that the sample mean is greater than 73?
16. The average weight of volleyball players is 170 lbs, with a standard deviation of 7 lbs. Fifteen percent of the time when a random sample of 42 volleyball players is tested, what is the value by which the sample average should exceed?
17. Average height of the students in a college is 5.7 ft., with a standard deviation of 0.5 ft. If a random sample of 46 students is taken, what is the probability that the sample will have an average height less than 5.5 ft.?
18. The mean and standard deviation of a population are 40 and 11, respectively. If a random sample of size 49 is drawn, what is the probability that the sample mean will be in the following?

    i. less than 38
    ii. more than 41
    iii. less than 44
    iv. more than 37
    v. between 36 and 42

19. The population proportion of nonvegetarian students is 0.20, and 60% of the time if a random sample is drawn from this population you get a sample proportion of vegetarian of 0.15 or more. How large was the sample drawn?

20. In a population the proportion of obese people is 0.60. In a sample of size 60, 55% of the time the sample proportion will be less than what value if samples are drawn randomly?
21. The average IQ of the students in a college is 98, with a standard deviation of 20. If a sample of 50 students is randomly selected from the college, what is the probability that the mean will be of the following?
    i. less than 92
    ii. more than 99
    iii. at least 95
    iv. between 89 and 104
22. Find the sample size required for estimating μ, given that $\sigma = 16$ and $E = 4$ at 99% confidence.
23. Determine the sample size required for estimating p for the given situations:
    i. E is within 0.1 of p, $\hat{p}$ is 0.45, and confidence level is 95%.
    ii. E is not more than 0.02, $\hat{p}$ is 0.32, and confidence level is 99%.
24. Distinguish between two-stage sampling and stratified random sampling.
25. Describe the following methods of sampling with suitable examples:
    i. Stratified sampling
    ii. Systematic sampling
    iii. Purposive sampling

ANSWERS

Check Your Progress

1. F	9. T	17. F	25. T	33. F	41. T	49. T
2. F	10. F	18. T	26. F	34. T	42. T	50. T
3. F	11. T	19. T	27. T	35. T	43. F	51. F
4. T	12. F	20. F	28. F	36. T	44. F	52. T
5. F	13. T	21. T	29. F	37. T	45. F	53. F
6. T	14. F	22. T	30. T	38. T	46. T	54. T
7. T	15. F	23. F	31. T	39. T	47. T	55. F
8. F	16. T	24. F	32. T	40. F	48. F	56. T

Practice Exercise

1.

	Male	Female
Undergraduate	1000	400
Postgraduate	300	100

2. i. $P(\bar{x} < 26.7) = 0.352$
   ii. $P(\bar{x} \geq 101.5) = 0.371$
   iii. $P(122 < \bar{x} < 124) = 0.051$
3. i. $P(\hat{p} \leq 0.31) = 0.1292$
   ii. $P(\hat{p} \leq 0.42) = 0.8790$
   iii. $P(\hat{p} \geq 0.39) = 0.2296$
   iv. $P(\hat{p} \geq 0.28) = 0.9268$
   v. $P(0.32 \leq \hat{p} \leq 0.40) = 0.6298$
4. $n = 168$
5. $n = 23$
6. $n = 28$

Chapter Exercise

9. i.

Sample without replacement:	42	40	37	32	46	49	35	50	45	31
Sample with replacement:	46	33	42	50	40	36	35	33	40	45

   ii. Mean estimate of vertical jump performance from the sample drawn without replacement = 40.7
   Mean estimate of vertical jump performance from the sample drawn with replacement = 40
   iii. SD estimate of vertical jump performance from the sample drawn without replacement = 6.8
   SD estimate of vertical jump performance from the sample drawn with replacement = 5.8

11. The distribution of population is negatively skewed, whereas the distribution of sample mean is close to a normal distribution. The following are all possible samples of size 2 along with their means.

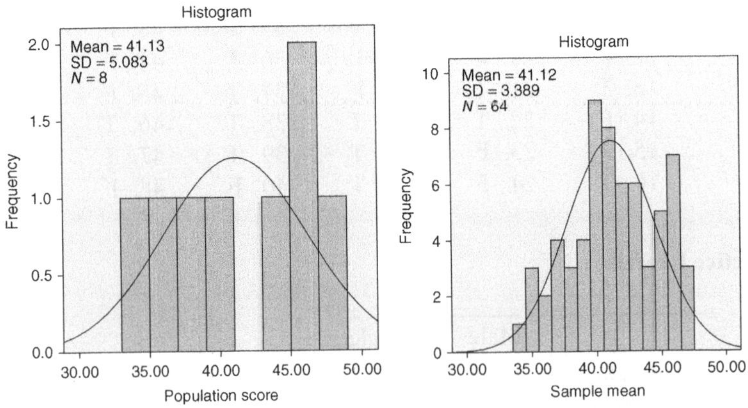

Sample of size 2		Mean	Sample of size 2		Mean	Sample of size 2		Mean
34	34	34	38	46	42	45	44	44.5
34	35	34.5	38	47	42.5	45	45	45
34	38	36	40	34	37	45	46	45.5
34	40	37	40	35	37.5	45	47	46
34	44	39	40	38	39	46	34	40
34	45	39.5	40	40	40	46	35	40.5
34	46	40	40	44	42	46	38	42
34	47	40.5	40	45	42.5	46	40	43
35	34	34.5	40	46	43	46	44	45
35	35	35	40	47	43.5	46	45	45.5
35	38	36.5	44	34	39	46	46	46
35	40	37.5	44	35	39.5	46	47	46.5
35	44	39.5	44	38	41	47	34	40.5
35	45	40	44	40	42	47	35	41
35	46	40.5	44	44	44	47	38	42.5
35	47	41	44	45	44.5	47	40	43.5
38	34	36	44	46	45	47	44	45.5
38	35	36.5	44	47	45.5	47	45	46
38	38	38	45	34	39.5	47	46	46.5
38	40	39	45	35	40	47	47	47
38	44	41	45	38	41.5			
38	45	41.5	45	40	42.5			

12. 0.7073
13. 42
14. 148.39
15. 0.0048
16. 171.12
17. 0.0034
18. i. 0.101
    ii. 0.2621
    iii. 0.9946
    iv. 0.972
    v. 0.8932
19. $n = 400$
20. 0.608
21. i. 0.0167
    ii. 0.3614
    iii. 0.8563
    iv. 0.9053

22. $n = 106$
23. i. $n \approx 10$
    ii. $n \approx 60$

FURTHER READING

1. Ards S, Chung C, Myers SL Jr. The effects of sample selection bias on racial differences in child abuse reporting. Child Abuse & Neglect 1999;23(12):1209; author reply 1211-5. PMID 9504213.
2. Bartlett JE II, Kotrlik JW, Higgins C. Organizational research: determining appropriate sample size for survey research. Information Technology, Learning, and Performance Journal 2001;19(1):43–50.
3. Berg S. Snowball Sampling–I. In: Samuel K, Campbell Read NB, Brani V, editors. Encyclopedia of Statistical Sciences. Hoboken, NJ: John Wiley and Sons, Inc.; 2006. p 7817–7821.
4. Dinov I, Christou N, Sanchez J. Central limit theorem: new SOCR applet and demonstration activity. Journal of Statistics Education (ASA) 2008;16(2).
5. Fritz S. "What is a Margin of Error?", Chapter 10. In: What is a Survey? Washington, D.C.: American Statistical Association; 2005. Accessed 2008 Jan 08.
6. Groves RM. Survey methodology. 2nd ed. USA: Wiley; 2009. ISBN 978-0-470-46546-2
7. Kish L. Survey Sampling. USA: Wiley; 1965. ISBN 0-471-48900-X.
8. Klartag B. A central limit theorem for convex sets. Inventiones Mathematicae 2007;168:91–131. DOI: 10.1007/s00222-006-0028-8 Also arXiv.
9. Kuehl RO. Design of experiments: Statistical principles of research design and analysis. 2nd ed. USA 2000. ISBN 978-0-534-36834-0
10. Lazarsfeld P, Fiske M. The "panel" as a new tool for measuring opinion. The Public Opinion Quarterly 1938;2(4):596–612.
11. Lucas SR. Beyond the existence proof: ontological conditions, epistemological implications, and in-depth interview research. Quality & Quantity 2012. DOI: 10.1007/s11135-012-9775-3.
12. Sarndal CE, Swenson B, Wretman J. J. Model assisted survey sampling. USA: Springer; 2003. ISBN 978 0 387 40620-6.
13. Scheaffer RL, Mendenhall W, Ott L. Elementary Survey Sampling. 5th ed. USA: BROOKS/COLE; 1995. ISBN 978-0-534-24342-5

7

STATISTICAL INFERENCE FOR DECISION-MAKING IN EXERCISE SCIENCE AND HEALTH

7.1 INTRODUCTION

In our day-to-day activities, we take decisions on different issues that are influenced by our experience. There are many situations in exercise science and health where decisions are required. Such decisions are taken by the coaches and players during games, administrators in organizing events, sports scientists in suggesting strategies to improve performance, and exercise scientists in prescribing fitness schedules. Whatever the area of decision-making, these decisions are taken on the basis of some observed phenomena. For instance, by looking at the activity pattern of randomly selected students in a school, one can draw a conclusion about the fitness culture among the entire student body in the school. In sports, decisions need to be taken quickly by the players during matches. For instance, in badminton, a player needs to return the shuttle served by the opponent. The decision regarding how to play the shuttle before the opponent begins to move is usually taken in a fraction of a second. The decision of the player is governed by his earlier experience. Although there is no standard way of making the decision, the process of decision-making can be structured by using certain scientific principles. The procedure of decision-making in inferring population characteristics on the basis of sample observations is known as *statistical inference*. Statistical inference can be broadly classified into two categories: theory of estimation and testing of hypothesis. These topics are discussed in detail in this chapter.

Statistics for Exercise Science and Health with Microsoft® Office Excel®, First Edition. J. P. Verma.

7.2 THEORY OF ESTIMATION

Theory of estimation deals with estimating population characteristics on the basis of sample observations. No doubt, studying every individual in a population provides a true picture of its characteristics. However, in most of the situations, the population is so large that it is impossible to investigate the entire population because of economical and timeliness considerations. Even if there are no such constraints, it is not advisable to study the whole population because it results in large nonresponse errors. Efficiency is accrued when the entire population is not included.

> **FACTS TO KNOW**
>
> Sample variance S^2 is an unbiased estimator of the population variance σ^2 whereas S is not

As a result of large nonresponse errors in the population study, the researcher always prefers to opt for a sample. In most situations, complete information on the population units may not be available, and therefore one may resort to sample study only. Consider a study in which it is required to know the fitness status of children in the age category of 14–16 years in a given state. If the researcher decides to draw a sample of children from different schools in the state, he will only be considering the children who study in some or the other school. What about those children who do not go to any of the schools? In such a situation, the researcher may not have a complete list of the population units; therefore, even if one decides to study the entire population it is not possible. Thus, invariably in all situations, a sample is used to study the population characteristics.

In sample studies, the most important issue is the reliability of the findings. This can be resolved to some extent by drawing a representative sample from the population of interest by using a proper sampling plan. Before investigating this issue further, let us see what parameters are usually required to know the nature of any population. Parameters such as mean, variance, and proportions of the population are usually estimated on the basis of the sample observations. Population parameters are estimated by an estimator. An estimator is a function of sample observation that gives the correct estimate of the population parameter. There may be a number of estimators that can estimate a population's characteristics, but the best estimator is the one that possesses all the characteristics of a good estimator. Estimation procedure can further be classified into two categories, namely, *point estimation* and *interval estimation*, depending on the way the population parameter is estimated.

7.3 POINT ESTIMATION

If a single value of the population parameter is estimated on the basis of a sample, then the procedure is known as point estimation. For instance, let us define all the intervarsity basketball players in the state as the population. To estimate their height, a random sample of basketball players is drawn. The mean height of this sample can be used to estimate the height of the players in the population. Here, sample mean becomes an estimator for estimating the population mean. Similarly, the median and mode can also be used as a point estimator for estimating the population mean. It is important to know which of these measures best represent the population mean and under what situation. Since sample mean is very frequently used to estimate the population mean, it has to be seen whether it possesses all the required characteristics of a good estimator. Similarly, to estimate population variance and population proportion, sample variance and sample proportion are used, respectively, as estimators. These estimators are computed from the sample values by using the following formulas:

$$\text{Estimator of population mean:}\quad \bar{x} = \frac{\sum x}{n} \tag{7.1}$$

$$\text{Estimator of population variance:}\quad s^2 = \frac{1}{n-1}\sum (x-\bar{x})^2 \tag{7.2}$$

where

n = the sample size,
x = the sample observations, and
$\bar{x}$ = the sample mean.

$$\text{Estimator of population proportion:}\quad \hat{p} = \frac{x}{n} \tag{7.3}$$

where

x = the frequency of occurrence of an attribute,
n = the number of total cases.

7.4 CHARACTERISTICS OF A GOOD ESTIMATOR

To estimate any population parameter, there can be many estimators. However, the best estimator is the one that is very close to the population parameter. An estimator is suitable if it possesses all the characteristics of a good estimator, namely, unbiasedness, consistency, efficiency, and sufficiency. Let us see what these characteristics are.

7.4.1 Unbiasedness

This property states that an average value of an estimator, which is used for estimating the population parameter, is equal to the population parameter. In estimating the population mean, the sample mean is an unbiased estimator while the median and mode are not.

Thus,

$$E(\overline{x}) = \mu \tag{7.4}$$

Similarly, sample variance is an unbiased estimator of the population variance because

$$E(s^2) = \sigma^2 \tag{7.5}$$

Since expected values of the sample mean and sample variance are equal to the population mean and population variance, respectively, these are known as unbiased estimators. Readers are advised to note that although sample variance is an unbiased estimate of the population variance, sample standard deviation (SD) is not an unbiased estimate of the population SD.

7.4.2 Consistency

This property indicates that as the sample size increases, the value of the estimator approaches the population parameter. The sample mean is a consistent estimator of population mean; hence,

$$\overline{x} \rightarrow \mu \text{ as } n \rightarrow \infty$$

7.4.3 Efficiency

An estimator is said to be efficient if its value does not differ much in different samples drawn from the same population. The best estimator would be the one that will have the least fluctuation in value in different samples drawn randomly from the same population. Out of the three estimators, mean, median, and mode, the mean has the least variance and is hence an efficient estimator.

7.4.4 Sufficiency

An estimator is said to be sufficient if it extracts all the information that is contained in the sample about the parameter. Since sample mean uses all the sample values in its computation while the mode and median do not, the sample mean is a sufficient estimator. Sufficiency is the most important property of an estimator.

7.5 THE *t*-DISTRIBUTION

The *t*-distribution was developed by the British statistician William S. Gosset. While publishing his first work on *t*-test, he used the pen name "Student." Therefore, the *t*-test is sometimes known as Student's *t*-test. The *t*-distribution is used to infer the population mean when the population SD is unknown and the distribution of the population is normal. The *t*-statistic is computed by

$$t = \frac{\overline{x} - \mu}{\frac{s}{\sqrt{n}}} \tag{7.6}$$

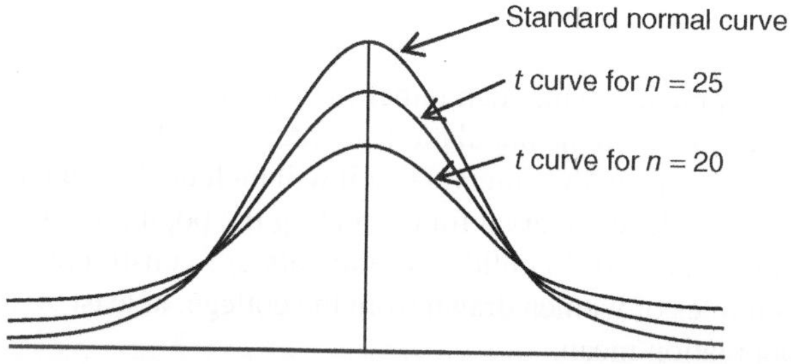

Figure 7.1 Comparison of the standard normal curve and t-distribution.

This formula is similar to that of the z-statistic, but the distribution takes different values. The t-table shown in Table A.7 in the appendix represents the probability distribution values and is useful for finding the value of t corresponding to different probability values in the tail. One of the main assumptions in using the t-statistic for testing of hypothesis is that the population is normally distributed. If the population distribution is not normal, then some nonparametric test may be used.

The t-distribution is a family of distributions because for different sample sizes, the shape of the t-distribution is different, as shown in Figure 7.1. The probability curve of the t-distribution is symmetrical at about $t=0$. By looking at the distribution in Figure 7.1, it is clear that the means of the t-distribution and the normal distribution are the same, but their variances differ. In fact, the variance of the t-distribution is more than that of the standard normal distribution; thus, the t-distribution is more flat on the top in comparison to the normal distribution. The most important feature of the t-distribution is that its shape differs at different degrees of freedom. Figure 7.1 shows that the t-distribution with 25 degrees of freedom is very close to the normal distribution, and as the sample size decreases the curve becomes more and more flat. However, as the sample size increases by 30 or more, it merges with the z-distribution. Since the shape of the t-distribution keeps changing as the sample size changes, the critical value of t also changes with the change in the sample size for a particular level of significance.

Since there are a large number of t-distributions corresponding to different sample sizes, a combined t-table has been presented for different degrees of freedom, showing the value of t corresponding to select probabilities in the tail. In the table, each line represents the t-values in the distribution corresponding to a particular degree of freedom. To find the t-value, one needs to know the degrees of freedom and the probability in the tail of the distribution.

7.6 INTERVAL ESTIMATION

In interval estimation, an exact value of the population parameter is not estimated; rather, a range is computed, which is supposed to include the population parameter with some degree of confidence. For instance, to estimate the flexibility of college-going women, a random sample of college-going women may be tested for their flexibility by using the sit and reach test. If the average flexibility of the women in the sample is 9.5 in., then rather than saying that the same would be the flexibility of the women in the population, an interval is obtained, say 9–10 in., and a confidence is attached to this interval that it will include the population flexibility. Thus, if a 90% confidence interval for estimating the population mean is obtained, it simply means that if 100 confidence intervals are constructed on the basis of 100 random samples of women drawn from the college, at least 90 intervals would include the population mean.

There are two issues with the confidence intervals. Firstly, why do we obtain confidence intervals instead of point estimates? Secondly, how do we construct these confidence limits and what is the theory that supports such confidence limits?

To answer the first issue, let us consider a study in which 25 women athletes were tested for their fat percentage as shown below:

Fat Percentage of the Women Athletes												
16	15	18	21	25	21	20	18	19	17	19	22	24
15	18	21	24	23	17	16	18	22	23	17	19	
Mean fat% = 19.52												

Let the three random samples of size 6 be drawn from this population and their mean fat percentage be computed as follows:

	Sample I			Sample II			Sample III		
	16	25	22	18	17	21	22	23	21
	18	25	22	20	21	19	25	19	24
Mean		21.33			19.33			22.33	

Now, to estimate the mean fat percentage of the population, 19.52, all the three samples provide different estimates, that is, 21.33, 19.33, and 22.33 percentages. In a real situation, none of these estimates would be equal to the population mean. These estimates would, most of the time, vary around the population mean. Thus, it may be more logical to construct an interval that will include the population mean with some degree of confidence.

The next question is, how to construct the confidence interval for a given population parameter. The answer to this question can be obtained by using the central limit theorem. As per the central limit theorem, if a random sample is drawn from a population having mean μ and variance σ^2, which may or may not be normal, then the distribution of sample mean tends to be normal with mean μ and variance σ^2/n, provided the sample is sufficiently large and drawn randomly from the population. As the sample size increases, the distribution of sample means becomes

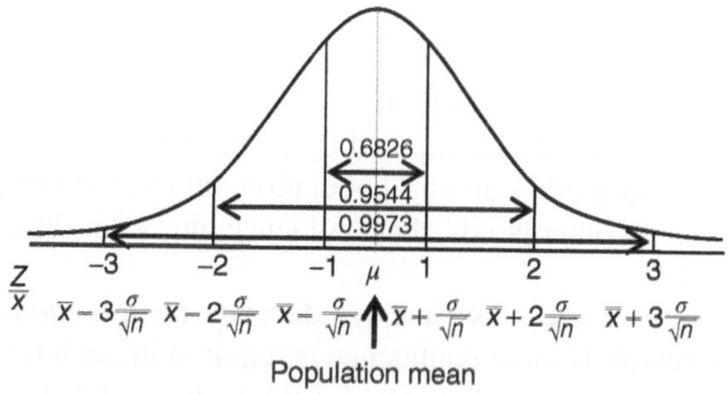

Figure 7.2 Normal distribution of the sample mean.

closer and closer to a normal distribution. Since for a sufficiently large sample the sample mean ($\bar{x}$) follows a normal distribution, the normal curve area property can be used to estimate the population mean on the basis of the sample mean. Let us consider the normal distribution of the sample mean as shown in Figure 7.2.

Since SD of the sample mean is the standard error of the mean and is given by

$$\mathrm{SE}(\bar{x}) = \frac{\sigma}{\sqrt{n}} \tag{7.7}$$

as per the normal distribution, there is 68.26% chance that the 1σ limit of the sample mean, that is,

$$\bar{x} - \frac{\sigma}{\sqrt{n}} \text{ to } \bar{x} + \frac{\sigma}{\sqrt{n}}$$

will include the population mean.

This means that if 100 such confidence intervals are constructed, then at least 68 intervals shall include the population mean. Similarly, 2σ and 3σ limits can be used to construct 95.44% and 99.73% confidence limits, respectively.

7.6.1 Factors That Affect the Confidence Interval

In the case of a large sample, the general formula for computing confidence interval for the population mean is given by

$$\bar{x} \pm Z_{\alpha/2}\mathrm{SE}(\bar{x}) \tag{7.8}$$

or

$$\bar{x} \pm Z_{\alpha/2}\frac{\sigma}{\sqrt{n}} \tag{7.9}$$

Looking at formula (7.9), it is clear that the confidence interval depends on the sample size n. As the sample size increases, the width of the confidence interval decreases. In other words, the confidence interval is inversely proportional to the square root of the sample size. If the sample size equals the population size, the sample mean and population mean will be the same, and in that case, the width of the confidence interval will become zero.

Since confidence interval is computed by using the value of σ in the formula (7.9), the more the variability among population values, the larger would be the confidence interval. In other words, the confidence interval is directly proportional to the *population* SD.

Lastly, the width of the class interval depends on the *choice of confidence* required in the interval. If more confidence is required in the interval, the value of $z_{\alpha/2}$ will become larger, which ultimately increases the confidence interval.

7.6.2 Confidence Intervals for Population Mean

Constructing a confidence interval for the population mean depends on whether the sample is large or small and whether the population SD is known or unknown. These cases have been discussed separately.

Case 1: Sample is large ($n \geq 30$) or population SD is known Most of the times, estimating the population mean is useful in exercise science and health research. For example, a community coach might want to estimate the average height of the basketball players in the city. If there are a large number of basketball players, direct calculation of the mean height may be practically impossible. Instead, a random sample of basketball players can be drawn, and the sample mean height may be used to estimate the population mean. Consider that a big fitness company opens up a new facility of sauna bath for its customers, and they do not know how much this facility would be used in a week. By taking a random sample of clients and calculating the mean hours the facility is proposed to be used by them per week, the company can estimate the average usage per week.

As per the central limit theorem, if a random sample of size n is drawn from the population having mean μ and SD σ, then the sampling distribution of the sample mean $\bar{x}$ is approximately normally distributed with mean μ and SD $\sigma/\sqrt{n}$, provided the sample is sufficiently large ($n \geq 30$) irrespective of the shape of the population distribution. If the population is normally distributed, then the sampling distribution of the sample mean $\bar{x}$ will always be normal even for a small sample size, provided the population SD is known. In the case of a large sample, even if the population SD is not known, the distribution of the sample mean would still be normal. Since for large samples, sample mean follows a normal distribution with SD $\sigma/\sqrt{n}$, the normal distribution property can be used to construct the confidence interval of the population mean. The general formula is given by

$$\bar{x} \pm Z_{\alpha/2}\text{SE}(\bar{x}) \tag{7.10}$$

or

$$\bar{x} \pm Z_{\alpha/2}\frac{\sigma}{\sqrt{n}} \tag{7.11}$$

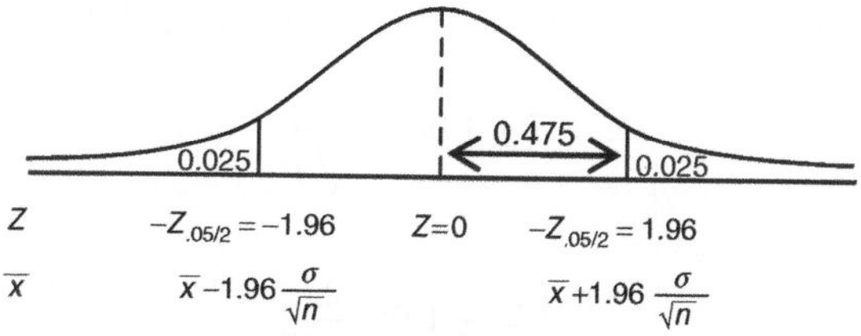

Figure 7.3 Sampling distribution of the sample mean.

where α is the error in the confidence interval. By deciding the error in the confidence limits, the desired confidence interval can be constructed by using the formula.

Thus, if the sample size is large ($n \geq 30$) or the population SD is known, in both the cases a 95% confidence interval for the population mean can be obtained by

$$\bar{x} \pm Z_{0.05/2}\frac{\sigma}{\sqrt{n}} \tag{7.12}$$

as shown in Figure 7.3. Since $Z_{0.05/2}$=1.96, the 95% confidence intervals for the population mean will become

$$\bar{x} \pm 1.96\frac{\sigma}{\sqrt{n}}$$

Similarly, 99% confidence limits for the population mean can be obtained by

$$\bar{x} \pm 2.58\frac{\sigma}{\sqrt{n}}$$

Example 7.1 A random sample of 35 athletes has a mean weight of 144 lb. Find the 95% confidence interval for the population mean weight of the athletes if the population SD is 22.

Solution: Since the population SD is known and the sample is large ($n \geq 30$), the 95% confidence interval for the population mean can be obtained by

$$\bar{x} \pm z_{0.05/2}\frac{\sigma}{\sqrt{n}}$$

Since it is required to find the 95% confidence interval, the critical region will lie in both the tails as shown in the figure. The area between the mean and the critical value that separates the critical region in both the tails is 0.475. By using this area and Table A.4, the critical value of z can be obtained as

$$z_{0.05/2} = 1.96$$

given that $n = 35$, $\bar{x} = 144$, and $\sigma = 22$.

Substituting these values, the 95% confidence interval for the population mean μ shall be

$$\bar{x} \pm 1.96 \times \frac{\sigma}{\sqrt{n}}$$

or

$$144 \pm 1.96 \frac{22}{\sqrt{35}}$$

or

$$144 \pm 7.28$$

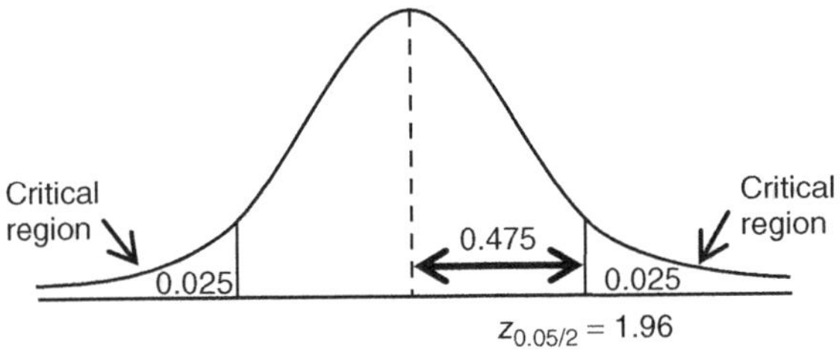

Thus, 95% confidence intervals for the population mean would be $(144 - 7.28$ to $144 + 7.28)$ or (136.72 to 151.28).

Case 2: The sample is small ($n < 30$) and population SD is not known In Case I, we have seen how to construct the confidence interval for estimating population mean by using the sample mean when the population SD is known or the sample is large. In most of the situations, while estimating population mean, the population SD is not known; therefore, in such situations, the methods used in Case I cannot be used. Consider a situation where a health scientist is interested in estimating the average fat percentage of the women employees in a bank. The bank is enormous in size, and a large number of employees may be women. To estimate the average fat percentage, the researcher has to draw a sample of women employees. Further, it is more likely that the population SD of the fat percentage may be unknown. In such a situation, the population mean fat percentage of the women employees may be estimated by constructing the confidence interval using the mean and standard deviation of the sample. Let us consider another situation in which an exercise scientist is interested in estimating the mean physical fitness index (PFI) of the students in a college but does not have any idea about the population SD. He will have to construct the confidence interval on the basis of the sample mean and sample SD.

Thus, in all situations where population SD is not known, the t-distribution is used to construct the confidence interval for estimating the population mean by using the sample mean and sample SD.

If a random sample of size n (<30) is drawn from a normal population where the population SD is not known, then the sampling distribution of the sample mean follows a t-distribution with mean μ and standard error $s/\sqrt{n}$, where s is the sample SD.

By using the t-distribution, the 95% confidence interval for the sample mean can be computed by the following formula:

$$\bar{x} \pm t_{0.05/2}(n-1)\mathrm{SE}(\bar{x}) \tag{7.13}$$

or

$$\bar{x} \pm t_{0.05/2}(n-1)\frac{s}{\sqrt{n}} \tag{7.14}$$

Similarly, 99% confidence limits of the sample mean would be obtained as

$$\bar{x} \pm t_{0.01/2}(n-1)\frac{s}{\sqrt{n}} \tag{7.15}$$

where the value of t is obtained from Table A.7 at the given level of significance, with $n-1$ degrees of freedom.

Example 7.2 A random sample of 20 athletes was selected and their heights were measured in centimeters. If the mean and SD of the sample were 171 and 5 cm, respectively, construct (i) 80% and (ii) 90% confidence limits for estimating the populations, mean height.

Solution:

i. As the population SD is unknown and the sample is small ($n < 30$), the 80% confidence interval for the mean can be obtained by

$$\bar{x} \pm t_{0.20/2}(19)\frac{s}{\sqrt{n}}$$

In finding the 80% confidence interval, the critical region will lie in both the tails as shown in the figure. The area between the mean and the critical value that separates the critical region in both the tails is 0.40. By using Table A.7, the critical value of t at 19 degrees of freedom can be obtained as

$$t_{0.20/2}(19) = 1.328$$

given that $n = 20$, $\bar{x} = 171$, and $s = 5$.

Substituting these values, the 80% confidence interval for the population mean μ shall be

$$\bar{x} \pm 1.328 \times \frac{s}{\sqrt{n}}$$

or

$$171 \pm 1.328 \frac{5}{\sqrt{20}}$$

or

$$171 \pm 1.48$$

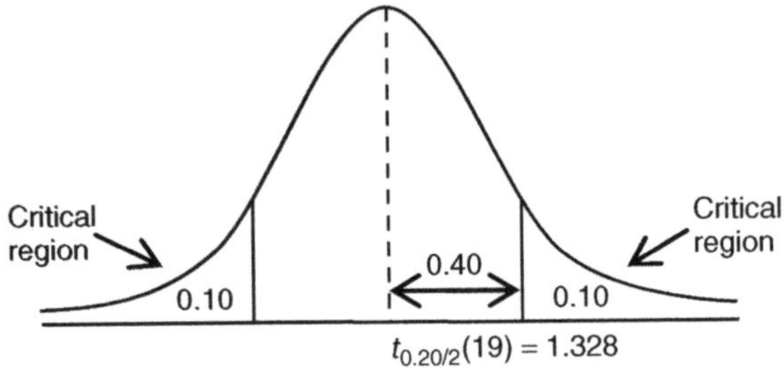

Thus, 80% confidence intervals for the population mean height would be (171 − 1.48 to 171 + 1.48) or (169.52 to 172.48).

ii. The 90% confidence interval for the population mean, when the population SD is unknown and sample is small ($n < 30$), is given by

$$\bar{x} \pm t_{0.10/2}(19) \frac{s}{\sqrt{n}}$$

In this case, the critical region shall be divided in both the tails as shown in the figure. The critical value of t with 19 degrees of freedom at significance level 0.10 can be obtained by using Table A.7.

$$t_{0.10/2}(19) = 1.729$$

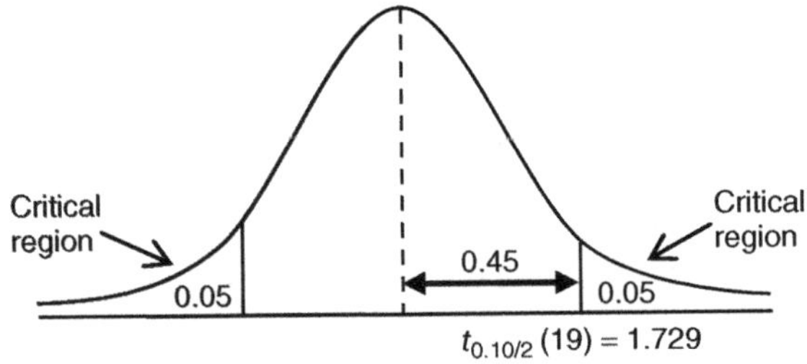

given that $n = 20$, $\bar{x} = 171$, and $s = 5$.

Substituting these values, the 90% confidence interval for population mean μ shall be

$$\bar{x} \pm 1.729 \times \frac{s}{\sqrt{n}}$$

or

$$171 \pm 1.729\frac{5}{\sqrt{20}}$$

or

$$171 \pm 1.93$$

Thus, the 90% confidence interval for the population mean height would be (171 − 1.93 to 171 + 1.93) or (169.07 to 172.93).

Example 7.3 The following are the push-up performance of the physically active students of a college:

x:	12	15	10	20	18	16	18	15	14	9	11

Assuming that the push-up performance is normally distributed, compute the 99% confidence interval to estimate the population mean.

Solution:

Since the population SD is unknown and sample size is small ($n < 30$), the 99% confidence interval for the mean can be obtained by

$$\bar{x} \pm t_{0.01/2}(10)\frac{s}{\sqrt{n}}$$

In finding the 99% confidence interval, the critical region will lie in both the tails as shown in the figure. The critical value of t with 10 degrees of freedom can be obtained by using Table A.7.

$$t_{0.01/2}(10) = 3.169$$

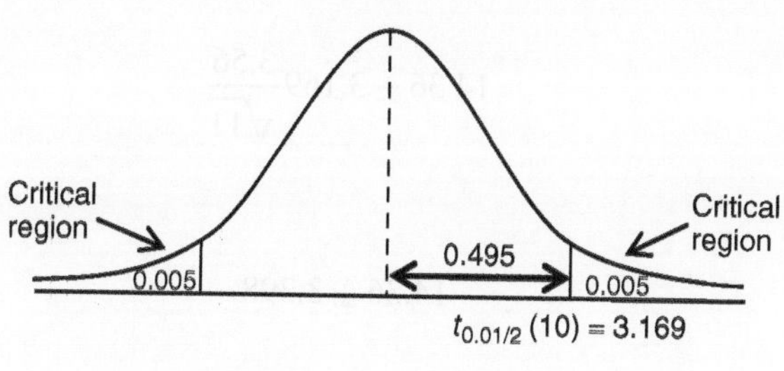

In order to compute the confidence interval, the sample mean and sample SD need to be computed first.

Computation of Mean and SD

x	x^2
12	144
15	225
10	100
20	400
18	324
16	256
18	324
15	225
14	196
9	81
11	121
$\sum x = 158$	$\sum x^2 = 2396$

$$\bar{x} = \frac{\sum x}{n} = \frac{158}{11} = 14.36$$

$$s = \sqrt{\frac{\sum x^2}{n-1} - \frac{\left(\sum x\right)^2}{n(n-1)}} = \sqrt{\frac{2396}{10} - \frac{158^2}{11 \times 10}} = 3.56$$

Since the sample size n is 11, substituting these values the 99% confidence interval for the population mean μ shall be

$$\bar{x} \pm 3.169 \times \frac{s}{\sqrt{n}}$$

or

$$14.36 \pm 3.169 \frac{3.56}{\sqrt{11}}$$

or

$$14.36 \pm 3.398$$

Thus, the 99% confidence interval for the population mean push-up would be (14.36 − 3.398 to 14.36 + 3.398) or (11 to 18).

7.6.3 Confidence Intervals for Population Proportion

If x is a binomial variate, the occurrence of which is a success and nonoccurrence is a failure, then the sample proportion of success $\widehat{p}$ follows a binomial distribution. However, if the sample is large, as per the central limit theorem the distribution of the sample proportion $\widehat{p}$ follows a normal distribution with mean p and SD $pq/\sqrt{n}$, where p is the population proportion and $q=1-p$. Even if the sample size is less than 30, the distribution of sample proportion $\widehat{p}$ follows a normal distribution provided $n \cdot \widehat{p} \geq 5$ and $n \cdot \widehat{q} \geq 5$.

Thus, if $\widehat{p}$ is the sample proportion, then

$$Z = \frac{\widehat{p} - p}{\sqrt{\dfrac{p \times q}{n}}} \text{ is distributed as } N(0, 1) \tag{7.16}$$

In general, the confidence interval for the population proportion with an α level of error is given by

$$\widehat{p} \pm z_{\alpha/2}\sqrt{\frac{p \times q}{n}} \tag{7.17}$$

If the population proportion p is not known, it may be estimated by $\widehat{p}$.

Thus, the 95% confidence interval for the population proportion can be obtained by computing the limits

$$\widehat{p} \pm 1.96\sqrt{\frac{\widehat{p} \times \widehat{q}}{n}}$$

The 99% confidence interval for the population proportion can be obtained by computing the limits

$$\widehat{p} \pm 2.58\sqrt{\frac{\widehat{p} \times \widehat{q}}{n}}$$

Example 7.4 On a particular day, out of 90 women visiting the health center 30% had an injury. Construct 95% and 99% confidence limits for the population proportion of women visiting the health center and having injuries.

Solution: Since the proportion of injuries reported $(\widehat{p})=0.3$, $q=0.7$, given that $n=90$ then 95% confidence limits for the population proportion is given by

$$\widehat{p} \pm z_{0.05/2}\sqrt{\frac{\widehat{p} \times \widehat{q}}{n}}$$

Since for a large sample proportion, $\widehat{p}$ follows a normal distribution, the critical value of z for 95% confidence limits from Table A.4 is

$$z_{0.05/2} = 1.96$$

Substituting the values, the confidence interval shall be

$$0.3 \pm 1.96 \times \sqrt{\frac{0.3 \times 0.7}{90}}$$

or

$$0.3 \pm 0.09$$

Thus, 95% confidence limits for the population proportion of the women reporting injuries are 0.21 to 0.39.

Similarly, 99% confidence limits for the population proportion are given by

$$\hat{p} \pm z_{0.01/2}\sqrt{\frac{\hat{p} \times \hat{q}}{n}}$$

The critical value of z for the 99% confidence limits from Table A.4 is

$$z_{0.01/2} = 2.58$$

Substituting the values, we get

$$0.3 \pm 2.58 \times \sqrt{\frac{0.3 \times 0.7}{90}}$$

or

$$0.3 \pm 0.125$$

Thus, 99% confidence limits for the population proportion of the women reporting injuries are 0.175 to 0.425.

Check Your Progress

Note: Tick the correct answer by using the sign ($\surd$).

	True	False
1. Parameters refer to the characteristics of a population.	-	-
2. An estimator is used to estimate the sample proportion from the sample observations.	-	-
3. The value of a consistent estimator approaches the value of the population parameter if the sample size increases.	-	-

4.	Population mean can be estimated by any of the estimators.	-	-
5.	Confidence interval increases if the variability in population decreases.	-	-
6.	An estimator is sufficient if it extracts all the information that is contained in the population about the sample.	-	-
7.	An estimator is good if it is unbiased.	-	-
8.	The expected value of a variable is equivalent to its mean value.	-	-
9.	Width of the class interval increases if the confidence required in the interval decreases.	-	-
10.	Interval estimation is meaningless if no confidence is attached to it.	-	-
11.	Theory of estimation refers to inferring sample characteristics.	-	-
12.	Sample SD is the unbiased estimator of the population SD.	-	-
13.	Sample mean is used to estimate the population proportion.	-	-
14.	In a small sample, the confidence interval of the mean is constructed by taking the degrees of freedom of t as $n-1$ irrespective of whether 95% or 99% confidence is required.	-	-
15.	The standard error of a sample mean is given by $\sigma/\sqrt{n}$.	-	-
16.	In case of a large sample, 95% confidence limits of the mean are obtained by taking the value of z as 2.	-	-
17.	An estimator is computed by the sample observations.	-	-
18.	An estimator is said to be the best if its value is equal to the sample statistic.	-	-
19.	In constructing the confidence limits of population mean, the value of α is divided in both the tails.	-	-
20.	The confidence interval is directly proportional to the population SD.	-	-
21.	A sample is said to be small if $n \leq 30$.	-	-
22.	The value of z can be used to construct the confidence interval of mean if the sample is large irrespective of whether the population SD is known or unknown.	-	-

23.	The Z-value can be used to construct the confidence interval of the population mean even if the sample is small, provided the population is normally distributed and the population SD is known.	-	-
24.	So long as the sample is small ($n<30$), the t-distribution can be used in constructing the confidence interval of population mean irrespective of the distribution of population.	-	-
25.	The t-distribution is a family of distributions.	-	-
26.	Sample variance is the unbiased estimator of the population variance.	-	-
27.	An efficient estimator has nothing to do with the consistency of its values in different samples drawn from the same population.	-	-
28.	In constructing the 99% confidence interval of population mean in a small sample, the value of $\alpha=0.01$ would lie in one tail only.	-	-
29.	The z-test can be used to construct confidence intervals for the population proportion if the sample size is sufficiently large so that $n\bar{p} < 5$.	-	-

PRACTICE EXERCISE

1. Construct 95% confidence intervals for the population mean by using the following sample information:

$$n = 49, \bar{x} = 15.7, \sigma = 9.8$$

2. A random sample of 16 women was tested for their vital capacity. If the mean and SD of the sample are 3.5 and 0.3 l, respectively, compute a 99% confidence interval for the population mean.
3. The mean muscular strength score of a random sample of 81 athletes was found to be 152 with an SD of 35. Construct a 99% confidence interval for the population mean. What size of the sample is required to estimate the mean within 6 of the true mean with the 99% confidence?
4. On a particular day, 110 persons attended the fitness program in a health park, out of which 45 were women. Construct 95% and 99% confidence limits for the population proportion of women visiting the health park for the exercise program.

5. In a random sample of 120 students in a college, 55 students are nonvegetarians. Use this information to calculate a 90% confidence interval of the population proportion. As the level of confidence increases and the other sample information remains unchanged, what happens to the confidence interval?

7.7 TESTING OF HYPOTHESIS

Testing of hypothesis is a procedure of decision-making about the population parameter(s) on the basis of sample information. It deals with testing some claim about the population parameter. For instance, if a coach claims that the average vertical jump performance of all the athletes in the college is 1.2 m, this assumption can be tested by taking a random sample of athletes and testing their performance on vertical jump. If the sample mean comes out to be 1.0 m, the issue is whether the difference of 0.2 m can be considered to be large enough to reject the claim of the coach or this difference is due to sampling error only. The procedure in testing of hypothesis uses the theory of statistical distribution to assess how much confidence the researcher has in rejecting or accepting the claim. A hypothesis is an assertion or claim about the population characteristic, which a researcher desires to verify. The choice of statistical test for testing a hypothesis depends on whether the hypothesis is parametric or nonparametric. A hypothesis is said to be parametric if parameters such as mean, proportion, or variance are used to construct it. The examples of parametric hypotheses are whether the average height of the nation basketball players is 6.1 ft. or the average weight of the women power lifters in the interuniversity is 160 lb. On the other hand, in nonparametric hypotheses, no such parameters are used. For instance, hypotheses such as basketball team A has more graceful movement in comparison to team B or boys are more imaginative than girls are known as nonparametric hypotheses. This chapter deals with only parametric hypothesis, whereas testing of nonparametric hypotheses are discussed in Chapters 10 and 11.

FACTS TO KNOW

To use any parametric test, the distribution of the population must be normal

FACTS TO KNOW

Null hypothesis is meant for rejection. The researcher intends to test its rejection in favor of the alternative hypothesis

In this chapter, testing of hypotheses for the population mean, population proportion, and population variance is discussed for single population and two populations only. A detail discussion is made to test various hypotheses by using Z, t, F, and χ^2 tests later in this chapter.

7.8 TYPES OF HYPOTHESIS

A hypothesis is an assumption, conjecture, or statement about certain things. It is an educated guess or proposition about some facts or natural phenomena. Hypotheses are framed for testing its correctness. The hypotheses can be scientific or statistical depending on how it is tested. If a hypothesis is tested by using some scientific investigations, then it is known as scientific hypothesis. For example, the hypotheses such as life exists on the planet, spicy food may cause pimples, or ultraviolet light may cause cancer are all examples of scientific hypotheses. On the other hand, if a hypothesis about some population parameter can be tested on the basis of sample information, then it is known as statistical hypothesis. To qualify a hypothesis to be a statistical hypothesis, one must be able to define the population, draw a sample, and test the sample for testing the hypothesis. However, in statistics, we are only concerned about the statistical hypothesis that can be tested on the basis of the sample data. As in this text only statistical hypotheses are discussed, liberty has been taken to call them hypotheses. In other words, hypothesis in this text refers to only statistical hypothesis.

A hypothesis is denoted by H. It can be written as H: $\mu = 15$. This simply means that population mean is equal to 15. Hypotheses are framed for testing population parameters and are tested on the basis of a random sample drawn from the population. A hypothesis can be simple or composite depending on whether it specifies all the parameters of the distribution . For instance, if the distribution of scores is normally distributed with an SD σ^2, then the hypothesis, H: $\mu = 15$ is a simple hypothesis whereas hypotheses such as H: $\mu \neq 15$, H: $\mu > 15$, or H: $\mu < 15$ are composite hypotheses. While testing the hypothesis for some population parameter, a researcher needs to frame two different types of hypothesis, namely, null hypothesis and alternative hypothesis.

7.8.1 Null Hypothesis

Null hypothesis can be defined as the hypothesis of no difference. In a single-group testing for the standing long jump performance, the null hypothesis might be H_0: $\mu = 82$. This means that the researcher is interested in verifying whether mean performance of long jump of a given population is equal to the specified value of 82 in. Two groups testing the null hypothesis refer to no difference between the two-group means and is written as H_0: $\mu_1 = \mu_2$. Corresponding to every null hypothesis, an alternative hypothesis is also constructed. Usually, the alternative hypothesis is of interest to the researcher and null hypothesis is used to test it. If on the basis of sample data null hypothesis is rejected, then the alternative hypothesis is accepted. Thus, null hypothesis is a via media for testing an alternative hypothesis. Another reason for constructing the null hypothesis is that under this assumption only the test statistic follows a particular distribution. The null hypothesis is never proved. It is made for rejection; therefore, on the basis of the sample data a researcher either rejects or fails to reject the null hypothesis.

7.8.2 Alternative Hypothesis

Alternative hypothesis is also known as *research hypothesis.* It is of interest to the researcher. A researcher first develops a research hypothesis, which is tested on the basis of the sample data or the results obtained in an experimental study. After constructing the alternative hypothesis, a null hypothesis is constructed. In fact, a researcher is required to develop both null and research hypotheses. If the null hypothesis is rejected, the research hypothesis is automatically accepted. The alternative hypothesis is denoted by H_1. Further, an alternative hypothesis may either be unidirectional or bidirectional. For instance, the researcher may frame a research hypothesis such as the average sit-ups performance of the athletes is more than 45(H_1: $\mu > 45$) or the average push-up performance of the women athletes is not equal to 25($H_1 : \mu \neq 25$). Testing of research hypothesis is based on proof of contradiction, that is, it is accepted only when the null hypothesis is rejected. Non-rejection of the null hypothesis leads to nonacceptance of the research hypothesis.

7.9 TEST STATISTIC

A test statistic may be considered as a random variable x whose value is tested against the critical value for testing the null hypothesis. It is a function of sample observations. A test statistic follows a particular sampling distribution under the assumption of null hypothesis, and on the basis of this distribution only decision about rejecting or not rejecting the null hypothesis is taken. A test statistic is computed by the following generalized formula for testing a population parameter:

$$\text{Test statistic} = \frac{\text{Statistic} - E(\text{Statistic})}{\text{SE(Statistic)}} \tag{7.18}$$

where statistic is the sample characteristic, E(statistic) is the expected value of the statistic and is equal to the population parameter, and SE(statistic) is the standard error of the statistic. In the case of a large sample ($n \geq 30$), most of the test statistic follows a normal distribution. This characteristic of the test statistic is due to the central limit theorem. For instance, in the case of a large sample, the test statistic z for testing the hypothesis concerning the population mean follows a standard normal distribution.

$$z = \frac{\bar{x} - E(\bar{x})}{\text{SE}(\bar{x})} = \frac{\bar{x} - \mu}{\sigma/\sqrt{n}} \sim N(0, 1) \tag{7.19}$$

In fact, a test statistic tells us how much sample statistic differs from the population parameter. Thus, in testing the hypothesis concerning population mean, the higher the value of test statistic z, the larger is the difference between the sample and the population mean. In other words, the larger the value of test statistic z, the more confident we are in saying that the sample mean differs from the population mean.

7.10 CONCEPT USED IN HYPOTHESIS TESTING

After constructing the research and null hypotheses, they are tested by using a test statistic, which follows certain known distributions under the assumption that the null hypothesis is true. Usually, the test statistics z, t, and F are used for testing parametric hypotheses, and under the assumption of null hypothesis these statistics follow z, t, and F distributions, respectively. The statistics z and t are used for testing the hypotheses concerning population mean, whereas F-statistic is used for population variance.

To show the concept in testing a null hypothesis, H_0: $\mu = 82$, let us assume that a random sample is drawn from a population that has mean μ and SD σ. If the sample is large ($n \geq 30$), then as per the central limit theorem the sample mean ($\bar{x}$) follows a normal distribution with mean μ and SD $\sigma/\sqrt{n}$. Since the sample mean ($\bar{x}$) follows a normal distribution, the standard normal variate, z, will also follow a standard normal distribution:

$$z = \frac{\bar{x} - \mu}{\sigma/\sqrt{n}} \sim N(0, 1) \tag{7.20}$$

Now, if the sample is drawn from a population having mean 82 (assuming null hypothesis is true), then by using the normal curve area property one can be 95.44% confident that the difference between the sample mean $\bar{x}$ and the population mean 82 is only due to sampling error so long as the sample mean $\bar{x}$ lies between $\bar{x} - 2\text{SE}(\bar{x})$ and $\bar{x} + 2\text{SE}(\bar{x})$ and no real difference exists. In that case, the null hypothesis will not be rejected. Similarly, one can be 95% confident that the difference between the sample mean and the population mean would be due to the sampling error so long as the sample mean lies between $\bar{x} - 1.96\ \sigma/\sqrt{n}$ and $\bar{x} + 1.96\ \sigma/\sqrt{n}$. However, if the sample mean $\bar{x}$ lies outside these limits, then one may conclude that the difference between the sample mean $\bar{x}$ and the population mean 82 is significant, and the null hypothesis is rejected with 95% confidence.

The next question is how to find the limits $\bar{x} - 1.96\ \sigma/\sqrt{n}$ to $\bar{x} + 1.96\ \sigma/\sqrt{n}$ for different variables as these will have different units leading to different shapes of the normal curve. To solve this issue, the z-statistic as mentioned in (7.20) is used to test the null hypothesis. Since $\bar{x}$ for any variable follows a normal distribution (for large sample $n \geq 30$), the statistic z as mentioned in (7.20) will also follow the standard normal distribution; therefore, the limits equivalent to $\bar{x} - 1.96\ \sigma/\sqrt{n}$ to $\bar{x} - 1.96\ \sigma/\sqrt{n}$ would be equal to -1.96 to 1.96 (because z has a mean 0 and SD 1). These limits have been shown in Figure 7.4.

To conclude, as per the empirical rule, 95% of all samples drawn from the population will have a sample mean that falls within 2-SDs of the mean; hence, it is unlikely (less than a 0.05 probability) that the sample will fall beyond 2-SDs from the population mean under the assumption of null hypothesis.

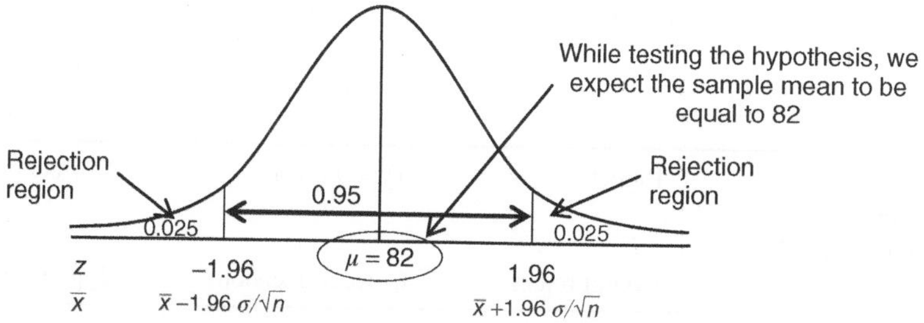

Figure 7.4 Showing sampling distribution of $\bar{x}$.

7.11 TYPE I AND TYPE II ERRORS

> **FACTS TO KNOW**
>
> Type I error is more dangerous because wrongly rejecting the null hypothesis compels a researcher to accept the wrong claim

A researcher tests the null hypothesis on the basis of a random sample drawn from the population of interest. For instance, if a researcher is interested in testing whether the flexibility of the men students in a sports college is 22 cm, then this hypothesis may be tested by drawing a random sample from the entire college. A random sample ensures that the sample truly represents the population and whatever conclusion is drawn on the basis of the sample may be correctly approximated to the population. Thus, by using an appropriate test statistic, a decision is taken about the rejection or nonrejection of the null hypothesis. As the decision about the population is taken on the basis of a small sample, there is always a chance that the researcher might commit a mistake. Thus, while taking a decision about the null hypothesis, two different kinds of errors may occur. The first error occurs if the null hypothesis is rejected when actually it is correct, whereas the second error occurs if the null hypothesis is not rejected when actually it is wrong. These two decisions are known as type I and type II errors, respectively. In addition to these two erroneous decisions, the other two decisions that a researcher can take are the correct decisions, namely, rejecting the null hypothesis when it is wrong and not rejecting the null hypothesis when it is true. Thus, there are four courses of action that a researcher can take about the null hypothesis for testing the population parameter on the basis of the sample. These four decisions can be summarized as shown in Table 7.1.

In the testing of a hypothesis, a researcher always tries to reduce both type I and type II errors. But for a fixed sample size, reduction in both type I and type II errors simultaneously is not possible because if one error is minimized, the other gets enhanced. One way to reduce both the errors simultaneously is to increase the sample size. In fact, this is not always possible in research studies because once the data are collected, the same has to be used by the researcher for drawing the inferences. Further, increasing the sample size will have an impact on economy

TABLE 7.1 Decision Options while Testing the Null Hypothesis

		Actual State of H_0	
		True	False
Researcher's decision about H_0	Reject	Type I error	Correct decision
	Do not reject	Correct decision	Type II error

and timeliness, as well as on the accuracy of the study. Moreover, by increasing the sample size, an experimenter loses control over the experiment because of which these errors get increased.

For a fixed sample size, the scope of reducing both the types of errors is limited and therefore the researcher identifies the more severe error out of the two and fixes it up at a desired level, and then tries to minimize the other error to a maximum possible extent. In research studies, type I error is generally considered to be more severe than type II error because wrongly rejecting a true null hypothesis forces the researcher to accept the research hypothesis that is actually wrong. For example, consider an experiment where it is desired to test whether the new conditioning program is superior to the existing program in improving cardiorespiratory endurance. The null hypothesis required to be tested in this case would be "The new conditioning program and existing conditioning program are equally effective" against the research hypothesis "The new conditioning program is more effective than the existing conditioning program." Now, if the null hypothesis is wrongly rejected, the research hypothesis shall be wrongly accepted, and it may be concluded that the new conditioning program is more effective in improving the cardiorespiratory endurance of students whereas actually it is not. Owing to the introduction of the faulty conditioning program in the college, the students may suffer. Since the type I error is a serious error, the researcher needs to decide its level in advance.

7.12 LEVEL OF SIGNIFICANCE

Level of significance is the probability of committing type I error and is denoted by α. This is the tolerance limit set by the researcher for wrongly rejecting the null hypothesis. As discussed earlier, type I error is more serious than the type II error; hence, it is set by the researcher at the lowest level in advance before conducting the research study. Usually, the level of significance is set as 0.05 or 0.01 in exercise science and health research. However, in the medical field where consequences of wrongly

FACTS TO KNOW

By fixing the level of significance, a researcher restricts the maximum possible error in accepting the wrong claim rejecting the null hypothesis is very high, the level of significance may be set at very low levels such as 0.001, 0001, or even 0.00001. Since the level of significance is a probability value, it is always written in fraction. Therefore, while rejecting the null hypothesis, the researcher may write a statement such as "hypothesis may be rejected at the significance level 0.05" or, alternately, he may write "hypothesis may be rejected at 5% level." By fixing the level of significance, the researcher ensures the maximum acceptable error in wrongly rejecting the null hypothesis in his study. In mathematical notation, the level of significance is written as

$$\alpha = \text{Prob}(\text{Rejecting } H_0/H_0 \text{ is true})$$

The above expression indicates the probability of rejecting the null hypothesis when actually it is true. Let us see what happens if a null hypothesis is rejected at the significance level 0.05. It simply means that if the study is conducted 100 times by drawing 100 random samples from the same population, then the null hypothesis may be wrongly rejected for a maximum of five occurrences. In other words, the researcher is 95% confident that the null hypothesis is correctly rejected.

7.13 POWER OF THE TEST

The power of a test is the efficiency of a test statistic in correctly rejecting the null hypothesis. It is denoted by $1-\beta$, where β is the probability of a type II error. In other words, β can be defined as the probability of nonrejection of H_0 when actually it is false. Mathematically, it is written as

$$\beta = \text{Prob}(\text{Nonrejection of } H_0/H_0 \text{ is false})$$

Thus, the power of a test can be computed as

$$\begin{aligned} \text{Power} &= 1-\beta \\ &= \text{Prob}(\text{Rejecting } H_0/H_0 \text{ is false}) \end{aligned}$$

In other words, the power of a statistical test tells how powerful the test is in rejecting the null hypothesis correctly. Thus, the power decides the robustness of a statistical test.

7.14 REJECTION REGION AND CRITICAL VALUE

Under the assumption of null hypothesis, the test statistic follows a normal distribution (for a sufficiently large sample) as shown in Figure 7.5. This distribution is divided into two regions, namely, nonrejection region and rejection region. Rejection region is that part of the distribution in which if the value of the test statistic

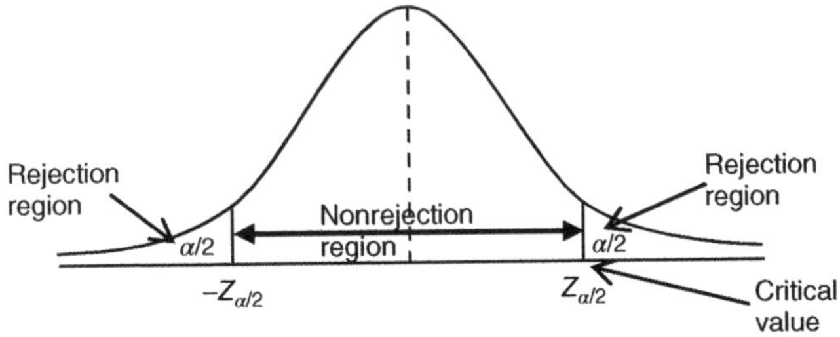

Figure 7.5 Distribution showing rejection region and critical value.

falls, the null hypothesis is rejected. A rejection region is also known as the critical rejection. The value of the statistic in the distribution that divides the sample space into nonrejection region and rejection region is known as critical value. Figure 7.5 shows the acceptance and rejection regions along with the critical value.

The size of the rejection region is determined by the level of significance (α), that is, how much error an investigator is willing to tolerate in wrongly rejecting the null hypothesis. If the test statistic falls in the rejection region, the null hypothesis H_0 is rejected and if it falls in the nonrejection region, one fails to reject the null hypothesis.

7.15 *p*-VALUE

p-Value can be defined as the probability of obtaining a test statistic at least as extreme as the one that was actually observed, assuming that the null hypothesis is true. It is associated with the test statistic. If a researcher decides for his study that the level of significance is 0.05 and if the *p*-value associated with the test statistic is smaller than 0.05, then the null hypothesis is rejected. Thus, the criterion in the testing of hypothesis is that so long as the *p*-value attached to the test statistic is smaller than 0.05 or 0.01 (if the researcher sets the level of significance as 0.01), the null hypothesis is rejected. The value of *p* decreases when the magnitude of the test statistic increases. Therefore, as the value of the test statistic increases, the probability of rejecting the true null hypothesis decreases. Let us see what happens if the *p*-value is not shown. In the case of a large significant value of the test statistic, the probability of wrongly rejecting the null hypothesis is very small, say, 0.001, but still the researcher states that the decision in rejecting the null hypothesis includes 5% error (as the level of significance was chosen as 0.05), which is logically not correct. The benefit of showing the *p*-value

FACTS TO KNOW

If assumptions in parametric tests are not fulfilled, the level of significance increases and the power of the test decreases with the test statistic in the result is that one can understand how much probability of error is attached in rejecting the null hypothesis. Now, two options are available to the researcher: first, he may fix up the level of significance in advance for his study and then take a decision depending on whether the test statistic falls in the critical region or not; second, the option is not to fix up the level of significance (α) before the study and take a decision on the basis of the p-value. However, one must understand the purpose of both α-value and p-value. The value α provides the maximum error limit that the researcher can tolerate in rejecting the null hypothesis when it is true, whereas p-value is the actual estimated error attached with the decision. Thus, the appropriate strategy for the researcher would be to assume the level of significance as 0.05 (or 0.01 as the case may be) and reject the null hypothesis so long as the p-value attached to the test statistic is less than 0.05. As most of the statistical packages calculate the value of p along with the test statistic, it is advisable to show this value also in the results. The p-value may be calculated for different statistics by using the free conversion software available on many sites such as http://www.danielsoper.com/statcalc3/calc.aspx?id = 8 or http://vassarstats.net/tabs.html.

7.16 ONE-TAILED AND TWO-TAILED TESTS

> **FACTS TO KNOW**
>
> At a given level of significance, if a null hypothesis is rejected for a two-tailed test, it will be rejected for the one-tailed test as well

Null hypothesis is always constructed along with the alternative or research hypothesis. Research hypothesis is the one in which the researcher is actually interested. The construction of a research hypothesis is based on some theoretical construct. Depending on whether the research hypothesis is unidirectional or bidirectional, a researcher decides to use the one-tailed or two-tailed test.

A statistical test is known as a *one-tailed test* if the null hypothesis is rejected only for values of the test statistic falling into one specified tail of its sampling distribution. In one-tailed tests, the direction is specified. For instance, a researcher may be interested in testing whether the population parameter is greater than or less than some value. In other words, the researcher is sure that after the experiment, the result can go only in one direction. If theory suggests that the effect of the experiment will be only in one direction, then in all such cases a one-tailed test should be used. Depending on the research hypothesis, one-tailed tests can be classified as right-tailed or left-tailed.

If the research hypothesis is to test whether the population parameter is more than some specified value, then such hypothesis is tested using a *right-tailed test*, and the entire rejection region shall lie in the right tail only. For example, in testing the research hypothesis that the exercise program will increase the bodily strength, the researcher would use the right-tailed test because theory suggests that after going through the exercise program the strength will either increase or may not increase but will never decrease. In this case, if the test statistic falls into the right rejection region, the null hypothesis shall be rejected and in turn an alternative hypothesis will be accepted.

On the other hand, if the research hypothesis is to test whether the population parameter is less than some specified value, then to test such hypothesis the test used is known as a *left-tailed test* and the entire rejection region shall lie in the left tail only. If the value of test statistic falls into the left rejection region, the null hypothesis shall be rejected. Consider a situation where the researcher is interested to test whether 100 m timing of athletes will decrease after attending an athletic training camp for 2 weeks. In this case, he would use the left-tailed test because all literature holds the fact that after attending the training camp the 100 m timings of athletes will either reduce or may not reduce but will never increase. In the worst-case scenario, even if for some reason such as noncooperation of the athletes in the sample or because of their indisposition the average timing of the 100 m event increases, it will not make any impact on the study as the researcher is only interested in testing whether the timing reduces after the camp. The rejection regions for testing the null hypothesis at an α level of significance in left-tailed and right-tailed tests are shown in Figure 7.6.

If a researcher is not sure of which way the results will go after an experiment, then he constructs the research hypothesis as bidirectional. For instance, in comparing the effect of two circuit training programs in improving the 400 m performance, the researcher is not sure as to which program would be better than others; he would construct the research hypothesis that the effect of two circuit training programs would not be the same in improving 400 m performance. To test such bidirectional hypothesis, the statistical test used is known as a two-tailed test. A statistical test is said to be a *two-tailed test* if the null hypothesis is rejected only for the value of the test statistic that falls into either tail of its sampling distribution. In two-tailed tests, no direction is specified. We are only interested in testing whether the population parameter is greater than or less than some value. If the test statistic falls into either of the critical regions (left side or right side), the null hypothesis would be rejected. The rejection of null hypothesis will lead to the acceptance of the research hypothesis.

In a *two-tailed test*, the critical region is divided in both the tails as shown in Figure 7.7. If the hypothesis is tested at an α level of significance, then the area

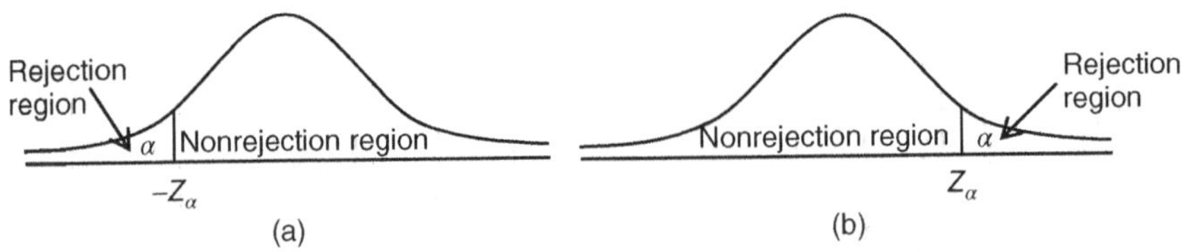

Figure 7.6 Showing rejection regions in (a) left-tailed test and (b) right-tailed test.

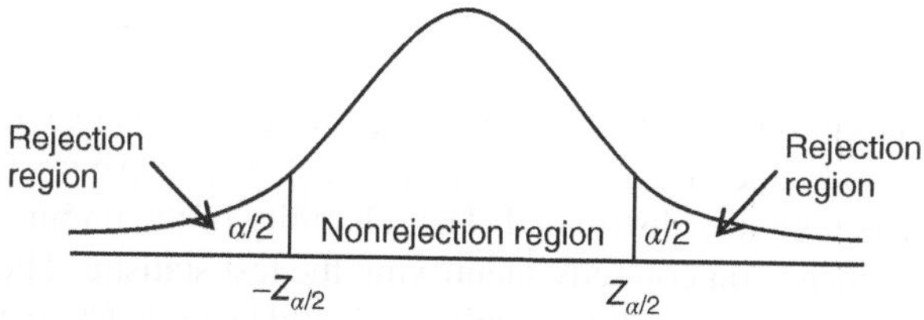

Figure 7.7 Distribution of rejection region in a two-tailed test.

of the rejection region in both the tails will become $\alpha/2$. Depending on whether or not the population SD is known, the distribution of the test statistic for testing the population mean follows z- or t-distribution, respectively. The statistical tables for z and t mentioned in the appendix provide critical values for both one- and two-tailed tests.

> **FACTS TO KNOW**
>
> As the degrees of freedom increase, the accuracy in estimating the population variance also increases

7.17 DEGREES OF FREEDOM

Degrees of freedom can be defined as the number of independent pieces of information used for estimating the population variance on the basis of sample information. The number of degrees of freedom can be considered as a measure of accuracy in representing the population by the sampled observations. The larger the number of degrees of freedom, the more confidence one has in saying that the sample is a true representative of the population. The degree of freedom is usually represented by the Greek letter mu (ν).

Mathematically, the number of degrees of freedom of an estimate is equal to the number of independent observations in the sample that are required to estimate the parameter minus the number of parameters estimated as intermediate steps in the estimation of the parameter itself. In general, each item being estimated costs one degree of freedom. The number of degrees of freedom can also be defined as the number of independent observations or pieces of information that are free to vary in computing a statistic.

The population variance can be estimated by the sample variance S^2. Let us see what the degree of freedom of S^2 is. Since S is computed from the sample of n observations its degrees of freedom should have been n, but because one degree of freedom is lost because in its computation the population mean is estimated by the sample mean, the degree of freedom for S^2 becomes $n-1$.

In the case of two samples, the pooled SD S is computed by using $n_1 + n_2$ observations. In computing the value of S, the two parameters μ_1 and μ_2 are estimated by $\bar{x}_1$ and $\bar{x}_2$; hence, the two degrees of freedom are lost and the degree of freedom for the pooled SD S is $n_1 + n_2 - 2$.

7.18 STRATEGY IN SELECTING THE TEST STATISTIC

To test different kinds of parametric hypotheses, several statistical tests such as z, t, F, and χ^2 are used. One of the main assumptions for these parametric tests is that the population is normally distributed. The reliability of the findings in the testing of hypothesis depends on correctly identifying the test statistic. There are specific situations under which different test statistics should be used. Choosing a statistical test depends on whether the researcher is interested in testing the hypothesis concerning a single group or two groups. However, there are specific guidelines that the researcher should follow in identifying a test statistic under these two situations.

In testing the hypothesis concerning a single group, the researcher must check whether he or she is required to test the hypothesis concerning the mean, proportion, or variance. If the hypothesis is regarding testing of mean, one should use the z-test for a single group, provided the population SD is known or the sample is large ($n \geq 30$). However, the z-test can also be used for testing the population mean even for a small sample ($n < 30$), provided the population is normally distributed and the population SD is known. Even if the population SD is not known, in the case of a large sample ($n \geq 30$), the z-test can still be used to test the hypothesis concerning population mean by using the sample SD.

The t-test is used for testing the hypothesis concerning population mean in the case of a small sample ($n < 30$) if the population SD is not known and the population is normally distributed.

In testing the hypothesis concerning population proportion, one should use the z-test for proportion if the sample is large. However, even if the sample is small, the z-test can be efficiently used for testing the population proportion, provided $n\hat{p} \geq 5$. On the other hand, if the hypothesis regarding the population variance is tested, the χ^2 test should be used. The scheme of identifying the test statistic in the case of one-sample testing is shown in Figure 7.8.

In two-group testing, the researcher should identify whether the hypothesis testing is about comparing means, proportions, or variances in the two groups. In comparing the means of the two groups, the z-test for the two samples should be used, provided the population SDs are known or the samples are large (both n_1 and $n_2 \geq 30$). However, the z-test can also be used to compare the means of the two populations if the samples are small, provided the population SDs are known and the populations are normally distributed.

In case the population variances are not known and the samples are small, the t-test should be used for comparing two independent sample means, provided the populations are normally distributed. However, if the samples are related, then paired t-test should be used for comparing the two sample means.

If hypothesis testing is for comparing two population proportions, then the z-test for proportion should be used if the sample is large. However, even if the samples are small, the z-test can be efficiently used for testing the equality of population proportions, provided $n_1\hat{p}_1 \geq 5$ and $n_2\hat{p}_2 \geq 5$, whereas in comparing variances of two populations, the F-test should be used. The scheme of identifying the test statistic in the case of two-sample testing is shown in Figure 7.9.

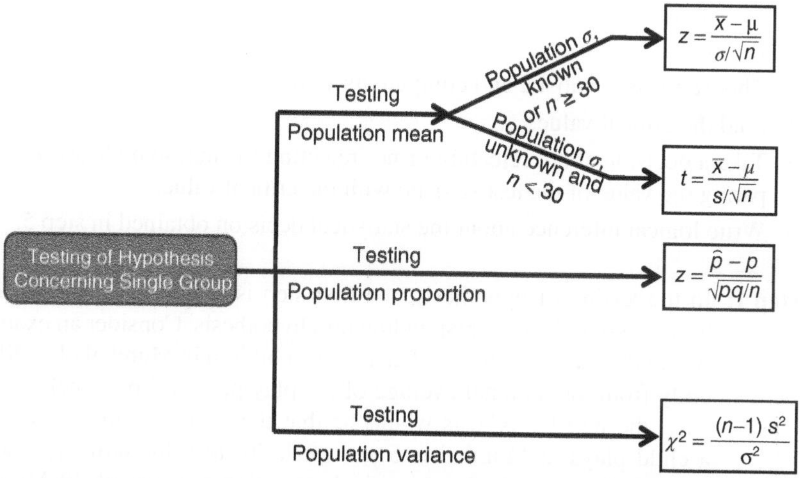

Figure 7.8 Strategy in selecting test statistic in single-group testing.

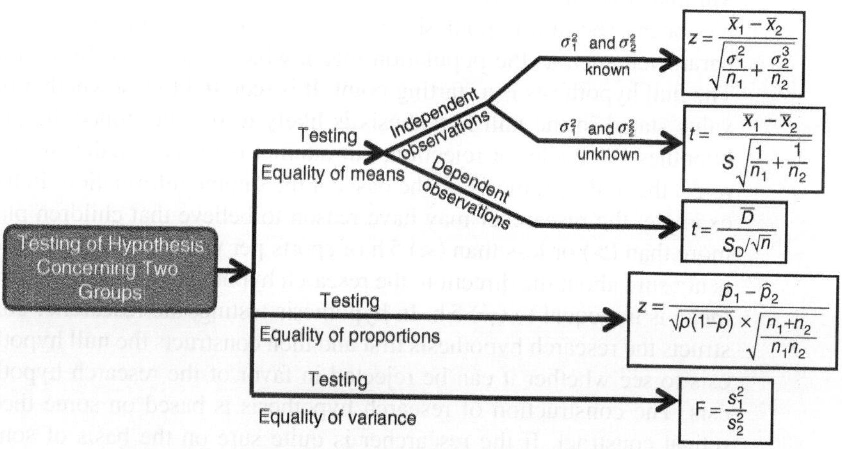

Figure 7.9 Strategy in selecting test statistic in two-group testing.

Remark The chi-square test is parametric as well as nonparametric as it is used for testing the significance of the population variance in the case of parametric data, whereas it is used for testing the significance of association between the two attributes and goodness of fit in the case of nonparametric data.

7.19 STEPS IN HYPOTHESIS TESTING

In the testing of hypothesis about population parameters, the following six steps are involved:

1. Construct research and null hypotheses.
2. Decide the level of significance at which the hypothesis needs to be tested.
3. Choose the test statistic and compute its value.
4. Find the critical value.
5. Take a decision about rejecting or not rejecting the null hypothesis by comparing the value of the test statistic with the critical value.
6. Write logical inference about the statistical decision obtained in step 5.

Step 1: In the testing of hypothesis, the first step is to construct the research hypothesis and the corresponding null hypothesis. Consider an example where the literature claims that average children in Mumbai play differently from the national average of 5 h play per child per week. In this case, the null hypothesis would be that the average number of hours a child plays in Mumbai is 5 per week. To test this null hypothesis, a researcher records the time (in hours) that a group of 30 Mumbai children, in a random sample drawn from among all the children in Mumbai, play sports. The mean obtained for these 30 children is a sample mean. The null hypothesis (H_0) is a statement about a population parameter, such as the population mean, which is assumed to be true. The null hypothesis is a starting point. It is required to test whether the value stated in the null hypothesis is likely to be true. Since the null hypothesis is made for rejection, our attempt is to see whether we can reject the null hypothesis on the basis of the sample information. In this example, the researcher may have reason to believe that children play more than (>) or less than (<) 5 h of sports per week. If the researcher is not sure about the direction, the research hypothesis can state that the mean is not equal to (≠) 5 h. In hypothesis testing, the researcher constructs the research hypothesis first and then constructs the null hypothesis to see whether it can be rejected in favor of the research hypothesis. The construction of research hypothesis is based on some theoretical construct. If the researcher is quite sure on the basis of some theory that the effect of the treatment on the dependent variable can only go in one direction, only then should he or she construct the research hypothesis as unidirectional (less than or more than type). In all other cases, the researcher should construct the research hypothesis as bidirectional. For instance, if it is desired to test the effect of 6 weeks of an aerobic exercise program on improving the cardiorespiratory endurance, it is quite logical to assume that there may or may not be significant improvement in the cardio but in no way will the exercise program deteriorate the cardio. In such a case, the researcher may construct his or her research hypothesis as H_1: $\mu_{\text{Post}} > \mu_{\text{Pre}}$, whereas the null hypothesis will be H_0: $\mu_{\text{Post}} = \mu_{\text{Pre}}$. In constructing the research hypothesis, the researcher's only concern is to verify whether the exercise program will improve the cardio significantly but even if due to some reasons such as noncooperation of the subjects in the sample or uncontrolled experimental situations, the researcher gets the findings that the cardio decreases after the exercise program, it will not bother the researcher as his or her intention is to test whether the exercise will improve the cardio or not. Consider another example where a researcher is interested in comparing the effect of two exercise programs of different intensities. In this case, the researcher is not sure whether any of the exercise programs is better than the others; therefore, he or she should construct the research hypothesis as a two-tailed hypothesis such as H_1: $\mu_{\text{Ex\_1}} \neq \mu_{\text{Ex\_2}}$ and the null hypothesis becomes H_0: $\mu_{\text{Ex\_1}} = \mu_{\text{Ex\_2}}$. To conclude, a researcher should always prefer a two-tailed hypothesis over a one-tailed hypothesis unless there is a strong evidence that the effect will be unidirectional. Otherwise also, at a particular level of significance, if a null hypothesis is rejected in a two-tailed test, then it will also be rejected in the one-tailed test.

Step 2: The second step is to decide the level of significance at which the researcher decides to test the null hypothesis. The decision about the level of significance depends on how sensitive it is for the researcher to reject the correct null hypothesis. Usually, in exercise science and health research, the level of significance is taken as either 0.05 or 0.01. In fact, by setting the level of significance, the researcher decides to allow the maximum error in wrongly rejecting the correct null hypothesis in the experiment.

Step 3: The next step is to identify the test statistic for testing the hypothesis. Depending on the types of hypothesis and conditions existing, the researcher needs to identify the test statistic and the computation is made by using the relevant formula. The guidelines given in Figures 7.8 and 7.9 may be used in this regard.

Step 4: Depending on whether the researcher uses the one-tailed or the two-tailed test, the critical value of the test statistic may be located in the relevant distribution table of the test statistic as shown in the appendix. This critical value is used to take the decision about rejecting or not rejecting the null hypothesis. Most of the time, a researcher uses either the z- or t-distribution in testing a hypothesis; therefore, let us see how to locate the critical value in these two distributions.

7.19.1 Finding the Critical Value in z-Test

The researcher uses either a one-tailed or a two-tailed test to test a hypothesis. In the case of testing a two-tailed hypothesis at the significance level 0.05, the critical region is divided in both the tails as shown in Figure 7.10.

The area between the mean and the critical value that separates the rejection region in both the tails is 0.475. By using this area and Table A.4, the critical value of $z_{0.05/2}$ can be obtained as 1.96.

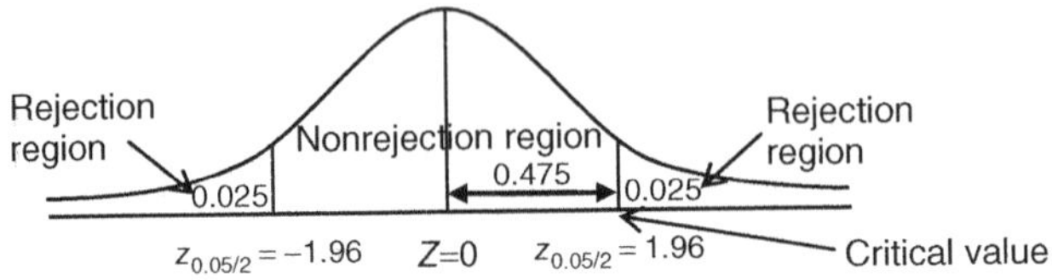

Figure 7.10 Showing critical regions in a two-tailed test at 5% level using z distribution.

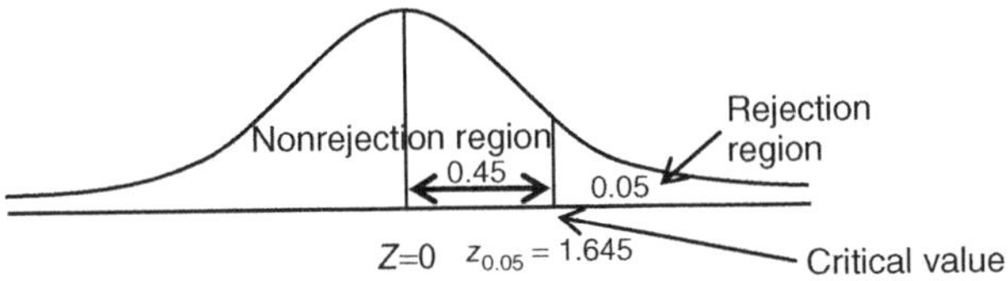

Figure 7.11 Showing the critical region in a one-tailed test at 5% level using z-distribution.

TABLE 7.2 Critical Value of z

Level of Significance	Two-Tailed Test	One-Tailed Test (Right-Tailed)	One-Tailed Test (Left-Tailed)
0.01	2.58	2.33	−2.33
0.05	1.96	1.645	−1.645
0.10	1.645	1.28	−1.28

On the other hand, if the hypothesis is tested by using a one-tailed test at the significance level 0.05, the entire critical region shall lie in one tail only. Figure 7.11 shows the critical region in a one-tailed test (right-tailed) at 5% level.

The area between the mean and the critical value that separates the rejection region in the right tail is 0.45. By using this area and Table A.4, the critical value of z can be obtained as 1.645.

Similarly, the critical value at other levels of significance may be obtained from the standard normal curve area table. However, the most frequently used levels of significance and their corresponding critical values in the z-distribution are shown in Table 7.2 for ready reference to the reader.

7.19.2 Finding the Critical Value in t-Test

The critical value of t can be obtained from the t-distribution table as given in Table A.7. Since for different sample sizes the shape of the t-distribution keeps changing, to locate the critical value of t you require degrees of freedom also along with level of significance α. The t-table in the appendix shows the critical values of t for

> **FACTS TO KNOW**
>
> The larger the value of the test statistic, the more confident the researcher is in rejecting the null hypothesis

TABLE 7.3 Cross-Section Table of *t*-Distribution

	Level of Significance for Two-Tailed Test				
df	0.2	0.1	0.05	0.02	0.01
1	3.078	6.314	12.71	31.82	63.66
2	1.886	2.92	4.303	6.965	9.925
3	1.638	2.353	3.182	4.541	5.841
4	1.533	2.132	2.776	3.747	4.604
5	1.476	2.015	2.571	3.365	4.032
6	1.44	1.943	2.447	3.143	3.707
7	1.415	1.895	**2.365**	2.998	3.499
8	1.397	1.86	2.306	2.896	3.355
9	1.383	1.833	2.262	2.821	3.25
	0.1	0.05	0.025	0.01	0.005
	Level of Significance for One-Tailed Test				

two-tailed as well as one-tailed tests. For a two-tailed test, the reader must see the level of significance in the top row, whereas for a one-tailed test the value of level of significance should be seen in the last row of the table. For easy understanding of the readers, a cross section of the *t*-distribution table is shown in Table 7.3. Now, if the sample size is 8, then for a two-tailed test at 0.05 level of significance, the critical value of *t* would be obtained by seeing the value of the degrees of freedom (8−1) in the first column and level of significance in the first row, the value of *t* at the cross-section point, 2.365, is the critical value.

Step 5: After computing the test statistic and locating the critical value from the table, a decision about the null hypothesis is taken as per the following strategy.

(i) In a two-tailed test

Reject null hypothesis H_0 if the calculated value of the test statistic (say $|z|$) > the critical value (say $z_{\alpha/2}$).

Do not reject H_0 if the calculated value of the test statistic (say $|z|$) ≤ critical value (say $z_{\alpha/2}$).

(ii) In a one-tailed test

Reject H_0 if Cal $Z > Z_\alpha$ for right-tailed test and Cal $Z < -Z_\alpha$ for left-tailed test.

Do not reject H_0 if Cal $Z \leq Z_\alpha$ for right-tailed test and Cal $Z \geq -Z_\alpha$ for left-tailed test.

If the null hypothesis is rejected, the test statistic is said to be significant, and otherwise insignificant. It may be noted that the null hypothesis is either rejected or not rejected. Nonrejection of the null hypothesis does not mean that the null hypothesis is accepted, as our only intention is to test whether the null hypothesis can be rejected or not. Thus, in case the researcher fails to reject the null hypothesis, it simply means that on the basis of the sample it is not possible to reject the null hypothesis in favor of the research hypothesis.

7.19.3 Testing with *p*-Value

The null hypothesis may be tested by using the *p*-value (significance value). Most of the statistical software provides the *p*-value in the output while applying the test of significance. In such cases, the decision on the null hypothesis is not taken by comparing the calculated value of the test statistic with that of the critical value. In fact, so long as the *p*-value is less than 0.05 (or 0.01 as the case may be), the null hypothesis is rejected and we say that the test statistic is significant.

Step 6: Finally, the inference is written on the basis of the decision taken about the null hypothesis in step 5. One must be careful in writing the inference if the null hypothesis is rejected. For instance, while testing the effect of exercise program on flexibility, the higher the score on sit and reach test, the better is the performance; whereas in testing the effect of circuit training program on the speed, the higher the score on 100 m timings, the lesser is the performance in speed.

7.20 ONE-SAMPLE TESTING

> **FACTS TO KNOW**
>
> If the distribution of a population is normal and the population SD is known, then the *z*-test can be used for any sample size

In one-sample testing, a claim about the population parameter is tested on the basis of a random sample drawn from the population of interest. Usually, hypotheses about the population mean, population proportion, and population variance are tested to answer some research questions. In this section, statistical tests such as *z*, *t*, and chi-square are discussed along with their assumptions for testing the significance of the null hypothesis. Few solved examples are also discussed to brief the reader about the procedure used in testing a hypothesis.

7.20.1 Test of Significance about a Population Mean with the *z*-Test (σ Known)

Testing of a hypothesis concerning population mean is the most frequent test used by a researcher. An exercise scientist might be interested in investigating whether an established norm for the average number of days one should do strength training is true for the students in college. Similarly, a sports researcher may like to investigate whether after renovating the infrastructure of a sports complex the average number of hours spent by people in the complex per day increases beyond 2 h per day. Other situations where the researcher might test the hypothesis of a single mean might be as follows:

1. A researcher may like to test whether the average hemoglobin count of women students in a college is more than 12 gm dl^{-1}.
2. A sports goods manufacturing company may wish to test whether the average play life of the cricket ball manufactured by them is more than 70 overs.
3. An athletic coach may be interested in testing whether the average timing of a sports person in a college on 100 m event is less than 12 s.

The z-test can be used for testing the hypothesis about the single population mean if the population SD is known or if the sample is large ($n \geq 30$). The z-test can be used even if the sample is small, provided the population SD is known and the population is normally distributed. The z-statistic is computed by using the formula in (7.21):

$$z = \frac{\bar{x} - \mu}{\sigma / \sqrt{n}} \tag{7.21}$$

The critical value of the z-statistic can be obtained from the standard normal curve area table in the appendix.

Example 7.5 It is given that the SD for the standing long jump performance in a population is 6.5 in. If a sample of 72 athletes drawn from this population has a mean standing long jump performance of 85 in., can it be concluded on the basis of this sample that the mean performance of the population is 82 in.? Test your hypothesis at the significance level 0.05.

Solution: In this problem, the sample is large ($n > 30$) and the population variance is known. To test the hypothesis that the population mean is equal to 85 in., the following steps shall be followed:

Hypothesis: Here, it is required to test whether the population mean is equal to 82, and therefore, the two-tailed test shall be used. The null and alternative hypotheses shall be as follows:

$$H_0\colon \mu = 82$$
$$H_1\colon \mu \neq 82$$

Level of Significance: 0.05

Test Statistic: Since the sample is large and the population variance is known, to test the above-mentioned null hypothesis, the z-test shall be used.

$$Z = \frac{\bar{x} - \mu}{\sigma / \sqrt{n}}$$

Given that $\bar{x} = 85$, $n = 72$, $\mu = 82$, and $\sigma = 6.5$. Substituting these values in the formula, the calculated z (Cal z) becomes

$$\text{Cal } z = \frac{85 - 82}{6.5/\sqrt{72}} = 3.92$$

$$\Rightarrow \text{Cal } |z| = 3.92$$

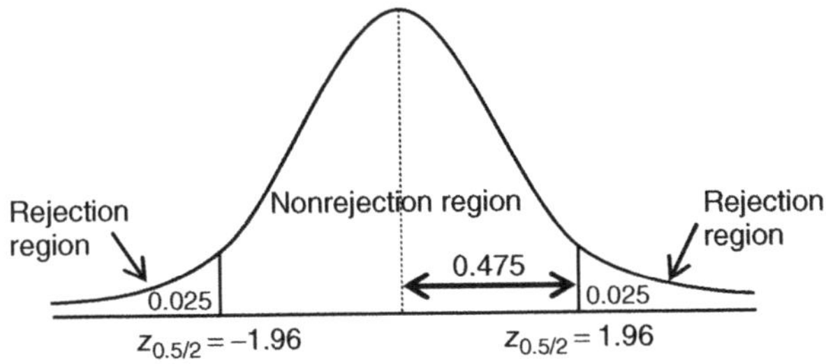

In the two-tailed test, the critical region lies in both the tails, and therefore in this problem, the critical region 0.05 is divided in both the tails as shown in the figure. The area between the mean and the critical value that separates the rejection region in both the tails is 0.475. By using this area and Table A.4, the critical value of z can be obtained as

$$z_{0.05/2} = 1.96$$

Since the absolute value of z is more than 1.96, H_0 may be rejected at the significance level 0.05.

Inference: Since H_0 has been rejected, it may be concluded that the population mean is not 82 in.

Example 7.6 In a physical education university, every year more than 600 students appear for the entrance examination for the bachelor degree program. The authorities claim that over the years, the average performance of these students on a 1.5 mile run test has been more than 16.5 min along with an SD of 2.3 min. If a random sample of size 120 drawn from these aspirants has a mean performance of 17.5 min, can it be concluded that the claim of the authorities is true? Test your hypothesis at the significance level 0.01.

Solution: Here, the sample is large ($n > 30$) and the population variance is known. To test the alternative hypothesis that the population mean is more than 16.5, the following steps shall be followed:

Hypothesis: Since it is required to test whether the population mean is more than 16.5, the one-tailed test (right-tailed) shall be used. The null and alternative hypotheses shall be as follows:

$$H_0\colon \mu = 16.5$$

$$H_1\colon \mu > 16.5$$

Level of Significance: 0.01

Test Statistic: Since the sample is large and the population variance is known, to test the above-mentioned null hypothesis the z-test shall be applied:

$$Z = \frac{\bar{x} - \mu}{\sigma/\sqrt{n}}$$

given that $\bar{x} = 17.5$, $n = 120$, $\mu = 16.5$, and $\sigma = 2.3$. Substituting these values in the formula, the calculated z (Cal z) becomes

$$\text{Cal } z = \frac{17.5 - 16.5}{2.3/\sqrt{120}} = 12.86$$

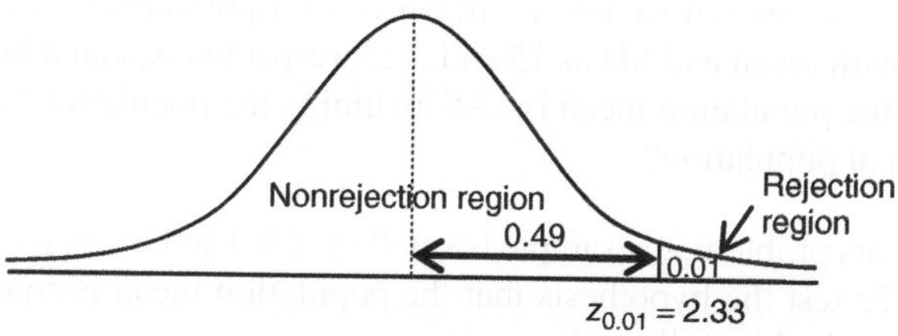

In a one-tailed test, the critical region lies in one tail only; therefore, in this right-tailed test the entire critical region 0.01 lies in the right tail as shown in the figure. The area between the mean and the critical value that separates the rejection region in the right tail is 0.49. By using this area and Table A.4, the critical value of z can be obtained as

$$z_{0.01} = 2.33$$

Since Cal z (12.86) is greater than 2.33, H_0 may be rejected at the significance level 0.01.

Inference: Since H_0 is rejected, it may be concluded that the population mean is higher than 16.5.

7.20.2 Test of Significance about a Population Mean with the t-Test (σ Unknown)

In most of the situations, when a researcher collects the data on the sample for testing the population mean, population SD is not known; in that case, the z-test cannot be used to test the hypothesis. In all cases where the population SD is not known, the t-test is used to test the hypothesis about single population mean, provided the distribution of population is normal and the sample is small ($n < 30$). The t-statistic is computed from the following formula:

$$t = \frac{\bar{x} - \mu}{s/\sqrt{n}} \tag{7.22}$$

where

$$\bar{x} = \frac{1}{n}\sum x_i \text{ and } s = \sqrt{\frac{1}{n-1}\sum (x_i - \bar{x})^2}$$

To find the critical value of t in one-sample test, the number of degrees of freedom is $(n - 1)$. The calculated value of the t-statistic is compared with the tabulated value of t at a certain level of significance with $(n-1)$ degrees of freedom to take the decision regarding rejecting or not rejecting the null hypothesis. In using the t-test, one must ensure that the population from which the sample has been drawn follows a normal distribution; population SD is unknown and the scores in the sample must be independent of each other.

Example 7.7 A random sample is drawn from a population. If the size of the sample is 18 with mean and SD as 15 and 3.25, respectively, can it be concluded at 1% level that the population mean is 13.5 assuming the population has been drawn from the normal population?

Solution: In this problem, the sample is small ($n < 30$) and the population variance is unknown. To test the hypothesis that the population mean is equal to 13.5, the following steps shall be followed:

Hypothesis: Here, it is required to test whether the population mean is equal to 13.5, and therefore, the two-tailed test shall be used. The null and alternative hypotheses shall be as follows:

$$H_0: \mu = 13.5$$

$$H_1: \mu \neq 13.5$$

Level of Significance: 0.01

Test Statistic: Since the sample is small and has been drawn from a normal population with population variance unknown, the above-mentioned null hypothesis can be tested by using the t-test:

$$t = \frac{\bar{x} - \mu}{S/\sqrt{n}}$$

given that $\bar{x} = 15$, $S = 3.25$, $n = 18$, and $\mu = 13.5$. Substituting these values in the formula, the calculated t (Cal t) becomes

$$\text{Cal } t = \frac{15 - 13.5}{3.25/\sqrt{18}} = 1.96$$

$$\Rightarrow \text{Cal } |t| = 1.96$$

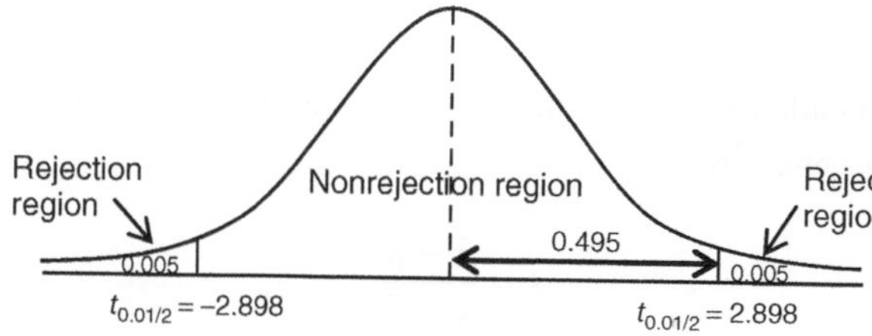

Here, the two-tailed test has been used; hence, the critical region 0.01 has been divided in both the tails as shown in the figure. The area between the mean and the critical value that separates the rejection region in both the tails is 0.495. By using Table A.7, the critical value of t for the two-tailed test with 17 degrees of freedom can be obtained as

$$t_{0.01/2}(17) = 2.898$$

Since absolute value of t is less than 2.898, H_0 is not rejected at the significance level 0.01.

Inference: Since H_0 has not been rejected, it may be concluded that the population mean is 13.5.

Example 7.8 The following set of data represents the weight of a random sample of 12 wrestlers (in pounds) drawn from a university:

180	190	185	200	178	192	196	181	175	186	189	195

Test the following hypotheses at 1% level assuming that the data were drawn from a normally distributed population.

$$H_0\colon \mu = 192, \quad H_1\colon \mu < 192$$

Solution: In this problem, the sample is small ($n < 30$) and the population variance is not known. To test the above-mentioned hypotheses the following steps shall be followed:

Hypothesis: The following hypotheses are required to be tested on the basis of the sample information.

$$H_0\colon \mu = 192$$

$$H_1\colon \mu < 192$$

Level of Significance: 0.01

Test Statistic: Since the sample is small and has been drawn from a normal population with the population variance unknown, the above-mentioned null hypothesis can be tested by using the t-test

$$t = \frac{\bar{x} - \mu}{S/\sqrt{n}}$$

In order to compute the value of t, the mean and SD need to be computed from the sample data:

Computation of Mean and SD

x	x^2
180	32,400
190	36,100
185	34,225
200	40,000
178	31,684
192	36,864
196	38,416
181	32,761
175	30,625
186	34,596
189	35,721
195	38,025
$\sum x = 2247$	$\sum x^2 = 421417$

$$\bar{x} = \frac{\sum x}{n} = \frac{2247}{12} = 187.25$$

$$S = \sqrt{\frac{\sum x^2}{n-1} - \frac{\left(\sum x\right)^2}{n(n-1)}} = \sqrt{\frac{421417}{11} - \frac{2247^2}{12(12-1)}}$$

$$= \sqrt{38310.64 - 38250.07} = 7.78$$

given that $n = 12$, $\mu = 192$, and the calculated value of mean and SD are $\bar{x} = 187.25$ and $S = 7.78$, respectively. Substituting these values, the calculated t (Cal t) becomes

$$\text{Cal } t = \frac{187.25 - 192}{7.78/\sqrt{12}} = -2.12$$

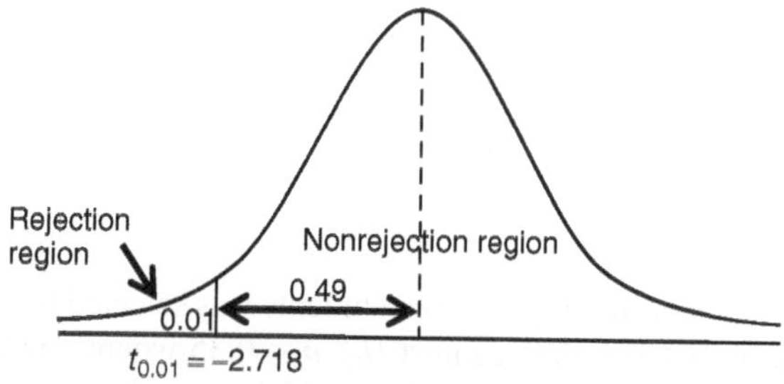

In one-tailed test, the entire critical region lies in one tail only. Since in this case a left-tailed test is used, the entire critical region 0.01 lies in the left tail only as shown in the figure. The area between the mean and the critical value that separates the rejection region in the left tail is 0.49. By using this area and Table A.7, the critical value of t with 11 df can be obtained as

$$t_{0.01} = -2.718$$

Since Cal t (−2.12) is more than −2.718 and it lies in the nonrejection region, H_0 is not rejected at the significance level 0.01.

Inference: Since H_0 has not been rejected, it may be concluded that the population mean is not less than 192.

7.20.3 Test of Significance about a Proportion

Researchers in the area of exercise science and health often use proportions to describe such aspects as girls' participation, injured athletes, defective sports equipments, smoker athletes, vegetarian sports persons, scholarships holders, and so on. Surveys often produce data expressed in proportion form, such as 0.20 of all the students go for physical activity or 0.75 of all the students in the college have participated in the intercollegiate competition. The researchers test hypothesis about such proportions to investigate whether such proportions have changed over a period of time in some way or the other. Consider an example where in a physical education university 0.20 of the students admitted were women for the last several years. Owing to the massive campaign by the university and change in government policy, a researcher may be interested in testing whether the proportion of women candidates admitted in the university has gone up.

In such cases, hypothesis regarding population proportion can be tested on the basis of the sample proportion by using the z-statistic as shown in formula (7.23). As per the central limit theorem, the test statistic z in formula (7.23) follows a normal distribution, provided the sample is sufficiently large such that $n\hat{p} \geq 5$ and $n\hat{q} \geq 5$:

$$z = \frac{\hat{p} - p}{\sqrt{pq/n}} \tag{7.23}$$

where

$\hat{p}$ = sample proportion
p = population proportion, $q = 1 - p$
n = sample size

Example 7.9 A random sample of 180 students was selected from a university to test the hypothesis H_0: $p = 0.35$ against H_0: $p < 0.35$ where p represents the proportion of smoker students in the population. If the sample proportion of smokers is 0.25, test the above-mentioned hypothesis at 5% level.

Solution: In this example, the sample size is large ($n > 30$) and the one-tailed hypothesis needs to be tested. The required hypotheses can be tested by using the z-test for proportion by following the below-mentioned steps.

Hypothesis: Since it is required to test whether population proportion is less than 0.35, a one-tailed test (left-tailed) shall be used. The null and alternative hypotheses shall be as follows:

$$H_0: p = 0.35$$

$$H_1: p < 0.35$$

Level of Significance: 0.05

Test Statistic: Since the sample is large, the hypothesis concerning population proportion shall be tested by using the following z-statistic:

$$z = \frac{\hat{p} - p}{\sqrt{pq/n}}$$

given that sample proportion ($\hat{p}$) = 0.25, population proportion (p) = 0.35, q = 0.65, and n = 180.

Substituting these values in the equation, the value of calculated z (Cal z) becomes

$$\text{Cal } z = \frac{0.25 - 0.35}{\sqrt{\dfrac{0.35 \times 0.65}{180}}} = \frac{-0.10}{0.0356} = -2.81$$

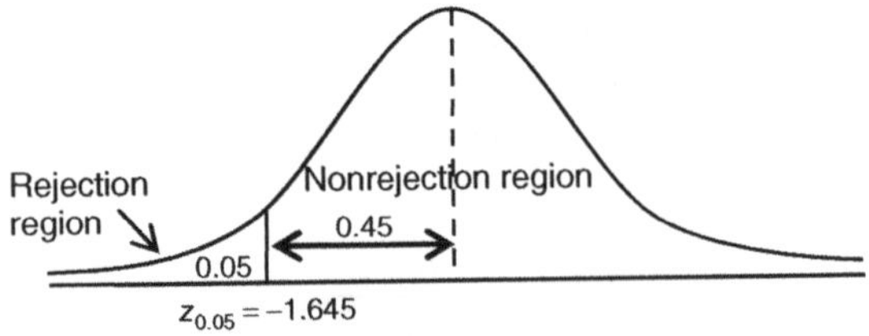

In the one-tailed test, the critical region lies in one tail only; therefore, in this left-tailed test the entire critical region 0.05 lies in the left tail as shown in the figure. The area between the mean and the critical value that separates the rejection region in the left tail is 0.45. By using this area and Table A.4, the critical value of z can be obtained as

$$z_{0.05} = -1.645$$

Since Cal z (−2.81) is less than −1.645 and lies in the rejection region, the null hypothesis is rejected at the significance level 0.05.

Inference: Since H_0 is rejected, it may be concluded that the population proportion is less than 0.35. In other words, the proportion of smokers in the population is less than 35%.

Example 7.10 It is claimed that in a sports college, 60% students prefer to have nonvegetarian food. To test this hypothesis, a sample of 220 students were randomly selected and were asked for their preferences on food. Sixty-five percent students in the sample preferred nonvegetarian food. Test whether the claim is true at 5% level.

Solution: In this example, the sample size is large and a two-tailed hypothesis needs to be tested. This hypothesis can be tested by using the z-test for proportion by following the below-mentioned steps.

Hypothesis: Since it is required to test whether population proportion is 0.60, a two-tailed test shall be used. The null and alternative hypotheses shall be as follows:

$$H_0: p = 0.60$$

$$H_1: p \neq 0.60$$

Level of Significance: 0.05

Test Statistic: Since the sample is large, the hypothesis concerning population proportion shall be tested by using the following z-statistic:

$$z = \frac{\hat{p} - p}{\sqrt{pq/n}}$$

given that sample proportion $\hat{p} = 0.65$, population proportion $p = 0.60$, $q = 0.40$, and $n = 220$.

Substituting these values in the formula, the value of calculated z (Cal z) becomes

$$\text{Cal } z = \frac{0.65 - 0.60}{\sqrt{\dfrac{0.60 \times 0.40}{220}}} = \frac{0.05}{0.0330} = 1.52$$

$$\Rightarrow \text{Cal } |z| = 1.52$$

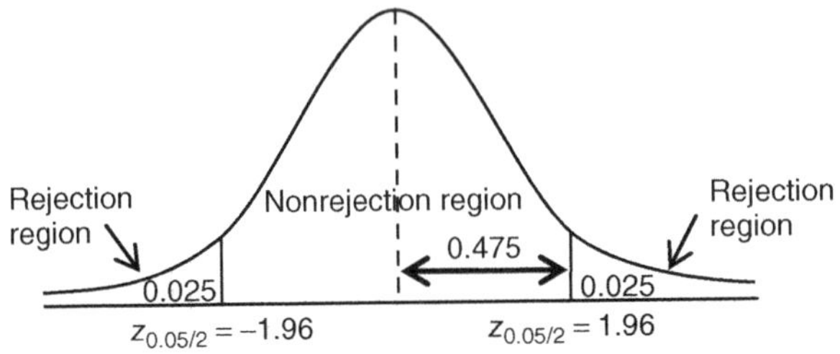

Since in a two-tailed test the critical region lies in both the tails, in this example the critical region 0.05 has been divided in both the tails as shown in the figure. The area between the mean and the critical value that separates the rejection region in the right as well as in left tails is 0.475. By using this area and Table A.4, the critical value of z can be obtained as

$$z_{0.05/2} = 1.96$$

Since the absolute value of z (=1.52) is less than 1.96, it lies in the nonrejection region and therefore null hypothesis is not rejected at the significance level 0.05.

Inference: Since H_0 is not rejected, the claim that 60% students prefer nonvegetarian food may be true.

7.20.4 Test of Significance about a Variance

Sometimes, the researcher needs to test a hypothesis concerning population variance. In sports engineering companies, sports goods are manufactured, which require to be consistent in dimensions. Suppose a company manufactures tennis balls that have specific parameters in terms of dimensions and bounce. Owing to the manufacturing process, the dimensions of these parameters may keep varying. The production manager can accept the product lot if the variation in these dimensions is within an acceptable limit. By testing the hypothesis for the variance of the dimension and bounce measurements, quality control people in the organization can monitor the variations in the quality of the product that are unacceptable.

To test the hypothesis concerning population variance, the test statistic χ^2 (chi-square) mentioned in formula (7.24) can be used.

$$\chi^2 = \frac{(n-1)s^2}{\sigma^2}, \text{d.f} = n - 1 \qquad (7.24)$$

In testing the significance of the test statistic, χ^2, its critical value can be obtained from Table A.11 in the appendix at $n-1$ degrees of freedom. The chi-square distribution is not symmetrical, and its shape varies according to the degrees of freedom. Using χ^2 test for testing the population variance is very sensitive to the assumption that the population is normally distributed. Therefore, one should be very cautious in using this method of testing population variance.

Example 7.11 For a normal population, test the hypothesis H_0: $\sigma^2 = 27$ against H_1: $\sigma^2 > 27$ at 5% level if $n = 25$, $s^2 = 24$.

Solution: Given that sample variance $s^2 = 24$, population variance, $\sigma^2 = 27$, $n = 25$, it is required to test the one-tailed hypothesis concerning population variance.

The hypothesis mentioned in the question can be tested by using the following steps.

Hypothesis: The following hypotheses need to be tested here:

$$H_0: \sigma^2 = 27$$
$$H_1: \sigma^2 > 27$$

Level of Significance: 0.05

Test Statistic: Since testing of hypothesis is for the population variance, the above-mentioned null hypothesis can be tested by using the following chi-square test statistic:

$$\chi^2 = \frac{(n-1)s^2}{\sigma^2}$$

with $\text{df} = n-1$.

Substituting the values of s^2, σ^2, and n in the above formula, the statistic becomes

$$\chi^2 = \frac{(25-1) \times 24}{27} = 21.33$$

Thus, Cal $\chi^2 = 21.33$.

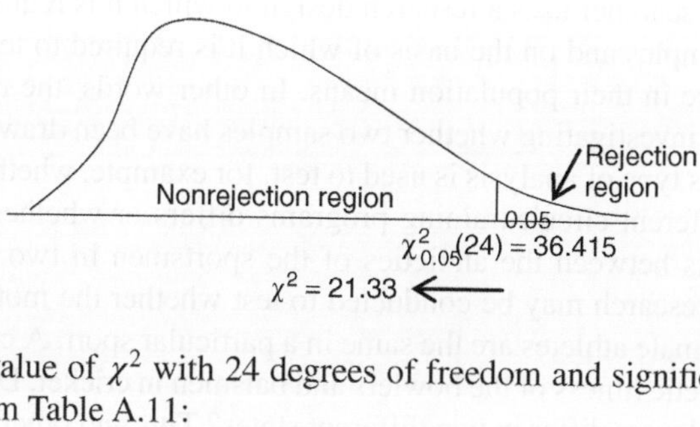

The tabulated value of χ^2 with 24 degrees of freedom and significance level 0.05 can be seen from Table A.11:

$$\chi^2_{0.05}(24) = 36.415$$

Since this is a one-tailed test, the rejection region is in the upper tail of the chi-square distribution as shown in the figure.

Since Cal $\chi^2 < 36.415$, H_0 may not be rejected at 5% level.

Inference: Since H_0 is not rejected, it may be concluded that the population variance is not more than 27.

7.21 TWO-SAMPLE TESTING

Most of the times, researchers are interested in comparing the effect of two different training programs or two groups on some characteristics, and therefore it is important to know how to draw inferences about the two populations. Several techniques shall be discussed for analyzing the data that come from two populations. In all, five different techniques are discussed to compare the means, proportions, and variances of the two groups. These techniques are discussed by using the z, t, and F statistics. Out of these five techniques, four techniques are used in a situation when the samples are assumed to be independent, whereas one technique is used when the samples are dependent. The concept of independent sample is that the subjects sampled in two groups are in no way related to each other. For instance, comparing the speed of basketball and soccer players, IQ of boys and girls, or flexibility of gymnasts and basketball players are all the examples of independent samples because in both the groups the subjects are different. On the other hand, related samples mean that the data in the two samples have been obtained on the same subjects or experimental units at different points of time or on different traits. For instance, in comparing the weight of the participants before and after the 6 weeks aerobic exercise program or comparing the sports infrastructure facilities at two points of time in the schools of a district, the samples are dependent because in both the groups, observations are obtained on the same subjects or experimental units.

7.21.1 Test of Significance about the Difference in Two Means with z-Test for Two Independent Samples (σ_1 and σ_2 Known)

Sometimes, a researcher uses a research design in which it is required to draw two independent samples and on the basis of which it is required to test whether there is any difference in their population means. In other words, the researcher might be interested in investigating whether two samples have been drawn from the same population. This type of analysis is used to test, for example, whether the effectiveness of two different circuit training programs differs or whether any significant difference exists between the anxieties of the sportsmen in two different sports. Psychological research may be conducted to test whether the motivation levels of the male and female athletes are the same in a particular sport. A coach might wish to compare athletic fitness of the bowlers and batsmen in cricket. Does the height of the volleyball players differ in two different states? This and other similar research questions can be answered by comparing the means of the two groups.

As per the central limit theorem, the difference in the two sample means, $\bar{x}_1 - \bar{x}_2$, follows a normal distribution with mean $\mu_{\bar{x}_1-\bar{x}_2}$ and SD $\sigma_{\bar{x}_1-\bar{x}_2}$ as given below, provided the samples are large (both n_1 and $n_2 \geq 30$) irrespective of the distribution of the populations:

$$\mu_{\bar{x}_1-\bar{x}_2} = \mu_1 - \mu_2 \tag{7.25}$$

$$\sigma_{\bar{x}_1-\bar{x}_2} = \sqrt{\frac{\sigma_1^2}{n_1} + \frac{\sigma_2^2}{n_2}} \tag{7.26}$$

Since $\bar{x}_1 - \bar{x}_2$, the difference of means in two independent samples is a normal variate, under the null hypothesis H_0: $\mu_1 - \mu_2 = 0$, the test statistic

$$Z = \frac{\bar{x}_1 - \bar{x}_2 - (\mu_1 - \mu_2)}{\mathrm{SE}(\bar{x}_1 - \bar{x}_2)} \tag{7.27}$$

or

$$Z = \frac{\bar{x}_1 - \bar{x}_2}{\sqrt{\frac{\sigma_1^2}{n_1} + \frac{\sigma_2^2}{n_2}}} \tag{7.28}$$

follows a standard normal distribution with mean 0 and SD 1.

Thus, if the samples are large, the test statistic z mentioned in formula (7.28) can be used to compare the means of the two independent samples irrespective of the distribution of the population, provided the sample is sufficiently large.

If the sample is small, the above formula of z can be used to test the means of the two independent groups, provided the populations are normally distributed and the SDs of the populations are known.

Example 7.12 Test the significance of the difference between the mean standing broad jump performance of the basketball players and swimmers from the following data. Test your hypothesis at 5% level.

Groups	n	Mean	σ
Basketball (A)	100	170 cm	10 cm
Swimming (B)	120	176 cm	12 cm

Solution: In this example, it is required to test the significance of the mean difference between the two groups; hence, the two-tailed test is used. Since the sample is large ($n > 30$) and the population variance is known, z-test for the two-sample test shall be used to test the required hypothesis by following the below-mentioned steps:

Hypothesis: Since it is required to test the significance of the mean difference, the following hypotheses need to be tested:

$$H_0\colon \mu_A = \mu_B$$

$$H_1\colon \mu_A \neq \mu_B$$

Level of Significance: 0.05

Test Statistic: Since the sample is large and the population variances are known, to compare the two group means the z-statistic mentioned below is used as a test statistic:

$$Z = \frac{\bar{x}_1 - \bar{x}_2}{\sqrt{\frac{\sigma_1^2}{n_1} + \frac{\sigma_2^2}{n_2}}}$$

Here, $\bar{x}_1 = 170$, $\bar{x}_2 = 176$, $\sigma_1 = 10$, $\sigma_2 = 12$, $n_1 = 100$, and $n_2 = 120$. Substituting these values in the formula, we get

$$\text{Cal } z = \frac{170 - 176}{\sqrt{\frac{10^2}{100} + \frac{12^2}{120}}} = -\frac{6}{1.483} = -4.05$$

$$\Rightarrow \text{Cal } |z| = 4.05$$

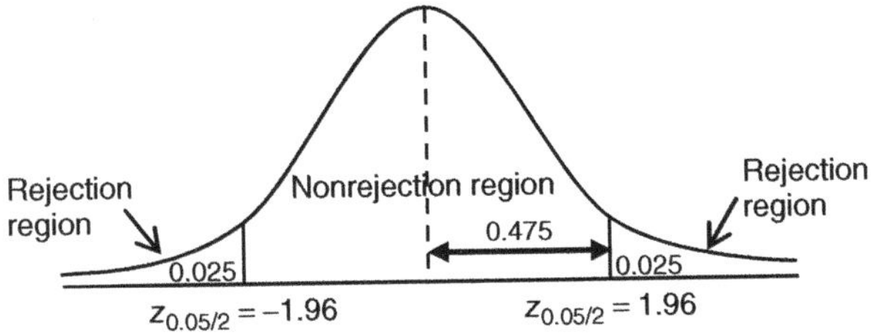

Since the hypothesis required to be tested is two-tailed, the critical region 0.05 has been divided in both the tails as shown in the figure. The area between the mean and the critical value that separates the rejection region in the right as well as the left tail is 0.475. By using this area and Table A.4, the critical value of z can be obtained as

$$z_{0.05/2} = 1.96$$

Since the absolute value of z (=4.05) is more than 1.96, H_0 may be rejected at the significance level 0.05.

Inference: Since H_0 has been rejected, the difference between the mean standing broad jump performance of the basketball players and swimmers is significantly different.

7.21.2 Test of Significance about the Difference in Two Means with *t*-Test (σ_1 and σ_2 Unknown)

In most of the situations, researchers do not know anything about the population SDs and what they have is the two samples of data. In that situation, the z formula mentioned in (7.21) is not valid. Testing of hypothesis in such situations where the population SDs are not known is discussed in this section. To test the hypothesis about the two population means when the population SDs are not known, two different types of t-tests are used depending on whether the samples are independent or dependent. Both these statistical tests assume that the populations from which these samples have been drawn are normally distributed. These two cases have been discussed in this section.

Case 1: Two-sample t*-test for independent samples* Researchers in exercise science and health are always striving for betterment in their approach. In doing so, the existing training program may be compared with the new program to see whether the training effect can be enhanced by the new approach. The researchers plan their experiment on certain subjects. If in an experimental design each individual subject can be randomly assigned to one and only one treatment group in comparing two treatments, it results in two independent samples. Such experiments may be conducted, for example, to see the effect of two conditioning programs on arm cardiorespiratory endurance, the effect of two stretching programs on flexibility, or the effect of two different intensities of aerobic programs on lung capacity. Besides investigating the effect of treatment on the dependent variable, other studies may be planned for comparing the means of two groups such as comparing arm length of tennis and squash players, or the abdomen strength of wrestlers and weight lifters. Similarly, a psychologist may like to know whether mental toughness is more in soccer players or hockey players. In such situations, the experiment results in two independent samples. Let us see how to test the hypothesis about the two population means in such a scenario.

If two random samples of sizes n_1 and n_2 having means $\bar{x}$ and $\bar{y}$ have been drawn from the two independent populations that are normally distributed and whose population SDs are not known, then under the assumption of null hypothesis, H_0: $\mu_x = \mu_y$ (population means are same), the statistic t as given in formula (7.29) follows a t-distribution with $(n_1 + n_2 - 2)$ degrees of freedom:

$$t = \frac{\bar{x} - \bar{y}}{S\sqrt{\dfrac{1}{n_1} + \dfrac{1}{n_2}}} \tag{7.29}$$

where S is the pooled SD of the two samples and is calculated as

$$S = \sqrt{\frac{1}{n_1 + n_2 - 2}\left(\sum_{i=1}^{n_1}(x_i - \bar{x})^2 + \sum_{j=1}^{n_2}(y_j - \bar{y})^2\right)} \tag{7.30}$$

After solving,

$$S = \sqrt{\frac{1}{n_1 + n_2 - 2}\left(\sum x_i^2 + \sum y_j^2 - n_1\bar{x}^2 - n_2\bar{y}^2\right)} \tag{7.31}$$

The t-statistic given by formula (7.29) is used to test the hypothesis about the two population means in a situation where the two population variances are unknown. This test would be valid for testing the hypothesis about the two population means only when the variances of the two populations are equal.

Example 7.13 In a basketball nursery, a coach wanted to investigate the best training angles out of the two for enhancing the shooting accuracy. Two groups of children were randomly selected. The first group was trained for shooting by using 45° angle, whereas the second group was trained by using the arm at 90° angle. After 4 weeks of training, the subjects were asked to take 20 attempts of shooting the basketball from a fixed distance. Successful shots were counted, and the scores obtained are shown in the following table. Given that the population variances of the two groups are nearly equal and the variable (shooting accuracy) is normally distributed, can it be concluded from the sample data that any one technique of training is more effective than the other in improving the shooting accuracy? Test your hypothesis at 5% level.

Shooting Scores										
Group A (45° angle):	10	9	11	8	5	13	10	7	8	
Group B (90° angle):	12	16	15	13	15	16	9	8	12	11

Solution: In this problem, it is required to test whether the two treatments, that is, training with 45° degree and with 90° degree angles, are equally effective in improving the shooting accuracy. To test this hypothesis, a two-tailed test is used. Here, the samples are (n_1, $n_2 < 30$), population variances are unknown, and the population variances of both the groups are nearly same. Under these conditions, the t-test for two independent samples is used to test the required hypothesis.

Hypothesis: To test whether the two treatments are equally effective, the following hypotheses need to be tested:

$$H_0\colon \mu_{45°} = \mu_{90°}$$

$$H_0\colon \mu_{45°} \neq \mu_{90°}$$

Level of Significance: 0.05

Test Statistic: Since population variances are unknown and samples are small, the t-statistic mentioned below is used as a test statistic to compare the two group means:

$$t = \frac{\bar{x} - \bar{y}}{S\sqrt{\frac{1}{n_1} + \frac{1}{n_2}}}$$

where

$$S = \sqrt{\frac{\sum x^2 + \sum y^2 - n_1\bar{x}^2 - n_2\bar{y}^2}{n_1 + n_2 - 2}}$$

To compute the *t*-value, the mean and variance of both the groups need to be computed from the following data.

Computation for *t* Value

45° Angle *x*	90° Angle *y*	x^2	y^2
10	12	100	144
9	16	81	256
11	15	121	225
8	13	64	169
5	15	25	225
13	16	169	256
10	9	100	81
7	8	49	64
8	12	64	144
	11		121
$\sum x = 81$	$\sum y = 127$	$\sum x^2 = 773$	$\sum y^2 = 1685$

$$\bar{x} = \frac{\sum x}{n} = \frac{81}{9} = 9$$

$$\bar{y} = \frac{\sum y}{n} = \frac{127}{10} = 12.7$$

$$S = \sqrt{\frac{773 + 1685 - 9 \times 9^2 - 10 \times 12.7^2}{9 + 10 - 2}}$$

$$= 2.61$$

Thus, $\bar{x} = 9$, $\bar{y} = 12.7$, $S = 2.61$, $n_1 = 9$, and $n_2 = 10$. Substituting these values in the formula, we get

$$\text{Cal } t = \frac{9 - 12.7}{2.61 \times \sqrt{\frac{1}{9} + \frac{1}{10}}} = -\frac{3.7}{1.199} = -3.09$$

$$\Rightarrow \text{Cal } |t| = 3.09$$

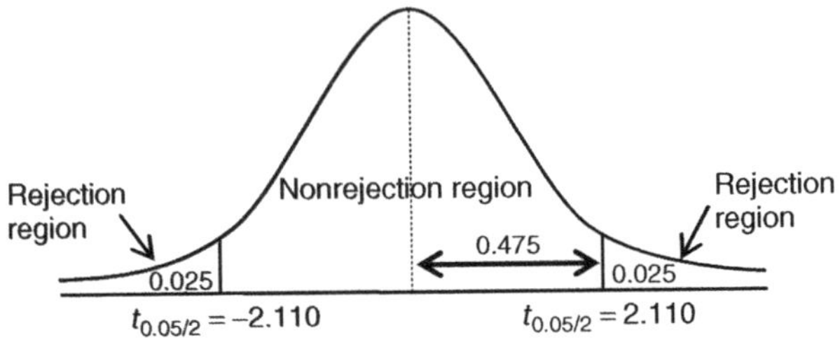

Since the hypothesis required to be tested is two-tailed, the critical region 0.05 has been divided in both the tails as shown in the figure. The area between the mean and the critical value that separates the rejection region in the right as well as the left tail is 0.475. By using this area and Table A.7, the critical value of t with 17(9 + 10 − 2)df can be obtained as

$$t_{0.05/2} = 2.110$$

Since the absolute value of Cal t is more than 2.110, H_0 may be rejected at the significance level 0.05.

Inference: Since H_0 has been rejected, it may be concluded that both the angles are not equally effective in improving the shooting accuracy. However, looking at the mean value of these treatment groups, it may be concluded that the training with 90° is more effective in comparison to that with 45° in improving the shooting accuracy.

Example 7.14 The following are the data on arm length obtained on badminton and table tennis players.

	Arm Length (cms)											
Badminton:	78	71	72	75	77	68	65	78	80	81	74	72
Table Tennis:	65	68	73	71	70	66	68	71	62	64	66	63

Can it be concluded that the arm length of the badminton players is more than that of the table tennis players? Given that the arm length is normally distributed and population variances of both the sports groups are nearly equal, test your hypothesis at the significance level 0.05.

Solution: In this problem, it is required to test whether badminton players have larger arm length in comparison to the table tennis players; hence the one-tailed test is used. Here, the samples are small, population variances are not known, arm length is normally distributed, and the population variances of both the groups are nearly the same. Under these conditions, to test the hypothesis, the t-test for two independent samples is used by following the below-mentioned steps:

Hypothesis: Since it is required to test whether arm length of the badminton players is more than that of table tennis players, the following hypotheses need to be tested:

$$H_0: \mu_{\text{Badminton}} = \mu_{\text{TableTennis}}$$

$$H_1: \mu_{\text{Badminton}} > \mu_{\text{TableTennis}}$$

Level of Significance: 0.05

Test Statistic: Since population variances are unknown and samples are small, the t-statistic mentioned below shall be used as a test statistic to compare the two group means:

$$t = \frac{\bar{x} - \bar{y}}{S\sqrt{\frac{1}{n_1} + \frac{1}{n_2}}}$$

where

$$S = \sqrt{\frac{\sum x^2 + \sum y^2 - n_1\bar{x}^2 - n_2\bar{y}^2}{n_1 + n_2 - 2}}$$

To compute the t-value, the mean of both the groups and pooled SD S need to be computed, which are shown in the following data.

Computation for t-Value

Badminton (x)	Table Tennis (y)	x^2	y^2
78	65	6084	4225
71	68	5041	4624
72	73	5184	5329
75	71	5625	5041
77	70	5929	4900
68	66	4624	4356
65	68	4225	4624
78	71	6084	5041
80	62	6400	3844
81	64	6561	4096
74	66	5476	4356
72	63	5184	3969
$\sum x = 891$	$\sum y = 807$	$\sum x^2 = 66417$	$\sum y^2 = 54405$

$$\bar{x} = \frac{\sum x}{n} = \frac{891}{12} = 74.25$$

$$\bar{y} = \frac{\sum y}{n} = \frac{807}{12} = 67.25$$

$$S = \sqrt{\frac{66417 + 54405 - 12 \times 74.25^2 - 12 \times 67.25^2}{12 + 12 - 2}}$$

$$= 4.23$$

Thus, $\bar{x} = 74.25$, $\bar{y} = 67.25$, $S = 4.23$, and $n_1 = n_2 = 12$. Substituting these values in the formula, we get

$$\text{Cal } t = \frac{74.25 - 67.25}{4.23 \times \sqrt{\frac{1}{12} + \frac{1}{12}}} = \frac{7}{1.727} = 4.053$$

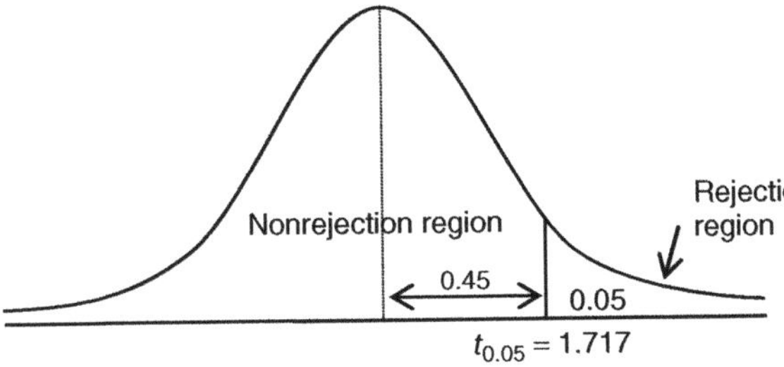

Since the hypothesis required to be tested is one-tailed (right), the entire critical region, 0.05, shall be in the right tail only as has been shown in the figure. The area between the mean and the critical value that separates the rejection region in the right tail is 0.45. By using this area and Table A.7, the critical value of t with 22 df can be obtained as

$$t_{0.05} = 1.717$$

Since the value of Cal t is more than 1.717, H_0 may be rejected at the significance level 0.05.

Inference: Since H_0 has been rejected, it may be concluded that the arm length of the badminton players is significantly larger than that of table tennis players.

Case 2: Paired t-*test for two dependent samples* In some of the experimental designs subjects serve as their own control; in that case, if the effects of two treatment conditions need to be compared, then the samples obtained would be dependent as the same subjects are tested in two treatment conditions. For instance, if an experimenter is interested in comparing the effect of some cooling down exercise with that of the autogenic relaxation technique on the recovery of athletes in a soccer match, the same subjects may be tested under these two treatment conditions so as to serve as their own control. Or, if the researcher is interested in seeing the impact of a circuit training program on dribbling accuracy, the same subjects would be tested for their dribbling performance before and after the circuit training program. In all such situations, the data obtained in the two groups shall be dependent. In these situations, the paired t-test is used to test the hypothesis about the population means by using the statistic t as mentioned in formula (7.32).

Let x_i and y_i $(i = 1, 2, \ldots, n)$ be the scores in the two samples that are related; then, under the null hypothesis H_0: $\mu_x - \mu_y = 0$ (no difference between the population means) the mean difference $\overline{D}$ between the two samples follows the t-distribution with $(n-1)$ degrees of freedom as given by formula (7.32):

$$t = \frac{\overline{D}}{S_D/\sqrt{n}} \tag{7.32}$$

where

$$\overline{D} = \frac{\sum D_i}{n}, D_i = y_i - x_i \forall i \tag{7.33}$$

and

$$S_D = \sqrt{\frac{1}{n-1}\sum_{i=1}^{n}(D_i - \overline{D})^2} = \sqrt{\frac{1}{n-1}\sum D_i^2 - \frac{\left(\sum D_i\right)^2}{n(n-1)}} \tag{7.34}$$

The t-test for testing the means of the two paired groups by using this t-statistic is known as a paired t-test. This paired t-test is used under the assumptions that the data in both the samples are related, sample sizes in both the samples are equal, each difference score, that is, $d_i = y_i - x_i$, is independent of the other, and these differences are normally distributed.

Example 7.15 A random sample of 10 women participated in a 4-week aerobic program. Their weight (in lbs) was measured before and after the program. The data obtained are shown in the following table. Assuming that the difference in weight is normally distributed, test the hypothesis whether the aerobic program was effective in reducing the weight. Test this hypothesis at the significance level 0.05.

Weight of the Women (in lbs)

Pre-testing:	130	136	128	118	144	151	136	120	132	140	142	138
Post-testing:	126	134	130	114	134	148	134	121	126	136	134	136

Solution: In this problem, it is required to test whether the aerobic program was effective in reducing the weight of the women participants. Since it is intended to test whether the mean weight of the participants after the aerobic program reduces significantly, the one-tailed test shall be used.

Hypothesis: The following hypotheses are required to be tested:

$$H_0: \mu_{\text{After}} = \mu_{\text{Before}}$$
$$H_1: \mu_{\text{After}} < \mu_{\text{Before}}$$

Level of Significance: 0.05

Test Statistic: Since the sample size is small ($n < 30$) and data in both the groups are related, the following t-statistic shall be used as a test statistic:

$$t = \frac{\overline{D}}{S_D/\sqrt{n}}$$

where

$$\overline{D} = \frac{\sum D_i}{n}$$

and

$$S_D = \sqrt{\frac{1}{n-1}\sum D_i^2 - \frac{\left(\sum D_i\right)^2}{n(n-1)}}$$

To compute the t-statistic, the mean difference $\overline{D}$ and SD S_D of the differences shall be computed first.

Computation of $\overline{D}$ and S_D

Computation of Mean and SD of the Differences for the Data on Weight (in lbs)

Pre-testing (X)	Post-testing (Y)	$D = Y - X$	D^2
130	126	−4	16
136	134	−2	4
128	130	2	4
118	114	−4	16
144	134	−10	100
151	148	−3	9
136	134	−2	4
120	121	1	1
132	126	−6	36
140	136	−4	16
142	134	−8	64
138	136	−2	4
		$\sum D = -42$	$\sum D^2 = 274$

$$\overline{D} = \frac{\sum D}{n} = \frac{-42}{12} = -3.5$$

$$S_D = \sqrt{\frac{1}{n-1}\sum D_i^2 - \frac{\left(\sum D_i\right)^2}{n(n-1)}}$$

$$= \sqrt{\frac{274}{12-1} - \frac{(-42)^2}{12\times(12-1)}}$$

$$= \sqrt{24.91 - 13.37}$$

$$= 3.397$$

Here, $n = 12$, $\overline{D} = -3.5$, and $S_D = 3.397$. Substituting these values in the formula, the calculated t (Cal t) can be obtained as

$$\text{Cal } t = \frac{\overline{D}}{S_D/\sqrt{n}}$$

$$= \frac{-3.5}{3.397/\sqrt{12}} = -3.57$$

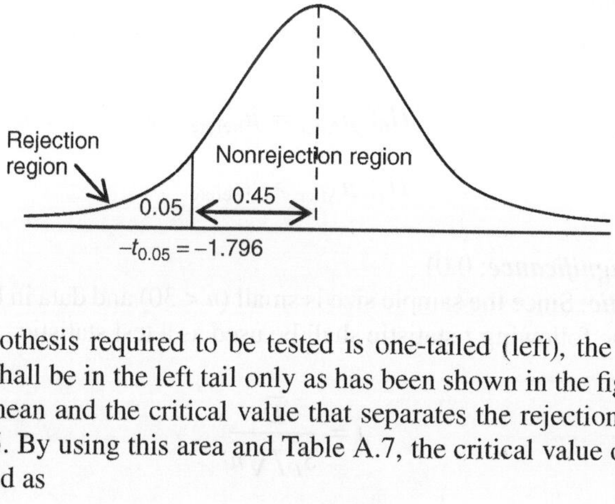

Since the hypothesis required to be tested is one-tailed (left), the entire critical region, 0.05, shall be in the left tail only as has been shown in the figure. The area between the mean and the critical value that separates the rejection region in the left tail is 0.45. By using this area and Table A.7, the critical value of t with 11 df can be obtained as

$$t_{0.05} = -1.796$$

Since the value of Cal t is less than -1.796, the test statistic t falls in the critical region; hence, H_0 may be rejected at the significance level 0.05.

Inference: Since H_0 has been rejected, it may be concluded that the aerobic program was effective in reducing the weight of the women participants.

Example 7.16 An 8-week fitness workout administered to each of 10 randomly chosen students resulted in the following increase in red blood corpuscles (RBCs) in millions per centimeter. Assuming the difference to be normally distributed, test whether the fitness workout was effective in enhancing the RBC count. Test your hypothesis at 1% level.

Increase in RBC
1.2
0.2
0
0.3
0.5
−0.1
0.3
0.9
1.1
0.2

Solution: Since it is required to see whether the fitness workout was effective in enhancing the RBC count, the one-tailed hypothesis shall be used in testing the required hypothesis.

Hypothesis: The following hypotheses are required to be tested:

$$H_0: \mu_{\text{After}} = \mu_{\text{Before}}$$

$$H_1: \mu_{\text{After}} > \mu_{\text{Before}}$$

Level of Significance: 0.01

Test Statistic: Since the sample size is small ($n < 30$) and data in both the groups are related, the following t-statistic shall be used as a test statistic:

$$t = \frac{\overline{D}}{S_D/\sqrt{n}}$$

where

$$\overline{D} = \frac{\sum D_i}{n}$$

and

$$S_D = \sqrt{\frac{1}{n-1}\sum D_i^2 - \frac{\left(\sum D_i\right)^2}{n(n-1)}}$$

To compute the t-statistic, the mean difference, $\overline{D}$, and SD, S_D, of the differences shall be computed first.

Computation of $\overline{D}$ and S_D

Here, data are given in the form of difference D_i (post-score−pre-score); the computation of $\overline{D}$ and S_D has been shown in the following table.

Computation for Paired t-Test

D = Post-score−Pre-score	D^2
1.2	1.44
0.2	0.04
0	0
0.3	0.09
0.5	0.25
−0.1	0.01
0.3	0.09
0.9	0.81
1.1	1.21
0.2	0.04
$\sum D = 4.6$	$\sum D^2 = 3.98$

$$\overline{D} = \frac{\sum D}{n} = \frac{4.6}{10} = 0.46$$

$$S_D = \sqrt{\frac{1}{n-1}\sum D_i^2 - \frac{\left(\sum D_i\right)^2}{n(n-1)}}$$

$$= \sqrt{\frac{3.98}{10-1} - \frac{(4.6)^2}{10 \times (10-1)}}$$

$$= \sqrt{0.442 - 0.235} = 0.455$$

Here, $n = 10$, $\overline{D} = 0.46$, and $S_D = 0.455$. Substituting these values in the formula, the calculated t (Cal t) can be obtained as

$$\text{Cal } t = \frac{\overline{D}}{S_D/\sqrt{n}}$$

$$= \frac{0.46}{0.455/\sqrt{10}} = 3.197$$

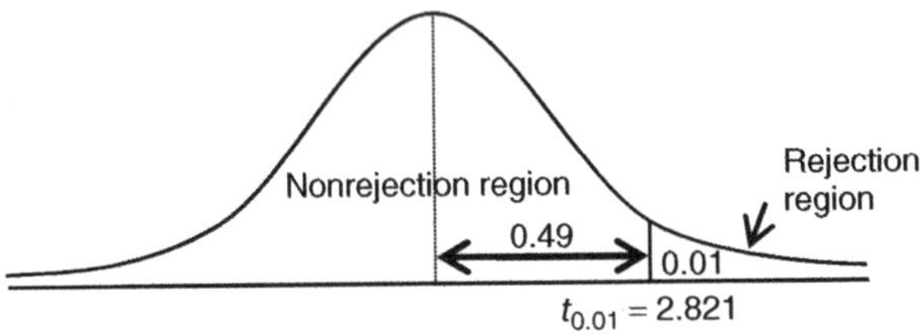

Since the hypothesis required to be tested is one-tailed (right), the entire critical region, 0.01, shall be in the right tail only as has been shown in the figure. The area between the mean and the critical value that separates the rejection region in the right tail is 0.49. By using this area and Table A.7, the critical value of t with 9df can be obtained as

$$t_{0.01} = 2.821$$

Since the value of Cal t is more than 2.821, the test statistic t falls in the critical region; H_0 may be rejected at the significance level 0.01.

Inference: Since H_0 has been rejected, it may be concluded that the fitness workout was effective in enhancing the RBC count of the participant.

7.22 TEST OF SIGNIFICANCE ABOUT TWO POPULATION PROPORTIONS

At times, the researcher is interested in drawing inferences about the difference in two population proportions. Such analysis can be used to compare the gender dominance in two different sports, studying the difference between male dopers in two different states, or comparing the proportion of males and females who qualify in the minimum muscular fitness test. In comparing such proportions in the populations, usually we use the statistic, $\hat{p}_1 - \hat{p}_2$, which is the difference in the sample proportions.

Let us assume that the two random samples of sufficiently large sizes n_1 and n_2 are drawn from the two independent populations having proportions as p_1 and p_2. If $\hat{p}_1$ and $\hat{p}_2$ are the sample proportions, then as per the central limit theorem the statistic $\hat{p}_1 - \hat{p}_2$ follows a normal distribution with mean $\mu_{\hat{p}_1-\hat{p}_2}$ and SD $\sigma_{\hat{p}_1-\hat{p}_2}$ as shown below:

$$\mu_{\hat{p}_1-\hat{p}_2} = p_1 - p_2 \quad (7.35)$$

$$\sigma_{\hat{p}_1-\hat{p}_2} = \sqrt{\bar{p} \cdot \bar{q}\left(\frac{1}{n_1} + \frac{1}{n_2}\right)} \quad (7.36)$$

where

$$\bar{p} = \frac{n_1\hat{p}_1 + n_2\hat{p}_2}{n_1 + n_2} \text{ and } \bar{q} = 1 - \bar{p} \quad (7.37)$$

Under the null hypothesis H_0: $p_1 = p_2$, the z-statistic as shown in formula (7.38) follows standard normal distribution, provided sample sizes are sufficiently large (each of $n_1.\hat{p}_1$, $n_1.\hat{q}_1$, $n_2.\hat{p}_2$ and $n_2.\hat{q}_2$ should be greater than 5).

$$Z = \frac{\hat{p}_1 - \hat{p}_2}{\sqrt{(\overline{p}.\overline{q})\left(\frac{1}{n_1} + \frac{1}{n_2}\right)}} \quad N(0, 1) \tag{7.38}$$

Thus, the z-statistic as shown in formula (7.38) can be used to test the hypothesis about the two population proportions, provided the samples are sufficiently large and are independent and randomly drawn from the populations.

Example 7.17 To assess hostel environment, a random sample of 190 boys and 95 girls was selected; out of the sample, 110 boys and 50 girls liked the environment. Do these data have sufficient evidence to conclude that the proportion of boys who were satisfied with the hostel is significantly higher than that of the girls? Test your hypothesis at 5% level.

Solution: Here, the proportion of the two groups needs to be compared. Further, it is required to test whether the proportion of boys who were satisfied with the hostel environment is higher than that of the girls; hence, the z-test for the difference of two proportions shall be used to test the one-tailed hypothesis.

Hypothesis: The hypotheses that are required to be tested are as follows:

$$H_0: p_1 = p_2$$

$$H_1: p_1 > p_2$$

where p_1 is the population proportion of the boys who were satisfied with the hostel facilities and p_2 is the population proportion of the girls who were satisfied with the hostel facilities.

Level of Significance: 0.05

Test Statistic: Since the sample is large and the proportions of the two groups need to be compared, the following test statistic shall be used to test the required hypothesis:

$$Z = \frac{\hat{p}_1 - \hat{p}_2}{\sqrt{p(1-p)} \times \sqrt{\frac{n_1 + n_2}{n_1 n_2}}}$$

where

$$p = \frac{n_1\hat{p}_1 + n_2\hat{p}_2}{n_1 + n_2}$$

Here, given that $n_1 = 190$ and $n_2 = 95$, p_1= proportion of boys who were satisfied with the hostel facilities in the sample = 110/190 = 0.58, p_2= proportion of girls who were satisfied with the hostel facilities in the sample = 50/95 = 0.53:

$$p = \frac{190 \times 0.58 + 95 \times 0.53}{190 + 95}$$

$$\Rightarrow p = 0.56$$

Substituting these values in the formula, we get

$$z = \frac{0.58 - 0.53}{\sqrt{0.56 \times (1 - 0.56)} \times \sqrt{\dfrac{190 + 95}{190 \times 95}}}$$

$$\Rightarrow z = \frac{0.05}{0.4964 \times 0.0686}$$

$$\Rightarrow \text{Cal } z = 1.47$$

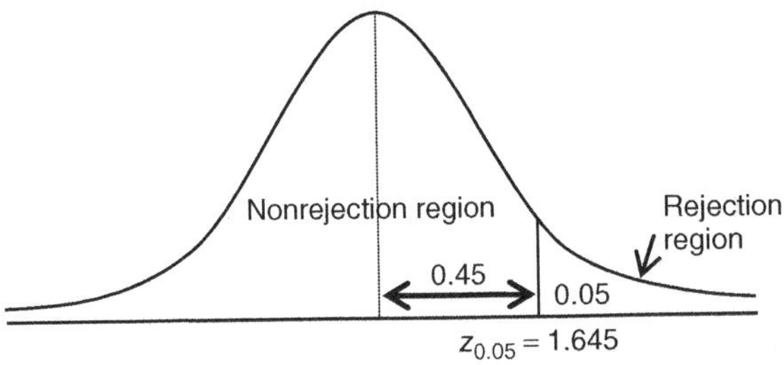

Since in one-tailed test the critical region lies only in one tail, in this example, the entire critical region 0.05 has been shifted in the right tail only as shown in the figure. The area between the mean and the critical value that separates the rejection region in the right tail is 0.45. By using this area and Table A.4, the critical value of z can be obtained as

$$z_{0.05} = 1.645$$

Since the value of z (=1.47) is less than 1.645, it lies in the nonrejection region and therefore the null hypothesis is not rejected at the significance level 0.05.

Inference: Since H_0 has not been rejected, it cannot be concluded that the proportion of boys who were satisfied with the hostel was significantly higher than that of the girls.

7.23 TEST OF SIGNIFICANCE ABOUT TWO POPULATION VARIANCES

In some situations, researchers are interested in testing the difference in the two population variances rather than the population means. For instance, a coach may be interested in knowing whether the variation in the height of men athletes is more than that of women athletes or the performance of the subjects in vertical jump among undergraduate and postgraduate students differs significantly. Let us see how to test the variances of the two groups in such situations.

Let us consider that the two samples $x_1, x_2, \ldots, x_{n_1}$ and $y_1, y_2, \ldots, y_{n_2}$ are drawn from two independent populations and that they are normally distributed. If σ_x^2 and σ_y^2 are the variances of the two populations, then under the null hypothesis, H_0: $\sigma_x^2 = \sigma_y^2$, the ratio of the sample variances follows F-distribution.

Thus,

$$F = \frac{S_x^2}{S_y^2} \tag{7.39}$$

is an F-distribution with (n_1-1, n_2-1) degrees of freedom where

$$S_x^2 = \frac{1}{n_1 - 1}\sum_{i=1}^{n_1} (x_i - \bar{x})^2 \text{ and } S_y^2 = \frac{1}{n_2 - 1}\sum_{j=1}^{n_2} (y_j - \bar{y})^2$$

The value of F can be obtained from Tables A.9 and A.10 at the desired level of significance (table values of F have been given only for 0.05 and 0.01 level of significance). The value of F at 0.05 level of significance and (n_1-1, n_2-1) degrees of freedom is obtained by identifying the value of F at the cross-section point while looking up n_1-1 in the first row and n_2-1 in the first column. The statistic F in formula (7.39) can be used to test the hypothesis about the two population variances, provided the populations from which the samples have been drawn are independent and normally distributed.

Example 7.18 A coach wanted to know whether women varied more than men in push-up performance. A sample of 12 women and 15 men among college athletes were tested for their push-up performance. The variance for the women was 9 and the variance for the men was 16. Can it be concluded at 5% level that the population variances for the push-up performance were significantly different in women and men?

Solution: In this problem, variances of the two groups are to be compared; hence, the F-test shall be used.

Hypothesis: The following hypotheses are required to be tested:

$$H_0\colon \sigma^2_{\text{Women}} = \sigma^2_{\text{Men}}$$
$$H_1\colon \sigma^2_{\text{Women}} \neq \sigma^2_{\text{Men}}$$

Level of Significance: 0.05

Test Statistic: Since it is required to compare the variances of the two groups, the following F-statistic shall be used to test the null hypothesis:

$$F = \frac{S_x^2}{S_y^2}$$

Sinces larger variance is present in the numerator, let x denote men and y denote women.

Here, it is given that $S_x^2 = 16$, n_1=15, and $S_y^2 = 9$, n_2= 12.

Substituting these values in the formula, we get

$$F = \frac{S_x^2}{S_y^2} = \frac{16}{9} = 1.78$$

Thus, Cal $F = 1.78$

To find the critical value of F, the degrees of freedom shall be (n_1-1, n_2-1) or (14, 11). Thus, by using Table A.9, the critical value of F shall be

$$F_{0.05}(14, 11) = 2.74$$

Since calculated $F(=1.78)$ is less than 2.74, the null hypothesis may not be rejected.

Inference: Since H_0 has not been rejected, it may not be concluded that the variation in the push-up performance is significantly different in men and women.

Remark: While locating the value of F in the table, n_1-1 (numerator df) degrees of freedom is to be seen in the first row and the value of n_2-1 (denominator df) degrees of freedom is to be seen in the first column.

Check Your Progress

Note: Tick the correct answer by using the sign (√).

	Truc	False
30. The χ^2 test is parametric as well as nonparametric.	-	-
31. The researcher must construct the research hypothesis along with null hypothesis.	-	-
32. If the value of α is 0, then the value of β is also 0.	-	-
33. All the hypothesis tests are based on the assumption that the null hypothesis is true.	-	-
34. The null hypothesis is a via media for testing a research hypothesis.	-	-

35.	A test statistic is not computed on the basis of the sample; rather, it is seen from the distribution table.	-	-
36.	A test statistic shows how much the sample statistic differs from the population parameter.	-	-
37.	Decision about using either one-tailed or two-tailed test is taken on the basis of the null hypothesis.	-	-
38.	The value of β can be outside the limits 0 and 1.	-	-
39.	The null hypothesis is never proved.	-	-
40.	The χ^2 test is used to test the hypothesis about the single population variance.	-	-
41.	A type II error is serious for the researcher as it wrongly accepts the false null hypothesis.	-	-
42.	The value of α lies between 0 and 1.	-	-
43.	The research and alternative hypotheses are two different types of hypothesis.	-	-
44.	Type I and type II errors both can be reduced simultaneously for a fixed sample size.	-	-
45.	Type I error and α represent the same thing.	-	-
46.	A research hypothesis may be unidirectional if the researcher is sure that the effect of the treatment can go only in one direction.	-	-
47.	In one-tailed (left) test if the hypothesis is tested at α level of significance, then the nonrejection area would be on the left side of the critical value.	-	-
48.	In case of large samples, the distribution of $\bar{x}_1 - \bar{x}_2$ follows a normal distribution.	-	-
49.	In testing the quality of sports goods, a type I error is a risk for the user whereas a type II error is a risk for the producer.	-	-
50.	$1-\alpha$ refers to the probability of not rejecting a null hypothesis when it is correct.	-	-
51.	The power of a test refers to the probability of rejecting H_0 when it is false.	-	-
52.	Critical region is the one in which if the test statistic falls the test statistic becomes insignificant.	-	-
53.	The p-value is the estimated significance level at which the null hypothesis may be rejected when it is true.	-	-
54.	Test of significance is used to test whether the research hypothesis can be rejected or accepted on the basis of the value of the test statistic value.	-	-

55.	"t" test is always used for testing of hypothesis about the population mean so long as the sample is small ($n < 30$).	-	-
56.	In testing of hypothesis the critical value of z will differ in one-tailed and two-tailed tests.	-	-
57.	If the level of significance is set at 0.05 for testing a hypothesis, then the null hypothesis may be rejected so long as the p-value is more than 0.05.	-	-
58.	If a two-tailed test is used at an α level of significance, then the nonrejection area would be equal to $1 - \alpha$.	-	-
59.	For sufficiently large samples, the difference of the two sample proportions $\hat{p}_1 - \hat{p}_2$ follows a normal distribution.	-	-
60.	For one-tailed and two-tailed tests, the total critical region would be α and $\alpha/2$, respectively, where α is the level of significance at which the hypothesis is tested.	-	-
61.	The degree of freedom is a measure of accuracy with which sample observations represent the population.	-	-
62.	If the sample sizes of two samples are n_1 and n_2 ($n_1 \neq n_2$), then the pooled standard deviation is the average of the two standard deviations.	-	-
63.	For a paired t-test, the degree of freedom is $n - 1$.	-	-
64.	In using a z-test for testing the hypothesis about two population proportions, no condition is imposed on the independence of the samples.	-	-
65.	In using the F-test in testing the hypothesis about two population variances, the critical value of F is obtained at (n_1, n_2) degrees of freedom.	-	-
66.	The degrees of freedom of S^2 is $n - 1$.	-	-
67.	The z-test can be used to test the hypothesis about the population mean even for a small sample ($n < 30$), provided the population is normally distributed and the population standard deviation is known.	-	-
68.	Since χ^2 test can be used for testing the hypothesis about a single population variance, it can also be used for testing two population variances.	-	-
69.	The z-test is used for testing the means of the two population means if any of the sample size n_1 or n_2 is more than 30.	-	-
70.	In a two-sample test, the critical value of t is obtained at $n_1 + n_2$ degrees of freedom.	-	-

71.	If the calculated value of test statistic is equal to critical value, H_0 is not rejected.	-	-
72.	Irrespective of whether t-test or z-test is used, the distribution of population should be normal if the sample size is less than 30.	-	-
73.	The z-test can be used in testing the hypothesis for two population proportions, provided the samples are large enough so that $np \geq 5$ and $nq \geq 5$.	-	-
74.	In using the t-test for testing the equality of two group means, no assumptions are made on the population variances so long as the sample is small and population variances are unknown.	-	-

PRACTICE EXERCISE

6. Test the hypothesis H_0: $\mu = 35$ against H_1: $\mu \neq 35$ where $\bar{x} = 32.4$, $\sigma = 5.6$, $n = 64$, and $\alpha = 0.05$.
7. A sample of 15 athletes drawn randomly from a college is tested for standing broad jump performance. The mean and SD of the sample are 5.6 ft and 0.5 ft, respectively. If the population is normally distributed, can it be concluded that the population mean is 5.2 ft? Test your hypothesis at 5% level.
8. It is claimed that in a university, 60% of students are nonsmokers. To test this hypothesis, a sample of 150 students were randomly selected and were asked about their smoking status. Fifty-four percent students in the sample reported that they were nonsmokers. Test the claim at 5% level.
9. The following is the information about the mean and variance of the sit-ups scores in two samples.

	$\bar{x}$	S	n
First Sample	24	6.2	12
Second Sample	21.5	5.5	16

Given that the sit-ups (x) is normally distributed and population variances are nearly equal, test the hypothesis H_0: $\mu_1 - \mu_2 = 0$ against H_1: $\mu_1 - \mu_2 > 0$ at 5% level.

10. The following is the difference in the fat percentage of 12 subjects measured before and after undergoing a fitness training program of 6 weeks.

Difference:	5	4	3	2	−1	8	6	−2	7	5	8	3

Assuming that the difference is normally distributed, do these data suggest that the fitness training program is effective in reducing the fat percentage? Test your hypothesis at the level of significance 0.05.

11. To assess the curriculum of a particular exercise science program, a random sample of 90 boys and 60 girls was randomly drawn, out of which 65 boys and 40 girls showed satisfaction with the contents. Do these data show enough evidence to conclude that the boys' proportion was significantly higher than that of the girls in expressing that the curriculum was good? Use a 5% level of significance.

12. By using the information in the following table, test the hypotheses H_0: $\sigma_1^2 = \sigma_2^2$ against H_1: $\sigma_1^2 < \sigma_2^2$ at 1% level by assuming that the populations are normally distributed.

	σ^2	n
First Sample	245	8
Second Sample	80	11

7.24 COMPUTING WITH EXCEL

7.24.1 Using Excel in Comparing Group Means

Excel can be used to compare the means of two groups in a situation where population variances are known as well as unknown. In this section, the use of Excel in applying the z-test, the t-test for two independent samples, and paired t-test for two dependent samples is discussed.

Remark The below-mentioned tests can be applied only if the Add-Ins "Analysis ToolPak" is already installed in your Excel. The readers can install this Add-Ins "Analysis ToolPak" in their Excel by following the procedure mentioned in Chapter 1.

7.24.2 z-Test for Comparing the Means of Two Samples

The z-test has already been discussed in detail earlier in this chapter and is used to compare the means of two groups in a situation where the population variances are known. In this section, the procedure for using Excel for applying the z-test is discussed by means of the following example.

Example 7.19 The following are the data on back strength (in kilogram) obtained on tennis and fencing players.

Back Strength in Kilograms												
Tennis:	79	85	82	78	97	85	75	78	85	82	76	78
Fencing:	75	78	74	70	68	66	69	72	66	68	69	65

On the basis of these data, can it be concluded that the back strength of the tennis players is higher than that of the fencing players, given that the back strength is normally distributed and the population variances for the tennis and fencing groups are 21.2 and 11.6, respectively? Test your hypothesis at the significance level 0.05.

Solution: Since the scores are normally distributed and the population SDs are known, the z-test is used to compare the means of the two groups. The following steps are used to apply the z-test in Excel:

1. Type the sample data of both the groups in the two columns A and B of the Excel sheet. The heading for both the variables may be written in the first cell of the column.
2. To compute the z-statistic, click the following commands in sequence in Excel to get the screen as shown in Figure 7.12.

Data ⟶ Data Analysis

3. Bring the scroll on the option **z-Test: Two Sample for Means** and then click **OK** in the screen as shown in Figure 7.12. This will take you to the screen as shown in Figure 7.13. You can now define the data range of both the samples.
4. Here, the data for the badminton group is written in column A and it occupies 13 cells in the column. This includes variable name as well. Thus, the range of the badminton variable would be $A1{:}A13$. Similarly, since the scores of the table tennis group have been written in column B and it occupies 13 cells of this column, its range would be $B1{:}B13$. Do the following steps to fill the entries in the screen shown in Figure 7.13.
   i. **Variable 1 Range**: $A1{:}A13$
      Variable 2 Range: $B1{:}B13$
   ii. **Variable 1 Variance(known)**: 21.2 (This is the variance of the first variable.)
   iii. **Variable 2 Variance(known)**: 11.6 (This is the variance of the second variable.)
   iv. Check **Labels** (because the heading for the data is written in the first cell).
   v. Write the value of α at which you want to test the hypothesis. In this example, it is taken as 0.05.

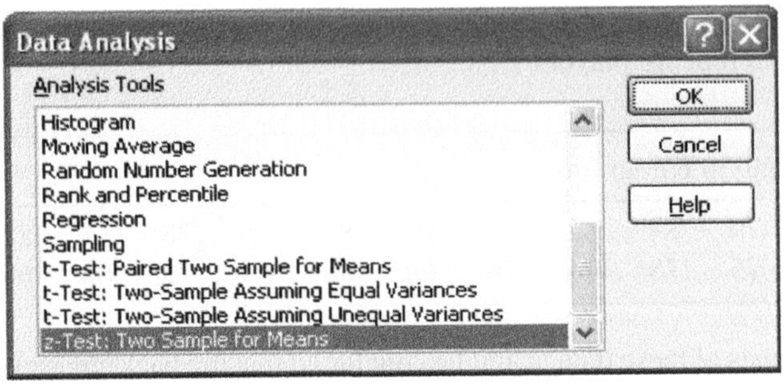

Figure 7.12 Command for applying the *z*-test for comparing two groups.

TABLE 7.4 ***z*-Test: Two Samples for Means**

	Badminton	Table Tennis
	Tennis	Fencing
Mean	81.67	70
Known variance	21.20	11.6
Observations	12.00	12
Hypothesized mean difference	0.00	
z	7.06	
$P(Z<=z)$ one tail	0.00	
z Critical one tail	1.64	
$P(Z<=z)$ two tail	0.00	
z Critical two tail	1.96	

vi. Fill the entry in the output range. The output can be obtained on the same Excel sheet, new worksheet, or new workbook. Here, the output is obtained on the same sheet starting from *A*15 onward, and therefore the following entry should be filled.
Output Range: *A*15

vii. Click **OK** to get the output as shown in Figure 7.14.

5. The output shown in Figure 7.14 can be formatted by formatting the cell entries of column 2. (Readers are advised to see the procedure discussed in Chapter 1 in this regard.) After the formatting, the results will look as shown in Table 7.4.

Since the calculated value of z (=7.06) is higher than 1.645, it may be concluded that the back strength of the tennis players is higher than that of the fencing players.

7.24.3 *t*-Test for Comparing Two Independent Samples

The *t*-test has been discussed earlier in this chapter and is used for comparing the means of two independent groups in a situation where the population variances are unknown. In this section, the procedure for using Excel for applying the *t*-test for two independent samples is discussed by means of the following example.

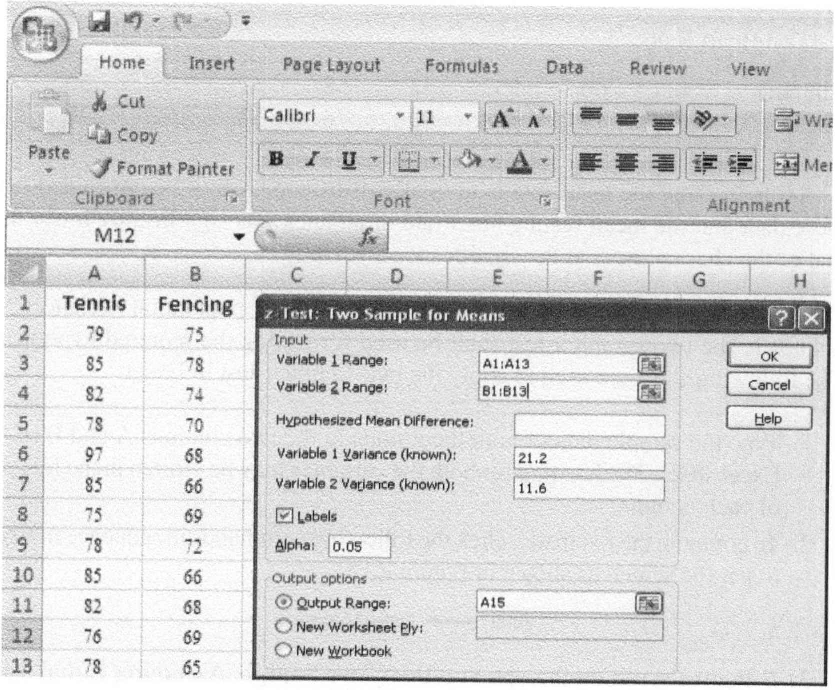

Figure 7.13 Options for applying *z*-test for comparing two groups.

15	z-Test: Two Sample for Means		
16			
17		*Tennis*	*Fencing*
18	Mean	81.66666667	70
19	Known Variance	21.2	11.6
20	Observations	12	12
21	Hypothesized Mean Difference	0	
22	z	7.056681087	
23	P(Z<=z) one-tail	8.52651E-13	
24	z Critical one-tail	1.644853627	
25	P(Z<=z) two-tail	1.7053E-12	
26	z Critical two-tail	1.959963985	

Figure 7.14 Outputs of *z*-test for comparing two groups.

Example 7.20 Scores on resting heart rate were recorded for two groups of male students in a college. Nine students in one group were the members of the college track and field team, whereas eight members of the other group were chess players. The resulting scores are shown in the following table:

Data on Heart Rate

Athletics	48	60	55	52	58	62	49	50	56
Chess		75	80	90	78	95	92	76	85

Assuming that the heart rate is normally distributed, can it be concluded from these data that the mean resting heart rate of athletes was significantly lower than that of the chess players at the significance level 0.05?

Solution: Since the samples are independent and the population variances are unknown, the two-sample t-test shall be used for testing the required hypothesis. The following steps are used to apply the two-sample t-test in Excel:

1. Type the sample data of both the groups in the two columns A and B of the Excel sheet. The heading for both the variables may be written in the first cell of each column.
2. To compute the t-statistic, click the following commands in sequence in Excel to get the screen as shown in Figure 7.15.

   Data → Data Analysis

3. Bring the scroll on the option ***t*-Test: Two Sample Assuming Equal Variances** and then click **OK** in the screen as shown in Figure 7.15. This will take you to the screen as shown in Figure 7.16. You can now define the range of both the sample data that need to be compared.
4. Here, the data for the athletics group are written in column A and it occupies 10 cells in the column. This includes the variable name as well. Thus, the range of the athletics variable would be *A*1:*A*10. Similarly, the scores of the chess group has been written in column B and it occupies 9 cells of this column; hence, its range would be *B*1:*B*9. Do the following steps to fill the entries in the screen shown in Figure 7.16.

   i. **Variable 1 Range**: *A*1:*A*10
   Variable 2 Range: *B*1:*B*9

   ii. Check **Labels** (because the heading for the data is written in the first cell).

   iii. Write the value of α at which you want to test the hypothesis. In this example, it is taken as 0.05.

   iv. Fill the entry in the output range. The output can be obtained on the same Excel sheet, new worksheet, or new workbook. Here, the output is obtained on the same sheet starting from *A*15 onward, and therefore the following entry should be filled.
   Output Range: *A*15

   v. Click **OK** to get the output as shown in Figure 7.17.

   vi. The output shown in Figure 7.17 can be formatted by formatting the cell entries of the columns 2 and 3 (Readers are advised to see the procedure

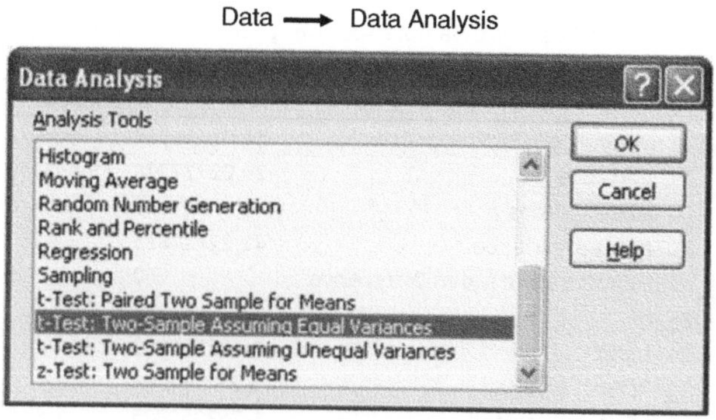

Figure 7.15 Command for applying *t*-test for comparing two independent groups.

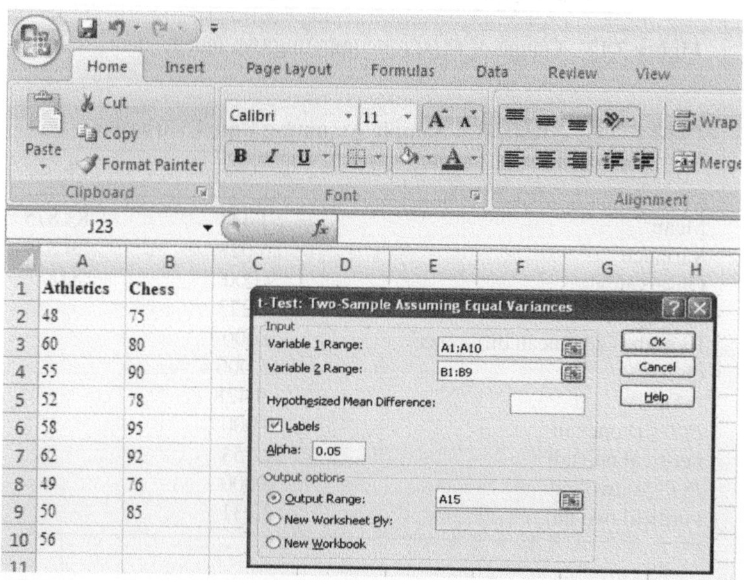

Figure 7.16 Options for applying *t*-test for comparing two independent groups.

discussed in Chapter 1 in this regard). After formatting, the results will look as shown in Table 7.5.

Since the calculated value of t (= −9.428) is less than −1.753, it may be concluded that the mean resting heart rate of athletes was significantly lower than that of the chess players at the significance level 0.05.

7.24.4 Paired *t*-Test for Two Dependent Samples

In the case of two dependent samples, the paired *t*-test is used to compare the means of the two groups. The procedure for applying the paired *t*-test by using Excel is discussed by means of the following example.

15	t-Test: Two-Sample Assuming Equal Variances		
16			
17		*Athletics*	*Chess*
18	Mean	54.44444444	83.875
19	Variance	25.02777778	59.839286
20	Observations	9	8
21	Pooled Variance	41.27314815	
22	Hypothesized Mean Difference	0	
23	df	15	
24	t Stat	-9.427715093	
25	P(T<=t) one-tail	5.39401E-08	
26	t Critical one-tail	1.753050325	
27	P(T<=t) two-tail	1.0788E-07	
28	t Critical two-tail	2.131449536	

Figure 7.17 Output of t-test for comparing two independent groups.

TABLE 7.5 ***t*-Test: Two-Sample Assuming Equal Variances**

	Athletics	Chess
Mean	54.444	83.875
Variance	25.028	59.839
Observations	9.000	8.000
Pooled variance	41.273	
Hypothesized mean difference	0.000	
df	15.000	
t stat	−9.428	
$P(T \leq t)$ one tail	0.000	
t critical one tail	1.753	
$P(T \leq t)$ two tail	0.000	
t critical two tail	2.131	

Example 7.21 Ten randomly selected sedentary men in the age category of 50–60 years were tested for their performance on positive breath-holding capacity (in seconds) before and after 4 weeks of the anulome vilome pranayama of 30 min duration every day for 5 days a week. The data obtained are shown below. Apply paired t-test to test the hypothesis as to whether the pranayama program was effective in enhancing the positive breath-holding capacity. Test your hypothesis at the significance level 0.01.

Data on Positive Breath-Holding Capacity (in Seconds)

Before:	40	43	46	41	40	46	42	41	40	42
After:	45	47	45	48	49	47	48	45	46	43

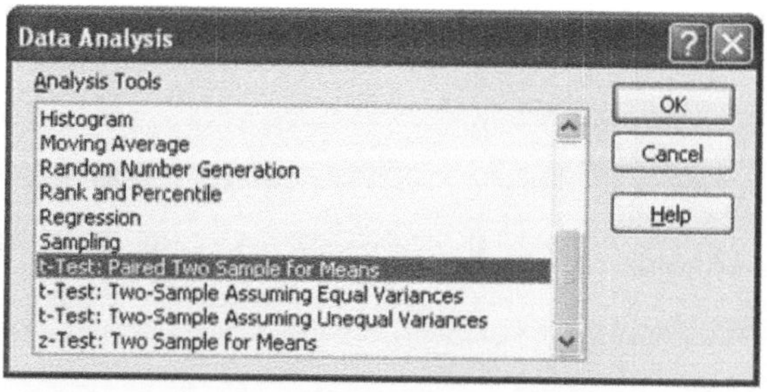

Figure 7.18 Command for applying paired *t*-test.

Solution: Since the samples are dependent and the variances are unknown, a paired *t*-test is used for testing the required hypothesis. The following steps are used to apply the paired *t*-test in Excel:

1. Type after and before test data in the two columns A and B of the Excel sheet. The heading for both the variables may be written in the first cell.
2. To compute the paired *t*-statistic, click the following commands in sequence in Excel to get the screen as shown in Figure 7.18.

   Data ⟶ Data Analysis

3. Bring the scroll on the option ***t*-Test: Paired Two Sample for Means** and then click **OK** in the screen as shown in Figure 7.18. This will take you to the screen as shown in Figure 7.19. You can now define the range of the data in both the groups that need to be compared.
4. Here, the data for the "After" testing group is written in column A and it occupies 11 cells in the column. This includes variable name as well. Thus, the range of the "After" variable would be *A*1:*A*11. Similarly, the scores of the "Before" testing group have been written in column B and it occupies nine cells of this column, its range would be *B*1:*B*11. Do the following steps to fill the entries in the screen shown in Figure 7.19.
   i. **Variable 1 Range**: *A*1:*A*11
      Variable 2 Range: *B*1:*B*11
   ii. Check **Labels** (because the heading for the data is written in the first cell).
   iii. Write the value of α at which you want to test the hypothesis. In this example, it is taken as 0.01.
   iv. Fill the entry in the output range. The output can be obtained on the same Excel sheet, new worksheet, or new workbook. Here, the output is obtained on the same sheet starting from *A*15 onward, and therefore the following entry should be filled.
      Output Range: *A*15
   v. Click **OK** to get the output as shown in Figure 7.20.
   vi. The output shown in Figure 7.20 can be formatted by formatting the cell entries of columns 2 and 3 (Readers are advised to see the procedure

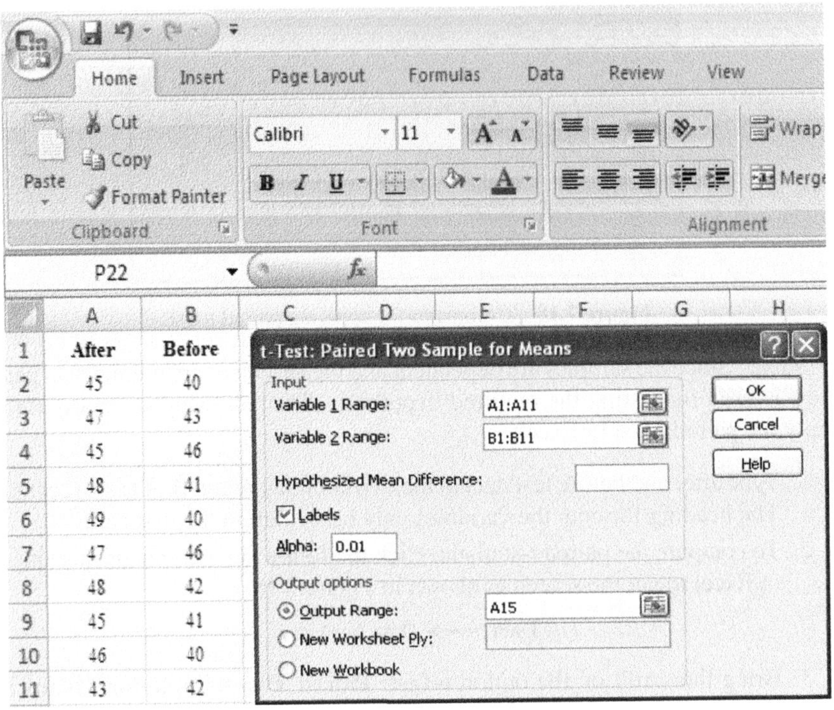

Figure 7.19 Options for applying paired *t*-test.

TABLE 7.6 *t*-Test: Paired Two Samples for Means

	After	Before
Mean	46.30	42.10
Variance	3.34	5.21
Observations	10.00	10.00
Pearson correlation	−0.11	
Hypothesized mean difference	0.00	
df	9.00	
t Stat	4.31	
$P(T \leq t)$ one-tail	0.00	
t Critical one-tail	2.82	
$P(T \leq t)$ two-tail	0.00	
t Critical two-tail	3.25	

discussed in Chapter 1 in this regard). After formatting, the results will appear as shown in Table 7.6.

Since the calculated value of t (= 4.31) is greater than 2.821, it may be concluded at 1% level that the pranayama was effective in enhancing the positive breath-holding capacity.

15	t-Test: Paired Two Sample for Means		
16			
17		*After*	*Before*
18	Mean	46.3	42.1
19	Variance	3.34444444	5.211111
20	Observations	10	10
21	Pearson Correlation	-0.11444552	
22	Hypothesized Mean Difference	0	
23	df	9	
24	t Stat	4.30659134	
25	P(T<=t) one-tail	0.00098576	
26	t Critical one-tail	2.82143792	
27	P(T<=t) two-tail	0.00197151	
28	t Critical two-tail	3.24983554	

Figure 7.20 Outputs of paired t-test.

IMPORTANT DEFINITIONS

Point estimation is the process of estimating a single value of the population parameter on the basis of the sample observations.

An estimator is said to be ***unbiased*** if its expected value is equal to the population parameter.

An estimator is said to be ***consistent*** if its value approaches the population parameter as the sample size increases to infinity.

An estimator is said to be ***efficient*** if its fluctuation is least in different samples drawn randomly from the same population.

An estimator is said to be ***sufficient*** if it extracts all the information that is contained in the sample about the parameter.

Interval estimation is the process of constructing a confidence interval that is supposed to contain the population parameter with some confidence.

The ***t-distribution*** is a family of probability distribution that is symmetrical, bell shaped, and similar to the standard normal curve but more flat at the top.

Testing of hypothesis is a procedure for testing a research hypothesis. Null hypothesis is used as a via media for testing the research hypothesis.

Null hypothesis is a hypothesis of no difference and is used to test the research hypothesis.

Alternative hypothesis is a research hypothesis that a researcher wants to verify.

A ***test statistic*** is a random variable x whose value is tested against the critical value for testing the null hypothesis.

Type I error can be defined as the error in rejecting the null hypothesis when it is correct.
Type II error can be defined as the error in not rejecting the null hypothesis when it is false.
Level of significance is the probability of committing type I error and is denoted by α.
Power of a test can be defined as the efficiency of a test statistic in rejecting the null hypothesis when it is wrong and is denoted by $1-\beta$.
Rejection region is that part of the distribution in which if the value of the test statistic falls, the null hypothesis is rejected. It is also known as the critical region.
The ***p-value*** can be defined as the estimated probability of rejecting the null hypothesis when it is true.
A statistical test is known as a ***one-tailed test*** if the null hypothesis is rejected only for values of the test statistic falling into one specified tail of its sampling distribution.
A statistical test is said to be a ***two-tailed test*** if the null hypothesis is rejected only for the value of the test statistic that falls into either tail of its sampling distribution.
The ***degrees of freedom*** can be defined as the number of independent pieces of information used for estimating the parameters or variability of the population on the basis of the sample statistic.

IMPORTANT FORMULAS

Estimator of population mean

$$\bar{x} = \frac{\sum x}{n}$$

Estimator of population variance

$$s^2 = \frac{1}{n-1}\sum (x-\bar{x})^2$$

Estimator of population proportion

$$\hat{p} = \frac{x}{n}$$

Unbiased estimator of population mean

$$E(\bar{x}) = \mu$$

Unbiased estimator of population variance

$$E(S^2) = \sigma^2$$

Standard error of sample mean

$$\text{SE}(\overline{x}) = \frac{\sigma}{\sqrt{n}}$$

Confidence interval for the population mean at an α level in a large sample

$$\overline{x} \pm Z_{\alpha/2}\text{SE}(\overline{x})$$

$$\overline{x} \pm Z_{\alpha/2}\frac{\sigma}{\sqrt{n}}$$

Confidence interval for the population mean at an α level in a small sample

$$\overline{x} \pm t_{\alpha/2}(n-1)\text{SE}(\overline{x})$$

$$\overline{x} \pm t_{\alpha/2}(n-1)\frac{s}{\sqrt{n}}$$

Confidence interval for the population proportion at an α level in a large sample

$$\hat{p} \pm z_{\alpha/2}\sqrt{\frac{p \times q}{n}}$$

Formula for constructing a test statistic

$$\text{Test statistic} = \frac{\text{Statistic} - E(\text{Statistic})}{\text{SE(Statistic)}}$$

The z-Statistic for testing the hypothesis about single mean

$$z = \frac{\overline{x} - E(\overline{x})}{\text{SE}(\overline{x})} = \frac{\overline{x} - \mu}{\sigma/\sqrt{n}}$$

Level of significance

$$\alpha = \text{Prob}(\text{Rejecting} H_0/H_0 \text{is true})$$

Power of a test

$$\begin{aligned}\text{Power} &= 1 - \beta \\ &= \text{Prob}(\text{Rejecting} H_0/H_0 \text{ is false})\end{aligned}$$

The t-statistic for testing the hypothesis about single mean

$$t = \frac{\bar{x} - \mu}{s/\sqrt{n}}$$

$$\bar{x} = \frac{1}{n}\sum x_i \quad \text{and} \quad s = \sqrt{\frac{1}{n-1}\sum (x_i - \bar{x})^2}$$

The z-statistic for testing the hypothesis about single proportion

$$z = \frac{\hat{p} - p}{\sqrt{pq/n}}$$

Chi-square test for testing the hypothesis about population variance in a single group

$$\chi^2 = \frac{(n-1)s^2}{\sigma^2}, \text{df} = n - 1$$

Mean and SD of the difference of two sample means

$$\mu_{\bar{x}_1 - \bar{x}_2} = \mu_1 - \mu_2$$

$$\sigma_{\bar{x}_1 - \bar{x}_2} = \sqrt{\frac{\sigma_1^2}{n_1} + \frac{\sigma_2^2}{n_2}}$$

The z-statistic for testing two independent samples (population SDs known)

$$Z = \frac{\bar{x}_1 - \bar{x}_2}{\sqrt{\frac{\sigma_1^2}{n_1} + \frac{\sigma_2^2}{n_2}}}$$

The t-statistic for testing the means of two independent samples (population SDs unknown)

$$t = \frac{\bar{x} - \bar{y}}{S\sqrt{\frac{1}{n_1} + \frac{1}{n_2}}}$$

$$S = \sqrt{\frac{1}{n_1 + n_2 - 2}\left(\sum x_i^2 + \sum y_j^2 - n_1\bar{x}^2 - n_2\bar{y}^2\right)}$$

The t-statistic for testing the means of two dependent samples

$$t = \frac{\bar{D}}{S_D/\sqrt{n}}$$

where

$$\overline{D} = \frac{\sum D_i}{n}$$

and

$$S_D = \sqrt{\frac{1}{n-1}\sum_{i=1}^{n}(D_i - \overline{D})^2}$$

$$= \sqrt{\frac{1}{n-1}\sum D_i^2 - \frac{\left(\sum D_i\right)^2}{n(n-1)}}$$

Mean and SD of the difference of two sample proportions

$$\mu_{\hat{p}_1 - \hat{p}_2} = p_1 - p_2$$

$$\sigma_{\hat{p}_1 - \hat{p}_2} = \sqrt{\overline{p}.\overline{q}\left(\frac{1}{n_1} + \frac{1}{n_2}\right)}$$

The z-statistic for testing the means of the two sample proportions

$$Z = \frac{\hat{p}_1 - \hat{p}_2}{\sqrt{(\overline{p}.\overline{q})\left(\frac{1}{n_1} + \frac{1}{n_2}\right)}}$$

where

$$\overline{p} = \frac{n_1\hat{p}_1 + n_2\hat{p}_2}{n_1 + n_2}$$

and

$$\overline{q} = 1 - \overline{p}$$

F-statistic for comparing the variances of two samples

$$F = \frac{S_x^2}{S_y^2}$$

where

$$S_x^2 = \frac{1}{n_1 - 1}\sum_{i=1}^{n_1}(x_i - \overline{x})^2$$

and

$$S_y^2 = \frac{1}{n_2 - 1}\sum_{j=1}^{n_2}(y_j - \bar{y})^2$$

KEY TERMS

F-test
p-value
t-test
z-test
alternative hypothesis
confidence interval
consistency
critical value
degrees of freedom
efficiency
hypothesis testing
interval estimation
level of significance
null hypothesis
one-tailed and two-tailed tests
point estimation
power of the test
rejection region
sufficiency
test
test of significance
type I and type II errors
unbiasedness

CHAPTER EXERCISE

1. What are the characteristics of a good estimator?
2. Discuss the factor that affects the confidence interval.
3. Write short notes on the following:
   i. Null and alternative hypotheses
   ii. Type I and type II errors
   iii. Test statistic
   iv. Level of significance and p-value
   v. One- and two-tailed tests
4. Discuss the procedure for testing a hypothesis.
5. Discuss the assumptions used in applying the t-test for two independent samples.
6. A sample of size 144 with mean 42 is drawn from a normal population having population variance 36. Construct 90% and 99% confidence limits of the population mean.
7. Construct 95% confidence interval to estimate the population mean with the following information: $\bar{x} = 35$, $\sigma = 5.5$, and $n = 49$.
8. A sample of 400 students is tested on 50 m dash. The mean and SD of the sample are 7.2 s and 0.15 s, respectively. Can it be concluded that the sample has been drawn from a large population having mean 7.32 s?
9. A sample of 100 athletes has a mean body fat percentage 13.53 and SD 4.52. Is the sample from a large population of mean fat percentage 14.14 and SD 4.52?

10. Construct an 85% confidence interval for estimating the population mean if a random sample of size 120 with mean 131 has been drawn from a population having population SD 25.
11. Using the below-mentioned sample information, construct the 90% confidence interval for estimating the population mean assuming that the population is normally distributed.

$$n = 18,\ \bar{x} = 25.2,\ s^2 = 28.5$$

12. Using the following sample information, construct 95% confidence interval for the population mean assuming that the population is normally distributed.

$$n = 22,\ \bar{x} = 45.5,\ s^2 = 142$$

13. Basal heart rates of 16 subjects were measured with mean and SD as 77 and 5, respectively. Assuming that the population from which the sample has been drawn is normally distributed, construct 95% and 99% confidence intervals for the population mean.
14. A random sample of 20 athletes was tested for aggression level. If the mean and SD of the aggression scores of the sample are 55 and 15, respectively, construct 95% and 99% confidence intervals for the population mean.
15. The following is the data obtained on a random sample of swimmers on positive breath-holding capacity. Assuming that the data have come from a normally distributed population, construct 99% confidence intervals for estimating the population mean.

Positive Breath-Holding Capacity (in Seconds)											
42	45	46	55	55	44	52	42	46	41	38	32

16. In a students center, out of 120 visitors 80 were reported to be women. Construct 99% confidence limits of the population proportion of women visiting the students center.
17. In a survey conducted in a city on college students, 550 students were selected, out of which 180 students were reported to be smokers. Use this information to construct a 95% confidence interval to estimate the population proportion of smokers among the college students in the city.
18. The following are the push-up performance of physically active students of a college:

12	15	10	20	18	16	18	15	14	9	11

Assuming that the push-up performance is normally distributed, compute a 90% confidence interval to estimate μ.

19. Assuming the data to be normally distributed, test the hypothesis H_0: $\mu = 16.5$ against H_1: $\mu \neq 16.5$ by using the following information: $\bar{x} = 19.2$, $\sigma = 2.3$, $n = 120$, and $\alpha = 0.01$.
20. Test the hypothesis H_0: $\mu = 102$ against H_1: $\mu < 102$ with the given information: $\bar{x} = 98$, $\sigma = 8.5$, $n = 72$, and $\alpha = 0.05$.
21. The SD for the data on weight of college students is known to be 81 lbs. A sample of 46 students drawn from the college has the mean weight 136 lbs. Test the hypothesis at 5% level that the population mean weight is 142 lbs.
22. The average height of the volleyball players who have participated in a senior national tournament was 175 cm. A random sample of 38 volleyball players had the average height of 165 cm. If the population SD was 10.5 cm, test your hypothesis to determine whether the sample can be considered to be drawn from the population who has participated in the senior national championships. Test your hypothesis with $\alpha = 0.05$.
23. A random sample of 48 gymnasts was drawn from a population and was tested for their speed of movement. The mean of the sample was 0.175 s. If the population SD was 0.02 s, can it be concluded that the sample was drawn from the population that had mean speed of movement 0.164 s? Test your hypothesis at 5% level.
24. A random sample of 100 school boys is tested on their sit-ups performance. The mean of the sample is 25. On the basis of this information, can it be concluded at 1% level that the sample has been drawn from the population having mean 28 and SD 5?
25. A random sample of size 16 has mean and SD as 24 and 2, respectively. Can this sample be considered to have been drawn from a population having mean 22. Test your hypothesis at 5% level by assuming that the population from which the sample has been drawn is normally distributed.
26. A random sample is drawn from a population. If the size of the sample is 18 with mean and variance as 15 and 6.25, respectively, can it be concluded at 1% level that the population mean is 12.5, assuming the sample has been drawn from the normal population?
27. A random sample of size 22 has $\bar{x} = 15.6$ and $s = 2.2$. On the basis of this information, test the following hypotheses if only 2% risk of committing a type I error is allowed and x is normally distributed.

$$H_0\text{: } \mu = 14.1, \quad H_1\text{: } \mu > 14.1$$

28. A random sample of 16 college basketball players had the mean vital capacity 3.51 with SD 0.41. Does this information support the assumption that all basket ball players of the college have mean vital capacity equal to 3.71?
29. The vertical jump performance of 10 randomly chosen college volleyball players (cm) are 64, 58, 62, 58, 60, 59, 50, 58, 65, and 59 and those of 10 randomly chosen college basketball players are 60, 48, 60, 68, 58, 59, 55, 65, 56, and 50. Test if the two groups differ significantly in relation to the performance on vertical jump.

30. The following set of data represents the weight of a sample of 12 wrestlers (in pounds) drawn from a university:

Weight in Pounds											
180	190	185	200	178	192	196	181	175	186	189	195

Test the following hypotheses at 1% level assuming that the data were drawn from a normally distributed population:

$$H_0\colon \mu = 192, \quad H_1\colon \mu < 192$$

31. A sports scientist claims that the average vital capacity of volleyball players is 4.21. To test his hypothesis, a random sample of 25 volleyball players is selected. The mean and SD of the sample are 3.9 and 0.221, respectively. Assuming that the vital capacity is normally distributed, can the claim be considered to be authentic at 5% level?
32. A sample of 11 basketball players was randomly selected among the senior national level players and their fat percentage in millimeters (mm) was measured, which is shown below. Assuming that the fat percentage is normally distributed in the population, can it be concluded at 1% level that the sample has been drawn from a population having mean fat percentage as 13.5 mm?

Fat Percentage (in Millimeter)	12	13	11	14	15	12	13	15	14	12	14

33. A random sample of 12 girls had the IQ scores 65, 120, 110, 100, 83, 98, 95, 98, 107, 102, 105, and 88. Assuming the population to be normally distributed, can it be concluded that the sample has been drawn from the population having mean 100?
34. The weights of a random sample of 10 male students in a class are found to be 125, 106, 122, 120, 121, 95, 101, 103, 125, and 132 lbs. Assuming the population to be normally distributed, is it reasonable to believe that the average weight is greater than 110 lbs? Test your hypothesis at $\alpha = 0.05$.
35. A random sample of 180 students was selected from a university to test the hypothesis $H_0\colon \overline{p} = 0.24$ against $H_1\colon \overline{p} > 0.24$. If the sample proportion of smokers is 0.31, test the hypotheses at 5% level.
36. In a survey, it is reported that 22% students like to watch a hockey match on the television. A hockey administrator believes that the figure is higher. To test this, a researcher selected a random sample of 430 students and they were asked as to which sport they like to see on the television. Out of the entire sample, 108 students preferred hockey. At the significance level 0.05, test the belief that the hockey viewers were more than 22%.

37. In a college, a sample of 280 students were asked about the liking or disliking of a classical concert. If 150 students liked the concert, can it be concluded that the concert would be liked by the students in general? Test your hypothesis at 1% level.
38. Test the hypothesis H_0: $\sigma^2 = 12$ against H_1: $\sigma^2 \neq 12$ at the significance level 0.05 for a sample of size $n = 18$, $s^2 = 9$, given that the distribution of the population is normal.
39. In the BPEd entrance examination, the variance among the marks obtained by the selected students during the past several years has been reported by the authorities as 82. To test this claim, a random sample of 14 students was selected and their entrance marks were noted, which are listed as follows:

Marks:	50	68	86	59	87	89	68	75	90	82	65	55	71	66

Can the claim be considered true at 5% level?
40. Test the hypothesis H_0: $\sigma^2 = 81$ against H_1: $\sigma^2 < 81$ at 5% level if $n = 19$, $s^2 = 78$, and the distribution of the population is normal.
41. By using the two sets of data shown in the table, test the hypothesis H_0: $\mu_1 - \mu_2 = 0$ against H_1: $\mu_1 - \mu_2 \neq 0$ at 10% level.

Sample	First	Second
$\bar{x}$	56	59
σ	6	7
n	35	32

42. The mean and SD of pull-ups score of 500 boys of class IX in a school are 6 and 2.5, respectively. Similarly, the mean and SD of pull-ups score of 600 boys of class X in the same school are 8 and 3.1, respectively. Is the difference in the mean pull-ups of the two classes significant at 5% level?
43. In order to draw a nutritional chart, it is desired to test whether basketball players are heavier than volleyball players. To test this hypothesis, two samples of athletes from the basketball and volleyball specialization groups have been randomly selected and their body weights are measured, which are shown in the following table.

Weights in lbs														
Volleyball	145	168	175	158	170	185	190	198	185	176	170	168	172	180
Basketball	146	165	156	150	175	170	165	155	180	168	170	177	167	160

Assuming that the weights in both the categories are normally distributed in the population, can it be concluded that the volleyball players are heavier than the basket ball players, given that the population variances for the data on weights in volleyball and basketball groups are 100 and 90, respectively? Test your hypothesis at the significance level 0.05.

44. A 4-week aerobic workout was given to 10 female subjects. Their hemoglobin contents were measured before and after the workout, which are shown in the following table:

Scores on Hemoglobin										
Before	15.2	11.8	12.8	11.7	13.4	13.8	13.9	12.2	12.6	12.6
After	15.1	12.4	15.6	15.4	15.2	14.4	16.2	12.4	15.8	12.4

Can it be concluded at the significance level 0.05 that aerobic workout in general increases the hemoglobin contents?

45. In order to compare the performance of basketball players and gymnasts on standing broad jump, two groups of athletes from these two sport groups were randomly selected and were tested for their performance on standing broad jump, which are shown in the following table:

Standing Broad Jump in Meters											
Basket ball:	2.75	2.40	2.45	2.60	2.63	2.10	2.10	2.21	2.70	2.80	2.70
Gymnastics:	2.45	2.75	2.85	2.80	2.70	2.18	1.90	1.95	1.85	1.80	2.10

Assuming that the population variances are nearly equal and the variable (standing broad jump) is normally distributed, test your hypothesis at the significance level 0.05, whether basketball player's performance on standing broad jump is higher than that of gymnasts.

46. Researchers are of the view that hockey is a more speedy game than volleyball. In order to test this assertion, two samples of athletes have been randomly selected from among the national level players of these two sports. These athletes have been tested for their performance on 100 m event and the timings in seconds have been recorded, which are shown in the following table.

100-m Performance in Seconds										
Hockey:	11.2	11.4	11.0	13.0	12.0	12.4	13.2	11.8	12.2	12.4
Basketball:	13.2	14.2	13.8	14.6	14.0	14.2	12.8	14.4	13.6	

Assuming that the population variances of the two groups are nearly equal and the variable (timings in 100 m) is normally distributed, can it be concluded that the researcher's view is correct? Test your hypothesis at the significance level 0.01.

47. The data shown in the following table indicate the resting respiratory rate (in count/min) of sedentary and active subjects in the age category of 30–40 years, given that the population variances of these two groups are nearly equal and the resting respiratory rate is normally distributed. Test the hypothesis at 1% level that the resting respiratory rate of the sedentary subjects is significantly higher than that of active subjects.

Resting Respiratory Rate (in count/min)										
Sedentary:	15	16	18	17	16	17	15	17	16	15
Active:	13	12	14	12	13	11	12	13	13	14

48. The data on shoulder width of the college boys after classifying them into high and low cardiorespiratory fitness groups are shown in the below-mentioned table. The population variance of these two groups is nearly equal and shoulder width is normally distributed.

Data on Shoulder Width in Centimeters	
High Cardio respiratory Fitness	Low Cardio respiratory Fitness
34	33
36	35
32	31
32	34
32	31
33	28
34	29
32	32
34	36
36	34
32	33
38	34
36	32
36	35
34	32

Can it be concluded that the students of the high cardiorespiratory fitness group have in general larger shoulder width than that of the students of the low cardiorespiratory fitness group? Test your hypothesis at 5% level.

49. The following scores represent the vertical jump performance in centimeters measured on high skilled and low skilled soccer players in two random samples. Assuming that the population variance in the two groups is nearly equal and the vertical jump performance is normally distributed, can it be concluded at 1% level that the vertical jump performance is better in high skilled soccer players in comparison to the low skilled?

Vertical Jump Performance in Centimeters	
High Skilled Group	Low Skilled Group
44	33
50	39
60	41
63	32
87	29
75	32
44	38
45	16
51	

50. An athletic coach wants to test the effectiveness of his circuit training program in improving agility. A random sample of 10 athletes was selected for the study. These subjects were tested for their performance on a 4 × 10 m shuttle run before and after a training program. The data so obtained are shown in the following table. Given that the difference in shuttle run performance before and after the training is normally distributed, test at the significance level 0.05 whether there is a significant increase in the shuttle run performance (decrease in the timings) after the circuit training program.

4 × 10 Shuttle Run Performance (in Seconds)											
Before training:	10.4	10.6	12.3	12.7	12.8	11.9	11.7	10.9	12.8	12.5	12.6
After training:	10.1	10.2	11.6	10.6	10.7	9.9	10.8	11.2	12.9	10.8	11.3

51. Twelve randomly selected sports school boys were tested for their performance on push-up before and after a 2-month intensive training program on fitness. The data obtained are as follows.

Push-Up Scores	
Initial	Final
18	21
20	22
20	23
26	28
13	18
19	22
22	28
9	12
15	16
16	18

Do these data provide evidence that the fitness program significantly improves the push-up performance? Test your hypothesis at 5% level by assuming the difference to be normally distributed.

52. Using the information given in the table, test the following hypotheses at the significance level 0.01, where x_1 and x_2 represent the number of occurrences of the event in the first group and second group, respectively.

$$H_0\colon p_1 - p_2 = 0, \quad H_1\colon p_1 - p_2 \neq 0$$

Samples	
First	Second
$n_1 = 600$	$n_2 = 500$
$X_1 = 225$	$X_2 = 190$

53. To investigate whether yoga is more popular among girls than among boys in the match practice option, a sample of 110 boys and 85 girls were asked for their choice. In this sample, 42 boys and 39 girls preferred yoga as a match practice option. At 1% level can it be concluded that the proportion of girls is significantly higher than that of boys in opting for yoga in match practice?

54. Following are the performance of students in statistics subjects in two sections of the master's degree class. Assuming that the populations are normally distributed, can it be concluded at 1% level that the population variance of Section A is higher than that of Section B?

Marks in Statistics Paper		
SN	Section A	Section B
1	55	65
2	90	80
3	65	70
4	60	72
5	75	62
6	58	66
7	85	75
8	88	72
9	58	68
10	68	66

55. In a study, 8 boys and 12 girls were tested for their fitness scores. The information obtained from these samples is shown in the following table where S_{Boys} and S_{Girls} represent the standard deviation of boys and girls, respectively.

Sample Statistics	
Boys	Girls
$S^2_{Boys} = 225$	$S^2_{Girls} = 81$
$n_1 = 8$	$n_2 = 12$

Test the hypothesis H_0: $\sigma^2_{Boys} = \sigma^2_{Girls}$ against H_1: $\sigma^2_{Boys} > \sigma^2_{Girls}$ at 5% level assuming that the populations are normally distributed.

ANSWERS

Check Your Progress

1. T	9. F	17. T	25. T	33. T	41. F	49. T	57. F	65. F	73. T
2. F	10. T	18. F	26. T	34. T	42. T	50. T	58. T	66. T	74. F
3. T	11. F	19. T	27. F	35. F	43. F	51. T	59. T	67. T	
4. F	12. F	20. T	28. F	36. T	44. F	52. F	60. F	68. F	
5. F	13. F	21. F	29. F	37. F	45. F	53. T	61. T	69. F	
6. F	14. T	22. T	30. T	38. F	46. T	54. F	62. F	70. F	
7. T	15. T	23. T	31. T	39. T	47. F	55. F	63. T	71. F	
8. T	16. F	24. F	32. F	40. T	48. T	56. T	64. F	72. T	

Practice Exercise

1. 95% confidence interval for population mean: 12.96 to 18.44.
2. 99% confidence interval for population mean: 3.28 to 3.72 l.
3. 99% confidence interval for population mean: 141.97 to 162.03, $n = 227$.
4. 95% confidence limits for population proportion: 0.318 to 0.502.
   99% confidence limits for population proportion: 0.289 to 0.531.
5. 90% confidence limits for population proportion: 0.383 to 0.533. With the increase in confidence level, confidence interval increases.
6. $z = 3.714$, H_0 is rejected.
7. $t = 3.098$, H_0 is rejected, population mean is not 5.2 ft.
8. $|z| = 1.5$, H_0 is not rejected. The claim is true.
9. $z = 1.1$, H_0 is not rejected. No difference between the sit-ups performance in the two groups.
10. $t = 4.30$, H_0 is rejected. The fitness training program is effective in reducing fat percentage.
11. $z = 0.65$, H_0 is not rejected. Boys' views were not different than that of girls on the curriculum.
12. $F = 3.06$, H_0 is not rejected.

Chapter Exercise

6. 90% confidence limits = 41.18 to 42.82, 99% confidence limits = 40.71 to 43.29.
7. 95% confidence interval = 33.46 to 36.54.
8. $|Z| = 16$, null hypothesis is rejected. Sample is not from the population having mean 7.32 s.
9. $|Z| = 1.35$, null hypothesis is not rejected. The sample is from the population having mean 14.14.
10. 85% confidence interval = 127.71 to 134.29.
11. 90% confidence interval = 23.01 to 27.39.
12. 95% confidence interval = 40.22 to 50.78.
13. 95% confidence interval = 74.34 to 79.66, 99% confidence interval = 73.32 to 80.68.
14. 95% confidence interval = 47.98 to 62.02, 99% confidence interval = 45.404 to 64.59.
15. 99% confidence interval = 38.76 to 50.90.
16. 99% confidence interval = 0.56 to 0.78.
17. 95% confidence interval = 0.29 to 0.37.
18. 90% confidence interval = 12.6 to 16.12.
19. $z = 12.86$, null hypothesis is rejected.
20. $z = -3.99$, null hypothesis is rejected.
21. $z = 0.50$, null hypothesis is not rejected. Population mean weight is 142 lbs.

22. $z=5.87$, sample has not been drawn from the population who have participated in the senior national championships.
23. $z=3.82$, null hypothesis is rejected. Sample has not been drawn from the population.
24. $z=6$, null hypothesis is rejected. Sample has not been drawn from the population.
25. $t=4$, null hypothesis is rejected. Sample has not been drawn from the population.
26. $t=5.94$, null hypothesis is rejected. Sample has not been drawn from the population.
27. $t=3.198$, null hypothesis is rejected at 2% level.
28. $|t|=2$, null hypothesis is not rejected; the average vital capacity of the college students is 3.71.
29. $t = 0.60$, null hypothesis is not rejected.
30. $t=-2.11$, null hypothesis is not rejected at 1% level.
31. $t=6.82$, null hypothesis is rejected. The claim is not true.
32. $t=0.797$, null hypothesis is not rejected. The sample has been drawn from the population.
33. $t=0.59$, null hypothesis is not rejected. The sample has been drawn from the population.
34. $t=1.26$, population mean is not greater than 110 lbs.
35. $z=1.88$, null hypothesis is rejected. The proportion of smokers in the university is greater than 0.24.
36. $z=1.50$, null hypothesis is not rejected. Hockey viewers were not more than 22%.
37. $z=1.34$, null hypothesis is not rejected. It cannot be concluded that the concert would be liked by the students in general.
38. $\chi^2 = 12.75$, null hypothesis is not rejected.
39. $\chi^2 = 26.88$, null hypothesis is rejected at 5% level.
40. $\chi^2 = 17.33$, null hypothesis is not rejected.
41. $z=1.875$, null hypothesis is not rejected.
42. $|Z| = 11.84$, the students of class IX and X differ significantly in their mean sit-ups performance.
43. $z=2.64$, null hypothesis is rejected at 5% level. Volleyball players are heavier than basketball players.
44. $t=3.25$, null hypothesis is rejected. Aerobic workout increases the hemoglobin contents.
45. $t=1.298$, null hypothesis is not rejected.
46. $t=-5.910$, null hypothesis is rejected. Hockey is a more speedy game than basketball.
47. $t=7.89$, null hypothesis is rejected. Respiratory rate of sedentary subjects is higher than that of active subjects.
48. $t=1.9$, null hypothesis is rejected. High cardio group has larger shoulder width.

49. $t = 4.21$, null hypothesis is rejected. Vertical jump is better in high skilled group.
50. $t = 3.78$, null hypothesis is rejected. Circuit training program is effective in increasing shuttle run performance.
51. $t = 6.36$, null hypothesis is rejected. Fitness program is effective in improving the push-up performance.
52. $|Z| = 1.5$, null hypothesis is rejected.
53. $z = 1.12$, null hypothesis is not rejected. Girls proportion is not higher than that of the boys in preferring yoga.
54. $F = 6.3$, null hypothesis is rejected. Section A is more variable than Section B.
55. $F = 2.78$, null hypothesis is not rejected.

FURTHER READING

1. Morris C, Ernest N. Neutral hypotheses, those of which the subject matter can never be directly proved or disproved, are very numerous in all sciences. In: An Introduction to Logic and Scientific Method. New York: Harcourt, Brace, and Company; 1934. p 375.
2. Adèr JH. Chapter 12: Modelling. In: Adèr HJ, Mellenbergh GJ, editors(with contributions by D.J. Hand). Advising on Research Methods: A Consultant's Companion. Huizen, The Netherlands: Johannes van Kessel Publishing; 2008. p 183–209.
3. Bickel PJ, Doksum KA. Mathematical Statistics: Basic and Selected Topics. I. 2nd (updated printing 2007) ed. London: Pearson Prentice-Hall; 2001.
4. Boneau CA. The effects of violations of assumptions underlying the t test. Psychological Bulletin 1960;57(1):49–64. DOI: 10.1037/h0041412.
5. Peirce CS. Illustrations of the logic of science VI: deduction, induction, and hypothesis. Popular Science Monthly 1878;13 Retrieved 2012 March 30.
6. Cox DR, Hinkley DV. Theoretical Statistics. Chapman & Hall; 1974. Section 7.2(iii).
7. de Levie R. Advanced Excel for Scientific Data Analysis. USA: Oxford University Press; 2004. ISBN 0-19-515275-1.
8. Lehmann EL. Testing Statistical Hypotheses. 2nd ed. New York: Springer Verlag; 1986. p 65 ISBN 0-387-94919-4.
9. Edgell SE, Noon SM. Effect of violation of normality on the t test of the correlation coefficient. Psychological Bulletin 1984;95(3):576–583. DOI: 10.1037/0033-2909.95.3.576.
10. Ferguson TS. A Course in Large Sample Theory. UK: Chapman & Hall; 1996. ISBN 0-412-04371-8.
11. Ferguson TS. An inconsistent maximum likelihood estimate. Journal of the American Statistical Association 1982;77(380):831–834JSTOR 2287314.
12. Fisher R. The nature of probability. Centennial Review 1958;2:261–274.
13. Fisher RA. The arrangement of field experiments. Journal of the Ministry of Agriculture of Great Britain 1926;33:503–513.
14. Newman JR. The world of mathematics. USA: DOVER PUBLICATIONS 1956. ISBN: 978-0-486-41151-4.

15. George GR. A Course in Mathematical Statistics. 2nd ed. USA: Elsevier Science & Technology Books 1997. ISBN: 978-0-12-599315-9.
16. Goodman SN. Toward evidence-based medical statistics. 1: the P value fallacy. Annals of Internal Medicine 1999;130:995–1004.
17. Halpin PF. Inductive inference or inductive behavior: Fisher and Neyman: pearson approaches to statistical testing in psychological research (1940–1960). The American Journal of Psychology 2006;119(4):625–653.
18. Harnett DL, Horrell JF. Data, Statistics, and Decision Models with Excel. USA: Wiley; 1998. ISBN 0-471-13398-1.
19. Hazewinkel M, editor. Student test. In: Encyclopedia of Mathematics. Netherlands: Springer; 2001. ISBN 978-1-55608-010-4.
20. Hubbard R, Parsa AR, Luthy MR. The spread of statistical significance testing in psychology: the case of the Journal of Applied Psychology. Theory and Psychology 1997;7(4):545–554. DOI: 10.1177/0959354397074006.
21. Huff D. How to Lie With Statistics. New York: Norton; 1993. ISBN 0-393-31072-8.
22. Kendall MG, Stuart DG. The Advanced Theory of Statistics. Vol 2: Inference and Relationship. London: Griffin; 1973. Section 20.4.
23. Lehmann EL, Romano JP. Testing Statistical Hypotheses. 3E ed. New York: Springer; 2005. ISBN 0-387-98864-5.
24. Liese F, Miescke K-J. Statistical Decision Theory: Estimation, Testing, and Selection. New York: Springer; 2008.
25. John AR. Mathematical Statistics and Data Analysis. 3rd ed. USA: Thomson/Brooks/Cole 2007. ISBN: 978-0-534-39942-9.
26. Moore D. Introduction to the Practice of Statistics. New York: W.H. Freeman and Co; 2003. p 426 ISBN 9780716796572.
27. Neyman J. On the problem of the most efficient tests of statistical hypotheses. Philosophical Transactions of the Royal Society of London Series A-Mathematical Physical and Engineering Sciences 1933;231(694–706):289–337. DOI: 10.1098/rsta.1933.0009.
28. O'Mahony M. Sensory Evaluation of Food: Statistical Methods and Procedures. USA: CRC Press; 1986. p 487 ISBN 0-8247-7337-3.
29. Optimal State Estimation: Kalman, H-infinity, and Nonlinear Approaches. XXXX. Dan Simon website.
30. Kent M. The Oxford dictionary of sports science & medicine. 3rd ed. UK: Oxford University Press 2007. ISBN: 978-0-19-921089-3.
31. Fisher RA. Statistical Methods for Research Workers. Vol. 1925. Edinburgh: Oliver and Boyd; 1925. p 43.
32. Rees DG. Essential Statistics. 4th ed. USA: Chapman and Hall/CRC; 2001. ISBN 1-58488-007-4 (Section 9.5).
33. Schervish M. Theory of Statistics. New York: Springer; 1996. p 218 ISBN 0-387-94546-6.
34. Sterne JAC. Sifting the evidence–what's wrong with significance tests? Physical Therapy August 2001;81(8):1464–1469.
35. Seidenfeld T. Philosophical Problems of Statistical Inference: Learning from R.A. Fisher. Netherlands: Springer-Verlag; 1979.

36. Lehmann E. Theory of point estimation. USA: Springer Verlag 1998. ISBN: 978-0-387-98502-2.
37. Kailath T, Sayed AH, Hassibi B. Linear Estimation. Upper Saddle River, NJ: Prentice-Hall; 2000. ISBN 978-0-13-022464-4.
38. Triola M. Elementary Statistics. 8th ed. Boston: Addison-Wesley; 2001. p 388 ISBN 0-201-61477-4.
39. Verma JP. Statistical Methods for Sports and Physical Education. New Delhi: Tata McGraw Hill Education; 2011.
40. Voinov VG, Nikulin MS. Unbiased Estimators and Their Applications. Vol.2: Multivariate Case. Netherlands: Kluwer Academic Publishers; 1996. ISBN 0-7923-3939-8.
41. Weiss NA. Introductory statistics. 9th ed. USA: Pearson Education 2012. ISBN: 978-0-321-69122-4.
42. Welch BL. The generalization of "Student's" problem when several different population variances are involved. Biometrika 1947;34(1–2):28–35. DOI: 10.1093/biomet/34.1-2.28. MR 19277.
43. Vincent WJ, Weir JP. Statistics in Kinesiology. 4th ed. Champaign, IL: Human Kinetics; 2012.
44. Zar JH. Biostatistical Analysis. New Jersey: Prentice Hall International; 1984. p 43–45G. Steed Jacaranda Wiley, Brisbane, Australia.

8

ANALYSIS OF VARIANCE AND DESIGNING RESEARCH EXPERIMENTS

8.1 INTRODUCTION

In Chapter 7, several techniques for testing hypotheses about the differences in two population means using two samples were discussed, but those techniques are not appropriate in comparing the means of three or more groups. This chapter deals with all such techniques that are used to analyze three or more samples in a situation where the data are measured on the interval or ratio scale.

The analysis of variance (ANOVA) is a statistical technique used for analyzing research designs in investigating different research questions. This technique focuses on analyzing the causes of variation in a dataset. In the ANOVA, the means of three or more groups are compared by testing the significance of the variance among the group means. If the variance among group means is significant, it indicates that the group means are different and the groups have not been drawn from the same population, whereas if the variance is not significant, one may conclude that the group means do not differ and the groups have been drawn from the same population.

In this chapter, the procedures involved in the one-way ANOVA, two-way ANOVA with one observation per cell, and two-way ANOVA with n observations per cell are discussed in detail by means of solved examples to analyze three basic research designs, namely, completely randomized design, randomized block design, and factorial designs. In addition to these designs, a separate section has been devoted to the analysis of covariance. Whatever design is used by the

Statistics for Exercise Science and Health with Microsoft® Office Excel®, First Edition. J. P. Verma.

researchers in their experiment, their data are analyzed by using the technique of ANOVA. It is therefore important for the readers to understand the basic concepts involved and the procedure used in testing different kinds of hypotheses.

8.2 UNDERSTANDING ANALYSIS OF VARIANCE

Analysis of variance is a group of statistical techniques used for analyzing the causes of variation in a dataset for comparing means of three or more groups. The total variation in the dataset is split into two components: variation due to assignable causes and variation due to unassignable causes. The group means are compared by comparing the between-group and within-group variances. According to Fisher, the ratio obtained by dividing the "between-group" variance by the "within-group" variance follows the F-distribution with $(r-1, n-r)$ degrees of freedom, where r is the number of groups and n is the total number of scores. If the F-ratio is significant, the variance among the group means becomes significant, and it is concluded that the group means differ significantly, otherwise they do not do so. Thus, the means of three or more groups are compared by using the ANOVA technique. This technique can also be used to compare the means of two groups, and thus the results of the ANOVA and t-test become identical. This is because the ANOVA is an extension of the t-test, or one may say that the t-test is a specific case of the ANOVA.

Before understanding the technique of ANOVA by means of an example, let us first understand what the difference between variation and variance is. Variation describes the spread of scores in a dataset, whereas variance is a measure of variation. The variance is calculated by finding the variation of scores around its mean value. In the ANOVA, we deal with sample data; therefore, the sample variance is computed to estimate the population variance. We use the sample variance as an estimate of the population variance because it is an unbiased estimator of the population variance. The sample variance is given by

$$S^2 = \frac{1}{n-1}\sum (x-\overline{x})^2$$

The term $\sum (x-\overline{x})^2$ is known as the *sum of squares* and $n-1$ is the degrees of freedom for the variance. Thus,

$$S^2 = \frac{\text{SS}}{\text{df}} = \frac{\text{Variation}}{\text{df}} = \text{MSS}$$

where MSS denotes the mean sum of squares and is equivalent to the variance of the data. In the ANOVA, the terms SS and MSS, which represent the variation and variance of the scores, respectively, are used frequently.

In order to understand the concept of between-group sum of squares and within-group sum of squares, let us consider the data on shooting accuracy in basketball obtained on college athletes in three different height categories as shown in Table 8.1. The coach is interested in knowing whether the shooting performance

TABLE 8.1 Data on Shooting Accuracy

	Height			
	Short	Medium	Tall	
	3	5	8	
	4	2	5	
	2	6	7	
	6	5	6	
	5	7	9	
Total	20	25	35	
Mean	4	5	7	Grand mean = 5.33

depends on the height of the athletes. In order to answer this research question, he tests the null hypothesis that the shooting performance in all the three height groups are the same against the alternative hypothesis that at least one group mean differs. Thus, the null hypothesis, which is tested by using the ANOVA is

$$H_0 : \mu_{\text{Short}} = \mu_{\text{Medium}} = \mu_{\text{Tall}}$$

against the alternative hypothesis that at least one group mean differs. It is evident from Table 8.1 that the scores are not the same. If we ask a simple question as to why these scores differ, one may immediately say that this is possibly because they come from different height groups. Thus, one of the reasons of variation of these scores may be the height factor (or between groups). But even in each height group (or within groups), the scores vary, and therefore this variation can be attributed to some unknown reasons. Thus, the total variation can be attributed to assignable causes and nonassignable causes. Assignable causes for variation are those that can be assigned by the researcher, such as height in this case, and nonassignable causes are those that cannot be assigned by the researcher (causes due to which variation occurs within each group). There may be various reasons, such as skill, arm strength, concentration, palm length, or eye–hand coordination, due to which the performance of shooting accuracy of the athletes within each group may differ. Since these causes are not known to the researcher, the variation because of unassignable causes is also known as *error variation* (or *within-group variation*). Since the total variation can be split into two components, namely, between-group variation and within-group variation, it is our endeavor to find out whether the variation because of groups is significant or not. Kindly note that the variation between groups is measured by computing the variance of the group means (4, 5, and 7) around the grand mean (5.33). On the other hand, the variation within groups is obtained by adding the variance within each of the three groups. The variance in the first group can be obtained by finding the variance of all the five scores in the first group (3, 4, 2, 6, and 5) around its mean 4. Similarly, variance of all the groups can be obtained. These computations have been shown in Example 8.1.

As mentioned earlier, the between-group and within-group variances are compared by using the F-test; hence, if the F-value is significant, it is concluded that the variance between the group means is significantly higher than that of the variance within groups, and one may infer that the group means are not equal. This is also logical because if the group means, in this example, that is, 4, 5, and 7 differ significantly, then obviously one should conclude that all three group means are not equal and that is what the F-test in the ANOVA does.

8.3 DESIGN OF EXPERIMENT

> **FACTS TO KNOW**
>
> In designing an experiment, the researcher should maximize the systematic variance, control the extraneous variance, and reduce the error variance

Design of experiment can be defined as a blueprint for organizing a research experiment for testing hypotheses to address some research questions in an efficient manner. It facilitates an experimenter in manipulating one or more independent variables, controlling the effect of extraneous variables, and reducing the error due to nonassignable causes. In an experimental design, we investigate the effect of an independent variable on some dependent variable. For instance, in testing the effect of a conditioning program on cardiorespiratory endurance, the conditioning program is the independent variable, whereas the cardiorespiratory endurance is the dependent variable. An independent variable may either be a treatment variable or a classificatory variable. A *treatment variable* is the one that the experimenter manipulates in the experiment. A *classificatory variable* is some characteristics of the subjects on the basis of which the experimental subjects can be classified. These characteristics are present in the subjects before the experiment is conducted and are not the result of the experimenter's manipulation.

If in an experiment, the effect of three different intensities of a conditioning program is to be seen on the cardiorespiratory endurance in male and female subjects, then, in this case, the two independent variables would be the conditioning program and sex, whereas the dependent variable would be the cardiorespiratory endurance. Here, the conditioning program is a treatment variable because the experimenter can manipulate its intensities, whereas the sex is a classificatory variable because this characteristic is present among the subjects before the experiment is conducted.

Manipulating the independent variable in an experiment depends on the nature of the study. Independent variables such as sex, height, weight, level of sports performance, type of sports the subjects play, or socioeconomic status are classificatory variables because these conditions existed before the experiment. The researchers cannot manipulate these conditions; therefore, they study the phenomenon of interest under several conditions of the classificatory variable. For example, an experimenter may be interested in comparing the flexibility among college-level athletes in three different sports, such as gymnastics, judo, and swimming. The interest of the researcher may be to see the effect of the nature of sport on flexibility. Here, the independent variable is the sport, which is a classificatory variable, and it is not being manipulated by the experimenter, whereas the phenomenon of interest is flexibility. On the other hand, some independent variables can be manipulated by the researcher. For example, in investigating the effect of aerobic exercise on lean body weight, the experimenter can manipulate the intensities of the aerobic program. He may take low, medium, and high intensity aerobic programs whose effects on lean body weight may be compared. Similarly, the effect of exercise duration on agility can be investigated by the researcher. In this case, the researcher may manipulate the duration of the exercise program, say, 15, 30, and 45 min in length.

In a research experiment, each independent variable may have different levels. For example, in the experiment studying the effect of the conditioning program on cardiorespiratory endurance among males and females, the two independent variables may have different levels. The conditioning program may have three levels (different intensities), whereas the sex has two levels (male and female). Decision about the number of levels of each independent variable in the study depends on the nature of the study and the resources available to the researcher.

The dependent variable in an experiment is also known as the *criterion variable* or *response variable*. This is the variable whose behavior under different treatment conditions interest the experimenter. In fact, the dependent variable is the response to the different levels of the independent variables.

> **FACTS TO KNOW**
>
> Design of experiments refers to cutting the error variance by using nonstatistical and statistical methods

The three basic designs that are discussed in this chapter are completely randomized design, randomized block design, and factorial design. Whatever experimental design is chosen by the experimenter, it is analyzed by a group of techniques known as the *analysis of variance*. Choice of the design depends on the nature of experimental material (subjects). In choosing the design, efforts should be made to reduce the error in the experiment while testing the hypothesis. This is done by maximizing the systematic variance through manipulating the independent variable; controlling the extraneous variance by controlling the extraneous variable either by randomization, matching, or including extraneous variables in the experiment; and reducing the error variance by experimental or statistical procedures.

8.4 ONE-WAY ANALYSIS OF VARIANCE

The one-way ANOVA is a method of comparing the means of three or more groups or treatments. In the one-way ANOVA, the effect of only one factor on the dependent variable is studied. The factor may have three or more levels, and the focus is to compare the means of the different groups. For example, in studying the effect of a weight-training program on the shot put performance, the researcher may choose three weight-training programs with different intensities, whose effect may be seen on the shot put performance. Here, the weight-training program becomes the independent variable having three levels and the shot put performance acts as the dependent variable. By applying the one-way ANOVA, the researcher compares the mean shot put performance in all the three treatment groups. The null hypothesis of no difference among the three group means is tested against the alternative hypothesis that at least one group mean differs. Once the null hypothesis of equality of group means is rejected, post hoc analysis is done to test the significance of difference between different pairs of group means. In the one-way ANOVA, group means are compared by comparing the between-group variability with within-group variability. This is done by computing the F-statistic, which is obtained by dividing the variance of between-group means by the variance of within-group means. According to Fisher, this F-statistic follows the F-distribution with $(r-1, N-r)$ degrees of freedom, where r is the number of groups and N is the total number of scores. According to central limit theorem, if the groups are drawn from the same population, the variance between the group means should be lower than the variance within the groups. Thus, a higher ratio (F-value) indicates that the samples are drawn from different populations. Let us study the procedure involved in the one-way ANOVA.

8.4.1 One-Way ANOVA Model

If there are r independent samples having $n_1, n_2, \ldots, n_r$ scores, respectively, and if Y_{ij} represents the jth score in the ith sample, then these scores in the one-way ANOVA model will be as shown in Table 8.2.

Here,

$N = n_1 + n_2 + \cdots + n_r$, the total of all the scores,

$G =$ grand total of all N scores, and

$R_i =$ total of all the scores in the ith sample.

TABLE 8.2 Arrangement of Scores in r Independent Groups

	Groups								
	1	2	–	–	i	–	–	r	
	Y_{11}	Y_{21}	–	–	Y_{i1}	-	-	Y_{r1}	
	Y_{12}	Y_{22}	–	–	Y_{j2}	-	-	Y_{r2}	
	–	–	–	–	–	–	–	–	
	Y_{1n_1}	Y_{2n_2}	–	–	Y_{in_i}	–	–	Y_{rn_r}	
Total	R_1	R_2	–	–	R_i	–	–	R_r	$G = R_1 + R_2 + \cdots + R_r$
Mean	$\overline{Y}_1$	$\overline{Y}_2$	–	–	$\overline{Y}_i$	–	–	$\overline{Y}_r$	

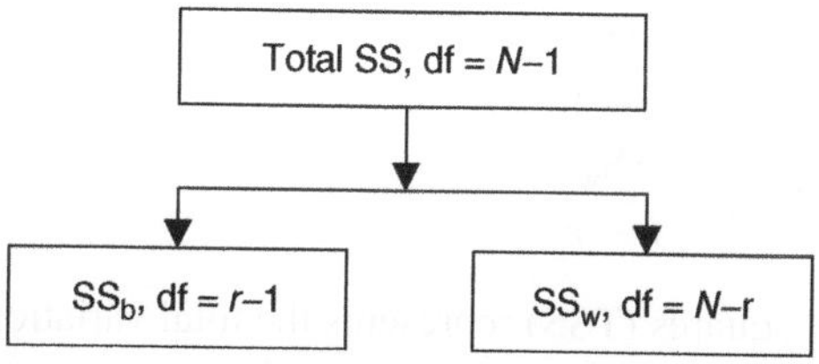

Figure 8.1 Distribution of variation and their associated degrees of freedom in the one-way ANOVA.

The total variability among the scores can be attributed to the variability between groups and the variability within groups. Thus, the model of the one-way ANOVA becomes

$$\text{TSS} = \text{SS}_\text{b} + \text{SS}_\text{w} \tag{8.1}$$

where TSS represents total variability among all the N scores, SS_b represents the variability between the groups, and SS_w is the variability within the groups. SS_b is also known as the *variability due to treatment* and SS_w as the *variability due to error*.

The splitting of total variations and their associated degrees of freedom is shown in Figure 8.1. The associated degrees of freedom are used to compute the mean sum of squares between the groups and within the groups.

The between-group and within-group variabilities are compared by comparing within-group and between-group variances using the F-test. The variances between the groups and within the groups are obtained by computing MSS_b and MSS_w, respectively. The procedure for computing various sums of squares and mean sums of squares along with the procedure involved in testing the hypothesis in the one-way ANOVA has been discussed later.

8.4.2 Procedure in One-Way ANOVA

In the one-way ANOVA, the following null hypothesis is tested against which the alternative hypothesis is that at least one mean differs.

$$H_0: \mu_1 = \mu_2 = \ldots = \mu_r$$

To test the above null hypothesis, the different sums of squares are computed as follows:

$$\text{TSS} = \sum_{i=1}^{r}\sum_{j=1}^{n_i}\left(Y_{ij} - \frac{G}{N}\right)^2 = \sum_i\sum_j Y_{ij}^2 - \frac{G^2}{N} \tag{8.2}$$

$$\text{SS}_\text{b} = \sum_i^r \frac{R_i^2}{n_i} - \frac{G^2}{N} \tag{8.3}$$

$$\text{SS}_\text{w} = \text{TSS}-(\text{SS})_\text{b} \tag{8.4}$$

$$\text{MSS}_\text{b} = \frac{\text{SS}_\text{b}}{r-1} \tag{8.5}$$

$$\text{MSS}_\text{w} = \frac{\text{SS}_\text{w}}{n-r} \tag{8.6}$$

The total sum of squares (TSS) represents the total variation present in the data and is equal to the total of the sum of squares between groups (SS_b) and sum of squares within groups (SS_w). SS_b represents the variation among the group means, whereas SS_w represents the variation within the group means. MSS_b represents the variance among the group means, whereas MSS_w represents the variance within the group means. Readers should note that the MSS_w is the sum of the variances of the scores in each of the groups.

After computing the sum of squares and mean sum of squares, the ANOVA table as shown in Table 8.3 is constructed for computing the F-statistic.

The critical value of F at 0.05 and 0.01 level of significance with $(r-1, N-r)$ degrees of freedom can be obtained by using Tables A.9 and A.10 in the appendix, respectively.

If calculated $F >$ tabulated $F_{0.05}(r-1, N-r)$, null hypothesis (H_0) is rejected,

and if calculated $F \leq$ tabulated $F_{0.05}(r-1, N-r)$, the null hypothesis (H_0) is not rejected.

Remark The sources of variations "between groups" and "within groups" are also known as *treatment* and *error*, respectively.

8.4.3 Post Hoc Tests

If the null hypothesis is rejected, at least one of the means will be different. Since the ANOVA does not tell us where the difference lies, post hoc tests are used to get a clear picture. There are several post hoc tests available that can be used, but Tukey's honestly significant difference (HSD) test and the least significant difference (LSD) test for equal sample sizes and Scheffe's test for unequal sample sizes are used more often by the researchers.

TABLE 8.3 ANOVA Table

Sources of Variation	df	SS	MSS	F-value
Between groups	$r-1$	SS_b	$\text{MSS}_\text{b} = \dfrac{\text{SS}_\text{b}}{r-1}$	$F = \dfrac{\text{MSS}_\text{b}}{\text{MSS}_\text{w}}$
Within groups	$N-r$	SS_w	$\text{MSS}_\text{w} = \dfrac{\text{SS}_\text{w}}{N-r}$	
Total	$N-1$	TSS		

In all the post hoc tests, a critical difference (CD) is calculated at a particular level of significance and if the difference of any pair of group means is higher than the CD, it is inferred that one mean is greater than the other. By comparing all pairs of group means, a conclusion is drawn as to which group mean is the highest. The computation of CD in different post hoc tests has been shown later.

LSD Test This test provides a CD that is used for comparing differences in all the pairs of means. The CD is computed as follows:

$$\text{Critical difference (CD)} = t_{0.05}(N-r) \times \sqrt{\frac{2}{n} \times \text{MSS}_\text{w}} \tag{8.7}$$

where r is the number of groups, n is the number of scores in each group, and N is the total number of scores.

Tukey's HSD Test The CD in the Tukey HSD test is given by

$$\text{CD} = q_{\alpha,r,N-r}\sqrt{\frac{\text{MSS}_\text{w}}{n}} \tag{8.8}$$

where r is the number of groups, N is the total number of scores, and q is the range statistic. The value of q at a particular significance level and $(r, N-r)$ degrees of freedom can be obtained from Table A.15 in the appendix.

Scheffe's Test

In Scheffe's test, different critical regions are computed for comparing different pairs of group means. Thus,

> **FACTS TO KNOW**
>
> Using multiple t-tests instead of one-way analysis of variance inflates the level of significance

CD for comparing the ith and jth group means

$$= \sqrt{(r-1)F_{0.05}(r-1, N-r)} \times \sqrt{\text{MSS}_\text{w}\left(\frac{1}{n_i} + \frac{1}{n_j}\right)} \tag{8.9}$$

where n_i and n_j represent the sample sizes of the ith and jth groups, respectively, and r and N are the number of groups and the total number of scores, respectively. The detailed procedure of the one-way analysis of variance in solving completely randomized design has been discussed in Example 8.1.

8.4.4 Assumptions in One-Way ANOVA

The following are the assumptions that need to be satisfied while using the one-way ANOVA:

1. All the samples have been drawn from the populations that are normally distributed.
2. The samples are independent of each other. In other words, the subjects are different in each group.
3. The observations in each group are independent of each other.
4. The populations from which the samples have been drawn have equal variance.

8.4.5 Using Multiple *t*-Tests Instead of One-Way ANOVA

In comparing two group means, it hardly matters whether you use the one-way ANOVA or *t*-test. In both these cases, you will get the same findings. It is because F and t are related by the formula, $F = t^2$. But this is valid only in the case of two groups. However, if the number of groups is more than two, the ANOVA procedure is more efficient than using several *t*-tests. In using multiple *t*-tests instead of the one-way ANOVA, the type I error increases while testing the hypothesis. Let us understand this fact by considering an example where three groups are compared. Instead of using the one-way ANOVA, if one decides to use multiple *t*-tests, then three *t*-tests need to be applied. If the hypothesis is tested at 0.05 significance level, then the probability of committing type I error in one *t*-test = 0.05; therefore, the probability of not committing type I error in one *t*-test = 1 − 0.05 = 0.95.

Since, probability of not committing type I error in all the three *t*-tests

$= 0.95 \times 0.95 \times 0.95 = 0.95^3$

$\Rightarrow$ P(Committing type I error in at least one of the three *t*-tests)

$= 1 - 0.95^3 = 0.1426$

Thus, we have seen that in applying three *t*-tests, although we had taken the significance level as 0.05, the actual level of significance has been inflated to 0.1426. This suggests that the one-way ANOVA is more efficient than multiple *t*-tests.

8.5 COMPLETELY RANDOMIZED DESIGN

The completely randomized design is the simplest design used by a researcher in a situation where the experimental subjects are homogeneous in nature in all aspects. In this design, the treatments are randomly allocated to the subjects. The

> **FACTS TO KNOW**
>
> The completely randomized design is used when the experimental subjects are homogeneous and the experimenter has full control over the experiment

completely randomized design is used when there is only one independent variable with three or more levels. Consider an experiment of investigating the effect of aerobic exercise on muscular endurance. The experimenter may choose three intensities of the aerobic exercise (low, medium, and high). These three treatments may be randomly assigned to the subjects. Here, the subjects need to be homogeneous in all aspects. In this design, it is not necessary to have an equal number of subjects in each group. The one-way ANOVA is used to analyze this design. The procedure in this design can be easily understood through Example 8.1.

8.5.1 Example of One-Way ANOVA for Solving a Completely Randomized Design

Example 8.1 It was observed by a coach that the athletes under him lacked flexibility. He developed three circuit training programs of different intensities (low, medium, and high). A completely randomized design was planned in which 31 subjects received the three treatments of circuit-training programs randomly. After 4 weeks of training, the flexibility (in angles) of these subjects was measured and the data so obtained are as shown in Table 8.4. Can it be concluded that any one circuit training program is more effective than others? Apply the one-way ANOVA to test the hypothesis at 1% level.

Solution: Since there is only one factor that affects the variability of scores, to analyze this completely randomized design, the one-way ANOVA shall be used.

TABLE 8.4 Flexibility (in Angles) Scores in Three Treatment Groups

	Circuit Training of Different Intensities			
	Low	Medium	High	
	58	60	47	
	49	64	45	
	59	59	54	
	50	61	50	
	48	57	48	
	49	62	45	
	52	63	49	
	53	58	48	
	47	59	46	
		64	48	
		65		
		66		
Group total	$R_1 = 465$	$R_2 = 738$	$R_3 = 480$	$G = R_1 + R_2 + R_3 = 1683$
Group mean	51.67	61.5	48	

The following null hypothesis is required to be tested at the significance level 0.01 against the alternative hypothesis that at least one of the group means differs.

$$H_0 : \mu_{\text{low}} = \mu_{\text{medium}} = \mu_{\text{high}}$$

Here,

$$\text{Number of groups} = r = 3$$

$$n_1 = 9,\ n_2 = 12,\ \text{ and } n_3 = 10$$

and

$$\text{Total number of scores} = N = n_1 + n_2 + n_3 = 31$$

Computation

$$\text{Correction factor (CF)} = \frac{G^2}{N} = \frac{1683^2}{31} = 91370.61$$

$$\text{Raw sum of squares (RSS)} = \sum_i \sum_j Y_{ij}^2$$

$$= (58^2+49^2+\cdots+47^2)+(60^2+64^2+\cdots+66^2)$$

$$+ (47^2 + 45^2 + \cdots + 48^2)$$

$$= 92759$$

$$\text{Total sum of square (TSS)} = \text{RSS} - \text{CF} = \sum_i \sum_j Y_{ij}^2 - \frac{G^2}{N}$$

$$= 92759 - 91370.61$$

$$= 1388.39$$

$$\text{Sum of squares treatment (SST)} = \sum_i \frac{R_i^2}{n_i} - \frac{G^2}{N}$$

$$= \frac{465^2}{9} + \frac{738^2}{12} + \frac{480^2}{10} - 91370.61$$

$$= 24025 + 45387 + 23040 - 91370.61 = 1081.4$$

$$\text{Sum of squares error (SSE)} = \text{TSS} - \text{SST} = 1388.39 - 1081.4$$

$$= 306.99$$

The values of different sums of squares are shown in Table 8.5. From Table A.10, the value of F at 1% level with df (2, 28) is 5.45. Since the calculated value of F (=49.33) is greater than tabulated F, the F-value is significant and the null

TABLE 8.5 ANOVA Table for the Data on Flexibility

Source of Variation	df	SS	MSS	F-value	Tabulated F
Treatment	$r-1=2$	1081.4	$\frac{1081.4}{2}=540.7$	49.33[a]	$F_{0.01}(2,28)=5.45$
Error	$N-r=28$	306.99	$\frac{306.99}{28}=10.96$		
Total	$N-1=30$	1388.39			

[a]Significant at 0.05 level.

hypothesis is rejected. Since the null hypothesis has been rejected, a post hoc test shall be done to compare the means of different groups.

Post Hoc Analysis

To find which group's flexibility is the best, a post hoc test shall be used. Since the sample size differs in each group, Scheffe's test shall be used for computing CD. In this test, different CDs are computed for comparing different pairs of means. The Scheffe's CD is computed as

$$\text{CD} = \sqrt{(r-1)F_{0.01}(2,28)} \times \sqrt{\text{MSS}_{\text{E}}\left(\frac{1}{n_i}+\frac{1}{n_j}\right)} \tag{8.10}$$

Since the hypothesis needs to be tested at 1% level, the CD has been computed at the significance level 0.01.

Thus,

CD for low and medium intensity groups

$$= \sqrt{(3-1)\times 5.45} \times \sqrt{10.96 \times \left(\frac{1}{9}+\frac{1}{12}\right)} = 4.82$$

CD for low and high intensity groups

$$= \sqrt{(3-1)\times 5.45} \times \sqrt{10.96 \times \left(\frac{1}{9}+\frac{1}{10}\right)} = 5.02$$

CD for medium and high intensity groups

$$= \sqrt{(3-1)\times 5.45} \times \sqrt{10.96 \times \left(\frac{1}{12}+\frac{1}{10}\right)} = 4.68$$

After listing the means and CDs in Table 8.6, the group means can be compared in pairs for a significant difference.

From Table 8.6, it is clear that the mean differences between the low and medium intensity groups as well as medium and high intensity groups are significant because they are higher than their corresponding CDs. However, there

TABLE 8.6 Post Hoc Comparison of Means Using Scheffe's Test

Means of Flexibility Scores in Different Groups				
Low	Medium	High	Mean Difference	CD at 1% Level
51.67	61.5		9.83[a]	4.82
51.67		48	3.67	5.02
	61.5	48	13.5[a]	4.68

[a]Significant at 0.01 level.

TABLE 8.7 Mean Score of Flexibility in Different Circuit Training Groups

Medium	Low	High
61.5	51.67	48

"└──┘" represents no significant difference between the means at 0.01 level.

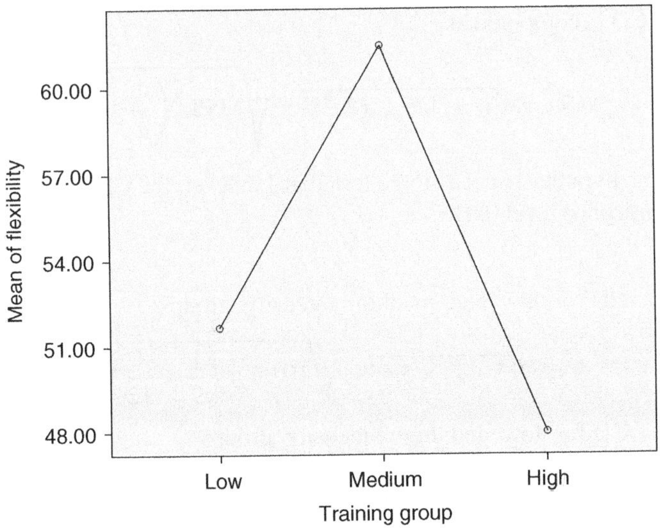

Figure 8.2 Mean plot of the flexibility in the three circuit training groups.

is no significant difference between the low and high intensity groups. By looking at their mean values, it may be inferred that the flexibility of the medium group is the highest, whereas the flexibilities of the low and high intensity groups are equal and significantly lower than that of the medium intensity group.

It may therefore be concluded that the medium intensity circuit training program is the best in improving the flexibility of the athletes. The above results have been shown graphically in Table 8.7.

Mean Plot

The mean flexibility of all the three treatment groups can be plotted as shown in Figure 8.2 to compare the effect of the three circuit training programs.

The mean plot clearly shows that the flexibility of the medium intensity circuit training program is the highest, whereas the flexibility of the athletes in the low intensity circuit training program is slightly higher than that of the high intensity group but this increase is not significant as shown in Table 8.6.

Check Your Progress

Note: Tick the correct answer by using the sign (√).

		True	False
1.	In the case of two groups, the one-way ANOVA and *t*-test will give the same results.	–	–
2.	In a completely randomized design, all the treatments are randomly allocated to the subjects.	–	–
3.	A randomized block design can be analyzed by using the one-way ANOVA.	–	–
4.	In the one-way ANOVA, the total degrees of freedom is computed as $N-2$.	–	–
5.	The Tukey HSD test is used when the sample size is the same in all the groups.	–	–
6.	The mean sum of squares is nothing but the variance.	–	–
7.	Variation and variance are one and the same.	–	–
8.	One of the conditions in the one-way ANOVA is that the samples must be randomly selected.	–	–
9.	If r groups are compared in a completely randomized design, then the degree of freedom for the between groups is $r-1$.	–	–
10.	In applying the one-way ANOVA, it hardly matters whether the population is normal or not, provided the sample is randomly drawn.	–	–
11.	In the one-way ANOVA, variance due to assignable causes is compared with the variance due to nonassignable causes.	–	–
12.	In the one-way ANOVA, if the F-ratio is not significant, it may still be possible in some situations that the means of any two groups may differ.	–	–
13.	The experimenter manipulates the independent variable so as to minimize the systematic variance.	–	–

14. The mean sum of squares is obtained by dividing the SS by the degrees of freedom.	–	–
15. Within-group sum of squares is also known as error.	–	–
16. In a completely randomized design, the one-way ANOVA is used for analysis.	–	–
17. Between-groups sum of squares explains the variance within each sample.	–	–
18. The extraneous variable can be controlled in a completely randomized design.	–	–
19. In the one-way ANOVA, SSE can be obtained by subtracting SST from TSS.	–	–
20. If in a completely randomized design N subjects are tested, then the total number of degrees of freedom is N.	–	–
21. In comparing three groups, it hardly matters whether we use the one-way ANOVA or multiple t-tests.	–	–
22. A classificatory variable can be manipulated by the experimenter.	–	–
23. If r samples having n scores in each are compared by the one-way ANOVA, then the degrees of freedom for tabulated F is $(r-1, N-r-1)$.	–	–
24. A treatment variable can be manipulated by the experimenter.	–	–
25. A dependent variable is the one in which the experimenter is interested.	–	–

PRACTICE EXERCISE

1. In a completely randomized design, the effect of aerobic exercise on flexibility was investigated. There were three treatment levels (three different intensities of the aerobic exercise) and a total of 31 subjects in the study. Fill up the entries in the following ANOVA table. Test the null hypothesis at 5% level.

Source of Variance	df	SS	MS	F
Treatment	?	64.34	?	?
Error	?	175.21	?	
Total	?			

2. Apply the one-way ANOVA on the following data of pull-ups performance obtained on the students of class XI and XII and compute the F-value.

XI:	4	5	6	3	4	2
XII:	8	9	6	7	8	5

Compare the calculated F-value with the critical value of F and decide whether the null hypothesis can be rejected at 5% level. Apply the t-test for independent samples and compare the t- and F-values. Is t^2 is equal to F?

3. The following are the number of double faults committed by the tennis players in three different teams. Apply the one-way ANOVA to test whether the average double faults are the same for all three teams. Test your hypothesis at 1% level.

Team A	3	4	5	7	6
Team B	2	3	4	1	7
Team C	6	7	5	8	8

8.6 TWO-WAY ANALYSIS OF VARIANCE (*N* OBSERVATIONS PER CELL)

The two-way ANOVA is an extension of the one-way ANOVA. In the two-way ANOVA model, the simultaneous effect of two factors on the dependent variable is studied. Each factor may have several levels. The two-way ANOVA is applied in two situations: first, where there is one observation per cell; second, where there is more than one observation per cell. In case there is more than one observation per cell, there should be an equal number of observations in each cell; otherwise, the analysis becomes very complicated. In a situation where the number of observations per cell is more than one, using the two-way ANOVA is more advantageous instead of doing two separate one-way ANOVAs because in addition to knowing the effect of two factors separately, one can also study the effect of interaction between the two factors on the dependent variable. Further, in the two-way ANOVA, the error variance can be reduced by introducing the second factor. In the two-way ANOVA, a researcher examines the effects of two factors on the dependent variable where both treatments have nominal-level measurements, For instance in all such studies where one investigates the effect of age and training duration on an athlete's performance, effect of training program and duration on a swimmer's performance, and effect of region and socioeconomic status on the attitude toward sports, both the treatment variables are measured on the nominal scale.

There may be several situations where the two-way ANOVA experiment can be planned. For example, in studying the effect of three different intensities of aerobic workout on weight reduction, one may select nutrition as another factor because nutrition may play a role in reducing the fat percentage. In framing this experiment as a two-way ANOVA, one can investigate three details: first, compare the effect of different aerobic workouts on fat reduction irrespective of nutrition (main effect of aerobic workout); second, compare the effect of nutrition in reduction of the fat, irrespective of the aerobic workout (main effect of nutrition); and third, test the significance of interaction between the aerobic workout and nutrition.

8.6.1 Advantages of Two-Way ANOVA

The two-way ANOVA model is more efficient than the one-way ANOVA for the following reasons:

1. In the two-way ANOVA, the effect of two factors on the dependent variable can be studied simultaneously unlike the one-way ANOVA where only one factor is investigated.
2. Because the total variability is split into two different factors and the interaction, the error variance is reduced compared to the one-way ANOVA.
3. In the two-way ANOVA, the effect of interaction between the two variables can be investigated simultaneously. This is not possible if, instead of the two-way ANOVA, two separate one-way ANOVAs are planned. However, the number of observations in each cell must be equal and more than one.
4. The two-way ANOVA also reduces computation as it includes several one-way ANOVAs.

8.6.2 Terminologies Used in Two-Way ANOVA

It is important to understand the meaning of different terminologies used in the two-way ANOVA. The following are the different terms used in the computation.

Factors Factors are the independent variables whose effect has to be investigated on the dependent variable. A factor may have different levels. In the two-way ANOVA, the effects of two factors are studied on a criterion variable. Each of the two factors may have two or more levels within it, and the degrees of freedom for each of the factors is one less than the number of levels.

Treatment Conditions The number of treatment conditions in a two-way ANOVA experiment is equal to the number of combinations of the levels in the two factors. For example, if factor A has 3 levels A_1, A_2, and A_3 and factor B has 2 levels B_1 and B_2, then there will be $3 \times 2 = 6$ different treatment conditions, namely, A_1B_1, A_1B_2, A_2B_1, A_2B_2, A_3B_1, and A_3B_2.

Main Effect The main effect is the effect of the first independent variable (or factor A) on the dependent variable across all the levels of the second independent variable (factor B). The interaction is ignored for this part. Just the rows or just the columns are used and not mixed. This is the part that is similar to the one-way ANOVA. Each of the variances calculated to analyze the main effects (rows and columns) are similar to that between variances. The degrees of freedom for the main effect can be obtained by subtracting 1 from its number of levels. For example, if factor A has r levels and factor B has c levels, then the degrees of freedom for factors A and B would be $r - 1$ and $c - 1$, respectively.

Simple Effect A simple effect is the effect of one independent variable in each level of the other factor. It is investigated by comparing the effect of all the levels of one factor in each of the levels of the other factor. The simple effect becomes meaningful when the interaction between the two factors is significant.

Interaction Effect The joint effect of two factors on the dependent variable is known as *interaction*. It can also be defined as the effect that one factor has on the other factor. The degrees of freedom for the interaction is the product of the degrees of freedom of both factors. If factors A and B have levels r and c, respectively, then the degrees of freedom for the interaction would be $(r - 1) \times (c - 1)$.

8.6.3 Two-Way ANOVA Model

Let us suppose that the effect of the two factors A and B on the criterion variable Y is to be investigated. Let us further suppose that factors A and B have levels r and c, respectively, with n scores in each cell, then these scores can be represented by the symbol Y_{ijk} as shown in Table 8.8,
where

Y_{ijk} = the kth score in the ith level of the row factor and the jth level of the column factor
T_{ij} = total of all the n scores in the (i, j)th cell
G = grand total of all the scores
R_i = total of all the scores in the ith level of factor A (row factor)
C_j = total of all the scores in the jth level of factor B (column factor)
N = total number of scores in the experiment and is equal to $n \times r \times c$.

In the two-way ANOVA, the total variability is equal to the sum of the variability due to rows (factor A), columns (or factor B), interaction (row × column), and error. Thus, the two-way ANOVA model becomes

$$\text{TSS} = \text{SSR} + \text{SSC} + \text{SSI} + \text{SSE}$$

where TSS is the total variability among all the N scores, SSR is the variability among the row means, SSR is the variability among the column means, SSI is the

TABLE 8.8 Format of Data in Two-Way ANOVA

		Column Factor B					
		1	–	j	–	c	Row Total
Row factor A	1	Y_{111}	–	Y_{1j1}	–	Y_{1c1}	
		Y_{112}	–	Y_{1j2}	–	Y_{1c2}	
		–	–	–	–	–	
		Y_{11n}	–	Y_{1jn}	–	Y_{1cn}	
		T_{11}	–	T_{1j}	–	T_{1c}	R_1
		–	–	–	–	–	
		–	–	–	–	–	
	i	Y_{i11}	–	Y_{ij1}	–	Y_{ic1}	
		Y_{i12}	–	Y_{ij2}	–	Y_{ic2}	
		–	–	–	–	–	
		Y_{i1n}	–	Y_{ijn}	–	Y_{jcn}	
		T_{i1}		T_{ij}		T_{ic}	R_i
		–	–	–	–	–	
		–	–	–	–	–	
	r	Y_{r11}	–	Y_{rj1}	–	Y_{rc1}	
		Y_{r12}	–	Y_{rj2}	–	Y_{rc2}	
		–	–	–	–	–	
		Y_{r1n}	–	Y_{rjn}	–	Y_{rcn}	
		T_{r1}	–	T_{rj}	–	T_{rc}	R_r
Column total		C_1		C_j	–	C_c	$G = \sum R_i = \sum C_j$

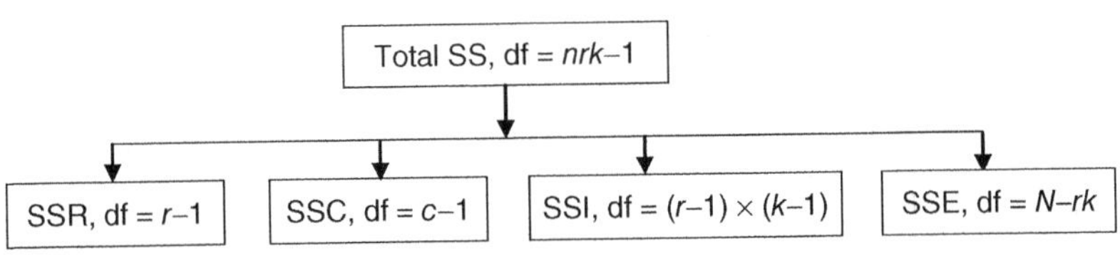

Figure 8.3 Distribution of variation and the associated degrees of freedom in the two-way ANOVA.

variability due to interaction, and SSE is the variability due to error. Figure 8.3 shows the splitting of the TSS along with their degrees of freedom. These degrees of freedom are used to compute the mean sum of squares of the row factor, column factor, and interaction.

In the two-way ANOVA model, it is assumed that the variability among the scores may be due to row, column, interaction (between row and column), and error factors. Since the variation in the dataset is explained by two factors as well as interaction, the reduction in error variance is greater in the two-way ANOVA compared to that of the one-way ANOVA design. This makes the two-way ANOVA design more efficient than the one-way ANOVA. In this model, we wish to test whether the effects of these factors are significant in explaining the variation in the data. The significance of these components is tested by means of the *F*-test. The procedure in computing the various sums of squares, mean sums of squares, and testing the hypotheses in the two-way ANOVA has been shown below.

8.6.4 Procedure in Two-Way ANOVA

In the two-way ANOVA, we wish to test the following hypotheses

Row effect: H_0: All row group means are equal
H_1: At least one row group mean differs

Column effect: H_0: All column group means are equal
H_1: At least one column group mean differs

Interaction effect H_0: Interaction effect between row and column factors is not significant
H_1: Interaction effect between row and column factors is significant

Row and column effects are known as *main effects*. Testing the significance of a main effect is meaningful only in a situation where the interaction effect is not significant. However, if the interaction is significant, then the simple effects are investigated. The simple effect of the row factor is tested by comparing the means of all the levels of the row factor in each level of the column factor and, similarly, the simple effects of the column factor is tested by comparing the means of all the levels of the column factor in each level of the row factor.

To test the above hypotheses, the *F*-test is used for the row factor, column factor, and interaction. The procedure for computing the *F*-statistic is similar to that discussed in the case of the one-way ANOVA. Let us see how to compute the various sums of squares and mean sums of squares in the two-way ANOVA:

$$\text{TSS} = \sum_{i=1}^{r}\sum_{j=1}^{c}\sum_{k=1}^{n}\left(X_{ijk} - \frac{G}{N}\right)^2 = \sum_{i}\sum_{j}\sum_{k}X_{ijk}^2 - \frac{G^2}{N} \tag{8.11}$$

$$\text{SSR} = \sum_{i=1}^{r}\frac{R_i^2}{nc} - \frac{G^2}{N} \tag{8.12}$$

$$\text{SSC} = \sum_{j=1}^{c}\frac{C_j^2}{nr} - \frac{G^2}{N} \tag{8.13}$$

$$\text{SSI} = \sum_{i=1}^{r}\sum_{j=1}^{c}\frac{T_{ij}^2}{n} - \frac{G^2}{N} - \text{SSR} - \text{SSC} \tag{8.14}$$

$$\text{SSE} = \text{TSS}-\text{SSR}-\text{SSC}-\text{SSI} \tag{8.15}$$

$$\text{MSS}_\text{R} = \frac{\text{SSR}}{r-1} \tag{8.16}$$

$$\text{MSS}_\text{C} = \frac{\text{SSC}}{c-1} \tag{8.17}$$

$$\text{MSS}_\text{I} = \frac{\text{SSI}}{(r-1)\times(c-1)} \tag{8.18}$$

TSS represents the total variation present in the data, SSR is the variation among the row group means, SSC is the variation among the column group means, SSI is the variation due to interaction, and SSE is the variation due to error. The degrees of freedom for row and column factors are $r - 1$ and $c - 1$, respectively, whereas the degrees of freedom for interaction and error are $(r - 1)(c - 1)$ and $N - rc$, respectively. These degrees of freedom are used to compute the various mean sums of squares.

MSS_R represents the variance among the row group means, MSS_C is the variance among the column group means, MSS_I is the variance due to interaction (between row and column factors), and MSS_E is the variance due to error.

After computing the above sums of squares and mean sums of squares, the ANOVA table as shown in Table 8.9 is developed for computing the F-statistic for different sources of variation.

Remark The TSS is additive in nature but the mean sum of squares is not.

Under the normality assumptions, the F-values computed in Table 8.9 follow an F-distribution. To test whether the F-value for the row factor is significant, its calculated F is compared with the tabulated F at $(r - 1, N - rc)$ degrees of freedom. For the column factor, tabulated F is seen at $(c - 1, N - rc)$ degrees of freedom, whereas for interaction, it is seen at $((r - 1)(c - 1), N - rc)$ degrees of freedom. These tabulated values of F can be obtained from Table A.9 or A.10, depending on whether the hypothesis is tested at 0.05 or at 0.01 significance level.

If calculated $F >$ tabulated F, null hypothesis (H_0) is rejected
and if calculated $F \leq$ tabulated F, the null hypothesis (H_0) is failed to be rejected.

TABLE 8.9 Two-Way Analysis of Variance Table

Source of Variation	df	SS	MSS	F
Row factor	$r-1$	SSR	$s_\text{R}^2 = \text{SSR}/(r-1)$	$s_\text{R}^2/s_\text{E}^2$
Column factor	$c-1$	SSC	$s_\text{C}^2 = \text{SSC}/(c-1)$	$s_\text{C}^2/s_\text{E}^2$
Interaction (row × column)	$(r-1)(c-1)$	SSI	$s_\text{I}^2 = \text{SSI}/(r-1)(c-1)$	$s_\text{I}^2/s_\text{E}^2$
Error	$N-rc$	SSE	$s_\text{E}^2 = \text{SSE}/(N-rc)$	
Total	$N-1$	TSS		

Once the F-statistic becomes significant, the post hoc test discussed in the one-way analysis may be used to analyze the main and simple effects. Since the sample size is the same, either the Tukey HSD or LSD post hoc test may be used for row, column, and interaction analysis. Applying the post hoc test for row and column facilitates us in analyzing the main effects and, for interaction analysis, provides us the simple effect. The CD for row, column, and interaction analyses by using the Tukey HSD post hoc test can be obtained as follows:

For row analysis

$$\text{CD} = q_{\alpha,r,N-rc}\sqrt{\frac{\text{MSS}_{\text{E}}}{nc}} \tag{8.19}$$

For column analysis

$$\text{CD} = q_{\alpha,c,N-rc}\sqrt{\frac{\text{MSS}_{\text{E}}}{nr}} \tag{8.20}$$

Row and column analyses provide information to the researchers in investigating the main effect. Row analysis provides us the information as to which row group mean is significantly different from others, whereas the column analysis reveals which of the column group means is significantly larger than others.

For interaction analysis

$$\text{CD} = q_{\alpha,r,N-rc}\sqrt{\frac{\text{MSS}_{\text{E}}}{n}} \tag{8.21}$$

Interaction analysis provides us with the information that will help study the simple effect. It facilitates comparison of all the row group means in each level of the column factor. Similarly, by using the same CD, all the column group means can be compared in each level of the row factor.

8.6.5 Assumptions in Two-Way Analysis of Variance

While using the two-way ANOVA, the following assumptions need to be satisfied.

a. The samples have been drawn from the normal population.
b. All the samples are independent. In other words, samples in each of the treatment conditions must be different.
c. The populations from which the samples have been drawn have equal variances.

8.7 TWO-WAY ANALYSIS OF VARIANCE (ONE OBSERVATION PER CELL)

The two-way ANOVA with one observation per cell is the specific case of the two-way ANOVA with n observations per cell. This analysis is used in solving randomized group design where the purpose of the researcher is to compare the effectiveness of different treatment conditions by including the extraneous variable in the design. The procedure for using this analysis can be seen in solution to Example 8.2. In this analysis, each cell has only one score. Only main effects of row and column factors can be studied in this design. Since there is only one score in each cell, there is no interaction. The assumptions of this design are similar to those in the two-way ANOVA design (with n observations per cell). One of the constraints of this design is that number of scores must be equal in each of the treatment groups.

8.7.1 Two-Way ANOVA Model (One Observation per Cell)

Let us suppose that the two factors A and B affect the criterion variable Y. In this design, the investigator is interested in studying the effect of one factor only, and the second factor is used to reduce the error variance. Of the two factors, one serves as the experimental variable, whereas the other is used as a blocking variable. Let the factor A represent the blocking variable having r blocks, factor B represent the experimental variable having c levels, and Y_{ij} represent the effect of the ith block and the jth treatment on the criterion variable; then the layout of the data will be as shown in Table 8.10,

where

$i =$ 1, 2, …, r (blocks)
$j =$ 1, 2, …, c (treatments)
$Y_{ij} =$ score in the ith level of row factor and the jth level of column factor
$G =$ grand total of all the scores
$R_i =$ total of all the scores in the ith level of factor A
$C_j =$ total of all the scores in the jth level of factor B
$N =$ total number of scores in the experiment and is equal to $r \times c$.

The total variability is equal to the sum of the variabilities due to rows (factor A), columns (or factor B), and error. Thus, the model becomes

$$\text{TSS} = \text{SSR} + \text{SSC} + \text{SSE}$$

TABLE 8.10 Layout of the Data in Two-Way ANOVA (One Observation per Cell)

		Column Factor B					
		1	–	j	–	c	Row Total
Row factor A	1	Y_{11}	–	Y_{1j}	–	Y_{1c}	R_1
	–	–	–	–	–	–	
	i	Y_{i1}	–	Y_{ij}	–	Y_{ic}	R_i
	–	–	–	–	–	–	
	r	Y_{r1}	–	Y_{rj}	–	Y_{rc}	R_r
Column total		C_1	–	C_j	–	C_c	$G = \sum R_i = \sum C_j$

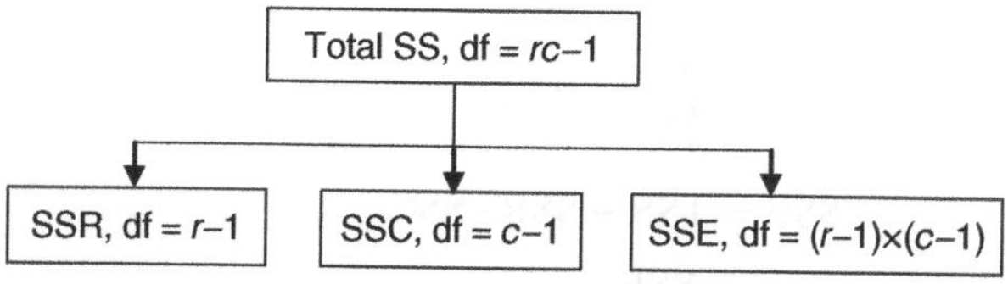

Figure 8.4 Distribution of variation and their associated degrees of freedom in the two-way ANOVA with one observation per cell.

where TSS is the total variability among all the *N* scores, SSR is the variability among the row means, SSC is the variability among the column means, and SSE is the variability due to error. Figure 8.4 shows the TSS and its components along with their degrees of freedom. These degrees of freedom are used to compute the mean sum of squares of the row and column factors.

In this ANOVA model, it is assumed that the variability among the scores may be due to the row factor (blocking), column factor (treatment), and the error factor. Since some of the variations within the groups have been explained by the row factor (blocking variable), reduction in error variance is more in this design compared to that in the one-way ANOVA design, making this design more efficient. In this model, we wish to compare the effect of different levels of treatment (column factor) only. However, the significance of row factor (blocking) simply tells whether blocking has improved the design, but this is not of interest to researchers for their experiment except in increasing the efficiency in testing the hypothesis. The significance of the *F*-value for the column factor (treatment) and row factor (blocking) can be tested in the same way as has been shown earlier. The following is the procedure for computing various sums of squares and mean sums of squares along with the procedure used in testing the hypothesis in the two-way ANOVA.

8.7.2 Procedure in Two-Way ANOVA (One Observation per Cell)

In this design, we wish to test the hypothesis

Column effect (treatment) H_0: All treatment group means are equal
H_1: At least one treatment group mean differs

The procedure for computing the *F*-statistic is similar to that described earlier. Let us see how to compute various sums of squares and mean sums of squares in testing the above hypotheses.

$$\text{TSS} = \sum_{i=1}^{r}\sum_{j=1}^{c}\left(Y_{ij} - \frac{G}{N}\right)^2 = \sum_{i}\sum_{j} Y_{ij}^2 - \frac{G^2}{N} \tag{8.22}$$

$$\text{SSR (Blocks)} = \sum_{i}^{r} \frac{R_i^2}{c} - \frac{G^2}{N} \tag{8.23}$$

$$\text{SSC (Treatment)} = \sum_{j=1}^{c} \frac{C_j^2}{r} - \frac{G^2}{N} \tag{8.24}$$

$$\text{SSE} = \text{TSS} - \text{SSR}-\text{SSC} \tag{8.25}$$

$$\text{MSS}_{\text{R}} = \frac{\text{SSR}}{r-1} \tag{8.26}$$

$$\text{MSS}_{\text{C}} = \frac{\text{SSC}}{c-1} \tag{8.27}$$

TSS represents the total variation present in the data, SSR is the variation among the row group (block) means, SSC is the variation among the column (treatment) group means, and SSE is the variation due to error. The degrees of freedom for row and column factors are $r - 1$ and $c - 1$, respectively, and that of error is $(r - 1)(c - 1)$. These degrees of freedom are used to compute various mean sums of squares.

MSS_{R} represents the variance among the row group (block) means, MSS_{C} is the variance among the column group (treatment) means, and MSS_{E} is the variance due to error.

After computing the above sums of squares and mean sums of squares, the ANOVA table as shown in Table 8.11 is constructed for computing the F-statistic for different sources of variation.

The significance of treatment and block can be tested by comparing their calculated F with the tabulated F at $(c - 1, (r - 1) \times (c - 1))$ and $(r - 1, (r - 1) \times (c - 1))$ degrees of freedom, respectively.

Once the F-statistic for treatment becomes significant, the post hoc test discussed in the one-way analysis may be used to analyze the treatment effects.

Since in this design only equal number of samples can be taken, the Tukey HSD or LSD post hoc test may be used for investigating which treatment group mean is significantly higher than others. However, no further action is required if the F-value for the block is significant. Significance of block indicates that the blocking has significantly reduced the error variance as a result of which the efficiency in the design has improved.

By using the Tukey HSD test, the CD for column (treatment) can be obtained as follows:

TABLE 8.11 Two-Way Analysis of Variance Table (One Observation per Cell)

Source of Variation	df	SS	MSS	F
Column (treatment)	$c - 1$	SSC	$s_{\text{C}}^2 = \text{SSC}/(c-1)$	$s_{\text{C}}^2/s_{\text{E}}^2$
Row (block)	$r - 1$	SSR	$s_{\text{R}}^2 = \text{SSR}/(r-1)$	$s_{\text{R}}^2/s_{\text{E}}^2$
Error (row × column)	$(r - 1) \times (c - 1)$	SSE	$s_{\text{E}}^2 = \text{SSE}/((r-1) \times (c-1))$	
Total	$rc - 1$	TSS		

For Column (Treatment) Analysis

$$\mathrm{CD} = q_{\alpha,r,(r-1)\times(c-1)}\sqrt{\frac{\mathrm{MSS_E}}{r}} \tag{8.28}$$

The application of this analysis has been shown in solving the randomized block design in Example 8.2. The term q represents the range statistic, the value of which can be obtained at an α level and $(r-1)(c-1)$ df from Table A.15.

8.8 RANDOMIZED BLOCK DESIGN

The randomized block design is used when the experimental subjects are not homogeneous. If three treatments need to be compared, then all the subjects under the study are divided into blocks of size 3 in such a manner that each block is homogeneous within itself. In each block, all the three treatments are randomly assigned. The experimenter needs to decide carefully the basis of making the blocks. Usually, blocking is done on the basis of a variable that is supposed to influence the criterion variable during the experiment.

For instance, in comparing the effect of three different types of circuit training programs on the long jump performance, one may decide to make blocks on the basis of the heights of the athletes. This is because the height of an athlete may have an impact on improving the long jump performance during an experiment. If the height is not controlled by blocking, its effect would be confounded in the performance of the long jump during the experiment, and one cannot say that the difference in the performance is only because of the circuit training program. The purpose of blocking is to reduce the error variance. By reducing the error variance, the efficiency is increased in testing the hypothesis. The two-way ANOVA with one observation per cell is used to analyze this design. The detailed computation can be understood by looking at the solution to Example 8.2.

> **FACTS TO KNOW**
>
> The randomized block design is used when one extraneous variable can be identified, which affects the criterion variable during experiment

8.8.1 Example of Two-Way ANOVA with One Observation per Cell for Solving Randomized Block Design

Example 8.2 A basketball coach wanted to investigate which elbow angle (45°, 90°, and free angle) is more appropriate to assess the shooting accuracy in converting the basket while performing the lap shot. The coach believed that height was a factor that might affect the lap shot performance in basketball; hence, height was taken as a blocking variable. Thus, a randomized block design was planned in which 30 randomly selected college athletes were first divided into 10 blocks so that the each block was homogeneous in relation to the height. The three

TABLE 8.12 Number of Basket Converted on the Lap Shot under Different Treatment Conditions

Subjects with Varying Heights	Angle of Release 45°	90°	Free Angle
1	6	12	5
2	5	14	6
3	4	11	7
4	6	10	8
5	7	9	4
6	3	12	5
7	4	7	6
8	5	8	3
9	8	12	7

treatment conditions were then randomly assigned to the subjects in each block. Thus, the subjects were asked to perform the lap shot in the first group with 45° angles, second group with 90° angles, and the third group with free angle. The data so obtained are shown in Table 8.12. Apply the two-way ANOVA (one observation per cell) to compare the effect of angles on the lap shot performance by removing the effect of the blocking variable, namely, height. Test your hypothesis at 5% level.

Solution: In this design, height is the blocking variable; hence, our primary aim is to see that after eliminating the effect of the height, whether there is any significant difference in the performance of the lap shot in three different groups. In other words, it is of interest to see whether any one angle is more suitable for shooting accuracy. Kindly note that the blocking variable is not of interest to the researcher; it is only used to reduce the error variance (Table 8.13).

TABLE 8.13 Number of Basket Converted on the Lap Shot under Different Treatment Conditions

Subject with Varying Heights	Angle of Release 45°	90°	Free Angle	Block Total
1	6	12	5	23
2	5	14	6	25
3	4	11	7	22
4	6	10	8	24
5	7	9	4	20
6	3	12	5	20
7	4	7	6	17
8	5	8	3	16
9	8	12	7	27
Group total	$R_1 = 48$	$R_2 = 95$	$R_3 = 51$	$G = R_1 + R_2 + R_3 = 194$
Group mean	5.33	10.56	5.67	

Thus, the null hypothesis that is required to be tested against the alternative hypothesis that at least one of the group mean differs is

$$H_0: \mu_{45°} = \mu_{90°} = \mu_{\text{Free\_angle}}$$

Here,

Number of treatment groups = $r = 3$ ($j = 1, 2, 3$; j represent the treatment group)
Number of blocks = $n = 9$ ($i = 1, 2, \ldots, 9$; i represent the block)
Total number of scores = $N = nr = 27$

Computation

$$\text{Correction factor (CF)} = \frac{G^2}{N} = \frac{194^2}{27} = 1393.93$$

$$\text{Raw sum of squares (RSS)} = \sum_j \sum_i Y_{ij}^2$$

$$= (6^2 + 5^2 + \cdots + 8^2) + (12^2 + 14^2 + \cdots + 12^2)$$
$$+ (5^2 + 6^2 + \cdots + 7^2)$$
$$= 1628$$

$$\text{Total sum of squares (TSS)} = \text{RSS} - \text{CF} = \sum_j \sum_i Y_{ij}^2 - \frac{G^2}{N}$$

$$= 1628 - 1393.93 = 234.07$$

$$\text{Sum of squares treatment (SST)} = \sum_j \frac{R_j^2}{n} - \frac{G^2}{N}$$

$$= \frac{48^2}{9} + \frac{95^2}{9} + \frac{51^2}{9} - 1393.93$$

$$= 256 + 1002.78 + 289 - 1393.93$$
$$= 153.85$$

$$\text{Sum of squares block (SSB)} = \sum_i \frac{B_i^2}{r} - \frac{G^2}{N}$$

$$= \frac{23^2}{3} + \frac{25^2}{3} + \frac{22^2}{3} + \frac{24^2}{3} + \frac{20^2}{3}$$
$$+ \frac{17^2}{3} + \frac{16^2}{3} + \frac{27^2}{3} - 1393.93$$
$$= 176.33 + 208.33 + 161.33 + 192 + 133.33$$
$$+ 133.33 + 96.33 + 85.33 + 243 - 1393.93$$
$$= 35.44$$

TABLE 8.14 ANOVA Table for the Data on Lap Shot

Source of Variation	df	SS	MSS	F-value	Tabulated F
Treatment	$r-1=2$	153.85	$\frac{153.85}{2}=76.93$	27.48[a]	$F_{0.05}(2,16)=3.63$
Block	$n-1=8$	35.44	$\frac{35.4}{8}=4.43$	1.58	$F_{0.05}(8,16)=2.59$
Error	$(r-1)(n-1)=16$	44.78	$\frac{44.78}{16}=2.799$		
Total	$N-1=26$	234.07			

[a]Significant at 0.05 level.

$$\begin{aligned}\text{Sum of squares error (SSE)} &= \text{TSS}-\text{SST}-\text{SSB}\\ &= 234.07-153.85-35.44\\ &= 44.78\end{aligned}$$

All the sum of squares computed have been listed in Table 8.14. From Table A.9, the value of F at 5% level with df (2,16) and df (8,16) can be noted as 3.63 and 2.59, respectively. Since the calculated value of F (=27.48) for treatment is greater than the tabulated value of F, the null hypothesis is rejected and we conclude that the F-value is significant. To find which angle of release is more useful in the lap shot performance, a post hoc comparison analysis shall be done. Readers may note that the F- ratio for the block is not significant. It is therefore clear that the blocking was not effective, and the assumption of the coach that the height may affect the performance of lap shot was not true. Even if the block F-ratio were significant, it would not have been discussed in the results as the block was not of interest to the experimenter. It is only used to reduce the error variance in order to correctly reflect the effect of treatment on the dependent variable.

Post hoc analysis

In order to know which angle is the most appropriate for the lap shot performance, the Tukey HSD test has been used because the sample sizes in all the treatment groups are equal.

Thus, the CD in the Tukey HSD test is given by

$$\text{CD} = q_{\alpha,r,N-r}\sqrt{\frac{\text{MSE}}{n}}$$

where

MSE = mean sum of square error

N = sample size

q = the range statistic, the value of which can be obtained at an α level and $(r-1)(c-1)$ df from Table A.15.

TABLE 8.15 Mean Score of Lap Shot in Three Different Treatment Groups

90°	Free Angle	45°	CD at 5% Level
10.56	5.67	5.33	1.91

"____" represents no significant difference between the means at 5% level.

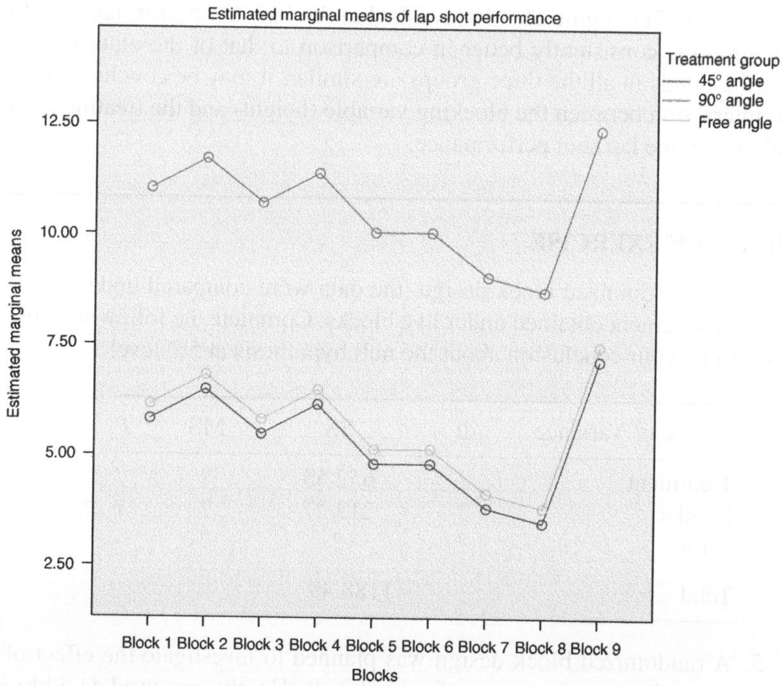

Figure 8.5 Mean scores on lap shot in all three treatment groups.

The value of q at 0.05 significance level and (3,16) degrees of freedom is 3.65 from Table A.15. Thus,

$$CD = 3.5\sqrt{\frac{2.6799}{9}}$$
$$= 1.91$$

Arranging means of the treatment groups in a descending order, each pair of group means can be compared for their significance. These means have been shown in Table 8.15.

It may be concluded from Table 8.15 that the performance of the lap shot with 90° angle is the best as this group mean is significantly higher than that of the remaining two treatment groups, whereas lap shot performance in the free angle as well as in 45° angle groups were equally good.

It may therefore be inferred that the 90° angle is the best for the lap shot performance in basketball.

Mean plot

The mean lap shot performance of all the three treatment groups has been plotted in Figure 8.5. This figure clearly reveals that the lap shot performance of the 90° angle group is consistently better in comparison to that of the other two groups. Since the trends in all the three groups are similar, it may be concluded that there is no interaction between the blocking variable (height) and the treatment (angles) in relation to the lap shot performance.

PRACTICE EXERCISE

4. In a randomized block design, the data were compared under five levels of treatment obtained under five blocks. Complete the following table and draw your conclusion about the null hypothesis at 5% level.

Source of Variance	df	SS	MS	*F*
Treatment	?	652.53	?	?
Blocks	?	212.27	?	?
Error	?	?	?	
Total		1188.49		

5. A randomized block design was planned to investigate the effect of age on push-up performance of school girls. Height was used as a blocking variable. Solve this design and test your hypothesis whether push-up performance of the girls was different in all the age groups. Apply a post hoc test to find which group's performance was the best. Test whether blocking was useful. Test your hypothesis at 1% level.

Push-Up Performance of the Girls

		Age		
		18	17	16
Block (Height)	1	12	8	6
	2	11	7	3
	3	13	6	4
	4	10	9	5

8.9 FACTORIAL DESIGN

> **FACTS TO KNOW**
>
> In the factorial design if the interaction effect is significant, then investigating main effects becomes meaningless

In the factorial design, the effect of two or more factors (treatments) on the criterion variable is investigated simultaneously. In this design, all the levels of one factor may be studied in each level of the other factor. If A and B are the two factors where factor A has two levels (A_1, A_2) and factor B has three levels (B_1, B_2, and B_3), then this design is known as a 2×3 factorial design. Thus, in a 2×3 factorial design, six treatments conditions ($A_1B_1, A_1B_2, A_1B_3, A_2B_1, A_2B_2, A_2B_3$) need to be compared; therefore, six random samples are selected. If experimenter decides to have 10 subjects in each treatment condition, then 60 ($=10 \times 2 \times 3$) subjects are randomly selected from the population of interest. By randomly allocating these six treatment conditions to the subjects, six treatment groups are formed. In this design, the main effect of both factors A and B are investigated along with the simple effect of each factor simultaneously.

In the randomized block design, only one factor is of interest to the experimenter, whereas the other factor (blocking variable) is used for reducing the within-group variability. On the other hand, in factorial design, the experimenter is interested in both factors. Another important feature of this design is that one can get an idea about the interaction effect between both the treatments.

8.9.1 Example of Two-Way ANOVA with *n* Observations per Cell for Solving Factorial Design

Example 8.3 An exercise scientist wanted to see the impact of exercise and the types of food on the fat percentage. Four levels of exercise (low, medium, high, and sedentary) and two levels of food (nonvegetarian and vegetarian) were chosen in the study, and therefore eight treatment (2×4) groups were required for the study. A factorial design was planned in which 40 women subjects were randomly chosen and divided into eight treatment groups. Exercise (four levels) and the Food (two levels) were the two factors in the study giving rise to the eight treatment conditions. These eight treatment conditions were randomly assigned to eight groups of subjects for 4 weeks to see their impact on the fat percentage. After the treatment period was over, the subjects were tested for their fat percentage, the data for which are shown in Table 8.16. Apply the two-way ANOVA to analyze the design and interpret your findings.

Solution: This is a factorial design with two factors: Exercise and Food. It is required to see the main effect of Exercise and Food on the fat percentage along with the interaction effect between them. Thus, the following hypotheses are required to be tested.

TABLE 8.16 Data on Fat Percentage

		Exercise Groups					
		Low	Medium	High	Sedentary	Total (R_i)	Mean
Food	Nonveg	17	12	15	24		
		15	15	18	20		
		20	17	12	28	370	18.5
		21	17	21	23		
		15	17	21	22		
		$T_{11} = 88$	$T_{12} = 78$	$T_{13} = 87$	$T_{14} = 117$		
	Veg	22	14	23	13		
		16	13	14	14		
		22	12	23	10	306	15.3
		13	13	13	17		
		10	10	18	16		
		$T_{21} = 83$	$T_{22} = 62$	$T_{23} = 91$	$T_{24} = 70$		
	Total (C_j)	171	140	178	187	$G = 676$	
	Mean	17.1	14.0	17.8	18.7		

Exercise effect: H_0: All Exercise group means are equal
H_1: At least one Exercise group mean differs

Food effect: H_0: Both Food group means are equal
H_1: Both Food group means are different

Interaction effect H_0: The interaction effect is not significant
H_1: The interaction effect is significant

Given

$r = 2$ (number of rows)
$c = 4$ (number of columns)
$n = 5$ (number of scores in each treatment group)
$N = nrc = 40$ (total number of scores)

$$\text{Correction factor (CF)} = \frac{G^2}{N} = \frac{676^2}{40} = 11424.40$$

$$\text{Raw sum of squares (RSS)} = \sum_{i=1}^{r}\sum_{j=1}^{c}\sum_{k=1}^{n} Y^2{}_{ijk}$$

$$= (17^2 + 15^2 + \cdots + 23^2 + 22^2)$$

$$+ (22^2 + 16^2 + \cdots + 17^2 + 16^2)$$

$$= 12192$$

$$\text{Total sum of squares (TSS)} = \text{RSS} - \text{CF} = \sum_{i=1}^{r}\sum_{j=1}^{c}\sum_{k=1}^{n} Y^2{}_{ijk} - \frac{G^2}{N}$$

$$= 12192 - 11424.40 = 767.6$$

$$\text{Sum of squares row (SSR)} = \sum_i \frac{R_i^2}{nc} - \frac{G^2}{N}$$

$$= \frac{370^2}{20} + \frac{306^2}{20} - 11424.40$$

$$= 6845 + 4681.8 - 11424.4$$

$$= 102.4$$

$$\text{Sum of squares column (SSC)} = \sum_j \frac{C_j^2}{nr} - \frac{G^2}{N}$$

$$= \frac{171^2}{10} + \frac{140^2}{10} + \frac{178^2}{10} + \frac{187^2}{10} - 11424.4$$

$$= 11549.4 - 11424.4$$

$$= 125$$

$$\text{Sum of squares interaction (SSI)} = \sum_{i,j} \frac{T_{ij}^2}{n} - \frac{G^2}{N} - \text{SSR} - \text{SSC}$$

$$= \frac{88^2}{5} + \frac{78^2}{5} + \frac{87^2}{5} + \frac{117^2}{5} + \frac{83^3}{5}$$

$$+ \frac{62^2}{5} + \frac{91^2}{5} + \frac{70^2}{5} - 11424.4 - 102.4 - 125$$

$$= 11800 - 11651.80$$

$$= 148.20$$

$$\text{Sum of squares error (SSE)} = \text{TSS} - \text{SSR} - \text{SSC} - \text{SSI}$$

$$= 767.6 - 102.4 - 125 - 148.20$$

$$= 767.6 - 375.6$$

$$= 392.0$$

In can be seen from Table 8.17 that computed values of F for row, column, and interaction are greater than the corresponding values of tabulated F at 5% level; hence, the null hypotheses for row, column, and interaction may be rejected at the significance level of 0.05. Post hoc comparison analysis shall be done for row,

TABLE 8.17 Two-Way ANOVA for the Data on Fat Percentage

Source of Variation	df	SS	MSS	Calculated F	Tabulated F
Row (food)	$r-1=1$	102.4	102.40	8.36[a]	$F_{0.05}(1,32)=4.15$
Column (exercise)	$c-1=3$	125	41.67	3.40[a]	$F_{0.05}(3,32)=2.90$
Interaction (food × exercise)	$(r-1)(c-1)=3$	148.20	49.40	4.03[a]	$F_{0.05}(3,32)=2.90$
Error	$N-rc=32$	392.0	12.25		
Total	$N-1=39$	767.6			

[a]Significant at 0.05 level.

column, and interaction separately for finding the main effect and simple effects of the factors by using the LSD test.

Main effects of the factors

The main effects become meaningful if the interaction is not significant. Since interaction is significant in this example, the analysis of main effects may be skipped by the researcher. However, in order to show the procedure, this analysis has been discussed here. The main effect of Exercise and Food shall be worked out by row and column post hoc analyses. Since the sample size is the same in all the treatment groups, the LSD test shall be used for comparison of group means.

Post hoc analysis for rows

$$\text{CD for rows} = t_{0.05}(32)\sqrt{\frac{2(\text{MSS})_E}{nc}}$$

$$= 2.04\sqrt{\frac{2\times 12.25}{5\times 4}}$$

$$= 2.26$$

Table 8.18 shows that the difference between the mean fat percentage of the non-vegetarian and vegetarian groups is greater than the CD at 5% level. Thus, it may be concluded that the mean fat percentage is higher in the nonvegetarian group in comparison to the vegetarian group when all the exercise groups are combined. This difference is shown graphically in the main plot as shown in Figure 8.6.

TABLE 8.18 Mean Fat Percentage of Food Groups (All Exercise Groups Combined)

Nonvegetarian	Vegetarian	CD at 5% Level
18.5	15.3	2.26

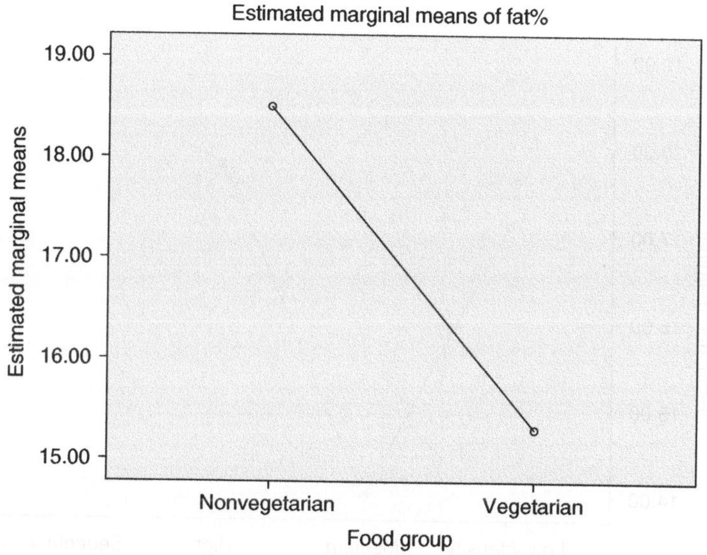

Figure 8.6 Mean plot of fat percentage scores in both food groups (all exercise groups combined).

TABLE 8.19 Mean Fat Percentage in Different Exercise Groups (Both Food Groups Combined)

Sedentary	High	Low	Medium	CD at 5% Level
18.7	17.8	17.1	14.0	3.19

"⎵" shows no significant difference between groups at 5% level.

Post hoc analysis for columns

$$\text{CD for columns} = t_{0.05}(32)\sqrt{\frac{2(\text{MSS})_E}{nr}}$$

$$= 2.04\sqrt{\frac{2 \times 12.25}{5 \times 2}}$$

$$= 3.19$$

Table 8.19 shows that the mean fat percentage is the same in the high exercise, low exercise, and sedentary groups. Further, mean values in these groups are significantly higher than that of the medium exercise group at 5% level when both food

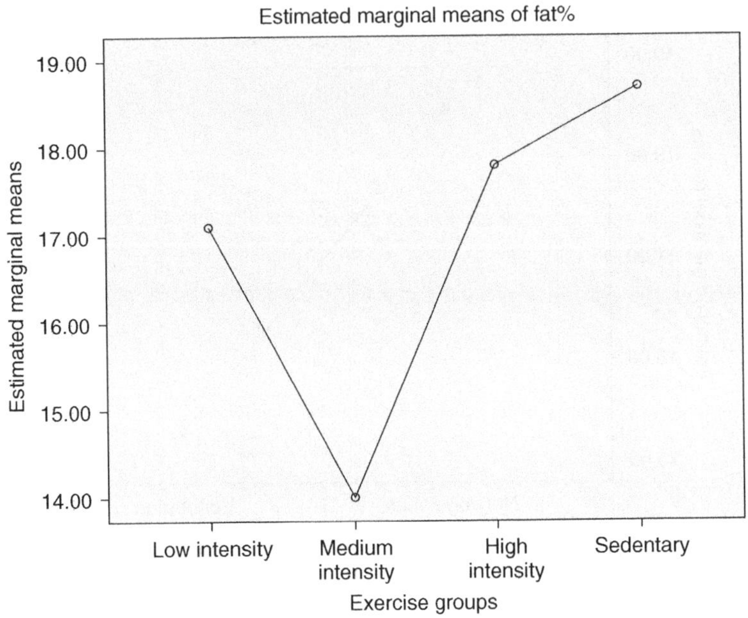

Figure 8.7 Mean plot of fat percentage scores in all four exercise groups (both food groups combined).

groups are combined. Mean plot of fat percentage of all the exercise groups when food groups are combined is shown in Figure 8.7.

Simple effects

Since interaction has been reported to be significant, investigating the simple effect is of great importance. The simple effect is a comparison of all the levels of one factor in each level with that of the other factor separately. For example, here the simple effect of Exercise is the comparison of mean fat percentage scores among all the levels of Exercise in the nonvegetarian groups with that of vegetarian groups separately. Similarly, the simple effect of Food is the comparison of mean fat percentage scores of nonvegetarian groups with that of vegetarian groups separately in each of the exercise groups. These simple effects shall be studied by using the LSD test in the post hoc analysis of the interaction, which is as follows:

Post hoc analysis for interaction

$$\text{CD for interaction} = t_{0.05}(32)\sqrt{\frac{2(\text{MSS})_\text{E}}{n}}$$

$$= 2.04\sqrt{\frac{2 \times 12.25}{5}}$$

$$= 4.52$$

TABLE 8.20 Mean Fat Percentage of Different Food Groups in Each Exercise Group

Exercise Group	Nonvegetarian	Vegetarian	CD at 5% Level
Low	17.6	16.6	4.52
Medium	15.6	12.4	4.52
High	17.4	18.2	4.52
Sedentary	23.4	14	4.52

"└──┘" shows no significant difference between groups at 5% level.

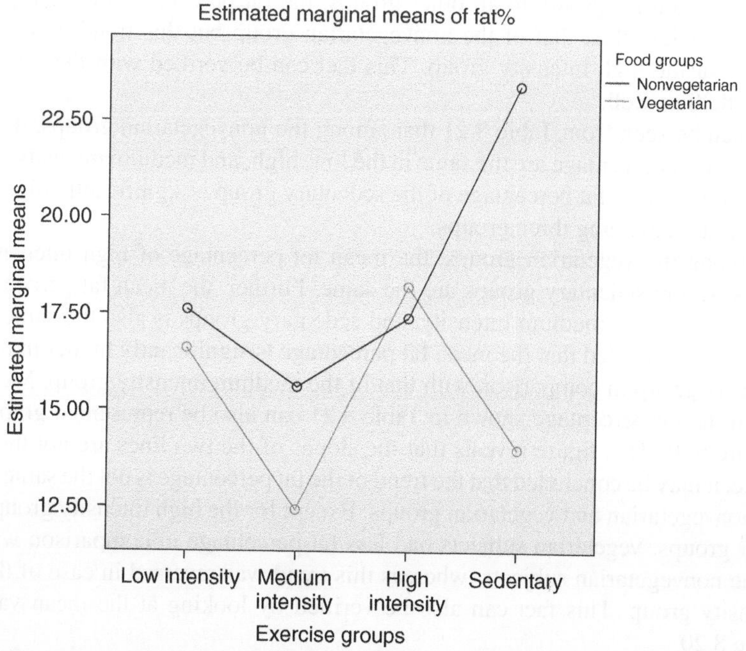

Figure 8.8 Comparison of mean fat scores between the vegetarian and nonvegetarian groups in each exercise group.

It can be seen from Table 8.20 that there is no difference between the fat percentage in the nonvegetarian and vegetarian groups in the low, high, and sedentary groups, whereas the difference is significant in the medium exercise group at 5% level. It may be concluded that among those who had undergone the medium intensity exercise program, the fat percentage was significantly higher in the nonvegetarian participants compared to that of vegetarian participants. The mean fat percentage of various groups as listed in Table 8.20 has been shown in Figure 8.8. The mean plot in Figure 8.8 shows that the slopes of all the lines are not the same;

TABLE 8.21 Mean Fat Percentage for Different Exercise Groups in Each Food Group

Food Group	Exercise Groups				CD at 5% Level
Nonvegetarian	23.4 (Sedentary)	17.6 (Low)	17.4 (High)	15.6 (Medium)	4.52
Vegetarian	18.2 (High)	16.6 (Low)	14 (Sedentary)	12.4 (Medium)	4.52

"_____/" shows no significant difference between groups at 5% level.

hence, the pattern of fat percentage in the nonvegetarian and vegetarian groups is not the same in all four exercise groups. It is clearly visible that except for the high intensity exercise group, in all other groups, the fat percentage of the vegetarian group was less than that of the nonvegetarian group but this trend was reversed in case of the high intensity group. This fact can be verified with the findings in Table 8.20 as well.

It can be seen from Table 8.21 that among the nonvegetarian groups, the mean values of fat percentage are the same in the low, high, and medium intensity groups. Further, the mean fat percentage of the sedentary group is significantly higher than that of the remaining three groups.

Among the vegetarian groups, the mean fat percentage of high intensity, low intensity, and sedentary groups are the same. Further, the mean fat percentage of the low intensity, medium intensity, and sedentary groups is also the same. Thus, it may be concluded that the mean fat percentage is significantly higher in the high intensity group in comparison with that of the medium intensity group. Mean values of the fat percentage shown in Table 8.21 can also be represented graphically (Figure 8.9). This figure reveals that the slopes of the two lines are not the same; hence, it may be concluded that the trend of the fat percentage is not the same among the nonvegetarian and vegetarian groups. Except for the high intensity group, in all other groups, vegetarian subjects had less fat percentage in comparison with that of the nonvegetarian subjects, whereas this trend was reversed in case of the high intensity group. This fact can also be verified by looking at the mean values in Table 8.20.

8.10 ANALYSIS OF COVARIANCE

Analysis of covariance is an extension of the ANOVA technique. This design is used to control the effect of an extraneous variable by adjusting the final scores on the criterion variable after the treatment is over. To control the effect of extraneous factors, subjects are randomly selected and treatments are randomly allocated to them. Such randomization makes the treatment groups homogeneous and enhances external and internal validity in findings. But on many occasions, it is not possible to make groups of subjects in accordance with the desired procedures. For instance, one may not have the choice to assign subjects to groups or treatments randomly

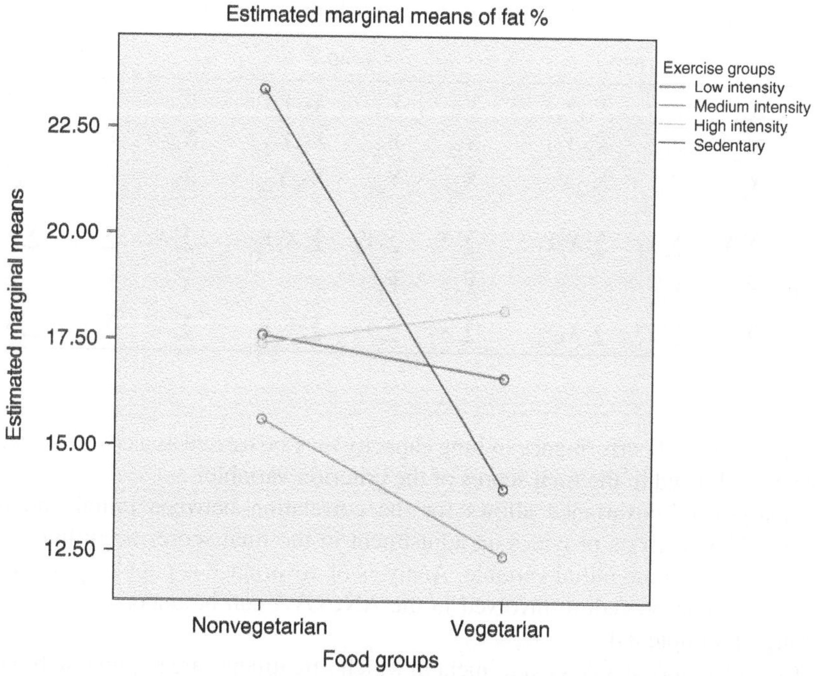

Figure 8.9 Comparison of mean fat scores among all four exercise groups in each of the two food groups.

and may be forced to take intact groups that are initially not homogeneous. These subjects in the intact groups may differ on some aspect that might affect the criterion variable during the experiment; hence, statistical control is necessary to reduce the experimental error due to such initial differences in the groups.

Thus, in any specific research situation, the individual variations that appear within the measures on the criterion variable are potentially correlated with some other factor. If the criterion variable is a measure of how well subjects learn swimming under three different methods of instructions, the potential correlates are likely to include parameters such as prior relevant learning, endurance, strength, motivation, self-discipline, and intelligence. These potential correlates are known as *covariates*. Analysis of covariance can be used to compare the effectiveness of these methods of instruction on learning swimming after removing the effect of the identified covariate.

In many experimental situations, it is difficult to identify the covariate that affects the criterion variable during the experiment. In that case, scores on the criterion variable before starting the experiment may serve as a covariate. For instance, let us consider an experiment in which it is required to investigate the comparative effect of three different physical fitness programs on the lung capacity of athletes. In this case, it is not possible to identify any covariate because there may be a number of parameters that might affect the lung capacity during treatments; therefore, in such

TABLE 8.22 Layout of the Data for the Analysis of Covariance

	Group 1			Group 2			Group r		
	X_{11}	Y_{11}	$X_{11}Y_{11}$	X_{21}	Y_{21}	$X_{21}Y_{21}$	X_{r1}	Y_{r1}	$X_{r1}Y_{r1}$
	X_{12}	Y_{12}	$X_{12}Y_{12}$	X_{22}	Y_{22}	$X_{22}Y_{22}$	X_{r2}	Y_{r2}	$X_{r2}Y_{r2}$
	X_{1n}	Y_{1n}	$X_{1n}Y_{1n}$	X_{2n}	Y_{2n}	$X_{2n}Y_{2n}$	X_{rn}	Y_{rn}	$X_{rn}Y_{rn}$
Sum	$\sum X_1$	$\sum Y_1$	$\sum X_1Y_1$	$\sum X_2$	$\sum Y_2$	$\sum X_2Y_2$	$\sum X_r$	$\sum Y_r$	$\sum X_rY_r$
Mean	$\overline{X}_1$	$\overline{Y}_1$		$\overline{X}_2$	$\overline{Y}_2$		$\overline{X}_r$	$\overline{Y}_r$	
SS	$\sum X_1^2$	$\sum Y_1^2$	$\sum X_1Y_1$	$\sum X_2^2$	$\sum Y_2^2$	$\sum X_2Y_2$	$\sum X_r^2$	$\sum Y_r^2$	$\sum X_rY_r$

situations, initial performance of lung capacity may be treated as a covariate whose effect is adjusted in the final scores of the criterion variable.

Analysis of covariance allows for the correlation between initial and final scores. This analysis provides an adjustment in the final scores according to the differences in some initial variable. Analysis of covariance is popularly written as *ANCOVA*. The procedure involved in the ANCOVA can be understood by going through Example 8.4.

Consider an ANCOVA experiment in which r treatments are required to be compared. These treatments have been randomly administered in r groups, each having n subjects. The subjects have been tested on some criterion variable before and after the treatments in all the groups. Let X_{ij} represent the jth score in the ith treatment group in the pre-testing and Y_{ij} represent the jth score in the ith treatment group in the post-testing. The layouts of the data in the pre- and post-testing groups have been shown in Table 8.22. Here, the pre-testing data serve as the covariate.

$\sum X_i$, $\sum Y_i$ and $\sum X_iY_i$ represent the ith group total in the pre-testing, post-testing, and cross product of pre- and post-testing, respectively. Similarly, $\overline{X}_i$ and $\overline{Y}_i$ represent the respective means of pre- and post-group scores in the ith treatment group.

The null hypothesis that is required to be tested here is

$$H_0 : \mu_{\text{Adj}Y_1} = \mu_{\text{Adj}Y_2} = \cdots = \mu_{\text{Adj}Y_r}$$

8.10.1 Steps in the Analysis of Covariance

1. *Correction factors*

$$C_x = \frac{\left(\sum x\right)^2}{N}$$

$$C_y = \frac{\left(\sum y\right)^2}{N}$$

$$C_{xy} = \frac{\sum x \sum y}{N}$$

where

$$\sum X = \sum X_1 + \sum X_2 + \ \ldots \ + \sum X_r$$
$$\sum Y = \sum Y_1 + \sum Y_2 + \ \ldots \ + \sum Y_r$$
$$\sum XY = \sum X_1Y_1 + \sum X_2Y_2 + \ \ldots \ + \sum X_rY_r$$

2. *TSS*

$$\text{TSS}_x = \sum X^2 - \text{C}_x$$
$$\text{TSS}_y = \sum Y^2 - \text{C}_y$$
$$\text{TSS}_{xy} = \sum XY - \text{C}_{xy}$$

where

$$\sum X^2 = \sum X_1^2 + \sum X_2^2 + \ \ldots \ + \sum X_r^2$$
$$\sum Y^2 = \sum Y_1^2 + \sum Y_2^2 + \ \ldots \ + \sum Y_r^2$$
$$\sum XY = \sum X_1Y_1 + \sum X_2Y_2 + \ \ldots \ + \sum X_rY_r$$

3. *Sum of squares due to treatment groups*

$$\text{SST}_x = \frac{(\sum x_1)^2 + (\sum x_2)^2 + \ldots + (\sum x_r)^2}{n} - C_x$$

$$\text{SST}_y = \frac{(\sum y_1)^2 + (\sum y_2)^2 + \ldots + (\sum y_r)^2}{n} - C_y$$

$$\text{SST}_{xy} = \frac{\sum x_1 \sum y_1 + \sum x_2 \sum y_2 + \ldots + \sum x_r \sum y_r}{n} - C_{xy}$$

4. *Sum of squares due to error*

$$\text{SSE}_x = \text{TSS}_x - \text{SST}_x$$
$$\text{SSE}_y = \text{TSS}_y - \text{SST}_y$$
$$\text{SSE}_{xy} = \text{TSS}_{xy} - \text{SST}_{xy}$$

5. *Adjusted sum of squares for Y* The purpose of this step is to adjust the post-testing scores y for the differences in the pre-testing scores x. $SS_{y.x}$ indicate that SS_y have been adjusted for any variability in y contributed by x.

   Let $y.x$ represent the adjusted value of y for x, then

$$TSS_{yx} = TSS_y - \frac{TSS_{xy}^2}{TSS_x} \tag{8.29}$$

$$SSE_{yx} = SSE_y - \frac{SSE_{xy}^2}{SSE_x} \tag{8.30}$$

   Sum of squares due to adjusted treatment means (post-testing)

$$SST_{y.x} = TSS_{y.x} - SSE_{y.x} \tag{8.31}$$

   The null hypothesis that the adjusted means in the post-testing groups are the same can be tested by testing the significance of $F_{y.x}$. If $F_{y.x}$ is greater than tabulated F at 0.05 significance level with $(r - 1, N - r - 1)$ degrees of freedom, the null hypothesis may be rejected; otherwise, we fail to reject the null hypothesis. Since the post mean is adjusted for the initial differences, 1 degree of freedom is lost and, therefore, the error degrees of freedom and total degrees of freedom shown in the ANCOVA table are $N - r - 1$ and $N - 2$, respectively (Table 8.23).

6. *Computation of correlation and regression coefficients* This additional step is useful for comparing the adjusted post means by using the post hoc test. To do so, the following correlation (r) and regression coefficients (b) are required to be computed:

$$r_{\text{total}} = \frac{TSS_{xy}}{\sqrt{TSS_x \times TSS_y}} \qquad b_{\text{total}} = \frac{TSS_{xy}}{TSS_x}$$

TABLE 8.23 Analysis of Covariance Table

Source of Variation	df	$SS_{y.x}$	$MSS_{y.x}$	$F_{y.x}$
Treatment	$r - 1$	$SST_{y.x}$	$s_{T_{Y.X}}^2 = \frac{SST_{y.x}}{r-1}$	$F_{y.x} = \frac{s_{T_{Y.X}}^2}{s_{E_{Y.X}}^2}$
Error	$N - r - 1$	$SSE_{y.x}$	$s_{E_{Y.X}}^2 = \frac{SSE_{y.x}}{N-r-1}$	
Total	$N - 2$	$TSS_{y.x}$		

$$r_{\text{between\_means}} = \frac{\text{SST}_{xy}}{\sqrt{\text{SST}_x \times \text{SST}_y}} \quad b_{\text{between\_means}} = \frac{\text{SST}_{xy}}{\text{SST}_x}$$

$$r_{\text{within}} = \frac{\text{SSE}}{\sqrt{\text{SSE}_x \times \text{SSE}_y}} \quad b_{\text{within}} = \frac{\text{SSE}_{xy}}{\text{SSE}_x}$$

When correlation among scores (r_{within}) is high and correlation among means ($r_{\text{among means}}$) is low, the ANCOVA will often result in significant F, and, in that case, the ANOVA fails to reveal significant differences among the post-group means (y). The magnitude of these two correlations may be used to decide whether the ANCOVA should be used or not.

7. *Calculation of adjusted post-group means* The following general formula gives the adjusted value of final means in all the groups:

$$M_{y.x} = M_y \ - b_{\text{within}} \ (M_x - \text{GM}_x) \tag{8.32}$$

$$\text{GM}_x = \frac{\bar{x}_1 + \bar{x}_2 + \ \dots \ + \bar{x}_r}{n} \tag{8.33}$$

where GM_x is the mean of all x scores, M_x and M_y represent the means of the x and y scores, respectively, for the group whose adjusted final mean is computed.

Thus, for the first group, the adjusted mean would be

$$M_{y_1.x_1} = \bar{Y}_1 - b_{\text{within}}(\bar{X}_1 - GM_x) \tag{8.34}$$

8. Testing the significance of the difference among adjusted post-group means:

$$\text{Critical difference at 0.05 level (CD)} = t_{0.05}(N - r - 1)\sqrt{\frac{2 \times \text{MSSE}_{y.x}}{n}}$$

$$= t_{0.05}(N - r - 1)\sqrt{\frac{2 \times S^2_{E_{y.x}}}{n}}$$

This CD is used to test the significant difference between all the paired adjusted post-group means as shown in Table 8.24. If the difference between any two adjusted post-group means is higher than this CD, the difference is significant, otherwise it is not. The procedure involved in the ANCOVA can be easily understood from Example 8.4.

TABLE 8.24 Group Means and Adjusted Final Means

Group size	Sample of x	Mean of x	Mean of y	Mean Adjusted $M_{y.x}$
1	n	$\overline{X}_1$	$\overline{Y}_1$	$M_{y_1.x_1}$
2	n	$\overline{X}_2$	$\overline{Y}_2$	$M_{y_2.x_2}$
3	n	$\overline{X}_3$	$\overline{Y}_3$	$M_{y_3.x_3}$
r	n	$\overline{X}_r$	$\overline{Y}_r$	$M_{y_r.x_r}$

Example 8.4 In an experiment, 32 college men basketball players were tested for their performance on the under-basket shot. Eight players were selected in each of the four groups: A, B, C, and D. Group A was given circuit training, group B, weight training, group C, a combination of weight and circuit training, whereas group D served as a control group in which no training was given. After 4 weeks of training, these groups were again tested for their performance on the under-basket shot. Apply the ANCOVA on the data shown in Table 8.25 to find out which training is the most effective.

Solution: The ANCOVA involves computations in the following steps:

1. *Total of all the four groups*

$$\sum x = 70 + 55 + 63 + 63 = 251$$

$$\sum y = 90 + 70 + 75 + 67 = 302$$

$$\sum xy = 813 + 505 + 635 + 560 = 2513$$

$$\sum x^2 = 638 + 415 + 543 + 527 = 2123$$

$$\sum y^2 = 1040 + 636 + 747 + 601 = 3024$$

2. *Correction factors*

$$C_x = \frac{(\sum x)^2}{N} = \frac{251^2}{32} = 1968.78$$

$$C_y = \frac{(\sum y)^2}{N} = \frac{302^2}{32} = 2850.13$$

$$C_{xy} = \frac{\sum x \sum y}{N} = \frac{251 \times 302}{32} = 2368.81$$

TABLE 8.25 Performance Score on Under-Basket Shot

	Circuit Training (*A*)			Weight Training (*B*)			Circuit × Weight Training (*C*)			Control (*D*)		
	x_1	y_1	x_1y_1	x_2	y_2	x_2y_2	x_3	y_3	x_3y_3	x_4	y_4	x_4y_4
	10	13	130	10	11	110	5	6	30	10	11	110
	12	14	168	5	7	35	5	7	35	8	7	56
	8	11	88	4	6	24	10	11	110	9	10	90
	9	12	108	6	8	48	7	8	56	7	7	49
	7	9	63	8	9	72	10	12	120	4	4	16
	6	8	8	5	10	50	6	8	48	6	8	48
	8	11	88	7	8	56	8	10	80	9	9	81
	10	12	120	10	11	110	12	13	156	10	11	110
Sum	70	90	813	55	70	505	63	75	635	63	67	560
Mean	8.75	11.25		6.88	8.75		7.88	9.38		7.88	8.38	
SS	638	1040		415	636		543	747		527	601	

3. *TSS*

$$\begin{aligned}\text{TSS}_x &= \sum X^2 - C_x\\ &= 2123 - 1968.78\\ &= 154.22\end{aligned}$$

$$\begin{aligned}\text{TSS}_y &= \sum Y^2 - C_y\\ &= 3024 - 2850.13\\ &= 173.87\end{aligned}$$

$$\begin{aligned}\text{TSS}_{xy} &= \sum XY - C_{xy}\\ &= 2513 - 2368.81\\ &= 144.19\end{aligned}$$

4. *Sum of squares due to treatment groups*

$$\begin{aligned}\text{SST}_x &= \frac{\left(\sum x_1\right)^2 + \left(\sum x_2\right)^2 + \left(\sum x_3\right)^2 + \left(\sum x_4\right)^2}{n} - C_x\\ &= \frac{70^2 + 55^2 + 63^2 + 63^2}{8} - 1968.78\\ &= 14.09\end{aligned}$$

$$\begin{aligned}\text{SST}_y &= \frac{\left(\sum y_1\right)^2 + \left(\sum y_2\right)^2 + \left(\sum y_3\right)^2 + \left(\sum y_4\right)^2}{n} - C_y\\ &= \frac{90^2 + 70^2 + 75^2 + 67^2}{8} - 2850.13\\ &= 39.13\end{aligned}$$

$$\begin{aligned}\text{SST}_{xy} &= \frac{\sum x_1 \sum y_1 + \sum x_2 \sum y_2 + \sum x_3 \sum y_3 + \sum x_4 \sum y_4}{n} - C_{xy}\\ &= \frac{70 \times 90 + 55 \times 70 + 63 \times 75 + 63 \times 67}{8} - 2368.81\\ &= 18.19\end{aligned}$$

5. *Sum of squares due to error*

$$\begin{aligned}\text{SSE}_x &= \text{TSS}_x - \text{SST}_x\\ &= 154.22 - 14.09\\ &= 140.13\end{aligned}$$

$$\text{SSE}_y = \text{TSS}_y - \text{SST}_y$$
$$= 173.88 - 39.13$$
$$= 134.75$$
$$\text{SSE}_{xy} = \text{TSS}_{xy} - \text{SST}_{xy}$$
$$= 144.19 - 18.19$$
$$= 126$$

6. *Adjusted sum of squares for y*

$$\text{TSS}_{yx} = \text{TSS}_y - \frac{\text{TSS}_{xy}^2}{\text{TSS}_x}$$
$$= 173.87 - \frac{144.19^2}{154.22}$$
$$= 39.06$$
$$\text{SSE}_{yx} = \text{SSE}_y - \frac{\text{SSE}_{xy}^2}{\text{SSE}_x}$$
$$= 134.75 - \frac{126^2}{140.13}$$
$$= 21.46$$
$$\text{SST}_{yx} = \text{TSS}_{yx} - \text{SSE}_{\text{yx}}$$
$$= 39.06 - 21.46$$
$$= 17.6$$
$$\text{Tabulated } F_{0.05}\,(3, 27) = 2.96$$

Since F_{yx} is greater than $F_{0.05}$ (Table 8.26), it may be concluded that the effects of all the treatments are not equal in improving the performance of the under-basket shot. In order to find which treatment is more effective, pairwise comparison of adjusted means of post-test data would be carried out (Tables 8.27 and 8.28).

TABLE 8.26 Analysis of Covariance Table for the Data on Under-Basket Shot

Source of Variation	df	$SS_{y.x}$	$MSS_{y.x}$	$F_{y.x}$
Treatment group means	4 − 1 = 3	17.60	5.87	$\frac{5.87}{0.79} = 7.43$
Error	32 − 4 − 1 = 27	21.46	0.79	
Total	30	39.06		

TABLE 8.27 Group Means and Adjusted Final Means

	Group	Sample Size	M_x	M_y	Adjusted Mean $M_{y.x}$
(*A*)	Circuit training	8	8.75	11.25	10.44
(*B*)	Weight training	8	6.88	8.75	9.62
(*C*)	Circuit × weight training	8	7.88	9.38	9.35
(*D*)	Control	8	7.88	8.38	8.35

7. *Regression coefficient*

$$b_{\text{within}} = \frac{\text{SSE}_{xy}}{\text{SSE}_x} = \frac{126}{140.13} = 0.899$$

8. *Calculation of adjusted y means*

$$\text{GM}_x = \frac{\bar{x}_1 + \bar{x}_2 + \bar{x}_3 + \bar{x}_4}{4} = 7.85$$

$$M_{y.x} = M_y - b_{\text{within}}(M_x - \text{GM}_x)$$

$$\text{Group A} \quad M_{y_1.x_1} = \bar{y}_1 - b_{\text{within}}(\bar{x}_1 - \text{GM}_x)$$
$$= 11.25 - 0.899(8.75 - 7.85)$$
$$= 10.44$$

$$\text{Group B} \quad M_{y_2.x_2} = \bar{y}_2 - b_{\text{within}}(\bar{x}_2 - \text{GM}_x)$$
$$= 8.75 - 0.899(6.88 - 7.85)$$
$$= 9.62$$

$$\text{Group C} \quad M_{y_3.x_3} = \bar{y}_3 - b_{\text{within}}(\bar{x}_3 - \text{GM}_x)$$
$$= 9.38 - 0.899(7.88 - 7.85)$$
$$= 9.35$$

$$\text{Group D} \quad M_{y_4.x_4} = \bar{y}_4 - b_{\text{within}}(\bar{x}_4 - \text{GM}_x)$$
$$= 8.38 - 0.899(7.88 - 7.85)$$
$$= 8.35$$

TABLE 8.28 Adjusted Means in Different Treatment Groups in Post-testing

Circuit Training (A)	Weight Training (B)	Circuit × Weight Training (C)	Control (D)	CD at 5% Level
10.44	9.62	9.35	8.35	0.91

"⌴" no significant difference exists between means at 0.05 level.

9. *Post hoc analysis using the LSD test* The CD has been computed by using the LSD test for comparing the adjusted post-group means.

$$\text{CD} = t_{0.05}(N - r - 1)\sqrt{\frac{2\text{MSE}_{y.x}}{n}}$$

$$= t_{0.05}(27)\sqrt{\frac{2 \times 0.79}{8}}$$

$$= 2/05\sqrt{\frac{2 \times 0.79}{8}}$$

$$= 0.91$$

Inference

Table 8.28 shows that treatments A and B are equally effective and also that treatments B and C are equally effective, whereas treatment D is the least effective. It is therefore concluded that if a choice has to be made out of the three treatments A, B, and C, treatment A should be preferred. In other words, the circuit training program may be recommended for improving the performance on the under-basket shot in general.

Check Your Progress

Note: Tick the correct answer by using the sign (√).

	True	False
26. In the factorial design, investigating main effects becomes meaningful if the interaction is significant.	–	–
27. The factorial design can be solved by using the two-way ANOVA.	–	–

28. In the randomized block design, the blocking factor is also investigated by using the post hoc test.	–	–
29. In the ANCOVA, the means of the treatment groups are adjusted for the covariate.	–	–
30. In the randomized block design, the samples may have different number of subjects.	–	–
31. In the factorial design, the simple effects are investigated only if the interaction is significant.	–	–
32. In the means plot, if the slopes of the lines are the same, then it indicates that the interaction is significant.	–	–
33. In the two-way ANOVA, the independent variables are also known as factors.	–	–
34. In the randomized block design with r blocks and c treatments, the total degree of freedom is obtained as $rc-2$.	–	–
35. The purpose of using an experimental design is to reduce the error variance.	–	–
36. The completely randomized design can be used only when the experimental subjects are homogeneous in all aspects.	–	–
37. Interaction can be tested in the two-way ANOVA with one observation per cell.	–	–
38. The randomized block design is usually solved with the two-way ANOVA with n observations per cell.	–	–
39. The randomized block design is more efficient than the completely randomized design.	–	–
40. In the two-way ANOVA with n observations per cell, the degree of freedom for error is $(r-1)(c-1)$.	–	–
41. Pre-testing scores cannot be used as a covariate in the ANCOVA design.	–	–
42. The TSS is additive in nature.	–	–
43. If calculated F is equal to the tabulated F, we may not reject the null hypothesis.	–	–
44. In the ANCOVA, the total degree of freedom is equal to $N-1$.	–	–
45. In the factorial design, one of the assumptions is that all the samples are independent.	–	–
46. In the two-way ANOVA, it is not necessary that the population variances are the same.	–	–
47. The randomized block design is used when an extraneous variable can be identified that is presumably associated with the criterion variable.	–	–
48. In the two-way ANOVA with one observation per cell, the error degree of freedom is $(r-1)(c-1)$.	–	–

49. The total mean sum of squares is additive in nature.	–	–
50. In the randomized block design, the block size must be equal to the number of treatments.	–	–
51. In a 3 × 4 factorial design, there are seven treatment groups.	–	–
52. Analysis of covariance is used when the subjects cannot be randomly chosen.	–	–
53. The blocking variable in a design is used to reduce the error variance.	–	–
54. In the randomized block design, interaction is meaningful.	–	–

PRACTICE EXERCISE

6. Explain the following factorial design. Write the number of independent and dependent variables in this design. How many levels are there for each treatment? Can the interaction be computed? Write the degrees of freedom for all sources of variation.

	Variable 1		
Variable 2	1	5	8
	5	4	8
	7	8	7
	6	9	8
	7	6	5
	8	6	4
	8	9	7
	6	4	5

7. Fill up the entries in the following two-way ANOVA table. Compute F-values and test their significance to draw conclusions about the hypotheses in main and interaction effects at 5% level.

Source of Variance	df	SS	MS	F
Row	4	65.35	?	?
Column	5	21.23	?	?
Interaction	?	?	?	?
Error	80	398.78	?	
Total		679.92		

8.11 COMPUTING WITH EXCEL

8.11.1 Solving Experimental Designs with Excel

Excel can be used to solve many experimental designs by means of the ANOVA analysis. The single-factor ANOVA is used in solving a completely randomized design (between-group design), the two-factor ANOVA without replication is used to solve a randomized group design, whereas the two-factor ANOVA with replication is used to solve a factorial design. All these designs have been explained in detail earlier in this chapter. In this section, the functionality of EXCEL in solving these three experimental designs shall be shown by means of three examples. The readers are advised to go through the relevant text in the chapter for interpretation of the findings obtained in these computations using Excel.

Remark The following analysis of variance design can be solved only if the Add-Ins "Analysis ToolPak" is already installed in your Excel. The readers can install this Add-Ins in their Excel by following the procedure described in Chapter 1.

Solving Completely Randomized Design (One-Way ANOVA) This design is used when the experimental subjects are homogeneous in nature. The one-way ANOVA is used to solve this design. In Excel, the single-factor ANOVA is used for solving the problems based on this design. The procedure involved in using Excel for computation in the single-factor ANOVA is discussed by means of the following example.

Example 8.5 In order to know the health risk of active, semi-active, and sedentary workers in an organization, their waist/hip ratio was calculated. The data are shown in Table 8.29.

Apply the one-way ANOVA to test the null hypothesis that the average waist/hip ratio of the three different types of workers is the same. Test your hypothesis at 5% level.

TABLE 8.29 Waist/Hip Ratio of the Workers

Active	Semi-active	Sedentary
0.96	0.99	1.3
0.98	1.1	1.5
0.92	1.3	1.6
0.92	1.2	1.4
0.91	1.1	1.5
0.92	0.95	1.8
0.98	0.99	1.7
0.97	0.97	1.6
0.88	1.2	1.8
0.88	1.3	1.3
0.80	1.5	
0.83		

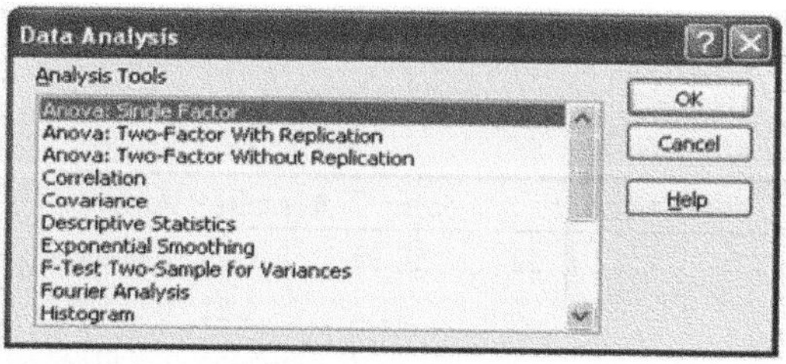

Figure 8.10 Command for applying the one-way ANOVA.

Solution: The procedure for applying the one-way ANOVA in case of equal and unequal sample sizes is the same. The following steps shall be used to apply the one-way ANOVA in Excel:

1. Type the data of all the three groups in the three columns A, B, and C of the Excel sheet. The headings for the three variables may be written in the first cell of each column.
2. To apply the one-way ANOVA, click the following commands in sequence in Excel to get the screen as shown in Figure 8.10.

   Data → Data Analysis

3. Bring the scroll on the option **Anova: Single Factor** and then click **OK** on the screen as shown in Figure 8.11. This will take you to the screen as shown in Figure 8.11. You can now define the data range of all the three samples.

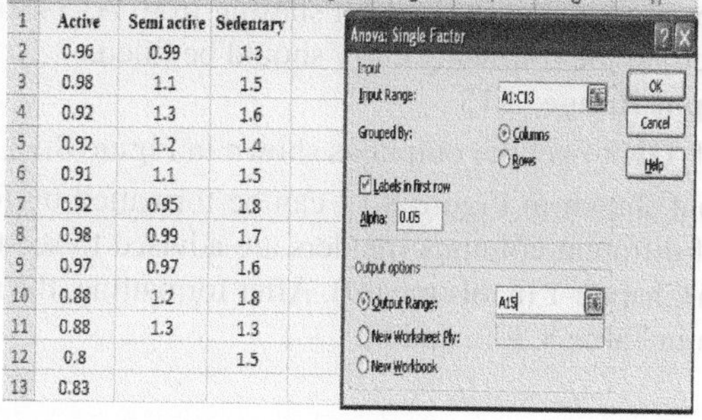

Figure 8.11 Options for applying the one-way ANOVA.

15	**Anova: Single Factor**						
16							
17	SUMMARY						
18	*Groups*	*Count*	*Sum*	*Average*	*Variance*		
19	Active	12	10.95	0.9125	0.003311		
20	Semi active	10	11.1	1.11	0.018067		
21	Sedentary	11	17	1.545455	0.030727		
22							
23							
24	ANOVA						
25	*Source of Variation*	*SS*	*df*	*MS*	*F*	*P-value*	*F crit*
26	Between Groups	2.37643561	2	1.188218	70.40627	4.67E-12	3.31583
27	Within Groups	0.50629773	30	0.016877			
28							
29	Total	2.88273333	32				

Figure 8.12 Output of the one-way ANOVA.

4. Here, all the data in the three groups are written in the first three columns A, B, and C of the Excel sheet. This includes variable names as well. Thus, the range of the entire dataset is from A1 to C13. Please note that cells B12, B13, and C13 are blank but you can go ahead. Do the following steps to fill the entries on the screen shown in Figure 8.11.
   i. **Input Range**: A1:C13
   ii. Check the "Column" option in the radio button **Grouped By**.
   iii. Check **Labels in first row** (because the heading for the data is written in the first cell of each variable).
   iv. Enter the value of α at which you want to test the hypothesis. In this example, it is taken as 0.05
   v. Fill the entry in the output range. The output can be obtained on the same Excel sheet, new worksheet, or new workbook. Here, the output is obtained on the same sheet starting from A15 location onward and, therefore, the following entry should be filled.
   Output Range: A15
   vi. Click **OK** to get the output as shown in Figure 8.12.
5. The output shown in Figure 8.12 can be formatted by formatting the cell entries of different columns (readers are advised to see the procedure discussed in Chapter 1 in this regard). After formatting, the results will appear as shown in Table 8.30(a and b).

TABLE 8.30 ANOVA: Single Factor

a. Summary

Groups	Count	Sum	Average	Variance
Active	12.000	10.95	0.913	0.003
Semi-active	10.000	11.1	1.110	0.018
Sedentary	11.000	17	1.545	0.031

b. ANOVA

Source of Variation	SS	df	MS	*F*	*p*-Value	*F* crit
Between groups	2.376	2	1.188	70.406	0.000	3.316
Within groups	0.506	30	0.017			
Total	2.883	32				

Since the calculated value of F (=70.406) is higher than 3.316, the null hypothesis that the average waist/hip ratio of the three different types of workers is the same is rejected at 5% level.

Solving Randomized Block Design (Two-Way ANOVA with One Observation per Cell) This design is used when the experimental subjects/material are not homogeneous in nature. The two-way ANOVA without replication is used to solve this design. In Excel, the two-factor ANOVA without replication is used for solving the problems based on this design. The procedure involved in using Excel for computation in the two-factor ANOVA without replication shall be discussed by means of the following example.

Example 8.6 A study was conducted to know the effect of circuit training programs on standing broad jump performance. The researcher believed that the height is a variable that might affect the performance of athletes during the training program. To control this variable, he decided to use the randomized block design by taking height as a blocking variable. In this design, each block consisted of three athletes, and all the three treatments were randomly allocated in each block. After treatment for 6 weeks, the performance of the athletes on standing broad jump was taken in meters. The data so obtained are shown in Table 8.31. Apply the two-way ANOVA without replication to solve this design and test the significance of the F-value at 5% level for the circuit training program.

Solution: This design shall be solved by the two-way ANOVA with one observation per cell. The following steps shall be used to solve the design in Excel:

TABLE 8.31 Scores of the Subjects on Standing Broad Jump Performance (*m*)

	Circuit Training		
Block	Low Intensity	Medium Intensity	High Intensity
1	1.8	2.5	2.1
2	2.1	2.6	2.7
3	1.9	2.8	2.0
4	1.85	2.75	1.9
5	1.7	2.6	2.25

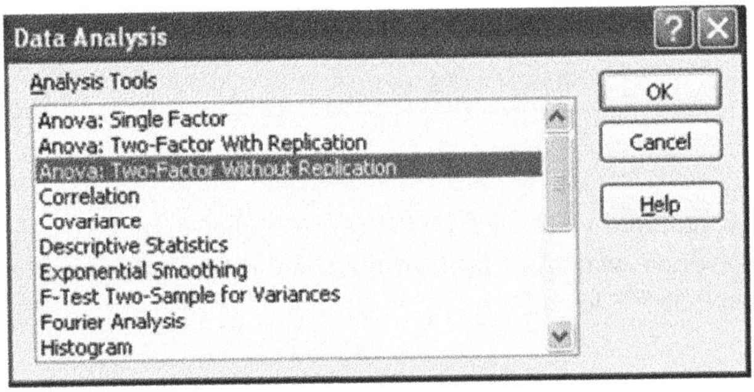

Figure 8.13 Command for applying the two-way ANOVA without replication.

1. Type the data of all the three groups in the three columns A, B, and C of the Excel sheet as shown in Figure 8.14. The headings for the three variables may be written in the first cell of each column. Each column represents the data in different circuit training groups, whereas each row represents a block.
2. To apply the two-way ANOVA without replication, click the following commands in sequence in Excel to get the screen as shown in Figure 8.13:

   Data → Data Analysis

3. Bring the scroll on the option **Anova: Two-Factor Without Replication** and then click **OK** on the screen as shown in Figure 8.13. This will take you to the screen as shown in Figure 8.14. You can now define the range of the data in samples.
4. Readers are advised to look at the format of data entry very carefully. Here, the range of the entire dataset is from A1 to D6. This range includes the names of the variables as well. Do the following steps to fill the entries on the screen shown in Figure 8.14.
   i. **Input Range**: A1:D6
   ii. Check **Labels** (since the headings have been included in the dataset).
   iii. Enter the value of α at which you want to test the hypothesis. In this example, it is taken as 0.05.

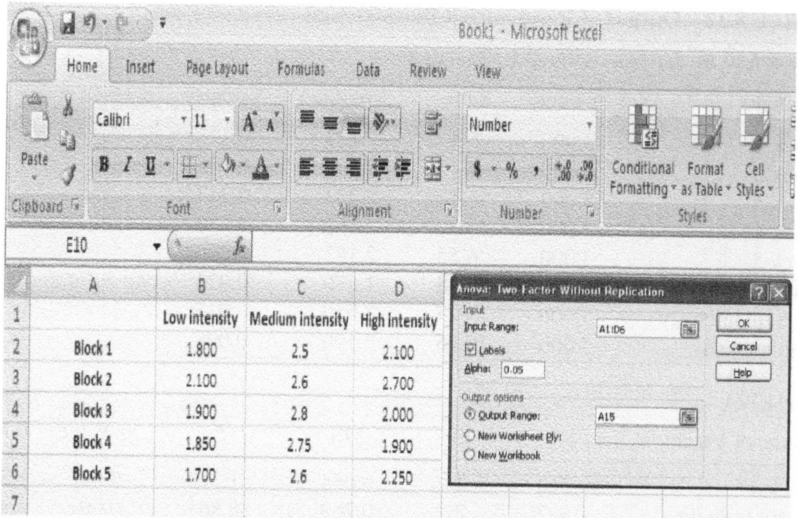

Figure 8.14 Options for applying the two-way ANOVA without replication.

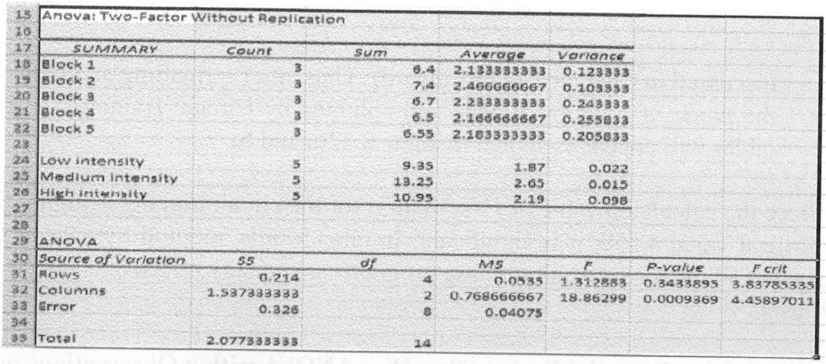

Anova: Two-Factor Without Replication

SUMMARY	Count	Sum	Average	Variance
Block 1	3	6.4	2.133333333	0.123333
Block 2	3	7.4	2.466666667	0.103333
Block 3	3	6.7	2.233333333	0.243333
Block 4	3	6.5	2.166666667	0.255833
Block 5	3	6.55	2.183333333	0.205833
Low intensity	5	9.35	1.87	0.022
Medium intensity	5	13.25	2.65	0.015
High intensity	5	10.95	2.19	0.098

ANOVA

Source of Variation	SS	df	MS	F	P-value	F crit
Rows	0.214	4	0.0535	1.312883	0.3433895	3.83785335
Columns	1.537333333	2	0.768666667	18.86299	0.0009369	4.45897011
Error	0.326	8	0.04075			
Total	2.077333333	14				

Figure 8.15 Output of the two-way ANOVA.

iv. Fill the entry in the output range. The output can be obtained on the same Excel sheet, new worksheet, or new work book. Here the output is obtained on the same sheet starting from A15 location onward and therefore the following entry should be filled.
Output Range: A15

v. Click **OK** to get the output as shown in Figure 8.15.

Remark In the ANOVA table, rows refer to the blocks, whereas columns refer to the treatments (the three different intensities of the circuit training program).

5. The output shown in Figure 8.15 can be formatted by formatting the cell entries of different columns (readers are advised to see the procedure

TABLE 8.32 Output of Randomized Block Design

a. ANOVA: Two-Factor without Replication

Summary	Count	Sum	Average	Variance
Block 1	3.000	6.4	2.133	0.123
Block 2	3.000	7.4	2.467	0.103
Block 3	3.000	6.7	2.233	0.243
Block 4	3.000	6.5	2.167	0.256
Block 5	3.000	6.55	2.183	0.206
Low intensity	5.000	9.35	1.870	0.022
Medium intensity	5.000	13.25	2.650	0.015
High intensity	5.000	10.95	2.190	0.098

b. ANOVA

Source of Variation	SS	df	MS	*F*	*p*-Value	*F* crit
Blocks	0.214	4	0.054	1.313	0.343	3.838
Circuit training	1.537	2	0.769	18.863	0.001	4.459
Error	0.326	8	0.041			
Total	2.077	14				

discussed in Chapter 1 in this regard). Thus, after formatting and replacing the name of rows by Blocks and columns by Circuit Training, the final tables will appear as shown in Table 8.32(a and b)

Since the calculated value of F (=18.863) for the circuit training is higher than the critical value 4.459, it is significant. In other words, the null hypothesis that states that all the three circuit training programs are equally effective is rejected at 5% level.

8.11.2 Solving Factorial Design (Two-Way ANOVA with *n* Observations per Cell)

This design is used when the effect of two factors on the dependent variable is required to be studied. In Excel, the two-factor ANOVA with replication is used for solving the problems based on this design. The procedure involved in using Excel for computation in the two-factor ANOVA with replication shall be discussed by means of the following example.

Example 8.7 Consider a factorial design in which it is desired to investigate the effect of 4 weeks of pranayama and aerobic exercises on the fat percentage of the male college students. Thirty male students were taken as subjects for the study. Three levels of pranayama (anulom–vilom, kapalbhati, and ujjayi) and two levels of aerobic exercise (high intensity and low intensity) were used in the experiment. The data on fat percentage obtained after implementing the treatments are shown in Table 8.33.

TABLE 8.33 Data on Fat Percentage

		Pranayama		
		Anumlom–Vilom	Kapalbhati	Ujjayi
Aerobic exercise	High intensity	16	14	17
		15	12	16
		16	13	14
		17	12	15
		17	14	16
	Low intensity	19	16	18
		16	14	20
		17	15	18
		14	15	13
		13	12	16

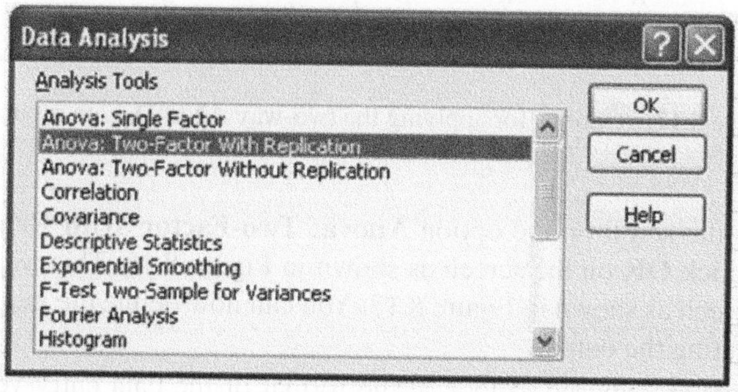

Figure 8.16 Command for applying the two-way ANOVA with replication.

Apply the two-way ANOVA and test the significance of the F-ratios for aerobic exercise, pranayama, and interaction at 5% level.

Solution: This design shall be solved by the two-way ANOVA with replication. The following procedure in Excel shall be used to get the output in this analysis.

1. Type the sample data of all the three groups in the three columns A, B, and C in the Excel sheet. The headings for the three variables may be written in the first cell of each column. Each column represents the data in different pranayama groups. The first five rows represent the data of high intensity aerobic exercise group, while next five rows represent the data of the low intensity aerobic exercise group.
2. To apply the two-way ANOVA, click the following commands in sequence in Excel to get the screen as shown in Figure 8.16:

   Data → Data Analysis

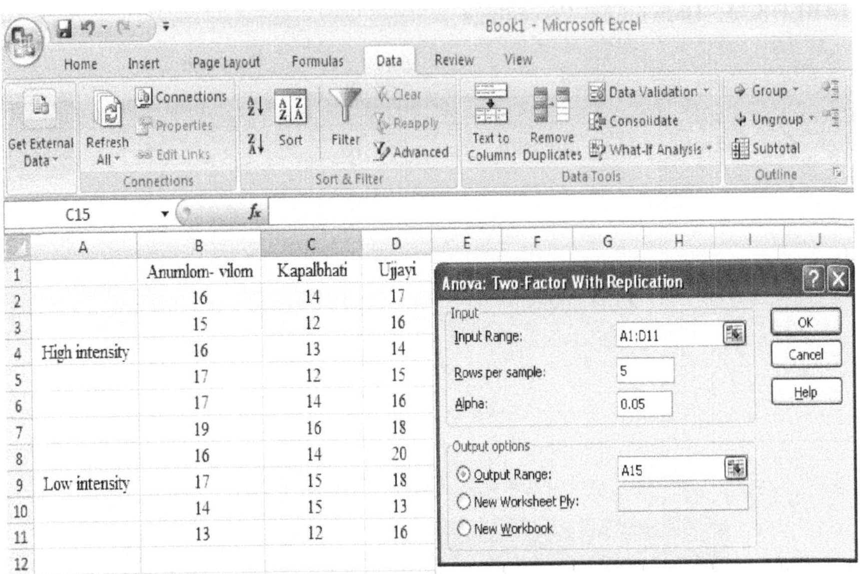

Figure 8.17 Options for applying the two-way ANOVA with replication.

3. Bring the scroll on the option **Anova: Two-Factor With Replication** and then click **OK** on the screen as shown in Figure 8.16. This will take you to the screen as shown in Figure 8.17. You can now define the range of data for generating the output.
4. Readers are advised to look at the format of the data entry very carefully. Here, the range of the entire dataset is from A1 to D11. This range includes the name of the variables as well. Do the following steps to fill the entries on the screen as shown in Figure 8.17.
   i. **Input Range**: A1:D11
   ii. **Rows per sample**: 5 (This indicates the number of row data in each of the column treatments.)
   iii. Enter the value of α at which you want to test the hypothesis. In this example, it is taken as 0.05.
   iv. Fill the entry in the output range. The output can be obtained on the same Excel sheet, new worksheet, or new workbook. Here, the output is obtained on the same sheet starting from the location A15 onward and, therefore, the following entry should be filled.
   Output Range: A15
   v. Click **OK** to get the output as shown in Figure 8.18.

Remark In the ANOVA table, sample refers to the row treatment (the two intensities of the aerobic exercises), whereas column refers to the column

	A	B	C	D	E	F	G
15	**Anova: Two-Factor With Replication**						
16							
17	SUMMARY	Anumlom- vilom	Kapalbhati	Ujjayi	Total		
18	*High intensity*						
19	Count	5	5	5	15		
20	Sum	81	65	78	224		
21	Average	16.2	13	15.6	14.933333		
22	Variance	0.7	1	1.3	2.9238095		
23							
24	*Low intensity*						
25	Count	5	5	5	15		
26	Sum	79	72	85	236		
27	Average	15.8	14.4	17	15.733333		
28	Variance	5.7	2.3	7	5.4952381		
29							
30	*Total*						
31	Count	10	10	10			
32	Sum	160	137	163			
33	Average	16	13.7	16.3			
34	Variance	2.888888889	2.011111111	4.2333333			
35							
36	ANOVA						
37	*Source of Variation*	*SS*	*df*	*MS*	*F*	*P-value*	*F crit*
38	Sample	4.8	1	4.8	1.6	0.218048	4.2596772
39	Columns	40.46666667	2	20.233333	6.7444444	0.0047392	3.4028261
40	Interaction	5.4	2	2.7	0.9	0.4198541	3.4028261
41	Within	72	24	3			
42							
43	Total	122.6666667	29				

Figure 8.18 Output of the two-way ANOVA with replication.

TABLE 8.34 Output of Factorial Design

a. Summary of Means

		Pranayama			
		Anumlom–Vilom	Kapalbhati	Ujjayi	Total
Aerobic exercise	High intensity	16.2	13	15.6	14.93
	Low intensity	15.8	14.4	17	15.73
	Total	16	13.7	16.3	

b. ANOVA: Two-Factor with Replication

Source of Variation	SS	df	MS	*F*	*p*-Value	*F* crit
Aerobic exercise	4.800	1	4.800	1.600	0.218	4.260
Pranayama	40.467	2	20.233	6.744	0.005	3.403
Interaction	5.400	2	2.700	0.900	0.420	3.403
Within	72.000	24	3.000			
Total	122.667	29				

treatments (the three types of pranayama, that is, Anulom–Vilom, Kapalbhati, and Ujjayi).

5. The output shown in Figure 8.18 can be formatted by formatting the cell entries of different columns (readers are advised to see the procedure

discussed in Chapter 1 in this regard). Further, a summary table for different means may be created by taking the entries from Figure 8.18. The two final tables as shown in Table 8.34(a and b) have been generated from this output.

Since the calculated value of F (=6.744) for the pranayama is higher than the critical value 3.403, it is significant. The other two F-ratios for aerobic exercise and interaction are not significant. It may, therefore, be concluded that the null hypothesis of all the three pranayama to be equally effective in reducing the fat percentage is rejected at 5% level.

IMPORTANT DEFINITIONS

Analysis of variance is a group of statistical techniques for comparing the group means by comparing the "between-group" variance with that of "within-group" variance.

Variation refers to the spread of scores in the dataset.

Variance is an index for measuring variation in the dataset.

The ***sum of squares*** is the sum of squared deviations of scores from their mean.

The ***mean sum of squares*** can be defined as an average of the sum of squares and is equal to the variance.

Design of experiment is a blueprint for organizing a research experiment for testing a hypothesis by facilitating the researcher in manipulating independent variables, controlling the extraneous variables, and reducing the error variance.

One-way analysis of variance is a statistical technique in which the effect of one factor on the criterion variable is investigated.

Post hoc tests are statistical tests used for comparing pairs of group means in the analysis of variance if the F-ratio is significant.

The ***completely randomized design*** is a statistical design for testing the hypothesis of equality of more than two group means when the experimental subjects are homogeneous in nature.

Two-way analysis of variance is a group of statistical techniques in which the effect of two factors on the criterion variable is studied simultaneously along with the interaction.

Factors are the independent variables whose effects on the dependent variable are investigated in the analysis of variance experiment.

Treatment conditions can be defined as the levels of the independent factor or combination of levels of the independent factors whose effects on the dependent variable are investigated.

The ***main effect*** is the effect of one independent variable (factor A) on the dependent variable across all the levels of the second independent variable (factor B).

The ***interaction effect*** can be defined as the joint effect of the two factors on the dependent variable.
The ***simple effect*** is the effect of one independent variable in each level of the other factor.
The ***randomized block design*** is a statistical design for testing the hypothesis of equality of more than two group means by using the blocking variable to reduce the error variance in the experiment.
The ***factorial design*** is a statistical design in which the main and simple effects are investigated simultaneously by using the two-way analysis of variance.
Analysis of covariance is a statistical design to compare the effect of different levels of an independent variable on the dependent variable by controlling the covariate that affects the dependent variable in the experiment.

IMPORTANT FORMULAS

Sample variance

$$S^2 = \frac{1}{n-1}\sum (x-\bar{x})^2$$

Sum of squares and mean sum of squares

$$S^2 = \frac{\text{SS}}{\text{df}} = \frac{\text{Variation}}{\text{df}} = \text{MSS}$$

Distribution of variation in the one-way ANOVA design

$$\text{TSS} = \text{SS}_\text{b} + \text{SS}_\text{w}$$

Formulas in the one-way ANOVA

$$\text{TSS} = \sum_{i=1}^{r}\sum_{j=1}^{n_i}\left(Y_{ij} - \frac{G}{N}\right)^2 = \sum_i\sum_j Y_{ij}^2 - \frac{G^2}{N}$$

Sum of squares between groups

$$\text{SS}_\text{b} = \sum_i^r \frac{R_i^2}{n_i} - \frac{G^2}{N}$$

Sum of squares within groups

$$\text{SS}_\text{w} = \text{TSS} - (\text{SS})_\text{b}$$

Mean sum of squares between groups

$$\text{MSS}_\text{b} = \frac{\text{SS}_\text{b}}{r-1}$$

Mean sum of squares within groups

$$\text{MSS}_\text{w} = \frac{\text{SS}_\text{w}}{n-r}$$

CD in the LSD test

$$\text{CD} = t_{0.05}(N-r) \times \sqrt{\frac{2}{n} \times \text{MSS}_\text{w}}$$

CD in the Tukey HSD test

$$\text{CD} = q_{\alpha,r,N-r}\sqrt{\frac{\text{MSS}_\text{w}}{n}}$$

CD in Scheffe's test
For i–j group means

$$\sqrt{(r-1)F_{0.05}(r-1, N-r)} \times \sqrt{\text{MSS}_\text{w}\left(\frac{1}{n_i} + \frac{1}{n_j}\right)}$$

Distribution of variation in the two-way ANOVA design (n scores per cell)

$$\text{TSS} = \text{SSR} + \text{SSC} + \text{SSI} + \text{SSE}$$

Formulas in the two-way ANOVA (n scores per cell)
Total sum of squares

$$\text{TSS} = \sum_{i=1}^{r}\sum_{j=1}^{c}\sum_{k=1}^{n}\left(X_{ijk} - \frac{G}{N}\right)^2$$

$$= \sum_{i}\sum_{j}\sum_{k} X_{ijk}^2 - \frac{G^2}{N}$$

Sum of squares due to the row factor

$$\text{SSR} = \sum_{i=1}^{r}\frac{R_i^2}{nc} - \frac{G^2}{N}$$

Sum of squares due to the column factor

$$\text{SSC} = \sum_{j=1}^{c} \frac{C_j^2}{nr} - \frac{G^2}{N}$$

Sum of squares due to interaction

$$\text{SSI} = \sum_{i=1}^{r} \sum_{j=1}^{c} \frac{T_{ij}^2}{n} - \frac{G^2}{N} - \text{SSR} - \text{SSC}$$

Sum of squares due to error

$$\text{SSE} = \text{TSS} - \text{SSR} - \text{SSC} - \text{SSI}$$

Mean sum of squares rows

$$\text{MSS}_\text{R} = \frac{\text{SSR}}{r-1}$$

Mean sum of squares columns

$$\text{MSS}_\text{C} = \frac{\text{SSC}}{c-1}$$

Mean sum of squares interaction

$$\text{MSS}_\text{I} = \frac{\text{SSI}}{(r-1) \times (c-1)}$$

For comparing row means

$$\text{CD by the Tukey HSD } q_{\alpha,r,N-rc}\sqrt{\frac{\text{MSS}_\text{E}}{nc}}$$

For comparing column means

$$\text{CD by the Tukey HSD } q_{\alpha,c,N-rc}\sqrt{\frac{\text{MSS}_\text{E}}{nr}}$$

For comparing simple effect

$$\text{CD} = q_{\alpha,r,N-rc}\sqrt{\frac{\text{MSS}_\text{E}}{n}}$$

Distribution of variation in the two-way ANOVA design (with one score per cell)

$$\text{TSS} = \text{SSR} + \text{SSC} + \text{SSE}$$

Formulas in the two-way ANOVA (one score per cell)
TSS

$$\text{TSS} = \sum_{i=1}^{r}\sum_{j=1}^{c}\left(Y_{ij} - \frac{G}{N}\right)^2 = \sum_i\sum_j Y_{ij}^2 - \frac{G^2}{N}$$

Sum of squares due to rows (blocks)

$$\text{SSR (Blocks)} = \sum_i^r \frac{R_i^2}{c} - \frac{G^2}{N}$$

Sum of squares of columns (treatments)

$$\text{SSC (Treatments)} = \sum_{j=1}^{c} \frac{C_j^2}{r} - \frac{G^2}{N}$$

Sum of squares of error

$$\text{SSE} = \text{TSS} - \text{SSR} - \text{SSC}$$

Mean sum of squares of rows (blocks)

$$\text{MSS}_\text{R} = \frac{\text{SSR}}{r-1}$$

Mean sum of squares of columns (treatments)

$$\text{MSS}_\text{C} = \frac{\text{SSC}}{c-1}$$

For comparing treatment groups

$$\text{CD by the Tukey HSD} = q_{\alpha,r,(r-1)\times(c-1)}\sqrt{\frac{\text{MSS}_\text{E}}{r}}$$

Formulas in analysis of covariance
Correction factors

$$C_x = \frac{\left(\sum x\right)^2}{N}$$

$$C_y = \frac{(\sum y)^2}{N}$$

$$C_{xy} = \frac{\sum x \sum y}{N}$$

where

$$\sum X = \sum X_1 + \sum X_2 + \ldots + \sum X_r$$

$$\sum Y = \sum Y_1 + \sum Y_2 + \ldots + \sum Y_r$$

$$\sum XY = \sum X_1 Y_1 + \sum X_2 Y_2 + \ldots + \sum X_r Y_r$$

Total sum of squares

$$\text{TSS}_x = \sum x^2 - C_x$$

$$\text{TSS}_y = \sum y^2 - C_y$$

$$\text{TSS}_{xy} = \sum xy^2 - C_{xy}$$

where

$$\sum X^2 = \sum X^2{}_1 + \sum X^2{}_2 + \ldots + \sum X^2{}_r$$

$$\sum Y^2 = \sum Y^2{}_1 + \sum Y^2{}_2 + \ldots + \sum Y^2{}_r$$

$$\sum XY = \sum X_1 Y_1 + \sum X_2 Y_2 + \ldots + \sum X_r Y_r$$

Sum of squares of treatment groups

$$\text{SST}_x = \frac{(\sum x_1)^2 + (\sum x_2)^2 + \ldots + (\sum x_r)^2}{n} - C_x$$

$$\text{SST}_y = \frac{(\sum y_1)^2 + (\sum y_2)^2 + \ldots + (\sum y_r)^2}{n} - C_y$$

$$\text{SST}_{xy} = \frac{\sum x_1 \sum y_1 + \sum x_2 \sum y_2 + \ldots + \sum x_r \sum y_r}{n} - C_{xy}$$

Sum of squares due to error

$$\text{SSE}_x = \text{TSS}_x - \text{SST}_x$$
$$\text{SSE}_y = \text{TSS}_y - \text{SST}_y$$
$$\text{SSE}_{xy} = \text{TSS}_{xy} - \text{SST}_{xy}$$

Adjusted sum of squares for Y

$$\text{TSS}_{y.x} = \text{TSS}_y - \frac{\text{TSS}_{xy}^2}{\text{TSS}_x}$$
$$\text{SSE}_{y.x} = \text{SSE}_y - \frac{\text{SSE}_{xy}^2}{\text{SSE}_x}$$
$$\text{SST}_{y.x} = \text{TSS}_{y.x} - \text{SSE}_{y.x}$$

Computation of correlation and regression coefficients

$$r_{\text{total}} = \frac{\text{TSS}_{xy}}{\sqrt{\text{TSS}_x \times \text{TSS}_y}}$$
$$r_{\text{between\_means}} = \frac{\text{SST}_{xy}}{\sqrt{\text{SST}_x \times \text{SST}_y}}$$
$$r_{\text{within}} = \frac{\text{SSE}}{\sqrt{\text{SSE}_x \times \text{SSE}_y}}$$
$$b_{\text{total}} = \frac{\text{TSS}_{xy}}{\text{TSS}_x}$$
$$b_{\text{between\_means}} = \frac{\text{SST}_{xy}}{\text{SST}_x}$$
$$b_{\text{within}} = \frac{\text{SSE}_{xy}}{\text{SSE}_x}$$

Calculation of adjusted post-group means

$$M_{y.x} = M_y - b_{\text{within}}(M_x - GM_x)$$
$$\text{GM}_x = \frac{\bar{x}_1 + \bar{x}_2 + \ldots.. + \bar{x}_r}{n}$$
$$M_{y_1.x_1} = \overline{Y}_1 - b_{\text{within}}(\overline{X}_1 - \text{GM}_x)$$

For comparing treatment groups

$$\text{CD in the LSD test} = t_{\alpha}(N - r - 1)\sqrt{\frac{2 \times \text{MSSE}_{y.x}}{n}}$$

KEY TERMS

analysis of covariance	design of experiment	post hoc tests
ANOVA	factorial design	randomized block design
completely randomized design	interaction effect	simple effect
	main effect	

CHAPTER EXERCISE

1. What are the important considerations an exercise scientist must keep in mind while designing an experiment?
2. What is meant by analysis of variance? What we do in it?
3. Write a short note on each of the following:
   i. Scheffe's test
   ii. The LSD test
   iii. The Tukey HSD test
4. What are the assumptions of the one-way ANOVA?
5. What happens if multiple t-tests are used instead of the one-way ANOVA?
6. Write a short note on each of the following:
   i. Completely randomized design
   ii. Randomized block design
   iii. Factorial design
7. Discuss how the degrees of freedom are distributed in CRD, RBD, and factorial designs.
8. Why is the randomized block design more efficient than the completely randomized design?
9. Discuss the advantages of the two-way ANOVA over the one-way ANOVA.
10. On the following data, apply the one-way analysis of variance.

X	23	21	24	26	24	21	20
Y	31	28	29	30	35	36	34
Z	32	34	37	36	33	37	32

Find the calculated F and compare it to the critical value of F to test the null hypothesis of no difference. Test your hypothesis at significance level 0.01.

11. Consider a situation in which a completely randomized design is used to study the effect of a weight training program on the physical fitness index. There are four treatment levels (four different intensities of the weight training program) and a total of 48 subjects in the study. Complete the following ANOVA table. Test the significance of the F-value at 5% level.

Source of Variation	SS	df	MS	F
Treatment	798.12	?	?	?
Error	?	?	?	
Total	1893.56			

12. A researcher wanted to develop criteria for talent identification in different sports. In order to find the effectiveness of height in different sports, the heights of the national level sportsmen in three different sports, namely, volleyball, swimming, and gymnastics were recorded. The data so obtained are as follows. Apply the one-way ANOVA to test the null hypothesis that the average height of the sportsmen in all the three sports is the same. Test your hypothesis at 5% level.

Height in Feet of Different Sportsmen

Volleyball	Swimming	Gymnastics
6.3	5.9	5.6
6.2	6.1	5.5
6.4	5.9	5.4
6.3	5.9	5.8
6.3	6.1	5.7
6.3	5.8	5.6
6.4	5.7	5.4
6.4	5.9	5.6
6.3	6	5.3
6.4	6.2	5.4
6.3	5.9	5.8
6.3	5.9	5.5

13. Following are the data on hemoglobin contents measured on the athletes in three different sports groups. Apply the one-way ANOVA and explain your findings at the significance level 0.05.

Data on Hemoglobin Content (in %)

Hockey	Volleyball	Football
14	14	14
15	12	13.5
13.5	14	13
15	12	14
14.5	13	14.5
13	12	14
14.5	12.5	15
14	12.5	13
14	12	
15.5		

14. A wrestling coach was interested in improving the shoulder strength of his athletes. He was interested in choosing the best out of three programs suggested to him. The data shown in the table represent the shoulder strength in the three treatment groups. Can it be concluded from the data on shoulder strength given in the following table that any one program is more effective than others? Test your hypothesis at the significance level 0.05.

Data on Shoulder Strength

Training Programs		
A	B	C
8	10	15
10	8	11
7	7	9
6	8	8
5	9	14
4	6	13
9	7	12
6	9	16
7	11	12
8	8	10

15. Following are data on the sit-ups performance obtained on the students of three schools. Apply one-way analysis of variance to find the school whose students' performance is better on sit-ups. Test your hypothesis at 5% level.

Data on Sit-Ups Performance

School		
A	B	C
12	16	9
10	12	12
11	14	8
9	15	11
8	9	9
12	11	8
11	10	10
7	13	
8		
13		

16. A basketball coach wanted to find out which training schedule out of circuit training, weight training, and a combination of circuit and weight training would be beneficial in improving the performance in front-shot. A completely randomized design was planned in which 40 college basketball players were randomly assigned four levels of the treatment schedule (circuit training, weight training, combination of circuit and weight training, and control). After they had undergone the treatment for 4 weeks, the subjects were tested for their performance on front-shot. The scores so obtained are shown below. Analyze this design and discuss your findings at the significance level 0.05.

Scores on Front-Shot

Training Schedule			
Circuit Training	Weight Training	Circuit × Weight Training	Control
20	10	17	3
12	15	18	4
8	20	12	10
12	7	23	8
17	8	20	3
20	10	18	12
8	12	16	13
10	18	21	5
10	14	21	14
12	9	12	3

17. To see the impact of warming-up duration on the performance of 100 m sprints, a completely randomized design was organized. Thirty college students were randomly assigned to three levels of treatments (15, 20, and

25 min warm-up programs). After the treatment, their performance on the 100 m sprint was recorded in terms of timings in seconds which is shown below.

Performance on 100 m (s)

Warming-Up Duration		
15 min	20 min	25 min
11.9	11.5	11.5
11.7	11.6	11.7
11.9	11.7	11.7
11.7	11.4	11.4
141.8	11.6	11.5
12.9	11.9	11.9
12.2	12	12
12.5	12	12
12.6	12.4	12.4
12.6	12.1	12.1

Apply one-way analysis of variance and test your hypothesis at 1% level. Comment on the suitability of the warming-up program in getting optimum performance on the 100 m sprint.

18. To know the effect of meditation on concentration, a complete randomized design was planned. Twenty-seven subjects were randomly chosen and three treatments of meditation (10, 15, and 20 min duration) were randomly assigned to these subjects in such a manner that each treatment was received by an equal number of subjects. The concentration score of the subjects was measured after 3 weeks of treatment and the scores so obtained are shown below.

Concentration Score After Meditation

10 min	15 min	20 min
21	31	32
18	28	25
19	30	33
21	27	28
28	25	30
26	32	30
25	30	35
20	28	27
18	26	28

Apply the one-way ANOVA to test the null hypothesis that all the three treatments are equally effective. Test your hypothesis at 5% level and if the null hypothesis is rejected, conclude which treatment is more effective.

19. Graduate and research degree programs are considered to be more academic than the undergraduate program. In order to compare the fat percentage of the male subjects in these courses, three random samples of male students from these courses, namely, research program, graduate, and undergraduate programs were randomly selected. These subjects were tested for their fat percentage, which is shown below.

Scores on Fat Percentage

Research Program	Graduate Program	Undergraduate Program
15	18	22
16	20	24
14	21	20
15	25	23
14	22	25
16	21	24
15	24	28
16	27	24
12	20	19
14	21	23

Apply the one-way ANOVA to test the null hypothesis that the fat percentage of the students in all the three categories is equal. Test your hypothesis at 5% level and if the *F*-ratio is significant, apply post hoc tests to discuss your findings.

20. Apply analysis of variance to analyze the following data obtained in a randomized block design. State the null and alternative hypotheses and test whether the null hypothesis can be rejected at the significance level 0.05.

		Treatment			
		1	2	3	4
Block	1	5	2	6	4
	2	6	3	7	5
	3	5	4	8	3
	4	4	1	5	4
	5	7	2	7	6
	6	6	3	9	5

21. A randomized block design has a treatment variable with three levels and a blocking variable with six blocks. Complete the following table. Test the null hypothesis at 1% level. Can it be concluded that the blocking has reduced the error variance significantly?

Source of Variance	SS	df	MS	F
Treatment	325.18	?	?	?
Blocks	369.36	?	?	?
Error	?	?	?	
Total	1188.49			

22. A survey was conducted to know whether the attitude of people differs toward sports in three different types of cities. The people were randomly selected from A1, B1, and B2 cities. A 25-point scale was developed to measure the attitude of the persons toward sports. On this scale, scoring 25 means that the attitude of the person toward sports is extremely positive and 1 indicates no attitude toward the sports at all. To control for differences in socioeconomic status, a blocking variable was taken using five different socioeconomic categories. The data are shown in the form of a randomized block design. At 5% level, test whether there is a significant difference in the mean responses of the attitude toward sports in the three types of cities.

Attitude Scores Toward Sports in Three Different Types of Cities

	Types of Cities		
Socioeconomic Status	A1	B1	B2
Upper	22	21	18
Upper middle	20	22	20
Middle	18	23	16
Lower middle	16	12	18
Lower	15	17	12

23. In a 3 × 2 factorial experiment with five observations per cell, the following incomplete two-way ANOVA table is obtained. With the existing information, complete the other entries in the table. Test the significance of different effects at 5% level.

Source of Variance	SS	df	MS	F
Row	502.45	?	?	?
Column	?	?	?	?
Interaction	403.34	?	?	?
Error	3523.12	?	?	
Total	6229.19			

24. In a two-way factorial design, the following data on lifestyle have been obtained. Use the two-way ANOVA to analyze the data at $\alpha = 0.05$. Discuss your findings by testing the significance of the F-ratio for both the treatments.

		Treatment 1		
		Delhi	Mumbai	Goa
	Male	56	45	74
		59	51	68
		62	58	72
Treatment 2				
	Female	65	56	62
		71	61	58
		68	58	62

25. In a 3 × 3 factorial design, the following data on shooting accuracy in basketball were obtained on 27 basketball players using three different distances and three different angles. Apply the two-way ANOVA to analyze the data and explain your findings at 5% significance level.

		Distance		
		5 ft.	10 ft.	15 ft.
Angle	45°	1	2	2
		4	6	4
		2	5	3
	90°	2	3	1
		2	5	6
		6	3	8
	180°	2	5	6
		6	2	4
		5	3	2

26. It is believed that the attitude toward fitness activity is affected by the gender of the person as well as their socioeconomic status. To test this belief, a study was planned to investigate the attitude of people toward fitness activity. The following data on attitude toward fitness activity of males and females in

different socioeconomic status were obtained. Apply the two-way ANOVA to test the main effects. Test the simple effects also if the interaction is significant. Test your hypothesis at 5% level.

Scores on Attitude Toward Fitness Activity

		Socioeconomic Status		
		Upper	Middle	Lower
Gender	Male	20	18	16
		22	16	18
		21	15	16
		20	15	16
		19	16	14
	Female	18	22	16
		16	20	15
		15	19	14
		18	21	16
		21	22	15

27. To study the effect of stance and knee angles on block jump performance, a 3×3 factorial experiment was planned. The study included three levels of the first treatment, stance (basic, wide, and narrow), and three levels of the second treatment, knee angles (90°, 115°, and 130°). Each combination of treatments was randomly allocated to the subjects. The performance of these subjects was measured on block jump under these treatment conditions. The data so obtained are shown below.

Data on Block Jump under Different Treatments

		Knee Angles		
		90°	115°	130°
		46	49	44
		44	42	40
	Basic	45	44	41
		56	49	50
		37	45	35
		47	46	45
		43	44	42
Stance	Wide	42	40	36
		53	53	52
		41	37	37
	Stance	47	47	43
		40	38	32
	Narrow	40	39	34
		55	56	52
		39	39	36

Apply the two-way ANOVA and explain your findings at $\alpha = 0.05$.

28. In an ANCOVA experiment, the pre- and post-scores on RBC count (measured in millions/μL of blood) obtained on athletes under four treatment conditions A, B, C, and D are shown in the following table. The four treatment conditions were the four different types of nutrition: A, low calorie nonvegetarian diet; B, high calorie nonvegetarian diet; C, low calorie vegetarian diet; and D, high calorie vegetarian diet.

Data on RBC Count (in Millions/μL of Blood in Four Treatment Conditions

	Treatment A		Treatment B		Treatment C		Treatment D	
S.N.	Pre	Post	Pre	Post	Pre	Post	Pre	Post
1	5.3	5.9	3.2	4.5	4.1	4.2	4.4	4.1
2	3.8	3.9	3.8	4.0	4.8	4.8	4.0	4.0
3	4.6	4.8	4.8	4.8	3.5	4.6	3.6	4.0
4	4.8	4.9	4.0	4.1	4.5	4.7	4.0	4.1
5	4.2	4.8	4.2	4.2	3.7	4.5	4.2	4.4
6	3.8	4.6	4.1	4.4	4.0	4.5	4.4	4.3
7	4.1	4.6	3.7	4.1	4.4	4.6	3.8	4.5
8	4.2	4.5	4.3	4.3	3.8	4.1	4.2	4.0
9	4.1	4.4	4.2	4.5	4.5	4.7	4.0	4.0
10	4.0	4.9	4.4	4.8	3.7	4.2	4.3	4.0

Apply the analysis of covariance on these data to test whether any one treatment is more effective than others in enhancing the RBC count. Test your hypothesis at $\alpha = 0.05$ and discuss the findings.

ANSWERS

Check Your Progress

1. T	10. F	19. T	28. F	37. F	46. F
2. T	11. T	20. F	29. T	38. F	47. T
3. F	12. F	21. F	30. F	39. T	48. T
4. F	13. F	22. F	31. T	40. F	49. F
5. T	14. T	23. F	32. F	41. F	50. T
6. T	15. T	24. T	33. T	42. T	51. F
7. F	16. T	25. T	34. F	43. T	52. T
8. T	17. F	26. F	35. T	44. F	53. T
9. T	18. F	27. T	36. T	45. T	54. F

Practice Exercise

1.

Source of Variance	SS	df	MS	F
Treatment	64.34	2	32.17	5.14
Error	175.21	28	6.26	
Total	239.55	30		

2. $t = 3.8$, $F = 14.4$, H_0 rejected.
3. $F = 4.568$, H_0 is significant.
   The double fault of player B is significantly less than that of player C. However, there is no significant difference between the double faults of the players B and A.
4. The null hypothesis is rejected.

Source of Variance	SS	df	MS	F
Treatment	652.53	4	163.13	8.06
Blocks	212.27	4	53.07	
Error	323.69	16	20.23	
Total	1188.49	24		

5. F for age = 27.75.
   a. Push-up performance of the girls in all the age categories was not same.
   b. The push-up performance of an age category of 18 years was the best.
   c. However, there was no difference between the push-up performance of age categories of 16 and 17 years.
   d. Since the F-value for the blocking was not significant, the blocking was not useful.
6. This is a 4 × 3 factorial design
   a. Number of independent variables = 2
   b. Number of dependent variables = 1
   c. Treatment 1 has 3 levels and Treatment 2 has 4 levels
   d. Yes, the interaction can be computed because there are 2 scores (more than 1) in each cell.

Source of Variation	df
Row	3
Column	2
Interaction (row×column)	6
Error	12
Total	23

7. Since F for rows is higher and as $F_{0.05}$ (4, 80) = 2.49, the row effect is significant. However, column and interaction effects are not significant.

Source of Variance	SS	df	MS	F
Row	65.35	4	16.34	3.28
Column	21.23	5	4.25	0.85
Interaction	194.56	20	9.73	1.95
Error	398.78	80	4.98	
Total	679.92	109		

Chapter Exercise

10. $F = 41.17$, reject the null hypothesis.

11.

Source of Variation	SS	df	MS	F
Treatment	798.12	3	266.04	10.69
Error	1095.44	44	24.896	
Total	1893.56	47		

$F = 10.69$, the null hypothesis is rejected.

12. $F = 109.78$, the null hypothesis is rejected. Volleyball players are taller and gymnasts are the shortest.
13. $F = 11.439$, the null hypothesis is rejected. H_b of hockey and soccer groups is the same and significantly higher than that of the volleyball group.
14. $F = 16.50$, the null hypothesis is rejected. Training C is the best and A and B are equally good but inferior to C.
15. $F = 4.56$, the null hypothesis is rejected. Training program C is the best.
16. $F = 9.72$, the null hypothesis is rejected. Circuit × weight training program is the best.
17. $F = 1.063$, the null hypothesis is not rejected.
18. $F = 17.341$, the null hypothesis is rejected. 15 and 20 min durations are equally effective and better than 10 min duration.
19. $F = 41.436$, the null hypothesis is rejected. Back strength of undergraduate and PG students are equal and better than that of Ph.D. students.
20. F for block = 3.56, F-value for treatment = 26.5
    The null hypothesis is rejected for treatment as well as block. Treatment 3 is the best.

21.

Source of Variance	SS	df	MS	F
Treatment	325.18	2	162.59	3.29
Blocks	369.36	5	73.872	1.496
Error	493.95	10	49.395	
Total	1188.49	17		

The F-values for treatment and block are insignificant. Blocking has not reduced error variance significantly.

22. F for cities = 0.88, F for block = 3.39. Both F-ratios are insignificant and the null hypothesis for city as well as for block cannot be rejected.

23.

Source of Variance	SS	df	MS	F
Row	502.45	2	251.23	1.71
Column	1800.28	1	1800.28	12.26
Interaction	403.34	2	201.67	1.37
Error	3523.12	24	146.797	
Total	6229.19	29		

Only the F-value for column is significant.

24. F for gender = 1.04, F for city = 15.2, F for interaction = 12.96. F-ratios for city and interaction are significant.
25. F for angle = 0.38, F for distance = 0.25, F for interaction = 0.61.
26. F for gender = 0.576, F for socioeconomic status = 15.81, F for interaction = 18.62.
27. F for stance = 0.39, F for knee angle = 1.54, F for interaction =0.076.
28. F for treatment = 5.97, the null hypothesis is rejected.

FURTHER READING

1. Addelman S. The generalized randomized block design. The American Statistician 1969;23(4):35–36. DOI: 10.2307/2681737JSTOR 2681737.
2. Addelman S. Variability of treatments and experimental units in the design and analysis of experiments. Journal of the American Statistical Association 1970;65(331):1095–1108. DOI: 10.2307/2284277JSTOR 2284277.
3. Aickin M, Gensler H. Adjusting for multiple testing when reporting research results: the Bonferroni vs Holm methods. The American Journal of Public Health 1996;86:726–728.

4. Ajit CT. Multiple comparisons in model I one-way ANOVA with unequal variances. Communications in Statistics - Theory and Methods 1977;6 Nr. 1:15–32. DOI: 10.1080/03610927708827466.
5. Anscombe FJ. The validity of comparative experiments. Journal of the Royal Statistical Society. Series A (General) 1948;111(3):181–211. DOI: 10.2307/2984159JSTOR 2984159. MR 30181.
6. van Belle G. Statistical Rules of Thumb. 2nd ed. Hoboken, N.J: John Wiley & Sons, Inc.; 2008. ISBN 9780470144480.
7. Box GE, Hunter WG, Hunter JS. Statistics for Experimenters: Design, Innovation, and Discovery. 2nd ed. Wiley; 2005. ISBN 0-471-71813-0.
8. Broota KD. Experimental Design in Behavioural Research. New Delhi: New Age International; 2006.
9. Caliński T, Kageyama S. Block designs: A Randomization approach, Volume I: Analysis. Lecture Notes in Statistics. 150. New York: Springer-Verlag; 2000. ISBN 0-387-98578-6.
10. Coakes SJ, Steed LG. SPSS : Analysis Without Anguish: Versions 7.0, 7.5, 8.0 for Windows. Brisbane, Australia: Jacaranda Wiley; 1999.
11. Cochran WG, Cox GM. Experimental Designs. 2nd ed. New York: John Wiley & Sons, Inc.; 1992. ISBN 9780471545675.
12. Cohen J. Statistical Power Analysis for the Behavior Sciences. 2nd ed. USA: Lawrence Erlbaum Associates, Incorporated ; 1988. ISBN 978-0-8058-0283-2.
13. Cox DR. Principles of Statistical Inference. Cambridge New York: Cambridge University Press; 2006. ISBN 9780521685672.
14. Dudoit S, van der Laan MJ. Multiple Testing Procedures with Application to Genomics. Springer; 2008.
15. Engqvist L. The mistreatment of covariate interaction terms in linear model analyses of behavioural and evolutionary ecology studies. Animal Behaviour 2005;70:967–971.
16. Betz F. Multiple Comparisons Using R. USA: Taylor & Francis; 2009. ISBN: 978-1-58488-574-0
17. Freedman D. Statistical Models: Theory and Practice. UK: Cambridge University Press; 2005. ISBN 978-0-521-67105-7.
18. Gates CE. What really is experimental error in block designs? The American Statistician 1995;49(4):362–363. DOI: 10.2307/2684574JSTOR 2684574.
19. Gelman A. Analysis of variance? Why it is more important than ever. The Annals of Statistics 2005;33:1–53. DOI: 10.1214/009053604000001048.
20. Gelman A. Variance, Analysis of The New Palgrave Dictionary of Economics. 2nd ed. Basingstoke, Hampshire New York: Palgrave Macmillan; 2008. ISBN 9780333786765.
21. Hayter AJ. The maximum familywise error rate of fisher's least significant difference test. Journal of the American Statistical Association 1986;81(396):1000–1004. DOI: 10.2307/2289074. edit.
22. Hinkelmann K. Design and Analysis of Experiments Set. I and II. 2nd ed. USA: Wiley; 2008. ISBN 978-0-470-38551-7.

23. Howell DC. Statistical Methods for Psychology. 7th ed. Belmont: Cengage Wadsworth; 2009.
24. Howell DC. Statistical Methods for Psychology. 5th ed. Pacific Grove, CA: Duxbury/Thomson Learning; 2002. ISBN 053437770X.
25. Jaccard J, Becker MA, Wood G. Pairwise multiple comparison procedures: a review. Psychological Bulletin 1984;96(3):589. DOI: 10.1037/0033-2909.96.3.589. edit.
26. Keppel G. Design and Analysis: A Researcher's Handbook. 3rd ed. Englewood Cliffs: Prentice-Hall, Inc.; 1991.
27. Keuls M. The use of the "studentized range" in connection with an analysis of variance. Euphytica 1952;1:112–122.
28. Kirk RE. Experimental Design: Procedures For The Behavioral Sciences. 3rd ed. Pacific Grove, CA, USA: Brooks/Cole; 1995.
29. Klockars AJ, Hancock GR. Scheffé's more powerful F-protected post hoc procedure. Journal of Educational and Behavioral Statistics 2000;25(1):13–19. DOI: 10.2307/1165310. edit.
30. Lehmann EL. Testing Statistical Hypotheses. John Wiley & Sons; 1959.
31. Lentner M, Thomas B. The generalized RCB design (Chapter 6.13). In: Experimental Design and Analysis. 2nd ed. P.O. Box 884 Blacksburg, VA: Valley Book Company; 1993. p 225–226ISBN 0-9616255-2-X.
32. Miller GA, Chapman JP. Misunderstanding analysis of covariance. Journal of Abnormal Psychology 2001;110(1):40–48.
33. Montgomery DC. Design and Analysis of Experiments. 8th ed. USA: John Wiley & Sons; 2012. ISBN 978-1-118-14692-7.
34. Miller RG. Simultaneous Statistical Inference. 2nd ed. New York: Springer Verlag; 1981. ISBN 0-387-90548-0.
35. Montgomery DC. Design and Analysis of Experiments. 5th ed. New York: John Wiley & Sons, Inc.; 2001. Section 3-2. ISBN 9780471316497.
36. Westfall PH, Young SS. Resampling-Based Multiple Testing: Examples and Methods for p-Value Adjustment. USA: Wiley; 1993. ISBN: 978-0-471-55761-6.
37. Raghavarao D, Padgett LV. Block Designs: Analysis, Combinatorics and Applications. Singapore: World Scientific; 2005. ISBN 981-256-360-1.
38. Rosenbaum PR. Observational Studies. 2nd ed. New York: Springer-Verlag; 2002. ISBN 978-0-387-98967-9.
39. Scheffé H. The Analysis of Variance. New York: John Wiley & Sons, Inc.; 1959.
40. Shadish WR, Cook TD, Campbell DT. Experimental and Quasi-experimental Designs for Generalized Causal Inference. Boston: Houghton Mifflin; 2001. ISBN 0-395-61556-9 Excerpts.
41. Stoline MR. The status of multiple comparisons: simultaneous estimation of all pairwise comparisons in one-way ANOVA designs. The American Statistician (American Statistical Association) 1981;35(3):134–141. DOI: 10.2307/2683979. JSTOR 2683979.
42. Street AP, Street DJ. Combinatorics of Experimental Design. Clarendon: Oxford University Press; 1987. p 400+xivISBN 0-19-853256-3.

43. Student. Errors of routine analysis. Biometrika 1927;19:151–164.
44. Tabachnick BG, Fidell LS. Using Multivariate Statistics. 5th ed. Boston: Pearson Education, Inc.; 2007.
45. Verma JP. Data Analysis in Management with SPSS Software. India: Springer; 2013.
46. Wilk MB. The randomization analysis of a generalized randomized block design. Biometrika 1955;42(1–2):70–79JSTOR 2333423.
47. Winkler RL, Hays WL. Statistics: Probability, Inference, and Decision. 2nd ed. New York: Holt, Rinehart and Winston; 1975. p 761.

9

UNDERSTANDING RELATIONSHIPS AND DEVELOPING REGRESSION MODELS

9.1 INTRODUCTION

Correlation refers to the relationship between two variables. It is a statistical technique through which one can show whether and how pairs of variables are strongly related. For example, height and shot put performance are related; a taller athlete tends to run faster than a shorter athlete. Correlation tells you how one variable changes when another variable increases or decreases. At times, finding a relationship becomes meaningful for researchers. The concept of correlation is used frequently by exercise and health scientists. For example, an exercise scientist may be interested in knowing the relationship between training load and VO_2 max; a sports scientist may want to know the relationship between sports performance and satisfaction level; a basketball coach may like to find the relationship between palm size and shooting accuracy; and a health scientist may want to investigate the relationship between protein intake and muscular strength. Knowledge about the relationships of different parameters with that of performance in any sport helps a coach to develop training strategies accordingly. For instance, by knowing the fact that shot put performance is related to shoulder strength, a coach will give priority to develop shoulder strength in his weight training program. If two variables are related to each other significantly, the value of one variable can be estimated with the help of the other with certain limitations. For instance, performance in the 50 m event may be estimated by knowing the reaction time of an athlete if a relationship exists between them. Similarly, the weight of a child can be estimated

Statistics for Exercise Science and Health with Microsoft® Office Excel®, First Edition. J. P. Verma.

by knowing the height. In this chapter, first, the issue of relationship between two variables is discussed; thereafter, the relationship among more than two variables will be examined in detail. Finally, the chapter ends with a detailed discussion on regression analysis for developing regression models.

9.2 TYPES OF RELATIONSHIP

The relationship between any two variables can be either of two types: linear or curvilinear. In a linear relation, the rate of increment in one variable with respect to the other is constant throughout the paired observations. Consider the data shown in Table 9.1. You can see that the rate of change in y, that is, Δy ($5 = 10 - 5$) with respect to the rate of change in x, that is, Δx ($2 = 4 - 2$), is the same. Since the rate of change of y corresponding to x, that is, $\Delta y/\Delta x$ is constant throughout the dataset, the relationship between y and x is linear.

The relationship is curvilinear if the rate of change of y with respect to x, that is, $\Delta y/\Delta x$ is not constant for all the pairs of the dataset. Consider the dataset shown in Table 9.2. Here, the rate of change of y with respect to x is different for different pairs of the data. For the first two pairs of the dataset, $\Delta y/\Delta x$ is 8/2, whereas for the last two pairs, it is 32/2.

The distinction between linear and curvilinear relationships can be made by looking at the equation representing them. In high school, you must have studied that the equation of a line is of the following form:

$$y = mx + c \tag{9.1}$$

TABLE 9.1 Data Showing Linear Relation

X	Y
2	5
4	10
6	15
8	20
10	25

TABLE 9.2 Data Showing Curvilinear Relation

X	Y
1	1
3	9
5	25
7	49
9	81

where m is the slope and c is the intercept on the y-axis. If, in an equation, the power of all the variables is at the most one, then it shows the linear relationship, whereas if the power of one of the variables is more than one, it shows a curvilinear relation. Owing to this criterion, the following equations can be categorized into linear and curvilinear categories.

Equations Showing	
Linear Relation	Curvilinear Relation
$y = 3x + 2$	$y = 3x^2 + 6$
$y = 1.2x + 3^2$	$y = 6x^3$

Linear and curvilinear relationships can be shown graphically as in Figure 9.1 (a and b). Since most behavioral parameters are related in a linear manner, only the linear relationship is discussed in this text. For learning about curvilinear relations, readers are advised to consult some other text on statistics.

9.3 CORRELATION COEFFICIENT

After knowing that the two variables are related to each other, one may be interested to know how strong this relationship is. For instance, shot put performance is related to arm strength as well as height. But the extent of these relationships may differ. In order to know whether arm strength is more strongly related with shot put performance or height, one needs to measure the relationships in terms of some numerical value. The product-moment correlation coefficient provides this numerical value for studying the linear relationship between any two variables. It is represented by the letter "r" and is computed by using formula (9.2). The product-moment correlation coefficient was developed by Karl Pearson and is referred to as the *Pearson r.* The suffixes x and y in the subscript of r indicate the variables between which the correlation is computed. Using the suffixes with r is optional.

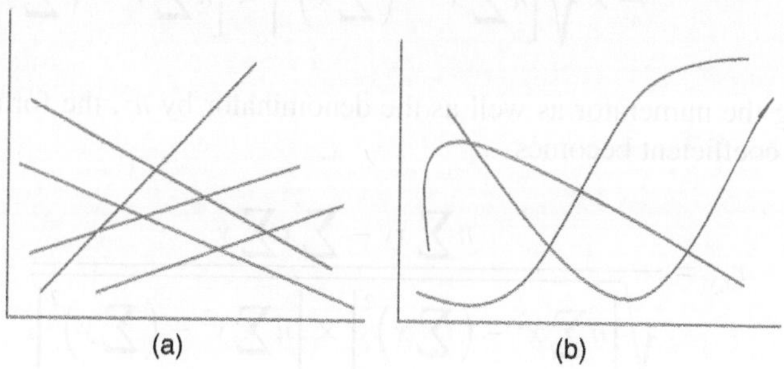

Figure 9.1 Different types of relationships: (a) linear relations and (b) curvilinear relations.

$$r_{x,y} = \frac{\text{cov}(x, y)}{\sqrt{\sigma_x \times \sigma_y}} \tag{9.2}$$

> **FACTS TO KNOW**
>
> The product-moment correlation coefficient does not explain the cause-and-effect relationship

Here, cov(x,y) represents the covariance between the variables x and y. Covariance can be defined as a measure of how much the two random variables vary together. A positive covariance between the arm strength and the shot put performance means that they move together. In other words, if a subject's score on arm strength is above its mean value, then the person's shot put performance tends to be above its mean value too. On the other hand, a negative covariance between the height and 100 m timings indicates that as the height increases the 100 m timings decrease. This can be understood as follows: if a subject's height is above its mean value, then his timings on 100 m tends to be below its mean value.

The symbols σ_x and σ_y represent the standard deviations of the variables x and y, respectively. As you know, the square of the standard deviation is known as *variance*. Let us see what the distinction between variance and covariance is. In fact, variance is a special case of covariance when the two variables are identical. Similar to standard deviation, variance too measures the variation of the scores on a single variable around its mean value.

Equation (9.2) can be simplified as follows:

$$r_{x,y} = \frac{E(xy) - E(x)E(y)}{\sqrt{\left[\frac{1}{n}\sum x^2 - \left(\frac{\sum x}{n}\right)^2\right] \times \left[\frac{1}{n}\sum y^2 - \left(\frac{\sum y}{n}\right)^2\right]}}$$

$$\Rightarrow \quad r_{x,y} = \frac{\frac{1}{n}\sum xy - \frac{1}{n}\sum x \frac{1}{n}\sum y}{\frac{1}{n^2} \times \sqrt{\left[n\sum x^2 - \left(\sum x\right)^2\right] \times \left[n\sum y^2 - \left(\sum y\right)^2\right]}}$$

Multiplying the numerator as well as the denominator by n^2, the formula for the correlation coefficient becomes

$$r_{x,y} = \frac{n\sum xy - \sum x \sum y}{\sqrt{\left[n\sum x^2 - \left(\sum x\right)^2\right] \times \left[n\sum y^2 - \left(\sum y\right)^2\right]}} \tag{9.3}$$

The product-moment correlation coefficient "r" can assume values between −1 and +1. Those interested in knowing how these limits have been derived may see the proof in the next section. Since only the linear relationship is discussed in this chapter, liberty has been taken to refer to the product-moment correlation coefficient simply as correlation coefficient. The product-moment correlation coefficient is also referred to as *zero-order correlation.* If the correlation coefficient is +1, it indicates that perfect positive linear correlation exists between the two variables. It happens if the increase (decrease) in the value of x results in the increase (decrease) in the value of y by the same amount on the z-scale. On the other hand, the value of r equal to −1 indicates perfect negative linear correlation between the variables. This situation arises if the increase (decrease) in the value of x results in the decrease (increase) in the value of y by the same amount on the z-scale. A value of r equal to zero indicates that the movement of the variable x has got nothing to do with that of the variable y. In research studies, one does not get these three extreme situations; rather, a trend is assessed on the basis of the plotted dataset. The plotting of the paired dataset in the $x - y$ plane is known as a ***scatter plot***. The three extreme situations, namely, r equal to +1, −1, or 0 can be shown in terms of the scatter plot in Figure 9.2(a–c).

The correlation coefficient "r" can be computed by using formula (9.3). In order to see the steps in computing "r", let us consider the following sets of scores on pull-ups and push-ups obtained on the five subjects.

Pull-Ups (x)	Push-Ups (y)
1	2
1	5
5	6
6	7
8	9
10	12

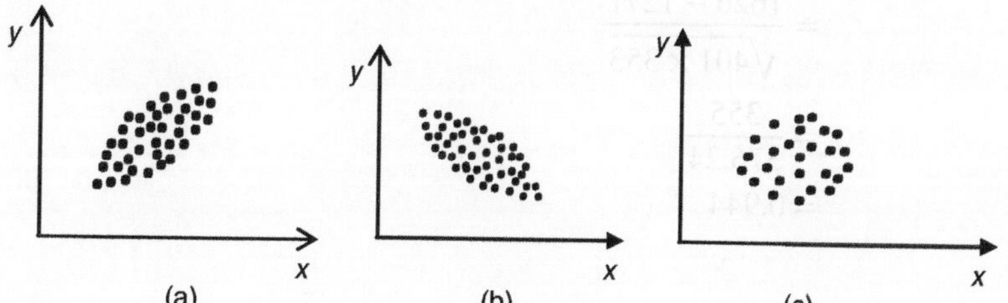

Figure 9.2 The scatter plots of the dataset for three extreme situations of correlations: (a) $r = +1$, (b) $r = -1$, and (c) $r = 0$.

TABLE 9.3 Computation of Correlation Coefficient

Pull-Ups x (1)	Push-Ups y (2)	x^2 (3)	y^2 (4)	xy (5)
1	2	1	4	2
1	5	1	25	5
5	6	25	36	30
6	7	36	49	42
8	9	64	81	72
10	12	100	144	120
$\sum x = 31$	$\sum y = 41$	$\sum x^2 = 227$	$\sum y^2 = 339$	$\sum xy = 271$

Steps in computing

a. Square each score of x in column 3.
b. Square each score of y in column 4.
c. Multiply each score of x by the corresponding score of y in column 5.
d. Add all the scores in each of the five columns to get the values of $\sum x$, $\sum y$, $\sum x^2$, $\sum y^2$, and $\sum xy$ respectively.
e. Substitute these totals in formula 9.3 (Table 9.3).

Here, $n = 6$ since the number of paired observations of x and y is 6:

$$r_{x,y} = \frac{n\sum xy - \sum x \sum y}{\sqrt{\left[n\sum x^2 - \left(\sum x\right)^2\right] \times \left[n\sum y^2 - \left(\sum y\right)^2\right]}}$$

$$= \frac{6 \times 271 - 31 \times 41}{\sqrt{[6 \times 227 - 31^2] \times [6 \times 339 - 41^2]}}$$

$$= \frac{1626 - 1271}{\sqrt{401 \times 353}}$$

$$= \frac{355}{376.24}$$

$$= 0.944$$

9.3.1 Testing the Significance of the Correlation Coefficient

After calculating the correlation coefficient between any two variables, one needs to know whether the obtained correlation is significant. In other words, what is the guarantee that the observed correlation coefficient has not been observed by chance? For instance, if the correlation is obtained between the height and the long jump performance on randomly chosen 20 athletes and if it is 0.52, can it be concluded that the observed correlation shall be obtained on most of the different randomly chosen samples? This problem can be answered by testing the significance of the computed correlation coefficient by the method described below.

Testing Significance The product-moment correlation can be tested for its significance by using the following *t*-statistic:

$$t = r\sqrt{\frac{n-2}{1-r^2}} \tag{9.4}$$

where *r* is the sample correlation and *n* is the sample size. This *t*-statistic follows the *t*-distribution with $n - 2$ degrees of freedom. By using this *t*-statistic, the following hypotheses can be tested:

$$H_0: \bar{r} = 0$$

$$H_1: \bar{r} \neq 0$$

where $\bar{r}$ is the product-moment correlation in the population. If the calculated value of *t* is greater than the tabulated value of *t* at some level of significance and $n - 2$ degrees of freedom, the null hypothesis may be rejected, otherwise it is failed to be rejected.

In the above example, $r = 0.52$ and $n = 20$. After substituting these values in formula (9.4),

$$t = 0.52\sqrt{\frac{20-2}{1-0.52^2}} = 2.58$$

From Table A.7 in the Appendix, the critical value of *t* at the significance level 0.05 with 18 degrees of freedom is 2.101. Since the calculated value of *t* is higher than 2.101, it may be concluded that the correlation coefficient of 0.52 is significant at 5% level.

Alternate Method The significance of the correlation coefficient can also be tested by comparing its value with that of the correlation coefficient required for its significance at 5% or 1% level with $n - 2$ degrees of freedom. These values have been shown in Table A.8. To test the significance of $r = 0.52$ between the height and long jump performance obtained on 20 athletes, the required value of *r* for its significance at 5% level and 18 (20 − 2) degrees of freedom can be seen from Table A.8, which is 0.444. Since the observed correlation coefficient 0.52 is greater than 0.444, it may be concluded that the correlation coefficient between height and long jump performance is significant.

9.3.2 Interpreting the Correlation Coefficient

If the correlation coefficient between the height and javelin throw obtained on 25 randomly chosen athletes is 0.49, what does it indicate? To interpret the correlation coefficient, you need to first test its significance at some desired level. Since the value of the correlation coefficient required for its significance at $\alpha = 0.05$ and 23 degrees of freedom for testing two-tail hypothesis is 0.396 (obtained from Table A.8), it may be concluded that the observed value of the correlation coefficient 0.49 is significant. It simply means that the correlation coefficient obtained from the random sample is not a chance occurrence and at least 95 times you will observe correlation coefficient greater than 0.396 out of 100 randomly drawn sample of athletes. The significance of the correlation coefficient ensures genuine relationship between the variables, but the question is how much variation in the performance of the dependent variable (javelin throw) is attributed to the independent variable (height). This is reflected by r^2, a term that is known as the *coefficient of determination*. The coefficient of determination indicates the percentage variance in the dependent variable that is explained by the independent variable. Thus, in this example, only 24.01% (= 0.49^2) variation of the athlete's javelin throw performance can be explained by the height.

9.3.3 Application of the Correlation Coefficient

Although the correlation coefficient does not explain the cause-and-effect relationship, it has several applications in research. The correlation coefficient r is used to estimate the dependent variable if the value of the independent variable is known. In simple regression, where one independent and one dependent variable are used to develop the regression line, the higher the correlation value, the better is the estimate of the dependent variable. Thus, 400 m performance can be efficiently estimated by using the leg strength rather than using reaction time. This is because leg strength is supposed to be highly related with the 400 m performance in comparison to the reaction time. In multiple regression analysis where the value of the dependent variable is estimated on the basis of more than one independent variable, regression coefficients are calculated by using the correlation coefficients only. In fact, partial and multiple correlations are computed by using different zero-order correlation coefficients.

The Pearson r is also used in testing the validity of a test. If a researcher has developed a regression equation for estimating the fat percentage on the basis of few skinfold measurements, then such a test can be validated by finding the correlation coefficient between the fat percentage obtained by the developed test and that obtained simultaneously by some standard procedure (such as underwater weighing) on the same set of subjects. The higher the correlation coefficient between these two sets of data, the better is the validity of the developed test. The Pearson r is also used in testing the reliability of the measurements by means of the test–retest method.

9.3.4 Effect of Change of Origin and Scale on the Correlation Coefficient

In comparative studies, the performance of athletes on 100 m and long jump cannot be compared owing to difference in the units of measurement, but there is no restriction in computing the correlation coefficient between them. This is because of the fact that the correlation coefficient is a pure number and does not depend on the unit of the variable. Since the correlation coefficient is free from change of units, it can be computed between any two variables having different units. In other words, the correlation coefficient is independent of the change of origin and scale. This fact shall be proved by means of the following example. Any score that is subtracted from each data item is known as the *origin*, and a score by which all the data are divided is known as the *scale*. Consider the two sets of data in Table 9.4:

$$r_{x,y} = \frac{n\sum xy - \sum x \sum y}{\sqrt{\left[n\sum x^2 - \left(\sum x\right)^2\right] \times \left[n\sum y^2 - \left(\sum y\right)^2\right]}}$$

$$= \frac{5 \times 2750 - 150 \times 125}{\sqrt{[5 \times 5500 - 150^2] \times [5 \times 4125 - 125^2]}}$$

$$= \frac{13750 - 18750}{\sqrt{5000 \times 5000}}$$

$$= \frac{-5000}{5000}$$

$$= -1$$

The value of the correlation coefficient is −1. Let us see what happens to the value of r if the following transformation is applied to x and y.

$$u = \frac{x - a}{h} \quad \text{and} \quad v = \frac{y - b}{k}$$

TABLE 9.4 Computation of the Correlation Coefficient

x	y	x^2	y^2	xy
10	45	100	2025	450
20	35	400	1225	700
30	25	900	625	750
40	15	1600	225	600
50	5	2500	25	250
$\sum x = 150$	$\sum y = 125$	$\sum x^2 = 5500$	$\sum y^2 = 4125$	$\sum xy = 2750$

TABLE 9.5 Computation of Correlation with the Transformed Variables

x	y	$u=\dfrac{x-30}{10}$	$v=\dfrac{y-25}{5}$	u^2	v^2	uv
10	45	−2	4	4	16	−8
20	35	−1	2	1	4	−2
30	25	0	0	0	0	0
40	15	1	−2	1	4	−2
50	5	2	−4	4	16	−8
		$\sum u=0$	$\sum v=0$	$\sum u^2=10$	$\sum v^2=40$	$\sum uv=-20$

Here, "*a*" and "*b*" are known as the *origins* and "*h*" and "*k*" are referred to as *scales*. Let us take $a = 30$, $b = 25$, $h = 10$, and $k = 5$. After transforming the variables x and y, the new variables have been worked out in Table 9.5.

$$r_{u,v} = \frac{n\sum uv - \sum u \sum v}{\sqrt{\left[n\sum u^2 - \left(\sum u\right)^2\right] \times \left[n\sum v^2 - \left(\sum v\right)^2\right]}}$$

$$= \frac{5 \times (-20) - 0}{\sqrt{(5 \times 10 - 0)(5 \times 40 - 0)}}$$

$$= \frac{-100}{\sqrt{50 \times 200}}$$

$$= \frac{-100}{\sqrt{10000}} = \frac{-100}{100} = -1$$

It can be seen that the value of correlation coefficient r_{uv} between the new transformed variables u and v is the same as r_{xy}. Thus, it is concluded that the change of origin and scale does not affect the correlation coefficient.

Remark The utility of the above concept lies in the fact that if the magnitude of the scores is high, it can be reduced by applying an appropriate transformation without affecting the value of the correlation coefficient.

9.3.5 Limitations of the Correlation Coefficient

In addition to its usefulness, the correlation coefficient has some limitations as well. One should carefully go through these limitations before making use of the correlation coefficient.

1. The correlation coefficient is suitable for interval or ratio data only and cannot be computed for ordinal or nominal data.

2. One of the main drawbacks of the correlation coefficient is that it does not explain the cause-and-effect relationship. In other words, one cannot be sure of the effect that one variable has on the other and vice versa. It may happen that there may be some other extraneous variable(s) that might affect one or both the variables under investigation. For instance, if the correlation coefficient between the height and shot put performance is 0.6, one cannot say with confidence that the taller athletes perform better on the shot put. It may be possible that enhanced performance in the shot put has been observed due to increased shoulder strength or the angle of release. Thus, one cannot be sure that height causes the shot put performance. Similarly, the reverse is also not true, as by enhancing the shot put performance, one cannot become taller.
3. Another limitation of the correlation coefficient is that it measures only linear relationships. If the two variables are related to each other in a curvilinear manner, then the correlation coefficient will give a wrong picture. To illustrate this fact, consider the following dataset of x and y.

x	y	x^2	y^2	xy
−2	4	4	16	−8
−1	1	1	1	−1
0	0	0	0	0
1	1	1	1	1
2	4	4	16	8
$\sum x = 0$	$\sum y = 10$	$\sum x^2 = 10$	$\sum y^2 = 34$	$\sum xy = 0$

$$r_{x,y} = \frac{5 \times 0 - 0 \times 10}{\sqrt{[5 \times 10 - 0^2] \times [5 \times 34 - 10^2]}} = 0$$

Here, the value of the correlation coefficient gives an impression that there is no relationship between x and y as the value of r is 0. But if you look into the scores of x and y, you can see that there is a perfect relationship between them as $y = x^2$. This dilemma can be solved by interpreting the correlation coefficient in the correct manner. Here, $r = 0$ indicates that there is no linear relationship between x and y, rather than interpreting that there is no relationship. The fact that the variables x and y are related by an equation $y = x^2$ indicates that the relationship between x and y is a curvilinear and not a linear one.

4. The correlation coefficient is very sensitive to outliers. Only one extreme pair of scores may give the wrong picture. For instance, the correlation coefficient between X: 1, 2, 3, 4, 5 and Y: 2, 4, 6, 8, 10 is +1, but if you add −80 to x and 90 to y then the correlation becomes −0.99.

Example 9.1 Following are the scores in two components of an AAHPER basketball skill test measured on 10 basketball players. Compute the product-moment correlation coefficient between these two test scores.

Under basket Pass (x)	Over arm Pass (y)
27	20
23	24
20	19
25	18
26	23
19	20
21	19
20	21
27	22
22	18

Solution: Here, $n = 10$. The values of x^2, y^2, and xy have been computed in the following table. The different column totals give the values of $\sum x$, $\sum y$, $\sum x^2$, $\sum y^2$, and $\sum xy$. Substituting these sums in the formula gives the value of the correlation coefficient.

Computation of the Correlation Coefficient

x	y	x^2	y^2	xy
27	20	729	400	540
23	24	529	576	552
20	19	400	361	380
25	18	625	324	450
26	23	676	529	598
19	20	361	400	380
21	19	441	361	399
20	21	400	441	420
27	22	729	484	594
22	18	484	324	396
$\sum x = 230$	$\sum y = 204$	$\sum x^2 = 5374$	$\sum y^2 = 4200$	$\sum xy = 4709$

$$r_{x,y} = \frac{n\sum xy - \sum x \sum y}{\sqrt{\left[n\sum x^2 - \left(\sum x\right)^2\right] \times \left[n\sum y^2 - \left(\sum y\right)^2\right]}}$$

$$= \frac{10 \times 4709 - 230 \times 204}{\sqrt{[10 \times 5374 - 230^2] \times [10 \times 4200 - 204^2]}}$$

$$= \frac{47090 - 46920}{\sqrt{[53740 - 52900] \times [42000 - 41616]}}$$

$$= \frac{170}{\sqrt{840 \times 384}} = \frac{170}{567.94} = 0.2993$$

Check Your Progress

Note: Tick the correct answer by using the sign ($\surd$).

	True	False
1. The Pearson "*r*" and product-moment correlation coefficient are different indexes for measuring relationship.	-	-
2. In a curvilinear relation, the rate of change of *y* with respect to *x* is constant throughout the dataset.	-	-
3. The value of *r* can be used in testing the validity of a test.	-	-
4. The correlation coefficient can be used for ordinal data.	-	-
5. The correlation coefficient is not causative in nature.	-	-
6. The equation $y = 5x + 6^2 - 7^2x$ indicates a curvilinear relation.	-	-
7. If the correlation is obtained with *n* samples, then its significant value can be obtained by using $n - 1$ degrees of freedom.	-	-
8. The covariance between the variables *X* and *X* is equivalent to the variance of *x*.	-	-
9. The expectation of *x*, that is, *E*(*X*), is same as the mean of *X*.	-	-
10. The value of covariance between *x* and *y* lies in between −1 and 1.	-	-
11. The value of correlation is always greater than 0.	-	-
12. In a linear relation, the rate of change of *y* with respect to *x*, that is, $\Delta y/\Delta x$ is constant.	-	-
13. The correlation coefficient between any two variables is unaffected if the units of both the variables are changed.	-	-

14. If the value of $r = 0.65$ between the height and weight is significant at 5% level, then it may be concluded that if 100 random samples are drawn, in at least 95 samples, the correlation between the height and weight would be 0.65 or more. - -
15. The correlation coefficient cannot be used for testing the reliability of a test. - -
16. The value of r^2 indicates the amount of variation in one variable explained by another variable. - -
17. The correlation coefficient is free from the change of origin but depends on the scale. - -
18. A scatter plot is the graph obtained by plotting the paired data on the x–y plane. - -
19. The slope of a line is equivalent to the rate of change of y with respect to x. - -
20. The coefficient of determination is the square of the correlation coefficient. - -
21. Although the correlation coefficient measures a linear relationship, it can also be used for measuring curvilinear relationships. - -
22. Outliers may reverse the sign of the correlation coefficient. - -

PRACTICE EXERCISE

1. Identify the dataset without computing whether the relationship between x and y is linear or curvilinear.

A		*B*		*C*		*D*		*E*	
x	y	x	y	x	y	x	y	x	y
2	3	45	3	1	1	2	12	1	55
4	5	48	9	3	8	2	16	2	57
6	8	51	15	5	27	2	18	3	59
8	20	54	21	7	64	2	20	4	61
10	35	57	27	9	125	2	22	5	63

2. Compute the product-moment correlation coefficient between the following two sets of scores.

X	Y
1	1
2	2
3	3
4	4
5	5

3. Compute the correlation coefficient for the following set of data and explain why the result is reversed with that of the correlation coefficient obtained in question 2.

X	Y
1	5
2	4
3	3
4	2
5	1

4. Compute the correlation coefficient r_{xy}. Also compute the correlation coefficient r_{uv} where $u = \frac{x-30}{10}$ and $v = \frac{y-15}{5}$. Check whether these two correlations are the same or different and give the reason.

X	Y
10	5
20	10
30	15
40	20
50	25

5. Following are the data on the upper arm length and lower arm length in centimeters obtained on eight athletes. Compute the correlation coefficient by appropriately changing the origins of x and y.

Upper Arm Length (*X*)	Lower Arm Length (*Y*)
34	50
33	52
33	48
32	43
31	45
30	44
32	45
34	49

9.4 PARTIAL CORRELATION

Partial correlation is a linear relation between two variables obtained after controlling the effect of other variables. Consider an experiment in which the heights and weights of 20 subjects belonging to different age categories ranging from 10 to 16 years were measured. If the correlation coefficient between height and weight was found to be 0.762, one may interpret it as high correlation. But the big issue is, can this correlation be considered as the actual relationship between the height and weight, especially in a situation where subjects were from the different age categories. It may be quite logical to conclude that the high magnitude of correlation was observed due to the fact that the subjects were from different developmental age categories. In other words, age affects both the variables height and weight because as the developmental age varies, both these variables also vary. Thus, to find the actual relationship between the height and the weight, the effect of age needs to be controlled. This can be done either by taking all the subjects in a particular age category or by controlling its effect statistically. While organizing a research study, it is difficult to manually control the effect of extraneous variables such as age, and hence a statistical procedure known as *partial correlation* is used in these situations. Partial correlation computes the linear correlation between two variables after controlling the effect of other variable(s). The partial correlation is denoted by the small letter "*r*" with a subscript in two parts. The subscript before the dot represents the variables between which the correlation is required to be computed and the variable(s) after the dot represents those variable(s) whose effects need to be controlled. If x_1, x_2, and x_3 represent the three variables, then the partial correlation between the variables x_1 and x_2 after controlling the effect of the third variable x_3 can be computed by the following formula:

$$r_{12.3} = \frac{r_{12} - r_{13}r_{23}}{\sqrt{1 - r_{13}^2}\sqrt{1 - r_{23}^2}} \tag{9.5}$$

The number of variables after the dot indicates the order of the partial correlation. Thus, the partial correlation $r_{12.3}$ is of the first order. Similarly, $r_{12.34}$ represents a second-order partial correlation as there are two variables after the dot. Using this principle, can you guess the order of the partial correlation $r_{12.34\ldots n}$? Do not be confused as the total number of variables in this correlation is n, of which only $n-2$ are after the dot; hence the order of this partial correlation would be $n-2$. The order of the product-moment correlation coefficient is zero because in this case no variable's effect is controlled.

Similar to $r_{12.3}$, other first-order correlations such as $r_{13.2}$ and $r_{23.1}$ can be computed by the formulas:

$$r_{13.2} = \frac{r_{13} - r_{12}r_{32}}{\sqrt{1-r_{12}^2}\sqrt{1-r_{32}^2}} \quad \text{and} \quad r_{23.1} = \frac{r_{23} - r_{21}r_{31}}{\sqrt{1-r_{21}^2}\sqrt{1-r_{31}^2}}$$

9.4.1 General Formula for Partial Correlation

In case of n variables, the maximum order of the partial correlation can be $n-2$. The generalized formula for the partial correlation of order $n-2$ is given by

$$r_{12.345\ldots n} = \frac{r_{12.34\ldots n-1} - r_{1n.345\ldots n-1}r_{2n.345\ldots n-1}}{\sqrt{1-r_{1n.345\ldots n-1}^2}\sqrt{1-r_{2n.345\ldots n-1}^2}} \tag{9.6}$$

If $n = 4$, formula (9.6) becomes the second-order partial correlation:

$$r_{12.34} = \frac{r_{12.3} - r_{14.3}r_{24.3}}{\sqrt{1-r_{14.3}^2}\sqrt{1-r_{24.3}^2}}$$

Similarly, putting $n = 5$ in formula (9.6), we get the third-order partial correlation, that is,

$$r_{12.345} = \frac{r_{12.34} - r_{15.34}r_{25.34}}{\sqrt{1-r_{15.34}^2}\sqrt{1-r_{25.34}^2}}$$

It can be seen from the above formulation that the partial correlation of any given order n can be expressed in terms of partial correlations of order $n-1$. As with product-moment correlation coefficient, the partial correlation also lies in between -1 to $+1$.

Example 9.2 In an experiment, the playing ability, height, and arm length were measured on 15 volleyball players. Product-moment correlations were computed among all the three variables as are shown in the following correlation matrix. Compute $r_{12.3}$ and $r_{13.2}$.

Correlation matrix among the variables

	x_1	x_2	x_3
x_1	1.00	0.67	0.75
x_2		1.00	0.94
x_3			1.00
	x_1: Playing ability	x_2: Height	x_3: Arm length

i. Since $r_{12.3} = \frac{r_{12}-r_{13}r_{23}}{\sqrt{1-r_{13}^2}\sqrt{1-r_{23}^2}}$, on substituting correlation values from the correlation matrix,

$$r_{12.3} = \frac{0.67 - 0.75 \times 0.94}{\sqrt{1-0.75^2}\sqrt{1-0.94^2}}$$
$$= \frac{0.67 - 0.705}{\sqrt{0.4375 \times 0.1164}}$$
$$= \frac{-0.035}{\sqrt{0.0509}} = -\frac{0.035}{0.226} = -0.15$$

ii. Since

$$r_{13.2} = \frac{r_{13} - r_{12}r_{32}}{\sqrt{1-r_{12}^2}\sqrt{1-r_{32}^2}}$$

on substituting the values of the correlation coefficients from the correlation matrix,

$$r_{13.2} = \frac{0.75 - 0.67 \times 0.94}{\sqrt{1-0.67^2}\sqrt{1-0.94^2}}$$
$$= \frac{0.75 - 0.6298}{\sqrt{0.55 \times 0.12}}$$
$$= \frac{0.1202}{\sqrt{0.066}} = \frac{0.1202}{0.2569} = 0.47$$

9.4.2 Limitations of Partial Correlation

While using and interpreting partial correlation, one should look for its limitations also, which are as follows:

1. Like the product-moment correlation coefficient, partial correlation too measures linear relationships only.

2. Even after controlling the effect of some of the extraneous variables, in computing partial correlation, one cannot be sure that it indicates the true linear relationship between the two variables as there may be some other causative variables whose effects might have not been controlled. For instance, if a partial correlation is computed between the swimming performance and height of the swimmers after controlling for cardiorespiratory endurance and back strength, one cannot be sure that the obtained partial correlation is indicative of the true relationship. This may be because of the fact that the swimming performance also depends on the shoulder strength and arm length, and the effects of these variables have not been controlled in computing the partial correlation. Thus, while computing partial correlation one must explore all such extraneous variables that might affect the relationship between two variables of interest.
3. A large sample must be taken to compute partial correlation for reliable assessment about the true relationship between two variables.

9.4.3 Utilities of Partial Correlation

Partial correlation is quite useful in research. It may help a researcher to identify the parameters that are strongly related with the performance according to their order of importance. Consider a situation where a researcher is interested in knowing the independent variables that are strongly related with the long jump performance (x_1) in order of their contribution. On the basis of a review of the literature, let us suppose that the researcher decides to study the three most important independent variables, namely, leg strength (x_2), reaction time (x_3), and angle of takeoff (x_4) in investigating the relationships with the long jump performance. By computing partial correlations between the long jump performance and each of these independent variables separately by controlling the effects of the remaining two variables, one can compare the relative strength of the linear relationship for deciding on the independent variable that contributes the most to long jump performance. For instance, if $r_{12.34} = 0.7$, $r_{13.24} = 0.3$, and $r_{14.23} = 0.6$, then it may be interpreted that the contribution of leg strength to long jump performance is 49% ($=0.7^2 \times 100$), which is the maximum, whereas the contribution of takeoff is 36% and that of back strength is 9% only. This information can give an insight to a coach in deciding the training schedule for developing these characteristics among the long jumpers according to the priority. One should concentrate only on those partial correlations that are found to be statistically significant. The significance of the partial correlation can be tested similarly to that of the product-moment correlation coefficient discussed earlier in this chapter. In research studies, the researcher must find the partial correlation between the criterion variable and those independent variables only that are found to be significantly related with it. Similarly, the effects of only those independent variables need to be controlled that are found to be significant with the criterion variable.

9.5 MULTIPLE CORRELATION

Multiple correlation is the correlation between a group of variables and a single variable not included in the group. It is used as an indicator of efficiency in predicting some criterion variable on the basis of some independent variables. Multiple correlation can be considered to be the correlation between the observed values of the criterion variable and its estimated values obtained on the basis of the independent variables. High multiple correlation indicates that the criterion variable can be efficiently predicted by the independent variables in the model. For instance, in developing a model for estimating the performance on the 100 m dash on the basis of independent parameters such as reaction time, stride length, leg length, and leg strength, the higher the value of the multiple correlation, the better would be the efficiency of estimation. Multiple correlation is represented by R with a subscript in two parts. The subscript preceding the dot represents the criterion or dependent variable, whereas the subscripts following the dot represent the independent variables. Thus, the multiple correlation between the variable x_1 and the group of variables including x_2 and x_3 can be computed by using the following formula:

$$R_{1.23} = \sqrt{\frac{r_{12}^2 + r_{13}^2 - 2r_{12}r_{13}r_{23}}{1 - r_{23}^2}} \tag{9.7}$$

Multiple correlation R can assume any value in the range 0 to +1. The square of multiple correlation (R^2) is known as the *coefficient of determination*. It represents the amount of variation in the dependent variable that can be explained by the independent variables together. Thus, in the above example, if R is 0.8, it simply indicates that 64% of the variability in the performance of 100 m dash can be explained by all four independent variables, namely, reaction time, stride length, leg length, and leg strength together.

Formula (9.7) is valid only if the total number of variables in the multiple correlation is 3. If the number of variables is more than three, the following generalized formula can be used:

$$R_{1.234\ldots n} = \sqrt{1 - (1 - r_{12}^2)(1 - r_{13.2}^2)(1 - r_{14.23}^2) \ldots (1 - r_{1n.234\ldots n-1}^2)} \tag{9.8}$$

Substituting the value of n in formula (9.8), the required multiple correlation can be obtained. Thus, if $n = 4$, the multiple correlation $R_{1.234}$ can be computed as

$$R_{1.234} = \sqrt{1 - (1 - r_{12}^2)(1 - r_{13.2}^2)(1 - r_{14.23}^2)}$$

Example 9.3 Using the following correlation matrix, compute $R_{1.34}$ and $R_{1.234}$.

Correlation Matrix

	x_1	x_2	x_3	x_4
x_1	1	0.7	0.42	−0.45
x_2		1	0.20	−0.19
x_3			1	−0.90
x_4				1

x_1: Standing broad jump x_2: Ponderal index x_3: Leg length x_4: Thigh length

Since

$$R_{1.34} = \sqrt{\frac{r_{13}^2 + r_{14}^2 - 2r_{13}r_{14}r_{34}}{1 - r_{34}^2}}$$

substituting values from the correlation matrix,

$$R_{1.34} = \sqrt{\frac{0.42^2 + (-0.45)^2 - 2 \times 0.42 \times (-0.45) \times (-0.90)}{1 - (-0.90)^2}}$$

$$= \sqrt{\frac{0.1764 + 0.2025 - 0.3402}{0.19}} = \sqrt{\frac{0.0387}{0.19}} = 0.45$$

In order to compute the value of $R_{1.234}$, let us see what needs to be computed first. Since

$$R_{1.234} = \sqrt{1 - (1 - r_{12}^2)(1 - r_{13.2}^2)(1 - r_{14.23}^2)}$$

to compute this multiple correlation, it is required to compute the following first- and second-order partial correlations first.

Required first-order partial correlations

$$r_{13.2} = \frac{r_{13} - r_{12}r_{32}}{\sqrt{1 - r_{12}^2}\sqrt{1 - r_{32}^2}} = \frac{0.42 - 0.7 \times 0.20}{\sqrt{1 - 0.7^2}\sqrt{1 - 0.20^2}} = 0.40$$

$$r_{14.2} = \frac{r_{14} - r_{12}r_{42}}{\sqrt{1 - r_{12}^2}\sqrt{1 - r_{42}^2}} = \frac{(-0.45)^2 - 0.7 \times (-0.19)}{\sqrt{1 - 0.7^2}\sqrt{1 - (-0.19)^2}} = 0.48$$

$$r_{43.2} = \frac{r_{43} - r_{42}r_{32}}{\sqrt{1 - r_{42}^2}\sqrt{1 - r_{32}^2}} = \frac{(-0.90)^2 - (-0.19) \times 0.20}{\sqrt{1 - (-0.19)^2}\sqrt{1 - 0.20^2}} = 0.88$$

Required second-order partial correlation

$$r_{14.23} = \frac{r_{14.2} - r_{13.2}r_{43.2}}{\sqrt{1 - r_{13.2}^2}\sqrt{1 - r_{43.2}^2}}$$

$$= \frac{0.48 - 0.40 \times 0.88}{\sqrt{1 - 0.40^2}\sqrt{1 - 0.88^2}} = \frac{0.13}{0.45} = 0.29$$

Thus,

$$R_{1.234} = \sqrt{1 - (1 - r_{12}^2)(1 - r_{13.2}^2)(1 - r_{14.23}^2)}$$

$$= \sqrt{1 - (1 - 0.7^2)(1 - 0.40^2)(1 - 0.29^2)}$$

$$= 0.78$$

Look at the following values of the correlations

$$R_{12} = 0.7$$

$$R_{1.23} = \sqrt{\frac{r_{12}^2 + r_{13}^2 - 2r_{12}r_{13}r_{23}}{1 - r_{23}^2}}$$

$$= \sqrt{\frac{0.7^2 + 0.42^2 - 2 \times 0.7 \times 0.42 \times 0.20}{1 - 0.20^2}}$$

$$= 0.75$$

$$R_{1.234} = 0.78$$

Here, as the number of variables keeps on increasing, the multiple correlation also keeps on increasing.

Remark

1. Multiple correlation is high if the correlation among independent variables is low.
2. A multiple correlation will not be less than the highest zero-order correlation between the independent and dependent variables.
3. Since multiple correlation is computed with product-moment correlations, this too measures only the linear relationship.

9.6 SUPPRESSION VARIABLE

There are instances where a variable does not show significant correlation with the dependent variable, but if it is combined with some variable it may produce higher multiple correlation. Such a variable is known as a *suppression variable*. The following example will illustrate this effect.

If $r_{12} = 0.4$, $r_{13} = 0$, and $r_{23} = 0.8$, then

$$R_{1.23} = \sqrt{\frac{r_{12}^2 + r_{13}^2 - 2r_{12}r_{13}r_{23}}{1 - r_{23}^2}}$$

$$= \sqrt{\frac{0.4^2 + 0 - 0}{1 - 0.8^2}} = \sqrt{\frac{0.16}{0.36}} = 0.67$$

It can be seen that the variable x_3 is not correlated with x_1 but when it is combined with the variable x_2 it produces a multiple correlation 0.67 that is higher than 0.40, the correlation between x_1 and x_2.

Check Your Progress

Note: Tick the correct answer by using the sign ($\surd$).

	True	False
23. In computing the partial correlation between height and weight, the effect of age can be controlled by taking all the subjects in the same age category.	-	-
24. Since in the partial correlation $r_{23.567}$, the number of variables before the dot is 2, the order of this partial correlation is 2.	-	-
25. The order of the partial correlation $r_{12.34...n}$ is n–2.	-	-
26. Partial correlation is always positive.	-	-
27. Even with a small sample, the partial correlation can assess the linear relationship accurately.	-	-
28. The amount of variability in x_1 explained by the variable x_2 can be assessed more accurately by $r_{12.3}^2$ in comparison to r_{12}^2.	-	-
29. The partial correlation of order n is computed by using the partial correlation of order n–2.	-	-
30. A multiple correlation can never be less than the highest zero-order correlation between the independent and dependent variables.	-	-

31. Multiple correlation is high if the correlation among independent variables is also high.	-	-
32. The order of the partial correlation $r_{12.345}$ is 5.	-	-
33. A suppression variable shows significant correlation with the dependent variable, but if it is combined with some variable it may reduce multiple correlation.	-	-
34. The value of the partial correlation $r_{34.5}$ is the same as $r_{43.5}$.	-	-
35. The value of the coefficient of determination is always positive.	-	-

PRACTICE EXERCISE

6. Compute the partial correlation between variables 1 and 2, keeping the third variable constant for the following data:

$$r_{12} = 0.6;\ r_{13} = 0.5;\ \text{and}\ r_{23} = 0.3$$

7. With the help of the following zero-order correlations, calculate the multiple correlation treating the first variable as dependent and the second and third as independent.

$$r_{12} = 0.85;\ r_{13} = 0.38,\ \text{and}\ r_{23} = 0.25$$

8. The correlations among height, weight, and calf girth are shown in the following correlation matrix. Compute the partial correlations $r_{13.2}$ and $r_{23.1}$.

Correlation Matrix

	X_1	X_2	X_3
X_1	1	0.8	0.4
X_2		1	0.6
X_3			1
	X_1: Height	X_2: Weight	X_3: Calf girth

9. Compute $R_{3.12}$ from the correlation matrix shown in question 8 and interpret your findings.

10. In a regression study for estimating fat percentage, the following data on fat percentage and skinfold measurement on abdomen and suprailiac were obtained.

Abdomen	Suprailiac	Fat
20	12	11
25	15	17
25	27	15
40	30	27
14	10	13
15	12	17
13	7	12

a. Compute the correlation matrix by calculating the intercorrelations among the variables.
b. Which predictor is the best for predicting the fat%? What is the correlation between the predictors?
c. Compute the multiple correlation using abdomen and suprailiac to predict fat%.
d. Compare the multiple correlation to the highest single zero-order correlation. Is there any difference?
e. Find the coefficient of determination. Is there any improvement by using both predictors rather than the best single one?

9.7 REGRESSION ANALYSIS

The procedure for developing a regression model for estimating a dependent variable on the basis of one or more independent variables is known as *regression analysis*. The association between dependent and independent variables is studied through the theory of regression and correlation. Sir Francis Galton (1822–1911), an English scientist, used the term regression for the first time while studying the resemblance between parents and children. In regression analysis, a regression equation is developed through which quantitative predications of one variable (dependent) is made from the values of one or more variables (independent). If regression analysis includes one dependent and only one independent variable, then it is known as *simple regression*, whereas if it includes more than one independent variable, it is referred as *multiple regression analysis*.

9.7.1 Simple Regression Analysis

In simple regression, an equation is developed by using one dependent variable and one independent variable, assuming that a relationship exists between the two. The regression equation is useful when other conditions are the same for the subjects. In an athletic training camp, where all the trainees have similar level of performance and training schedules, a coach may be interested in knowing the impact of practice duration on the performance of an athlete. It is assumed that all other variables influence all trainees in a similar manner except the practice duration. Let us see how the regression equation is developed between the dependent variable y and the independent variable x. You must be aware of the slope–intercept form of the equation of the line which is as follows:

$$y = mx + c$$

where m represents the slope and c represents the intercept of the line on the y-axis.

Let us consider N datapoints (x_1,y_1), (x_2,y_2), …, (x_N,y_N) in the population for which the regression line is to be developed for estimating the value of y on the basis of x. The developed regression equation for the line shall be of the form

$$\hat{y} = \beta_0 + \beta_1 x \tag{9.9}$$

where

$\hat{y}$ = the estimated value of y
β_0 = the population intercept (regression constant)
β_1 = the population slope (regression coefficient)

The line given by Equation (9.9) should be that which provides the best aggregates of all the datapoints in the population. To understand the procedure of how this line is obtained, let us plot the datapoints on the x–y plane as shown in Figure 9.3.

Equation (9.9) has been obtained on the basis of all the N datapoints in the population. But for any particular value of the dependent variable y_i

$$y_i = \beta_0 + \beta_1 x_i + \varepsilon_i \tag{9.10}$$

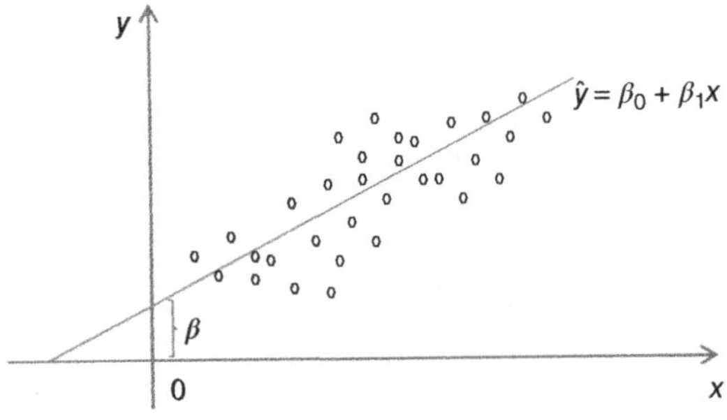

Figure 9.3 Plotting the data and the line of best fit.

where

y_i = value of the dependent variable for the ith subject
x_i = value of the independent variable for the ith subject
β_0 = the population intercept (regression constant)
β_1 = the population slope (regression coefficient)
ε_i = error of estimation for the ith subject

In exercise science and health research, regression lines are mostly developed by using the sample data and not the population data. Therefore, β_0 and β_1 are not attainable and must be estimated by using the sample statistics b_0 and b_1, respectively. Hence, the regression line contains the sample intercept of y (b_0) and sample slope b_1, which can be written as

$$\hat{y} = b_0 + b_1x \tag{9.11}$$

and any specific value of the dependent variable y_i in the sample will be equal to

$$y_i = b_0 + b_1x_i + \varepsilon_i \tag{9.12}$$

There can be infinite number of lines with different intercepts and slopes that can pass through the sample points, but the line of best fit will be the one that provides the least sum of the squared deviations of the observed and estimated values of y. This is known as the *method of least squares*, which is used in developing the regression equation. The method of least square uses the concept of calculus to calculate the values of the intercept (regression constant) and slope (regression coefficient) that provide the best fitted line for estimating the value of y on the basis of x. Thus, if there are n sample points $(x_1,y_1), (x_2,y_2), \ldots, (x_n,y_n)$, then the sample regression line will be the line of the best fit for which the deviation of all the observed scores y_i from their estimated scores $\hat{y}_i$ is the least. In other words, the sum of the squared deviations of all the observed scores of y_i from their estimated values $\hat{y}_i$ as calculated below should be minimum.

$$S^2 = \sum_{i=1}^{n} (y_i - \hat{y}_i)^2 = \sum_{i=1}^{n} \varepsilon_i^2 = \sum_{i=1}^{n} (y_i - b_0 - b_1x_i)^2 \tag{9.13}$$

Thus, it is required to find the values of b_0 and b_1 so that the value of S^2 is minimized. The values of these constants can be obtained by differentiating equation (9.13) first with respect to b_0 and then with respect to b_1 and equating the results to zero.

Thus,

$$\frac{\partial S^2}{\partial b_0} = -2\sum_{i=1}^{n}(y_i - b_0 - b_1x_i) = 0$$

and

$$\frac{\partial S^2}{\partial b_1} = -2\sum_{i=1}^{n} x_i(y_i - b_0 - b_1x_i) = 0$$

Solving these equations,

$$\sum_{i=1}^{n}(y_i - b_0 - b_1x_i) = 0$$

$$\sum_{i=1}^{n}x_i(y_i - b_0 - b_1x_i) = 0$$

By expanding the summation and rearranging the terms, the above two equations can be written as

$$b_1\sum_{i=1}^{n}x_i + nb_0 = \sum_{i=1}^{n}y_i \tag{9.14}$$

$$b_1\sum_{i=1}^{n}x_i^2 + b_0\sum_{i=1}^{n}x_i = \sum_{i=1}^{n}x_iy_i \tag{9.15}$$

These two equations are known as *normal equations* with two unknown coefficients b_0 and b_1. On solving these equations, the values of b_0 and b_1 can be obtained as follows:

$$b_0 = \frac{\sum y\sum x^2 - \sum x\sum xy}{n\sum x^2 - \left(\sum x\right)^2} \quad \text{and} \quad b_1 = \frac{n\sum xy - \sum x\sum y}{n\sum x^2 - \left(\sum x\right)^2}$$

Thus, by using the values of b_0 and b_1 in equation (9.11), the line of best fit can be obtained. In other words, the sum of squared deviations of the scores of the dependent variable y from its estimated values would be least if the regression line is developed by using the slope b_1 and intercept b_0.

Alternate Formula of Intercept and Slope The regression equation for estimating the value of the dependent variable on the basis of independent variable as shown by equation (9.11) can also be written as

$$\hat{y} - \bar{y} = b_1(x - \bar{x}) \tag{9.16}$$

where

$x =$ value of the independent variable
$\hat{y} =$ estimated value of the dependent variable
$\bar{x} =$ mean of the independent variable

$\bar{y} =$ mean of the dependent variable
$b_1 =$ slope of the sample data

Equation (9.16) can be rearranged to show the regression line in the form of intercept and slope:

$$\hat{y} = b_1 x + \bar{y} - b_1 \bar{x}$$

This can be written as

$$\hat{y} = b_0 + b_1 x$$

where

$$b_0 = \bar{y} - b_1 \bar{x} \text{ and } b_1 = r\frac{\sigma_y}{\sigma_x}$$

Here, σ_x and σ_y denote the standard deviation of x and y, respectively, and r is the correlation coefficient between x and y. The slope b_1 can further be simplified as shown below:

$$\begin{aligned} b_1 &= r\frac{\sigma_y}{\sigma_x} \\ &= \frac{\text{cov}(x, y)}{\sigma_x \sigma_y} \times \frac{\sigma_y}{\sigma_x} = \frac{\text{cov}(x, y)}{\sigma_x^2} \\ &= \frac{\sum (x - \bar{x})(y - \bar{y})}{\sum (x - \bar{x})^2} \\ \Rightarrow \quad b_1 &= \frac{\sum xy - \frac{1}{n}\left(\sum x\right)\left(\sum y\right)}{\sum x^2 - \frac{\left(\sum x\right)^2}{n}} \end{aligned}$$

The numerator of the slope b_1 is the sum of squares of xy and is denoted by SS_{xy}.

$$SS_{xy} = \sum (x - \bar{x})(y - \bar{y}) = \sum xy - \frac{1}{n}\left(\sum x\right)\left(\sum y\right)$$

The denominator of the slope b_1 is the sum of the squares of x and is denoted by SS_{xx}.

$$SS_{xx} = \sum (x - \bar{x})^2 = \sum x^2 - \frac{1}{n}\left(\sum x\right)^2$$

Thus, the alternative formula for the slope can be expressed as

$$b_1 = \frac{SS_{xy}}{SS_{xx}} \tag{9.17}$$

Since

$$b_0 = \bar{y} - b_1\bar{x}$$

$$\Rightarrow \quad b_0 = \frac{\sum y}{n} - b_1\frac{\sum x}{n} \tag{9.18}$$

To calculate the intercept (b_0), the value of the slope (b_1) should be calculated first. Thus, in developing the equation of the regression line for estimating y on the basis of x, the coefficients b_0 and b_1 can also be calculated by using formulas (9.17) and (9.18), respectively.

Computing Intercept and Slope in a Simple Regression Analysis Consider a situation where a researcher wishes to predict the lean body weight on the basis of the height only. To solve this problem, it is required to investigate what other variables are related to the lean body weight. Since some of the variables that might contribute to the lean body weight are weight, fat mass, abdomen girth, and thigh girth, these variables should be similar for all the athletes taken in the sample in order to estimate their lean body weight accurately on the basis of height only. Thus, to estimate the lean body weight on the basis of height only, suppose a sample of 11 athletes are selected from the same sport having similar age, body build, and the level of participation so as to reduce the influence of the extraneous variables. These subjects are tested for their height and lean body weight, and the data so obtained are shown in Table 9.6.

These data shall be used to construct a regression model to estimate the lean body weight on the basis of the height. To construct the regression equation, the intercept and slope can be calculated by first computing the terms: $\sum x$, $\sum y$, $\sum xy$, and $\sum x^2$. Computation of these terms has been shown in Table 9.7.

TABLE 9.6 Athletes' Data

Height (cm)	LBW (lbs)
191	162.5
186	136.0
191	163.5
188	154.0
190	149.0
188	140.5
191	157.3
190	154.0
189	151.5
192	160.5
188	147.5

TABLE 9.7 Computation for the Slope and the y-Intercept

Height (cm) x	LBW (lbs) y	x^2	xy
191.0	162.5	36481.00	31037.50
186.0	136.0	34596.00	25296.00
191.5	163.5	36672.25	31310.25
188.0	154.0	35344.00	28952.00
190.0	149.0	36100.00	28310.00
188.5	140.5	35532.25	26484.25
193.0	157.3	37249.00	30358.90
190.5	154.5	36290.25	29432.25
189.0	151.5	35721.00	28633.50
192.0	160.5	36864.00	30816.00
187.0	147.5	34969.00	27582.50
$\sum x = 2086.5$	$\sum y = 1676.8$	$\sum x^2 = 395818.75$	$\sum xy = 318213.15$

Since we know that

$$b_1 = \frac{SS_{xy}}{SS_{xx}} \text{ and } b_0 = \frac{\sum y}{n} - b_1 \frac{\sum x}{n}$$

$$SS_{xy} = \sum xy - \frac{1}{n}\left(\sum x\right)\left(\sum y\right)$$

$$= 318213.15 - \frac{1}{11} \times 2086.5 \times 1676.8 = 154.68$$

$$SS_{xx} = \sum x^2 - \frac{1}{n}\left(\sum x\right)^2 = 395818.75 - \frac{1}{11} \times 2086.5^2 = 47.64$$

$$\text{Slope} = b_1 = \frac{154.68}{47.64} = 3.247$$

$$\text{Intercept} = b_0 = \frac{1676.8}{11} - 3.247 \times \frac{2086.5}{11} = -463.461$$

Thus, the regression equation can be constructed by substituting the values of the y intercept b_0 and slope b_1:

$$y = -463.461 + 3.247x \tag{9.19}$$

Let us see how this regression equation is interpreted. Here, the slope is 3.247, which means that for every unit increase in x (every centimeter increase in the height), there is a 3.247 lbs increase in lean body weight of an individual. The y-intercept is the point where the line crosses the y-axis. In regression analysis, usually the y-intercept is meaningless. However, in multiple regression analysis, it may be used to test the effectiveness of the independent variables used in the model.

> **FACTS TO KNOW**
>
> The regression model provides a more accurate estimate if its assumptions are true

Analyzing the Residuals The regression line is usually developed on the basis of the historical data that are available with the researcher. To test whether the regression line so developed is a good fit or not, the value of the dependent variable $\hat{y}$ is estimated corresponding to each scores of the independent variable by using the regression equation. A difference of observed and estimated value of y, that is, $(y - \hat{y})$ is computed for each dataset. Each difference between the actual value and the estimated value shows the error of the regression line at a given point. This difference $(y - \hat{y})$ is known as a *residual*. Thus, residuals are estimates of the regression errors. It is the sum of the squares of these residuals that is minimized to construct the best fit regression line.

Table 9.8 shows the residuals for each pair of the data on height and lean body weight. The estimated values of y are obtained by inserting the values of the independent variable in the regression line developed above. For instance, for $x = 188$, $\hat{y} = -463.461 + 3.247 \times 188 = 146.975$.

From Table 9.8, the maximum and minimum residuals are seen to be −8.0985 and 0.537, respectively. In estimating the lean body weight, the regression line produces the maximum error of 8.0985 lbs when the height of an individual is 188.5 cm and the minimum error of 0.537 lbs when the height is 192 cm. These residuals tell us about the best and worst cases in estimating the dependent variable using the regression equation. It can be seen that the sum of the residuals is approximately zero. The sum of the residual is always zero except for the rounding-off error.

TABLE 9.8 Computation of Residuals

Height (cm) x	LBW (lbs) y	$\hat{y}$	$y - \hat{y}$
191.0	162.5	156.7160	5.7840
186.0	136.0	140.4810	−4.4810
191.5	163.5	158.3395	5.1605
188.0	154.0	146.9750	7.0250
190.0	149.0	153.4690	−4.4690
188.5	**140.5**	**148.5985**	**−8.0985**
193.0	157.3	163.2100	−5.9100
190.5	154.5	155.0925	−0.5925
189.0	151.5	150.2220	1.2780
192.0	**160.5**	**159.9630**	**0.5370**
187.0	147.5	143.7280	3.7720
			$\sum(y - \hat{y}) = 0.0055$

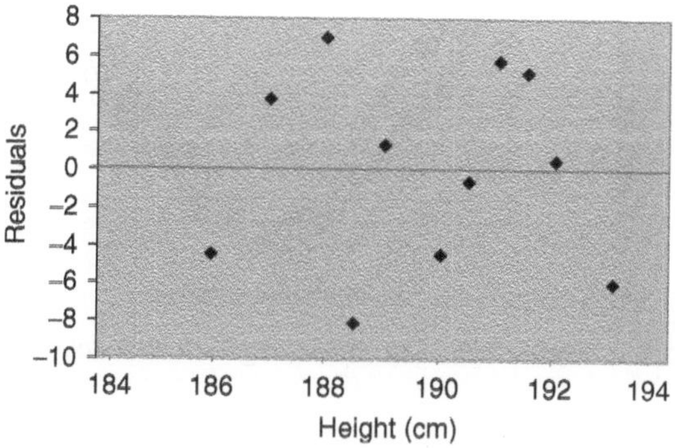

Figure 9.4 Residual plot for the data on lean body weight and height.

These residuals can also be used to find the outliers in the dataset. If the residual is extreme for some datapoints, then it must be checked for error. The error may occur during feeding the data or wrongly recording the data. The outliers must be checked in developing the regression analysis because they unnecessarily drag the regression line toward them.

Residual Plot The nature of the residuals can be studied by plotting them as ordered pairs $(x_i, y - \hat{y})$. The residuals are usually plotted along y-axis and the independent variable along the x-axis. In the residual plot, the movement of residuals can be seen as x increases. This residual plot can be used to test the assumptions in the regression analysis. The residual plot for the data in Table 9.8 is shown in Figure 9.4. The pattern of the residuals is random. However, the correct picture of the residual plot can be obtained only when a large dataset is used in the regression analysis.

Testing Assumptions in the Regression Model In regression analysis, certain assumptions need to be fulfilled. In the absence of these assumptions, the estimation of the dependent variable from the regression line may not be accurate. One must ascertain that the following assumptions have been met before developing the regression model.

1. The regression model is linear in nature.
2. The errors are independent.
3. The error terms are normally distributed.
4. The error has a constant variance.

One can have an idea about whether the above assumptions have been meted out or not by looking at the residual plot. If the residual plot obtained in the regression analysis similar to that in Figure 9.5, the assumption that the regression model is linear does not hold true.

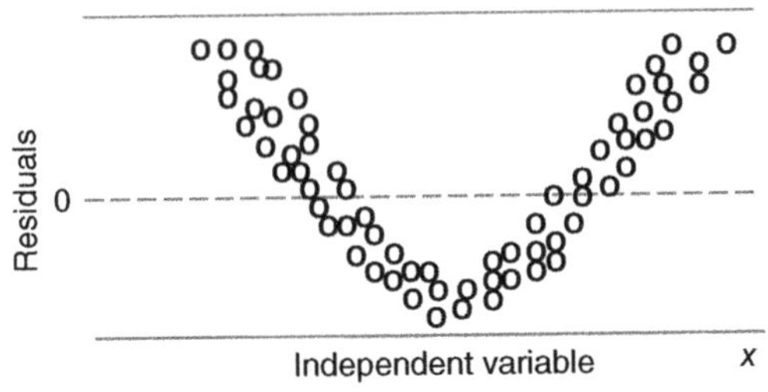

Figure 9.5 Curvilinear regression model.

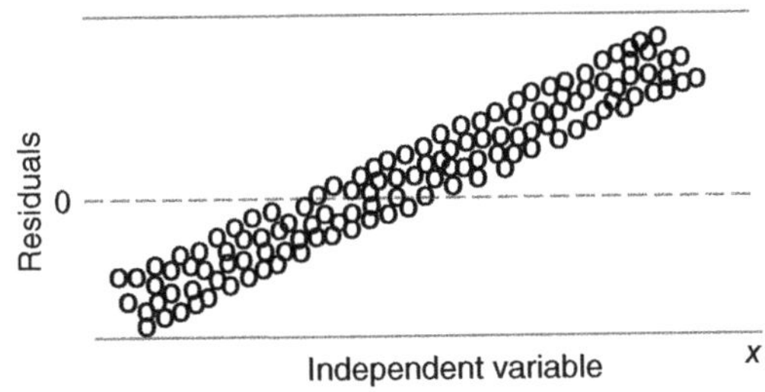

Figure 9.6 The error terms are related.

You may note that for low and high values of x, the residuals are positive and for middle values they are negative. This graph of the residuals is parabolic and not linear; therefore if you get the graph similar to this, the assumption of linearity will not hold true.

The assumption of independence of errors means that serial correlation should not occur between a given error term and itself over various time intervals. In other words, each error term should be independent of the error term next to it. In Figure 9.6, the error terms are not independent of each other because here the value of the residual is the function of the residual value preceding it. For example, a small positive residual occurs next to a small positive residual and a larger positive residual occurs next to a large positive residual.

The normality of residual terms can be tested by means of the normal plot (Q–Q plot). This plot can be obtained by using any of the statistical software. Figure 9.7 shows the plot of the residuals obtained by the Statistical Package for the Social Sciences (SPSS). The more the number of data close to the line, the better is the fit.

The assumption that the errors have constant variance is known as *homoscedasticity*. The meaning of this assumption is that the variations among the error terms are similar at different points of x. In other words, variation among the residuals for the higher, middle, and lower values of x should be similar. In Figure 9.8, the variance among the error terms is lower for small values of x and higher for greater values of x. This violates the assumptions of homoscedasticity. If this assumption

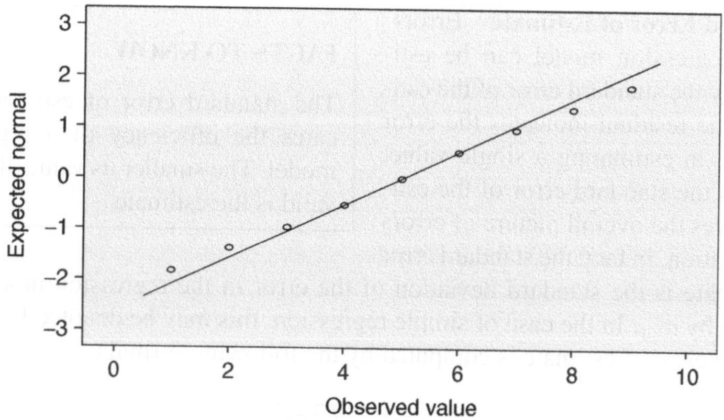

Figure 9.7 Normal Q–Q plot of the residuals.

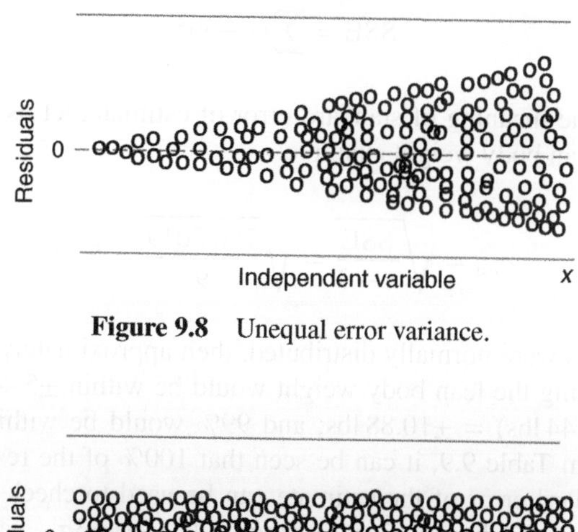

Figure 9.8 Unequal error variance.

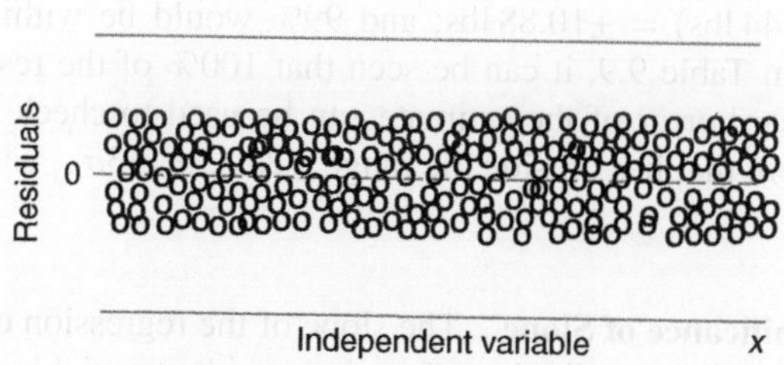

Figure 9.9 Healthy residual plots.

is not satisfied, then the regression equation will give an inaccurate estimate of the dependent variable.

If all the four assumptions of the regression model are satisfied, then the residual graph should look similar to the pattern shown in Figure 9.9. This is a healthy residual plot where the assumptions of linearity, independence of errors, normality of error terms, and homoscedasticity principle hold true.

> **FACTS TO KNOW**
>
> The standard error of estimate indicates the efficiency of a regression model. The smaller its value, the more valid is the estimate

Standard Error of Estimate Errors in the regression model can be estimated by the standard error of the estimate. The residual indicates the error involved in estimating a single value, whereas the standard error of the estimate gives the overall picture of errors in estimation. In fact, the standard error of estimate is the standard deviation of the error in the regression model and is denoted by σ_{est}. In the case of simple regression, this may be denoted by $\sigma_{y.x}$. The standard error of estimate is computed by the following formula:

$$\sigma_{\text{est}} = \sqrt{\frac{\text{SSE}}{n-2}} \tag{9.20}$$

where

$$\text{SSE} = \sum (y - \hat{y})^2$$

To understand the meaning of standard error of estimate, let us calculate σ_{est} for the data in the lean body weight example:

$$\sigma_{\text{est}} = \sqrt{\frac{\text{SSE}}{n-2}} = \sqrt{\frac{266.5019}{9}} = 5.44$$

If the error terms were normally distributed, then approximately 68% of the error terms in estimating the lean body weight would be within ±5.44 lbs; 95% would be within ±2(5.44 lbs) = ±10.88 lbs; and 99% would be within ±3(5.44 lbs) = ±16.32 lbs. From Table 9.9, it can be seen that 100% of the residuals are within $2\sigma_{\text{est}}$. The standard error of the estimate can be used to check the outlier in the dataset. Any score that lies outside the range $\pm 2\sigma_{\text{est}}$ or $\pm 3\sigma_{\text{est}}$ can be treated as an outlier.

Testing the Significance of Slope The slope of the regression equation indicates the importance of the contribution of an independent variable in estimating the value of the dependent variable. It is therefore important to test the significance of the slope in developing the regression equation. If the slope is not significant at any desired level for any independent variable, there is no point including it in the regression model. Let us first see how to test the hypothesis for the significance of the slope. The hypotheses that need to be tested are as follows.

$$H_0: \beta_1 = 0$$
$$H_1: \beta_1 \neq 0 \tag{9.21}$$

TABLE 9.9 Computation of Standard Error of Estimate

Height (cm) x	LBW (lb) y	$y-\hat{y}$	$(y-\hat{y})^2$
191.0	162.5	5.7840	33.454656
186.0	136.0	−4.4810	20.079361
191.5	163.5	5.1605	26.630760
188.0	154.0	7.0250	49.350625
190.0	149.0	−4.4690	19.971961
188.5	140.5	−8.0985	65.585702
193.0	157.3	−5.9100	34.928100
190.5	154.5	−0.5925	0.351056
189.0	151.5	1.2780	1.633284
192.0	160.5	0.5370	0.288369
187.0	147.5	3.7720	14.227984
		$\sum(y-\hat{y}) = 0.0055$	$\sum(y-\hat{y})^2 = 266.5019$

Here, β_1 is the population slope. It is required to test whether this population slope β_1 is significant on the basis of the sample slope b_1, calculated from the sample. Significance of this regression coefficient is tested by the following t-statistic:

$$t = \frac{b_1 - \beta_1}{\mathrm{SE}(b_1)} \tag{9.22}$$

where

$$\mathrm{SE}(b_1) = \frac{\sqrt{\frac{\sum(y-\hat{y})^2}{n-2}}}{\sqrt{\sum(x-\bar{x})^2}} \tag{9.23}$$

The expression for $\mathrm{SE}(b_1)$ can further be simplified as

$$\mathrm{SE}(b_1) = \frac{\sqrt{\frac{\sum(y-\hat{y})^2}{n-2}}}{\sqrt{\sum x^2 - \frac{\left(\sum x\right)^2}{n}}}$$

If the computed value of t in equation (9.22) is greater than the tabulated t at certain desired level of significance with $(n-2)$ degrees of freedom, then the null hypothesis in (9.21) is rejected and it is concluded that the slope is significant.

In the example of lean body weight, $b_1 = 3.25$, $\sum x = 2086.5$, $\sum x^2 = 395818.75$, and $\sum (y - \hat{y})^2 = 266.5019$

$$\text{SE}(b_1) = \frac{\sqrt{\dfrac{\sum (y-\hat{y})^2}{n-2}}}{\sqrt{\sum x^2 - \dfrac{\left(\sum x\right)^2}{n}}} = \frac{\sqrt{\dfrac{266.5019}{11-2}}}{\sqrt{395818.75 - \dfrac{2086.5^2}{11}}} = \frac{5.4416}{6.90191} = 0.788$$

$$t = \frac{b_1}{\text{SE}(b_1)} = \frac{3.25}{0.788} = 4.12$$

The tabulated value of t at significance level 0.05 and at 9 degrees of freedom (from Table A.7) is 2.262. Since the calculated t is greater than the tabulated t, the null hypothesis may be rejected; it may be concluded that the slope is significant and the variable height is a useful predictor in the regression model.

The significance of the slope can be tested directly by the t-value obtained in the output by using any statistical software package. The regression analysis output for the data of the lean body weight example using SPSS software has been shown in Table 9.10.

You may note that the t-value calculated above is same as that obtained in the SPSS output. Similarly, the value of the slope and intercept computed in the example are also the same as that shown in the output, except for the slight difference due to approximating fractional values.

Testing the Significance of the Model If the slope in a simple regression is significant, it indicates that the independent variable is worth including in the regression model. Next, we need to see whether the model as a whole is significant or not. The significance of the model can be tested by computing the F-value for the regression. If the F-value is significant, then the model is significant and it can be used for estimating the value of the dependent variable on the basis of the independent

TABLE 9.10 Regression Analysis Output for the Lean Body Weight Data

	Unstandardized Coefficients		Standardized Coefficients		
Model	B	Std. Error	Beta	t	Sig.
1 (Constant)	−463.468	149.559		−3.099	0.013
Height	3.247	0.788	0.808	4.118	0.003

Dependent Variable: Lean body weight $R = 0.808$, $R^2 = 0.653$, Adjusted $R^2 = 0.615$

variable(s). Since in simple regression only one independent variable is used, the value of F can be obtained by simply squaring the "t" value obtained while testing the significance of the slope (regression coefficient). Since the value of t in the lean body weight example is 4.12, the value of F would be

$$F = t^2 = 4.12^2 = 16.9744$$

While doing regression analysis by using any statistical package, the value F is automatically calculated, but to understand the procedure, let us see as to how it is computed.

In regression analysis, the dependent variable (y) is estimated on the basis of independent variable(s); therefore, the total variability in the dependent variable is the sum total of the two components as shown by the following model:

$$\text{Total variability in } Y = \text{variability due to regression} + \text{variability due to error}$$

or

$$\begin{aligned}\text{Total SS(TSS)} &= \text{sum of squares due to regression (SSR)}\\ &\quad + \text{sum of squares due to error in regression (SSE)}\end{aligned}$$

Thus,

$$\text{TSS} = \text{SSR} + \text{SSE} \tag{9.24}$$

These terms can be computed by the following formulas:

$$\text{TSS} = \sum (y - \bar{y})^2 \tag{9.25}$$

$$\text{SSR} = \sum (\hat{y} - \bar{y})^2 \tag{9.26}$$

$$\text{SSE} = \sum (y - \hat{y})^2 \tag{9.27}$$

Let us calculate various terms required for computing the F-value in the example on lean body weight. These computations are shown in Table 9.11.

$$\text{TSS} = \sum (y - \bar{y})^2 = 768.74$$

$$\text{SSE} = \sum (y - \hat{y})^2 = 266.5$$

$$\text{SSR} = \text{TSS} - \text{SSE} = 502.24$$

$$\text{MSR} = \text{SSR}/c = 502.24/1 = 502.24 \quad [c : \text{number of independent variable}]$$

$$\text{MSE} = \text{SSE}/(n - c - 1) = 266.5/(11 - 1 - 1) = 29.61 \quad [n : \text{sample size}]$$

$$F = \frac{\text{MSR}}{\text{MSE}} = \frac{502.24}{29.61} = 16.96, \quad F_{0.05}(1, 9) = 5.12$$

TABLE 9.11 Computation of the Terms for the *F*-Value

Height (cm) x	LBW (lb) y	$\hat{y}$	$(y-\bar{y})$	$(y-\bar{y})^2$	$y-\hat{y}$	$(y-\hat{y})^2$
191.0	162.5	156.7160	10.06	101.28	5.78	33.45
186.0	136.0	140.4810	−16.44	270.15	−4.48	20.08
191.5	163.5	158.3395	11.06	122.40	5.16	26.63
188.0	154.0	146.9750	1.56	2.44	7.02	49.35
190.0	149.0	153.4690	−3.44	11.81	−4.47	19.97
188.5	140.5	148.5985	−11.94	142.48	−8.10	65.59
193.0	157.3	163.2100	4.86	23.65	−5.91	34.93
190.5	154.5	155.0925	2.06	4.26	−0.59	0.35
189.0	151.5	150.2220	−0.94	0.88	1.28	1.63
192.0	160.5	159.9630	8.06	65.02	0.54	0.29
187.0	147.5	143.7280	−4.94	24.37	3.77	14.23
	$\bar{y} = 152.44$			$\sum(y-\bar{y})^2 = 768.74$		$\sum(y-\hat{y})^2 = 266.5$

Remark MSR is the mean sum of squares due to regression, and MSE is the mean sum of squares due to error in regression.

Since calculated value of F is greater than tabulated F, the model as a whole is significant. You may note that the calculated value of F is the same as that calculated above by squaring the t-value except for the rounding-off error. All standard statistical software packages provide the ANOVA table as a part of the standard output while performing regression analysis. Table 9.12 is the ANOVA table provided by the SPSS software in its output for the data of the lean body example. You may note that the F-value for the regression shown in the table is same as that calculated above.

In simple regression, where only one independent variable is used in developing the regression line, the significance of the regression coefficient is equivalent to the significance of the entire regression model. However, this differs in the case of multiple regression as many independent variables are used in the model.

TABLE 9.12 ANOVA Table for the Lean Body Weight Data

Model	Sum of Squares	df	Mean Square	Facts to Know	Sig.
2 Regression	502.244	1	502.244	16.961	0.003
Residual	266.502	9	29.611		
Total	768.745	10			

a. Predictors: (Constant), Height
b. Dependent Variable: LBW

Coefficient of Determination (R_2)

In simple regression, the coefficient of determination R^2 is similar to r^2. In regression analysis, it can be defined as the proportion of variation in the dependent variable accounted for by the independent variable(s) in the regression model. It can take any value between 0 and 1. If R^2 is 1, it indicates that 100% variation in the dependent variable can be explained by all the variables in the regression model, whereas the value of 0 indicates that there is no relationship between the predictor variables and dependent variable. The value of R^2 can be calculated from the ANOVA table generated by any of the statistical packages while doing the regression analysis. R^2 is calculated by the following formula:

> **FACTS TO KNOW**
>
> R^2 explains the percentage variability in the dependent variable as explained by the independent variable(s) in the model

$$R^2 = \frac{\text{SSR}}{\text{SS}_{yy}} = 1 - \frac{\text{SSE}}{\text{SS}_{yy}} \tag{9.28}$$

where SSR is the sum of squares due to regression, SSE is the sum of squares due to regression error, and SS_{yy} is the total sum of squares (TSS). In the lean body weight example, SSR = 502.24 and SS_{yy}=768.74.

Thus

$$R^2 = \frac{502.24}{768.74} = 0.653$$

It can be seen from Table 9.10 that the value of R^2 computed by the SPSS is the same as that computed here. This simply indicates that the 65.3% variation in the lean body weight can be explained by the height variable.

Example 9.4 In a study, the heights of 20 boys and their fathers were recorded and the following statistics were calculated on the data obtained.

Statistics of Height Data

	Father x	Son y
Mean	170	175
SD	2.5	2.0
r	.6	

Construct a regression line and estimate the expected height of a son if his father's height is 172 cm.

Solution: Here, y is to be estimated when x is 172. Thus, it is required to develop a regression equation of y on x which can be written as

$$\hat{y} - \bar{y} = b_1(x - \bar{x})$$

where

$$b_1 = r\frac{\sigma_y}{\sigma_x}$$

Substituting the values of $\bar{x}$, $\bar{y}$, r, σ_x, and σ_y

$$\hat{y} - 175 = 0.6 \times \frac{2}{2.5}(x - 170)$$

$$\hat{y} = 0.48x - 0.48 \times 170 + 175$$

$$\Rightarrow \qquad \hat{y} = 0.48x + 93.4$$

Since $x = 172$,

$$\hat{y} = 0.48 \times 172 + 93.4 = 175.96$$

Thus, corresponding to the father's height of 172 cm, the son's height would be 175.96 cm.

Example 9.5 In a study, the heights (in centimeters) and weights (in kilograms) of 25 badminton players were measured. The mean and standard deviation were calculated for these variables along with the correlation coefficient between them. The statistics so calculated are shown in the following table. Construct the regression equation for estimating the weight by using the height as a predictor. What would be the predicted weight of a badminton player if his height is 168 cm?

Anthropometric Measurements on the Badminton Players

	Height x	Weight y
Mean	175	58
SD	3.2	4.0
r		0.75

Solution: In this problem, the weight (y) is to be estimated if the height (x) is known. Thus, it is required to develop a regression equation of y on x. The regression equation can be constructed by using the following equation:

$$\hat{y} - \bar{y} = b_1(x - \bar{x})$$

where

$$b_1 = r\frac{\sigma_y}{\sigma_x}$$

Substituting the values of $\overline{x}$, $\overline{y}$, r, σ_x, and σ_y

$$\hat{y} - 58 = 0.75 \times \frac{4}{3.2}(x - 175)$$

$$\hat{y} = 0.9375x - 0.9375 \times 175 + 58$$

$$\Rightarrow \quad \hat{y} = 0.9375x - 106.0625$$

Given that $x = 168$, $\hat{y} = 0.9375 \times 168 + 106.0625 = 51.44$.

Thus, if the height of a badminton player is 168 cm, his estimated weight would be 51.44 kg.

Example 9.6 Six sportsmen were tested for their body weight x (in kilograms) and body fat y (in percentage). Develop a regression line for estimating the body fat.

Body Weight (in kg)	Body Fat (in %)
85	14.5
75	13.5
82	15.5
86	15
81	14
88	16

Do the following:

a. Test the significance of the regression coefficient at the significance level 0.05.
b. Compute the standard error of estimate and interpret your findings.
c. Compute r^2 and interpret it.

Solution:

i. *Developing the regression line* To develop a regression line for estimating the fat percentage (y) on the basis of body weight (x), it is required to compute $\sum x$, $\sum y$, $\sum x^2$, and $\sum xy$.

Computation for the Regression Equation

Body Weight (in kg) x	Body Fat (in %) y	x^2	y^2	xy
85	14.5	7225	210.25	1232.5
75	13.5	5625	182.25	1012.5
82	15.5	6724	240.25	1271
86	15	7396	225	1290
81	14	6561	196	1134
88	16	7744	256	1408
$\sum x = 497$	$\sum y = 88.5$	$\sum x^2 = 41275$	$\sum y^2 = 1309.75$	$\sum xy = 7348$

Since

$$b_1 = \frac{SS_{xy}}{SS_{xx}} \text{ and } b_0 = \frac{\sum y}{n} - b_1\frac{\sum x}{n}$$

$$SS_{xy} = \sum xy - \frac{1}{n}\left(\sum x\right)\left(\sum y\right) = 7348 - \frac{1}{6} \times 497 \times 88.5 = 17.25$$

$$SS_{xx} = \sum x^2 - \frac{1}{n}\left(\sum x\right)^2 = 41275 - \frac{1}{6} \times 497^2 = 106.83$$

$$\text{Slope} = b_1 = \frac{17.25}{106.83} = 0.1615$$

$$\text{Intercept} = b_0 = \frac{88.5}{6} - 0.1615 \times \frac{497}{6} = 1.3724$$

Thus, the regression equation can be constructed by substituting the values of the intercept b_0 and slope b_1 in the following equation:

$$y = b_0 + b_1 x$$

$$\Rightarrow \quad y = 1.3724 + 0.1615x$$

or

$$\text{Body fat in \%} = 1.3724 + 0.1615 \text{ (Body weight in kg)}$$

Since the regression coefficient $b_1 = 0.1615$, it indicates that if the body weight of the sportsmen is increased by 1 kg, the body fat would increase by 0.1615%.

ii. *Testing the significance of the regression coefficient* The null hypothesis that needs to be tested is given by

$$H_0 : \beta_1 = 0$$

against

$$H_1\colon \beta_1 \neq 0$$

Here, β_1 is the population slope. It is required to test whether β_1 is significant on the basis of the sample slope $b_1 = 0.1545$, computed from the sample. Significance of this regression coefficient can be tested by using the following t-statistic:

$$t = \frac{b_1 - \beta_1}{\mathrm{SE}(b_1)}$$

where

$$\mathrm{SE}(b_1) = \frac{\sqrt{\frac{\sum (y-\hat{y})^2}{n-2}}}{\sqrt{\sum (x-\bar{x})^2}} = \frac{\sqrt{\frac{\sum (y-\hat{y})^2}{n-2}}}{\sqrt{\sum x^2 - \frac{\left(\sum x\right)^2}{n}}}$$

Computation for the Residual, Standard Error, and r^2

Body Weight (in kg) x	Body Fat (in %) y	$\hat{y}$	$y-\hat{y}$	$(y-\hat{y})^2$
85	14.5	15.0999	−0.5999	0.35988001
75	13.5	13.4849	0.0151	0.00022801
82	15.5	14.6154	0.8846	0.78251716
86	15.0	15.2614	−0.2614	0.06832996
81	14.0	14.4539	−0.4539	0.20602521
88	16.0	15.5844	0.4156	0.17272336
$\sum x = 497$	$\sum y = 81$		$\sum (y-\hat{y}) = -0.0001$	$\sum (y-\hat{y})^2 = 1.59$

Here, $b_1 = 0.1615$, $\sum x = 497$, $\sum x^2 = 41275$, and $\sum (y-\hat{y})^2 = 1.59$

$$\mathrm{SE}(b_1) = \frac{\sqrt{\frac{\sum (y-\hat{y})^2}{n-2}}}{\sqrt{\sum x^2 - \frac{\left(\sum x\right)^2}{n}}}$$

$$= \frac{\sqrt{\frac{1.59}{6-2}}}{\sqrt{41275 - \frac{497^2}{6}}} = \frac{0.6305}{10.336} = 0.061$$

Substituting the value of SE(b_1),

$$t = \frac{b_1}{\mathrm{SE}(b_1)} = \frac{0.1615}{0.0610} = 2.65$$

The tabulated value of t at significance level 0.05 and 4 degrees of freedom is 2.776 (from Table A.7). Since the calculated t is less than the tabulated t, the null hypothesis is failed to be rejected. It may therefore be concluded that the slope is not significant.

iii. *Computing the standard error of estimate* The standard error of estimate is given by

$$\sigma_{\mathrm{est}} = \sqrt{\frac{\sum (y-\hat{y})^2}{n-2}} = \sqrt{\frac{1.59}{4}} = 0.630$$

Since one of the assumptions of the regression analysis is that the error term is normally distributed, it can be interpreted that while estimating the body fat from the body weight, approximately 68% of the error terms (residuals) would be within ±0.630%, 95% would be within ±2(0.630%) = ±1.260% and 99% would be within ±3(0.630%) = ±1.890%.

iv. *Computing R^2*

$$R^2 = 1 - \frac{\mathrm{SSE}}{\mathrm{SS}_{yy}}$$

$$= 1 - \frac{\sum (y-\hat{y})^2}{\sum y^2 - \frac{\left(\sum y\right)^2}{n}}$$

$$= 1 - \frac{1.59}{1309.75 - \frac{88.5^2}{6}}$$

$$= 1 - \frac{1.59}{4.375} = 0.637$$

Check Your Progress

Note: Tick the correct answer by using the sign (√).

	True	False
36. In simple regression, there can be two independent variables in the model.	-	-
37. The value b_1 is known as the y-intercept and b_0 is known as the slope.	-	-

38. In simple regression analysis, significance of β_1 indicates the predictability of the independent variable.	-	-
39. In simple regression analysis, if the model is significant, it does not necessarily mean that the regression coefficient is also significant.	-	-
40. In regression analysis, the line of best fit is the one for which the sum of squared deviations of y from its estimated value is maximum.	-	-
41. A residual can be calculated by $\overline{y} - \hat{y}$.	-	-
42. The regression coefficient b_1 can be computed by SS_{xy}/SS_{xx}.	-	-
43. The residuals can be defined as the estimates of the regression error.	-	-
44. The term heteroscedasticity refers to the constant variance of the errors.	-	-
45. The value β_1 is known as population regression coefficient, whereas b_1 is known as sample regression coefficient.	-	-
46. The assumptions of regression analysis can be tested by using the residual plot.	-	-
47. In regression analysis, the variation among the error terms should be different at different points of the independent variable.	-	-
48. In the least squares method, the sum of the squared deviations of all the observed scores y_i from their estimated values $\hat{y}_i$ is minimized.	-	-
49. In regression analysis, each error term should depend on the error term next to it.	-	-
50. A residual is the difference between the observed and estimated values of y.	-	-
51. The regression coefficient b_1 can also be calculated from σ_y/σ_x.	-	-
52. In regression analysis, there should not be any serial correlation among the residual and itself over various time intervals.	-	-
53. The formula for computing the standard error is $\sqrt{SSE/(n-1)}$.	-	-
54. One of the assumptions in simple regression analysis is that the error ε_i is normally distributed.	-	-

55. The standard error of estimate is the standard deviation of residuals. - -
56. Residuals can be used to find the outliers. - -
57. The regression constant b_0 can be calculated by $\bar{y} - b_1\bar{x}$. - -
58. In simple regression, the residual plot is obtained by plotting the residual along the x-axis and the independent variable along the y-axis. - -
59. One of the assumptions of regression analysis is that the errors are independent. - -
60. The mean of the residuals is 1. - -
61. The normality of the residuals can be tested by using the Q–Q plot. - -
62. The standard error of estimate is the error involved in estimating a single value. - -
63. The SSE is computed as $\sum(y - \hat{y})^2$. - -
64. If R^2 is 0.637, it can be interpreted that 63.7% variation in the dependent variable can be explained by the independent variables. - -

PRACTICE EXERCISE

11. In a regression analysis, if the value of multiple correlation is 0.85 what is the efficiency of prediction of the regression model?
12. While doing regression analysis, if the multiple correlation is reported to be 0.94, what would be the efficiency of the predicting model?
13. The regression equation for the data mentioned below is $\hat{y} = 28.33 - 0.54x$

X	Y
4	30
8	25
15	18
24	12
35	7
44	4
55	2

Find the residuals and graph the residual plot. Do these data violate any of the assumptions of regression analysis?

14. Find the regression equation for estimating Y by using the following data and compute the residuals.

X	Y
10	6
18	8
14	5
16	7
9	4
15	9

15. Draw a residual plot on the basis of the following data and indicate which of the assumptions for the regression are not followed. Compute the standard error of estimate.

X	$y-\hat{y}$	$(y-\hat{y})^2$
3	8	64
4	4	16
5	−1	1
6	−13	169
7	−3	9
8	3	9
9	7	49
10	11	121

16. The regression line developed for predicting the fat percentage of college boys on the basis of their weights is $\hat{y} = -19.5 + 0.5x$.

Weight x	Fat%y	$\hat{y}$	$(y-\hat{y})^2$	x^2	y^2
63	13	12	1	3969	169
68	14	14.5	0.25	4624	196
70	15	15.5	0.25	4900	225
64	12	12.5	0.25	4096	144
62	11	11.5	0.25	3844	121
69	16	15	1	4761	256

The estimated value of y has been computed by using the regression line. Compute the following on the basis of the information in the above table.

a. standard error of estimate
b. standardized regression coefficient
c. R^2 and adjusted R^2
d. t-value for testing the significance of the regression coefficient at 5% level

9.8 THE MULTIPLE REGRESSION MODEL

In most situations, the dependent variable cannot be estimated by using only one independent variable, and in such situations the regression model is developed by using more than one independent variable. For instance, estimating fat percentage on the basis of weight alone may be less reliable than estimating it with the help of weight as well as waist circumference. The regression model may be further improved if hip circumference is also added as a predictor along with weight and waist circumference. The regression analysis in which more than one independent variable is used for developing the regression model is known as *multiple regression analysis*. Conceptually, multiple regression analysis is similar to simple regression; the only difference is that in multiple regression more than one independent variable is used for estimation as against one independent variable in simple regression. However, computation becomes very tedious in multiple regression analysis. If y is the dependent variable and $x_1, x_2, x_3, \ldots, x_c$ are the c independent variables in the population, then the multiple regression equation is written as follows:

$$\hat{y} = \beta_0 + \beta_1 x_1 + \beta_2 x_2 + \ldots + \beta_c x_c \tag{9.29}$$

where

$\hat{y}$ = estimated value of dependent variable y in the population
β_0 = population regression constant
β_1 = population partial regression coefficient for x_1
β_2 = population partial regression coefficient for x_2
β_3 = population partial regression coefficient for x_3
β_c = population partial regression coefficient for x_c

Here, the β_i's are population partial regression coefficients and are similar to the full regression coefficient β in the simple regression (bivariate) model. Since in simple regression, a single independent variable is the sole predictor, β_1 is known as the *full regression coefficient*, whereas in a multiple regression model, many independent variables are used as predictors, hence the β_i's are known as *partial regression coefficients*. The partial regression coefficient β_i represents the amount of increase in the dependent variable y with one unit increase in the independent variable x_i if all other independent variables are held constant. In multiple regression, the dependent variable is also known as the *response variable*.

In almost all research studies, the multiple regression model is developed by using sample data, hence the population regression coefficients $\beta_1, \beta_2, \ldots, \beta_c$ are estimated by the sample regression coefficients $b_1, b_2, \ldots, b_c$, respectively. Thus, in multiple regression analysis, it is required to develop the best-fitted model for the sampled data as shown by equation (9.30):

$$\hat{y} = b_0 + b_1x_1 + b_2x_2 + \ldots + b_cx_c \tag{9.30}$$

where

$\hat{y}$ = estimated value of dependent variable, y, in the sample
b_0 = sample regression constant
b_1 = estimate of regression coefficient for x_1
b_2 = estimate of regression coefficient for x_2
b_3 = estimate of regression coefficient for x_3
b_c = estimate of regression coefficient for x_c

Any specific sample value y_i can be written as follows:

$$y_i = b_0 + b_1x_1 + b_2x_2 + \ldots + b_cx_c + \varepsilon_i \tag{9.31}$$

where ε_i is the error of prediction for y_i. The regression constant and regression coefficients $b_0, b_1, \ldots, b_c$ are determined in such a manner so that the sum of squared deviations of the dependent variable y from its estimated value $\hat{y}$ for all the n scores in the sample is minimized, that is, S^2, as shown below, needs to be minimized.

$$S^2 = \sum_{i=1}^{n} (y_i - \hat{y}_i)^2 = \sum_{i=1}^{n} \varepsilon_i^2 = \sum_{i=1}^{n} (y_i - b_0 - b_1x_1 - b_2x_2 - \ldots - b_cx_c)^2 \tag{9.32}$$

The procedure of finding these constants so that the S^2 is minimized shall be shown by using a model with two independent variables.

9.8.1 Procedure for Developing the Regression Equation with Two Independent Variables

In developing a regression equation for estimating a dependent variable, y, on the basis of two independent variables x_1 and x_2 in the sample, the constants b_0, b_1, and b_2 are determined in such a manner that S^2 given below is the least. For this reason, the procedure used in developing the regression equation is known as the *least squares method.*

$$S^2 = \sum_{i=1}^{n} \varepsilon_i^2 = \sum_{i=1}^{n} (y_i - b_0 - b_1x_1 - b_2x_2)^2$$

Differentiating S^2 with respect to b_0, b_1, and b_2 and equating the results to zero will give the following normal equations.

$$\sum y = b_0 n + b_1 \sum x_1 + b_2 \sum x_2 \tag{9.33}$$

$$\sum x_1 y = b_0 \sum x_1 + b_1 \sum x_1^2 + b_2 \sum x_1 x_2 \tag{9.34}$$

$$\sum x_2 y = b_0 \sum x_2 + b_1 \sum x_1 x_2 + b_2 \sum x_2^2 \tag{9.35}$$

These are the three equations with three unknowns b_0, b_1, and b_2. Solving these equations shall provide the values of b_0, b_1, and b_2 for which S^2 would be the least. Using the values of these constants, the regression equation can be constructed as shown in equation (9.36):

$$\hat{y} = b_0 + b_1x_1 + b_2x_2 \tag{9.36}$$

Computing regression coefficients and regression constants in developing a multiple regression model is tedious if attempted manually, and therefore statistical packages are invariably used in the analysis.

9.8.2 Developing a Multiple Regression Model

To understand the procedure in developing a multiple regression model, let us consider the data on standing broad jump obtained on college athletes. It was desired to know the independent variables that contribute to the performance of standing broad jump. Many variables were explored, and finally it was decided to develop a regression model by taking the three independent variables, namely, height, leg length, and leg strength. The data on these variables along with the performance on standing broad jump of 10 college athletes are shown in Table 9.13.

Many statistical software packages can be used for multiple regression analysis. All these packages provide the same results in different formats. Table 9.14 gives the outputs of the multiple regression analysis obtained by using the SPSS software for the data shown in Table 9.13. The sequence of commands in SPSS for regression analysis after making the data file is as follows:

Analyze ⟶ Regression ⟶ Linear

TABLE 9.13 Athletes' Data for Estimating Standing Broad Jump

Standing Broad Jump (m) y	Leg Length (cm) x_1	Leg Strength (kg) x_2	Height (cm) x_3
2.80	101	68	168
1.87	92	52.5	156
2.65	98	69	160
2.85	103	69	173
1.98	**96**	**50**	**168**
2.50	100	70	165
1.99	91	55.5	155
2.80	101	68.5	178
1.82	91	54	156
2.18	92	65	160

TABLE 9.14 Regression Analysis Output for the Standing Broad Jump Data

Part I: Regression Coefficients with Corresponding t-Test

Model	Unstandardized Coefficients		Standardized Coefficients		
	B	Std. Error	Beta	t	Sig.
2 (Constant)	−4.013	0.805		−4.988	0.002
leg length	0.050	0.011	0.558	4.549	0.003
leg strength	0.025	0.006	0.487	3.967	0.005

Dependent Variable: Standing broad jump

Part II: Excluded Variables

Model	Beta in	t	Sig.
Height	0.081	0.456	0.664

Part III: ANOVA Table

Model	Sum of Squares	df	Mean Square	F	Sig.
2 Regression	1.500	2	0.750	71.486	0.000
Residual	0.073	7	0.010		
Total	1.574	9			

Predictors: (Constant), leg length, leg strength
Dependent Variable: standing broad jump

Part IV: Model Summary

R	*R* Square	Adjusted *R* Square	Std. Error of the Estimate
0.976	0.953	0.940	0.1024411871

After selecting the dependent and independent variables from the data file, check the options "R squared change" and "Descriptive" by clicking the tag **Statistics**. Click **OK** to proceed further. Click the **Method** tag to select the option "Stepwise." Click **OK** to get the output. The detailed procedure for multiple regression analysis using SPSS can be seen in the book (Verma, 2011).

You may note from Part I of the output shown in Table 9.14 that only two variables, namely, leg length and leg strength have been retained in the model, whereas height has been excluded. Thus, by using the values of $b_0 = -4.013$, $b_1 = 0.050$, and $b_2 = 0.025$, the regression equation as shown in equation (9.37) can be developed.

$$\hat{y} = -4.013 + 0.050x_1 + 0.025x_2 \tag{9.37}$$

Let us see for leg length (x_1) = 96 cm and leg strength (x_2) = 50 kg, what is the estimated value of the standing broad jump (y).

$$\hat{y} = -4.013 + 0.050 \times 96 + 0.025 \times 50 = 2.037 \text{ m}$$

It can be seen from Table 9.13 that for these values of leg length and leg strength, the actual value of standing broad jump is 1.98 m. Thus, the residual for this dataset is 0.057 m (2.037 − 1.98). In other words, 0.057 m is the error in estimating the standing broad jump performance of an athlete whose leg length is 96 cm and leg strength is 50 kg.

Let us see what the regression constant and regression coefficients of x_1 and x_2 indicate. The regression constant −4.013 is the y-intercept. Describing the y-intercept is meaningless. It is meaningless to say that the standing broad jump performance would be −4.013 if an athlete's leg length and leg strength are zero.

The coefficient for the leg length (x_1) is 0.050. This indicates that by increasing the leg length by 1 cm, the standing broad jump would increase by 0.050 m if the leg strength is held constant.

The coefficient for the leg strength (x_2) is 0.025. This means that by increasing the leg strength by 1 kg, the standing broad jump would increase by 0.025 m if the leg length is held constant.

In many statistical software packages, the regression constant and partial regression coefficients are named as *unstandardized coefficients*.

9.8.3 Standardized Regression Coefficients

> **FACTS TO KNOW**
>
> Standardized regression coefficients indicate the relative importance of independent variables in the model

In a multiple regression model, different independent variables have different units and therefore by comparing the magnitudes of the regression coefficients of different independent variables, it is not possible to infer as to which variable is the most important for the model. In other words, by looking at these coefficients, one cannot find the relative importance of the independent variables in the regression model in estimating the dependent variable. To solve this problem, standardized partial regression coefficients are computed for each of the independent variables. The regression equation so obtained by using the standardized partial regression coefficients is known as the *regression equation in the standardized form*. These standardized partial regression coefficients are nothing but the partial correlations of the dependent variable and corresponding variable after eliminating the effect of other variables in the model. The standardized multiple regression equation in which two independent variables x_1 and x_2 are used for estimating the dependent variable y can be represented as follows:

$$z_y = r_{y1.2}z_1 + r_{y2.1}z_2 \tag{9.38}$$

Here, the variables are in the standard score form. Since these partial regression coefficients can assume values between −1 and 1 and are free from units, the relative importance of the independent variables for the model can be known by comparing the magnitudes of these coefficients. In SPSS, these partial regression coefficients are known as *standardized coefficients*.

It can be seen from the SPSS output in part I of Table 9.14 that the standardized coefficients for the leg length (0.558) is more than that of the leg strength (0.487); hence, one can say that the leg length is more important in comparison to leg strength in predicting the standing broad jump performance of an athlete by the developed regression model.

9.9 DIFFERENT WAYS OF TESTING A REGRESSION MODEL

The regression model can be developed for any set of data, provided the dependent and independent variables are measured at least on an interval scale. However, if the independent variables are measured on a categorical scale also, then that can also be used in the model by creating a dummy variable. Once the regression model is developed, it is required to be tested as to how far it fits into the dataset. Testing the model for its efficiency can be done in many ways as discussed below.

9.9.1 Testing the Significance of Overall Model

In multiple regression analysis, the significance of the model is tested by using the F-ratio calculated in the ANOVA table. Here, the variation due to regression is compared with the variation due to error (residual). The analysis of variance model for testing the significance of the regression model is given by

$$\text{TSS} = \text{SSR} + \text{SSE}$$

where TSS is the total sum of squares of the dependent variable y, which is obtained by $\text{TSS} = \sum (y - \bar{y})^2$, SSR is the sum of squares due to regression obtained by $\text{SSR} = \sum (\hat{y} - \bar{y})^2$, and SSE is the sum of the squares due to residuals obtained by $\text{SSE} = \sum (y - \hat{y})^2$. The detailed procedure for computing these sums of squares has already been shown while discussing simple regression analysis. In testing the significance of the overall model, the hypotheses that are required to be tested are as follows:

$$H_0\colon \beta_1 = \beta_2 = \dots = \beta_c = 0$$

$$H_1\colon \text{At least one regression coefficient } \neq 0$$

To test the null hypothesis, the F-value is computed. If this value is significant, H_0 is rejected and it is interpreted that there is at least one independent variable that has significant predictability in the model. On the other hand, if the researcher fails to reject the null hypothesis, it shows that no independent variable has a significant predictability in the model.

In the standing broad jump example, the value of F is 71.486 as shown in the SPSS output part III in Table 9.14. This F-value is significant because its significance value is 0.000, which is less than 0.05. Thus, it may be concluded that the regression model (9.37) is significant.

9.9.2 Testing the Significance of Regression Coefficients

In multiple regression analysis, the significance of each regression coefficient is tested by using the t-test. The procedure for testing has been discussed in detail in simple regression analysis. The hypotheses that are tested in multiple regression analysis for the significance of regression coefficients are as follows:

$$H_0\colon \beta_1 = 0 \;\; H_0\colon \beta_2 = 0 \;\; H_0\colon \beta_3 = 0$$

$$H_1\colon \beta_1 \neq 0 \;\; H_1\colon \beta_2 \neq 0 \;\; H_1\colon \beta_3 \neq 0$$

Almost all standard statistical software packages provide the values of t for testing the significance of individual regression coefficients. In the standing broad jump example, the values of t for all the three variables have been shown in the SPSS output parts I and II. The value of t for height (0.456) is not significant; however, the t-values of leg length (4.549) and leg strength (3.967) are significant because their significance values are 0.003 and 0.005, respectively. Since the t-values for the leg length and leg strength are significant, they are included in the model. Since the larger the value of t, more significant is the predictability of that variable, the leg length has more predictability in comparison to leg strength in predicting the lean body weight. Only those variables are kept in the regression model for which the t-values are significant; therefore, the variables such as leg length and leg strength have been included in the regression model, whereas height has not.

9.9.3 Analyzing the Residuals

A residual is the difference between the observed and estimated values of the dependent variable y. It is computed by $y - \hat{y}$. The computation of residuals for the standing broad jump example has been shown in Table 9.15. The estimated value for each score of y has been obtained by using the regression equation (9.37).

Thus, for leg length $(x_1) = 92$ m and leg strength $(x_2) = 52.5$ kg, the estimated value of standing broad jump $(\hat{y})$ would be

$$\hat{y} = -4.013 + 0.050x_1 + 0.025x_2 = -4.013 + 0.050 \times 92 + 0.025 \times 52.5 = 1.8995$$

It can be seen from Table 9.15 that the maximum and minimum residuals are 0.237 and 0.012, respectively. These two residuals are the worst and best cases in estimation. The residuals can be used to find the outliers through the residual plot.

In case of simple regression, the residual plot is obtained by plotting the residuals against the independent variable x, but in multiple regression, it is obtained by plotting the residuals against the estimated value $\hat{y}$ of the dependent variable y because it involves multiple independent variables.

The assumptions of multiple regression are similar to that of simple regression. The residual plot can be used to test the assumptions of multiple regression. The residual plot in Figure 9.10 shows that the variation of residuals is not same at the

TABLE 9.15 Computation of Residuals

Standing Broad Jump (m) y	Leg Length (cm) x_1	Leg Strength (kg) x_2	Estimated Value $\hat{y}$	Residuals $y - \hat{y}$	$(y - \hat{y})^2$
2.80	101	68.0	2.7370	0.0630	0.00396900
1.87	92	52.5	1.8995	−0.0295	0.00087025
2.65	98	69.0	2.6120	0.0380	0.00144400
2.85	**103**	**69.0**	**2.8620**	**−0.0120**	**0.00014400**
1.98	96	50.0	2.0370	−0.0570	.00324900
2.50	**100**	**70.0**	**2.7370**	**−0.2370**	**0.05616900**
1.99	91	55.5	1.9245	0.0655	0.00429025
2.80	101	68.5	2.7495	0.0505	0.00255025
1.82	91	54	1.8870	−0.0670	0.00448900
2.18	92	65	2.2120	−0.0320	0.00102400
					$\sum(y - \hat{y})^2 = 0.07819875$

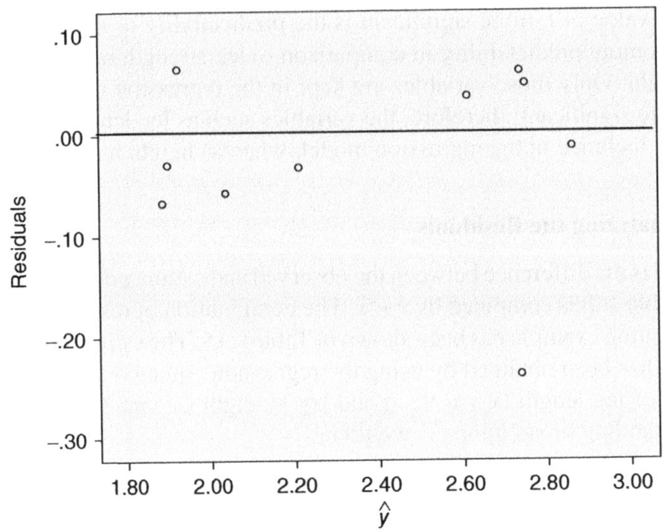

Figure 9.10 Residual plots for the standing broad jump example.

lower and higher ends of the estimated values of the dependent variable y. However, it is difficult to draw any conclusion with this plot because the sample size is too small. If the variation becomes too high at different points, then one can suspect violation of the homoscedasticity assumption.

The normal probability plot of the residuals shown in Figure 9.11 reveals that the residuals are not close to the straight line; this suggests the nonnormality of the

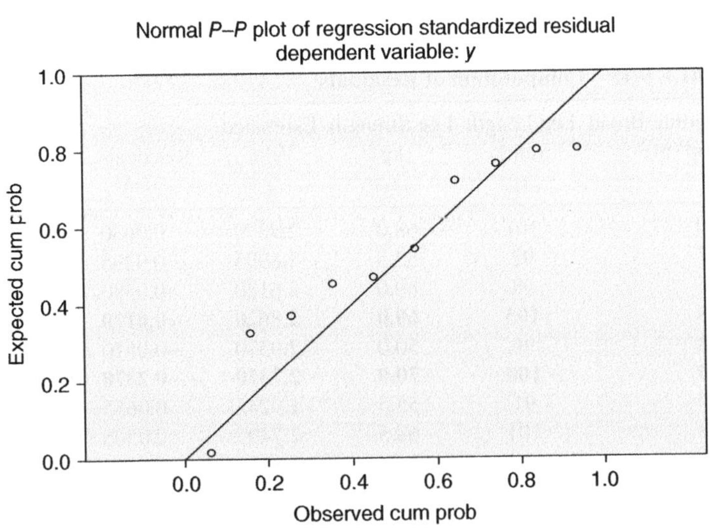

Figure 9.11 Normal probability plot of the residuals.

TABLE 9.16 Tests for Normality

	Kolmogorov–Smirnov			Shapiro–Wilk		
	Statistics	df	Sig.	Statistic	df	Sig.
Residuals	0.208	10	0.200*	0.842	10	0.046

*Significant at 5% level.

residuals. However, it is difficult to draw any conclusion on the basis of such a small sample. If these points are close to the line, then it is considered that the residuals are normally distributed. However, normality can be tested by using more stringent tests such as the Shapiro–Wilk or Kolmogorov–Smirnov tests. For residuals to be normally distributed, the Shapiro–Wilk test must be insignificant. In Table 9.16, this test is significant as its significance value is 0.046, which is less than 0.05; hence, it may be concluded that the residual plots are nonnormal, which is a violation of the assumption in multiple regression analysis. The Shapiro–Wilk test is more appropriate for a small sample size ($n < 50$) but can also be used for sample sizes as large as 2000, whereas the Kolmogorov–Smirnov test is more suitable for large samples. For this reason, the Shapiro–Wilk test is widely used to assess normality.

The output in Shapiro–Wilk test for normality can be obtained in SPSS by using the following sequence of commands:

Analyze ⟶ Descriptive ⟶ Explore

9.9.4 Standard Error of the Estimate

The standard error of the estimate is the standard deviation of the residuals in multiple regression analysis. The standard error describes the error in prediction. If the assumptions of normality for the error in multiple regression holds true, one can have an idea about the error range. The standard error can also be used to identify the outliers in the dataset. The standard error of estimate in multiple regression analysis is obtained by the following formula:

$$\sigma_{\text{est}} = \sqrt{\frac{\text{SSE}}{n - c - 1}} \tag{9.39}$$

Where n is the sample size and c is the number of independent variables used in developing the regression line. The SSE is obtained by

$$\text{SSE} = \sum (y - \hat{y})^2$$

Since in the standing broad jump example, only two variables leg length (x_1) and leg strength (x_2) have been used to estimate the standing broad jump performance (y), the value of c is 2.

From Table 9.15,

$$\text{SSE} = \sum (y - \hat{y})^2 = 0.07819875$$

$$\sigma_{\text{est}} = \sqrt{\frac{0.07819875}{10 - 2 - 1}} = 0.106$$

This value of the residual is the same as that obtained in the SPSS output in part IV of Table 9.14 except for the rounding-off error. One of the assumptions of the regression analysis is that the error terms are normally distributed with mean zero; hence, approximately 68% of the error terms (residuals) would be within $0 \pm 1\sigma_{\text{est}}$. Similarly, around 95% of the error terms would be within $0 \pm 2\sigma_{\text{est}}$, and 99% of the error terms would be within $0 \pm 3\sigma_{\text{est}}$.

In this example, the range of the residuals is 0.012–0.237 m, and the standard error of the estimate, $\sigma_{\text{est}} = 0.106$. If the errors were normally distributed, then approximately 68% of the error terms would be within $\pm$ 0.106 m and 95% would be within ± 2 (0.106 m) = 0.212 m. Looking at the residuals in the table, it can be seen that only one error term is outside the range $\pm 2\sigma_{\text{est}}$. It is up to the researcher to decide the range of the error beyond which the data item is considered to be an outlier. Thus, if one decides to identify an item of data to be an outlier if the error term corresponding to it is outside the 2σ limits, then the sixth data ($y = 2.50$, $x_1 = 100$, and $x_2 = 70.0$) may be considered to be the outlier in this example. Further, it is up to the researcher to make himself satisfied whether the data identified in this manner is actually an outlier or may be considered as genuine. It is very essential to check the outliers in the dataset because one or two extreme outliers may drag the regression line toward them, as a result of which the model becomes erroneous.

9.9.5 The Coefficient of Determination (R^2)

The square of the multiple correlation is known as the *coefficient of determination*, R^2. It can be defined as the proportion of variation in the dependent variable y, as explained by all the independent variables in the model. The value of R^2 can be anything between 0 and 1. If R^2 is 1, it indicates that 100% variation of the dependent variable can be explained by all the independent variables together in the model and if the value of R^2 is 0, which means no relationship exists between the predictor variables and the dependent variable. In a regression analysis, R^2 can be calculated by the following formula:

$$R^2 = \frac{\text{RSS}}{\text{TSS}} = 1 - \frac{\text{SSE}}{\text{TSS}} \tag{9.40}$$

While developing the regression model for the standing broad jump example, the SPSS produced the F-value in the ANOVA table as shown in Table 9.14. Let us examine this table again here.

Here, SSR =1.500 and TSS =1.574, and therefore $R^2 = \frac{1.500}{1.574} = 0.95299$.

This indicates that 95.299% of the variation in the standing broad jump performance is accounted for by the two independent variables leg length and leg strength in the model.

Since R^2 is an indicator of the proportion of variation that is accounted for by all the independent variables in the model, it can be considered as the efficiency of the model. R^2 can be used to find the improvement in the regression model by including other independent variables or by applying a different transformation if the variables are not linear. For instance, if a regression model has been developed to estimate the lean body weight on the basis of weight, forearm circumference, and wrist circumference, and R^2 is 0.7921, it simply indicates that 79.21% of the variation of the lean body weight can be explained by all the three independent variables together, namely, weight, forearm circumference, and wrist circumference. Now, if the researcher is interested in improving this model so that a more accurate estimate of the lean body weight can be estimated, then some more related independent variables may be included in the model. To decide as to which variable will improve the explainability of the dependent variable, one may look for an increase in the value of R^2. If by including the hip circumference, the value of R^2 increases by 0.8649, then one can say that there is an improvement in the model as R^2 has enhanced from 79.21% to 86.49%. However, this increase in R^2 may be tested for its significance.

Sometimes, the model is significant but none of the variable's regression coefficients may be significant. In such cases, the researcher may try a transformation such as X_1 / X_2, $X_1 \times X_2$ or $X_1 - X_2$ and see whether R^2 can be enhanced or not.

9.9.6 Adjusted R^2

In developing a regression model, each time a new variable is entered, R^2 increases. However, sometimes, adding a new variable does not add significant information to the model but still the value of R^2 increases. Because of this, the value of R^2 calculated in the regression model is inflated and needs to be corrected. The corrected value is known as adjusted R^2 and is computed as follows:

$$\text{Adjusted } R^2 = 1 - \frac{\text{SSE}/(n-c-1)}{\text{TSS}/(n-1)} \tag{9.41}$$

In fact, adjusted R^2 is an improvement over R^2 that adjusts for the number of explanatory independent variables in a model. Unlike R^2, adjusted R^2 will increase only if the new variable improves the model more than would be expected by chance.

$$\text{In this example, adjusted } R^2 = 1 - \frac{\text{SSE}/(n-c-1)}{\text{TSS}/(n-1)} = \frac{0.073/(10-2-1)}{1.574/(10-1)}$$

$$= \frac{0.010429}{0.174889} = 0.940$$

Thus, interpretation of explained variability in the model should be made on the basis of adjusted R^2 instead of R^2. Therefore, in reality, 94% variability in the standing broad jump performance can be explained by the two variables, leg length and leg strength, in the model developed on the basis of the data in the sample.

9.9.7 Testing the Significance of R^2

After computing the value of R^2, it is required to be tested for its significance. Since R^2 is actually the proportion of variation of dependent variable, y, as explained by all the independent variables together in the model, the significance of the model is the same as the significance of R^2. Thus, if the F-value in the ANOVA table is significant, both R^2 and the model will be significant.

In regression analysis, if you increase the number of predictors, the value of R^2 increases but whether this increase is significant or not can be tested by using the F-test. Let us suppose that the two models consists of c_1 and c_2 ($c_1 < c_2$) predictors with coefficient of determinations R_1^2 and R_2^2, respectively. The hypotheses to be tested are given as follows:

$$H_0: R_1^2 = R_2^2$$
$$H_1: R_1^2 \neq R_2^2$$

The null hypothesis can be tested by using the F-statistic.

$$F = \frac{(R_2^2 - R_1^2)/(c_2 - c_1)}{(1 - R_2^2)/(n - c_2 - 1)} \tag{9.42}$$

If calculated F is greater than F from the table at the significance level 0.05 and degrees of freedom $(c_2 - c_1, n - c_2 - 1)$, then the null hypothesis may be rejected and one may conclude that adding the new predictor has improved the model efficiency. However, if you fail to reject the null hypothesis, then it may be concluded that the increase in R^2 is not significant and adding new predictor may not improve the efficiency of the model.

Example 9.7 In a regression analysis, two models were developed for estimating the lean body weight on the basis of sample size 80. The first model consisted of three predictors, weight, forearm circumference, and wrist circumference with $R_1^2 = 0.7921$, whereas the second model consisted of four predictors, weight, forearm, wrist, and hip circumference with $R_2^2 = 0.8649$. Can it be concluded that R_2^2 is significantly higher than R_1^2 at the significance level 0.05?

Solution: Here, $R_1^2 = 0.7921, R_2^2 = 0.8649, c_1 = 3, c_2 = 4$, and $n = 80$. The hypotheses that need to be tested are

$$H_0: R_1^2 = R_2^2$$
$$H_1: R_1^2 \neq R_2^2$$

Substituting the values in the formula,

$$F = \frac{(R_2^2 - R_1^2)/(c_2 - c_1)}{(1 - R_2^2)/(n - c_2 - 1)} = \frac{(0.8649^2 - 0.7921^2)/(4-3)}{(1 - 0.8649^2)/(80 - 4 - 1)} = \frac{0.1206296}{0.0033593} = 35.91$$

From Table A.9, we obtain $F_{0.05}(4-3, 80-4-1) = F_{0.05}(1, 75) = 3.97$.

Since calculated F is more than the tabulated F, H_0 may be rejected at the level of significance 0.05. Thus, it may be concluded that R_2^2 is significantly higher than R_1^2, and hence the second model is an improvement over the first model.

9.10 LAW OF DIMINISHING RETURNS

While developing regression models for estimating a dependent variable, the value of R increases as the new independent variable is introduced in the model. The increase in the multiple correlations in different models follows a specific pattern whereby maximum increase occurs at the inclusion of the second independent variable in the model, and this increase keeps on decreasing as the number of independent variables keeps on increasing in the model. This trend of increase in the multiple correlation is known as the *law of diminishing returns*. To understand this fact, let us consider a study in which a regression model is required to be developed for estimating the lean body weight (x_1) of an individual on the basis of different independent variables such as weight (x_2), waist (x_3), hip circumference (x_4), forearm circumference (x_5), and wrist circumference (x_6). If different models are developed by including the most desirable independent variable every time, then the multiple correlation will also increase in succession as shown in Table 9.17. It can be seen from this table that the maximum increase of 0.18 in the multiple correlation occurs at the first instance when the second independent variable x_5 is added in the model; thereafter this increase keeps on decreasing every time a new independent variable is added, and finally it increases only 0.01 on adding the variable x_3.

TABLE 9.17 Different Models for Estimating Lean Body Weight

Model	Independent Variables Selected	Multiple Correlation (R)	Successive Increase in R
1	x_2	0.62	
2	x_2, x_5	0.80	0.18
3	x_2, x_5, x_6	0.89	0.09
4	x_2, x_5, x_6, x_4	0.93	0.04
5	x_2, x_5, x_6, x_4, x_3	0.94	0.01

x_1 : Lean body weight x_2 : Weight x_3 : Waist
x_4 : Hip circumference x_5 : Forearm circumference x_6 : Wrist circumference

9.11 DIFFERENT APPROACHES IN DEVELOPING MULTIPLE REGRESSION MODELS

The regression model is developed either for exploratory or confirmatory studies. In exploratory studies, the researcher is not aware of the relationship of different predictors with the dependent variable; therefore, as many predictors as possible are taken to develop the best model by selecting those variables for which the regression model becomes most efficient for prediction. On the other hand, in confirmatory studies, an already developed regression model is tested for its validity for the defined samples in the present context. For developing a regression model in exploratory studies, different methods such as *stepwise*, *forward*, or *backward* methods are used in SPSS, whereas in confirmatory studies, the *enter* method is used in which all the independent variables in the study are used to develop the model. The multiple regression model is developed by using computer software only because the procedure involved in it is very tedious and is not possible by manual calculation. Any of the methods can be used by choosing the appropriate option in the statistical software package. A brief description of these methods is given below.

9.11.1 Stepwise Regression

In stepwise regression, the model is developed step by step. If there are c independent variables $x_1, x_2, \ldots, x_c$ and a regression model is required to be developed for estimating the dependent variable y, then in the first step, the most significant independent variable is identified and a regression equation is developed by using this identified variable for estimating y. To find the first most contributing independent variable, a simple regression is developed by taking the dependent variable and each of the independent variables separately. The t-values are computed for the independent variable in each of the c regression models. The independent variable for which the absolute t-value is the largest is identified as the first variable to be included into the regression model. Let us say this independent variable is x_1, then the first model will be as follows.

$$\hat{y} = b_0 + b_1x_1$$

If none of the t-values is found to be significant, the search will stop by saying that no independent variable was included into the model.

To identify the second independent variable to be included in the model, all possible regression equations are developed with two independent variables at a time in which one variable is x_1, the one which is selected in the first step. The absolute t-value is examined for all the $c - 1$ remaining independent variables for significance in conjunction with the first variable. A variable for which the absolute t-value is the highest is identified as the second independent variable to be included into the model, say, this variable is x_2. Thus, the model will become

$$\hat{y} = b_0 + b_1x_1 + b_2x_2$$

At this stage, the significance of the first variable is also tested by means of using the t-value. If the variable x_1 is found to be insignificant, this will be removed from the model and a search will be on for the next independent variable. If none of the remaining $c - 1$ independent variables is found to be significant, the process will terminate with one variable in the model selected in the first step. This process will go on till all the variables in the study are tested for their significance by using the t-values. After testing all the independent variables in this way, a final model is achieved consisting of identified predictors which together explain the maximum variability of the dependent variable. The special feature of this method is that a variable that has already been selected in the model is tested again and again each time a new variable is introduced into the model. Quite often it happens that a variable may be included in the model at one stage but may be out of the model in subsequent stages. Stepwise regression is generally used to develop regression models because of its efficiency.

9.11.2 Forward Regression

In forward regression also, the model is developed in steps, the way it is done in the case of stepwise regression. But in this case, a variable once selected in the model cannot be out of the model in the subsequent stages. The variables selected by using forward regression are different from that of stepwise regression in some situations.

9.11.3 Backward Regression

In backward regression, the first model is developed by using all the variables in the study. Thereafter, the regression coefficients for all the independent variables are tested for their significance by calculating the t-values. If the absolute value of t of a variable is least and insignificant, the variable is dropped from the model and a new model is developed by taking the remaining $c - 1$ independent variables. In the second step, again the t-values are computed for each of the $c - 1$ independent variables in the model and the variable for which the absolute t-value is insignificant and least is dropped. This process is repeated till the t-values for all the independent variables in the model are significant. Usually, this method is not used because the researcher may not have sufficient samples to run the analysis.

9.11.4 Enter Method

In this method, only a single regression model is developed by using all the independent variables in the study. By computing the t-values for each of the independent variables, one can know whether all the variables have significant predictability or not. This method is generally used when an already developed regression model is tested for its efficiency and robustness for another sample. Efficiency of the model is tested in this method by looking at the value of R^2 computed in it.

Check Your Progress

Note: Tick the correct answer by using the sign ($\surd$).

	True	False
65. The stepwise regression method is used in exploratory studies.	-	-
66. In multiple regression analysis, the dependent variable is also known as the response variable.	-	-
67. In the enter method of regression analysis, only those variables that are found significant are included in the model.	-	-
68. The standard regression coefficient in multiple regression analysis is nothing but the partial correlation.	-	-
69. In forward regression, once the variable is selected in the first stage, it may be out of the model in the subsequent stages.	-	-
70. The significance of the F-value in multiple regression analysis indicates that the variables included in the model have significant predictability.	-	-
71. The SSR in regression analysis is computed by $\sum(\hat{y}-\bar{y})^2$.	-	-
72. In multiple regression analysis, the higher the value of the b coefficient, the better is the predictability of that independent variable.	-	-
73. The value of adjusted R^2 increases only if the new variable improves the model genuinely rather than by chance.	-	-
74. In multiple regression analysis, the higher the value of the standardized regression coefficient, the better is the predictability of the corresponding variable.	-	-
75. The Shapiro–Wilk test is more appropriate for testing the normality of residuals in large samples.	-	-
76. In multiple regression analysis, if c is the number of independent variables, the standard error of the estimate is computed by $\sqrt{SSE/(n-c)}$.	-	-
77. The enter method of regression analysis is used in confirmatory studies.	-	-

78.	The standardized regression coefficient can have values only between 0 and +1.	-	-
79.	Significance of the F-value in multiple regression analysis does not mean that the R^2 is also significant.	-	-
80.	In stepwise regression, the independent variable selected in the model at one stage can be out of the model at any subsequent stage.	-	-

PRACTICE EXERCISE

17. In a regression study conducted on 30 employees, job satisfaction was estimated on the basis of the employee's fitness index, nutritional status, and hygiene. The following output was generated by the computer.

Regression Coefficients with Corresponding t-Test

	Unstandardized Coefficients		Standardized Coefficients		
Model	B	Std. Error	Beta	t	Sig.
1 (Constant)	−119.275	31.114		−3.834	0.019
Nutritional status	4.04	1.276	0.563	3.166	0.034
Fitness index	3.43	0.780	0.785	4.398	0.012
Hygiene status	0.25	0.734	0.065	0.339	0.751

Dependent Variable: Job Satisfaction

ANOVA table

Model	Sum of Squares	df	Mean Square	F	Sig.
1 Regression	785.882	3	261.961	12.626	0.017*
Residual	82.993	4	20.748		
Total	868.875	7			

Model Summary

R	R^2	Adjusted R^2	Std. Error of the Estimate
0.951	0.904	0.833	4.56

Answer the following questions:

a. How many predictors are there in this model?
b. Comment on the overall significance of the model.
c. Discuss the t-ratios for the regression coefficients and their significance.
d. Develop the regression equation and interpret the meaning of the regression coefficient.
e. Which predictor is the most useful?
f. What is the role of standardized coefficients?
g. Interpret the meaning of standard error of the estimate.
h. Compute R^2 from the ANOVA table and verify whether it is 0.904.
i. Interpret the adjusted R^2. Is the R^2 significant?
j. From the information in these tables, what recommendations would you make about the predictor variables in the model?

9.12 COMPUTING WITH EXCEL

9.12.1 Computing Correlation Matrix in Excel

Excel can be used to compute the correlation matrix for investigating the relationship among different variables. The commands in Excel can be used to compute correlation between any two variables and among many variables simultaneously. The procedure involved in using Excel for computing the correlation matrix shall be discussed by means of the following example.

Remark The problems based on correlation and regression analysis can only be solved if the Add-Ins "Analysis ToolPak" is already installed in your Excel. The readers can install this Add-Ins in their Excel by following the procedure mentioned in Chapter 1.

Example 9.8 Data in Table 9.18 represent the score on different body parameters. Compute r for each pair of data and determine between which two parameters the maximum correlation exists.

TABLE 9.18 Data on Body Parameters

Chest Girth X	Arm Girth Y	Arm Length Z
86	33	75
82	27	72
88	31	77
86	28	73
81	29	71
83	27	69

Solution: The following steps shall be used to compute the correlation matrix in Excel:

1. Type the data of all three variables in the three columns A, B, and C of the Excel sheet. The heading for all the three variables may be written in the first cell of each column.
2. To find the correlation matrix, click the following commands in sequence in Excel to get the screen as shown in Figure 9.12.

   Data ⟶ Data Analysis

3. Bring the scroll on the option **Correlation** and then click **OK** in the screen as shown in Figure 9.12. This will take you to the screen as shown in Figure 9.13. You can now define the data range of all the three samples.
4. Here, all the data in the three groups have been entered in the first three columns A, B, and C of the Excel sheet. This includes variable names as well. Thus, the range of the entire dataset is from A1 to C6. Do the following steps to fill the entries in the screen shown in Figure 9.13.
   i. **Input Range**: *A*1:*C*6
   ii. Check the radio button **Grouped By** "Column" (Since the data have been typed columnwise.)
   iii. Check **Labels** (because the heading for the data is written in the first cell of each variable).

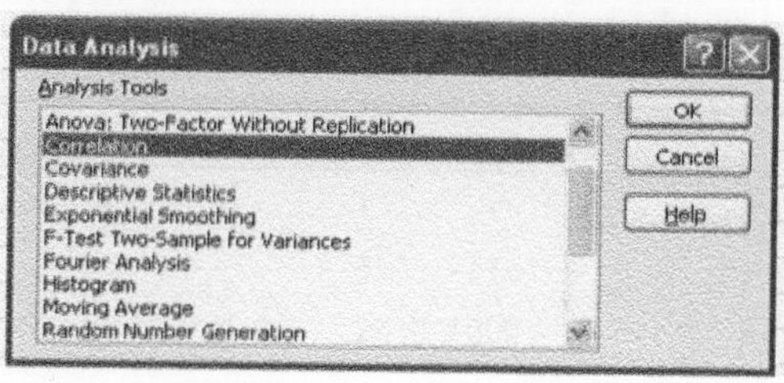

Figure 9.12 Command for computing the correlation matrix.

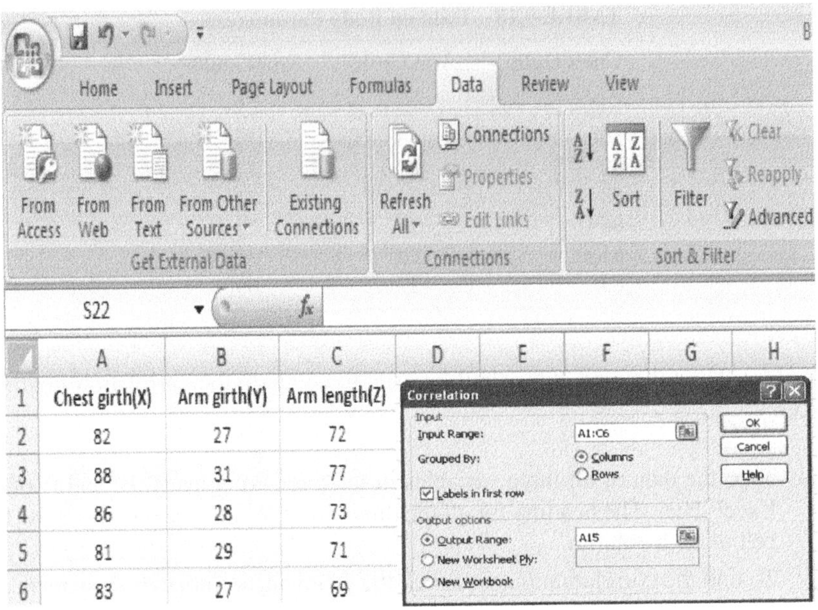

Figure 9.13 Options for computing the correlation matrix.

iv. Fill the entry in the output range. The output can be obtained on the same Excel sheet, new worksheet, or new workbook. Here, the output is obtained on the same sheet starting from location *A*15 onward and therefore the following entry should be filled.

Output Range: *A*15

v. Click **OK** to get the output as shown in Figure 9.14.

5. The output shown in Figure 9.14 can be formatted by formatting the cell entries of different columns. (Readers are advised to see the procedure discussed in Chapter 1 in this regard.) After formatting, the results will appear as shown in Table 9.19

Looking to the correlation matrix, it may be inferred that the highest correlation exists between arm length and arm girth.

15		Chest girth(X)	Arm girth(Y)	Arm length(Z)
16	Chest girth(X)	1		
17	Arm girth(Y)	0.614940046	1	
18	Arm length(Z)	0.809370258	0.815895751	1

Figure 9.14 Output of the correlation matrix.

TABLE 9.19 Correlation Matrix

	Chest girth (X)	Arm girth (Y)	Arm length (Z)
Chest girth (X)	1.00		
Arm girth (Y)	0.61	1.00	
Arm length (Z)	0.81	0.82	1

9.12.2 Regression Analysis with Excel

Excel can be very effectively used for regression analysis. Problems on simple and multiple regressions can be solved by using the Excel. Excel generates various outputs in regression analysis, which can be used to test the significance of the regression model and regression coefficients and develop the regression equation. It also generates the value of adjusted R^2, which is used for assessing the efficiency of the model. The procedure involved in using Excel for regression analysis shall be discussed by means of the following example.

Example 9.9 The data shown in Table 9.20 were recorded on college men. The fat percentage was measured by using standard equipment, whereas other measurements were obtained by using the equipment of anthropometry. Apply regression analysis to estimate the fat percentage on the basis of the three independent variables: height (in cm), weight (in lbs), and Axilla skinfold (in mm).

TABLE 9.20 Data on Physical Parameters

Fat% (Y)	Height (X_1) (cm)	Weight (X_2) (lbs)	Axilla (X_3) (mm)
23.2	177	181.94	16
7.2	177	124.08	6
27.5	182	209.22	24
12.5	171	130.46	5
15.7	168	137.06	6
12.5	171	141.68	5.2
10.6	166	129.14	5.8
21.9	171	155.1	13.8
16.8	175	137.28	9.5
13.6	178	144.54	5
9.1	171	130.68	6
11.7	181	148.28	6
12.1	172	141.9	5.5
8.6	180	143	6
13.8	163	113.3	6.2

Solution: The following steps shall be used in applying the regression analysis in Excel:

1. Type the data of all four variables in four columns A, B, C, and D of the Excel sheet. The heading for all four variables may be written in the first cell of each column.
2. To do the regression analysis, click the following commands in sequence in Excel to get the screen as shown in Figure 9.15.

   Data ⟶ Data Analysis

3. Bring the cursor on the option **Regression** and then click **OK** in the screen as shown in Figure 9.15. This will take you to the screen as shown in Figure 9.16. You can now define the data range of all the variables.
4. Here, all the data in the four groups have been written in the first four columns A, B, C, and D of the Excel sheet. This includes variable names as well.

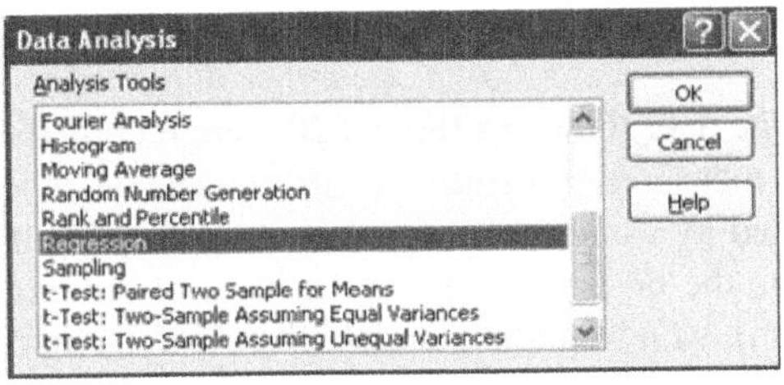

Figure 9.15 Command for regression analysis.

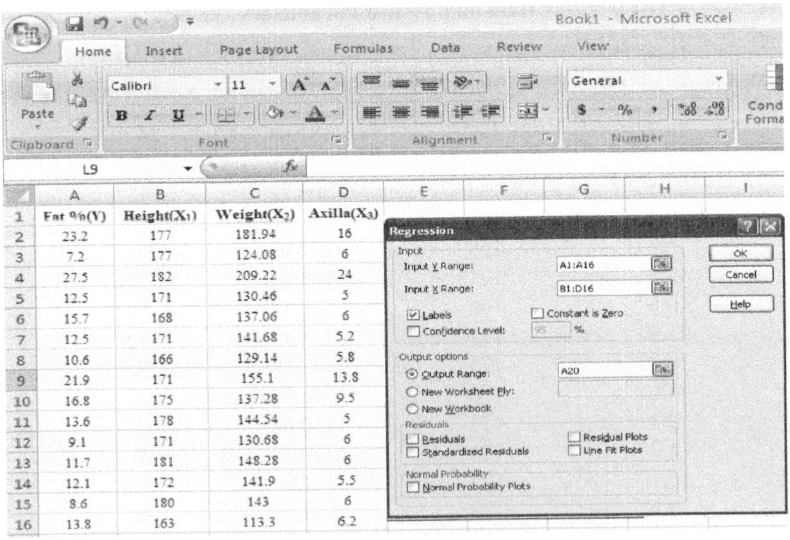

Figure 9.16 Options for regression analysis.

Since the variable in column A is the dependent variable, the input range of Y (dependent variable) is $A1{:}A16$. All three independent variables have been written in the columns of B, C, and D; hence, the input range of all the independent variables X is $B1{:}D16$. Do the following steps to fill the entries in the screen as shown in Figure 9.16.

i. **Input Y Range**: *A*1:*A*16
ii. **Input X Range**: *B*1:*D*16
iii. Check **Labels** (because the heading for the data is written in the first cell of each variable).
iv. Fill the entry in the output range. The output can be obtained on the same Excel sheet, new worksheet, or new workbook. Here, the output is obtained on the same sheet starting from location A15 onward, and therefore the following entry should be filled.
v. **Output Range**: *A*15
vi. Click **OK** to get the output as shown in Figure 9.17.

5. The output shown in Figure 9.17 can be formatted by formatting the cell entries of different columns (readers are advised to see the procedure discussed in Chapter 1 in this regard). After formatting and selecting only relevant details of the third table in Figure 9.17, the final results will appear as shown in Table 9.21 (a–c).

Since the p-values for the regression coefficients associated with height and axilla skinfold are less than 0.05, the t-values for these variables are significant. In other words, height and axilla skinfolds have significant predictability in estimating the fat percentage. On the other hand, the t-value for the regression coefficient associated with weight is not significant, hence this will not be included in the model. Thus, a regression equation can be developed by using the regression constant and

20	SUMMARY OUTPUT								
21									
22	*Regression Statistics*								
23	Multiple R	0.936922885							
24	R Square	0.877824492							
25	Adjusted R Square	0.844503899							
26	Standard Error	2.26406944							
27	Observations	15							
28									
29	ANOVA								
30		*df*	*SS*	*MS*	*F*	*Significance F*			
31	Regression	3	405.1312186	135.0437395	26.34480391	2.54254E-05			
32	Residual	11	56.3861147	5.126010427					
33	Total	14	461.5173333						
34									
35		*Coefficients*	*Standard Error*	*t Stat*	*P-value*	*Lower 95%*	*Upper 95%*	*Lower 95.0%*	*Upper 95.0%*
36	Intercept	52.73945639	21.62531662	2.438783085	0.032893606	5.142455443	100.3364573	5.142455443	100.3364573
37	Height(X1)	-0.354311671	0.151836314	-2.33351074	0.039623098	-0.688501145	-0.0201222	-0.688501145	-0.020122196
38	Weight(X2)	0.124679953	0.073354042	1.69970119	0.117253923	-0.036771205	0.286131111	-0.036771205	0.286131111
39	Axilla(X3)	0.616807038	0.274115766	2.250169871	0.045876238	0.013482305	1.220131771	0.013482305	1.220131771

Figure 9.17 Output in regression analysis.

TABLE 9.21 Output of the Regression Analysis

a. Summary Output

Regression Statistics	
Multiple R	0.937
R^2	0.878
Adjusted R^2	0.845
Standard error	2.264
Observations	15.000

regression coefficients of the variables height and axilla skinfold. The equation so developed is as follows:

$$Y\ (\text{Fat\%}) = 52.739 - 0.354X_1\ (\text{Height}) + 0.617X_3\ (\text{Axilla})$$

b. ANOVA

	df	SS	MS	F	Significance F
Regression	3.000	405.131	135.044	26.345	**0.000**
Residual	11.000	56.386	5.126		
Total		14.000	461.517		

c. t-Table for regression coefficients

	Coefficients	Standard Error	t-Stat	P-value
Intercept	52.739	21.625	2.439	**0.033**
Height (X_1)	−0.354	0.152	−2.334	**0.040**
Weight (X_2)	0.125	0.073	1.700	0.117
Axilla (X_3)	0.617	0.274	2.250	**0.046**

IMPORTANT DEFINITIONS

The ***product-moment correlation coefficient*** is an index of linear relationship that measures linear relationship between any two variables. It is also known as the *Pearson r*.

Covariance can be defined as the measure of how much two random variables x and y vary together.

Partial correlation measures the linear relation between the two variables after controlling the effect of other variables.

Multiple correlation is the correlation between the observed values of the criterion variable and its estimated values obtained on the basis of some of the independent variables.

A variable is said to be the ***suppression variable*** if it does not show a relationship with the criterion variable, but after combining with some other variable, its effect becomes significant in estimating the criterion variable.

Simple regression analysis is a procedure for determining the equation of a line for estimating the value of the dependent variable on the basis of only one predictor variable.

Multiple regression is a procedure of determining the equation of a line for estimating the value of the dependent variable on the basis of more than one predictor variable.

The ***residuals*** are the estimates of regression error and are obtained by finding the difference of observed and estimated values $(y-\hat{y})$ of the dependent variable.

The assumption of ***homoscedasticity*** means that the errors have constant variance.

The ***standard error of the estimate*** is the standard deviation of error terms (residual) that provides the overall picture of the errors in estimation.

The ***coefficient of determination*** R^2 is defined as the proportion of variation in the dependent variable accounted for by the independent variable(s) in the regression model.

Adjusted R^2 is an improvement over R^2 and can be defined as the proportion of variation in the dependent variable accounted for by the independent variable(s) after adjusting for the number of explanatory independent variables in the regression model.

The ***unstandardized regression coefficients*** are the sample partial regression coefficients that are used to develop the regression line.

The ***standardized regression coefficients*** are nothing but the partial correlation coefficients obtained in the multiple regression analysis and are used for comparing the effectiveness of the independent variables in the model.

The ***law of diminishing returns*** states that the increase in multiple correlation keeps on decreasing every time an independent variable is added in the regression model.

Stepwise regression is a technique of developing a regression line step by step by finding the most suitable combination of predictors in the model, wherein at each step, all the predictors selected in previous steps are tested again for their significance and may be out of the model if found insignificant.

Forward regression is a technique of developing a regression line step by step by finding the most suitable combination of predictors in the model, wherein the predictors selected previously remain in the model always.

Backward regression is a technique of developing a regression line wherein a full regression model is developed by taking all the independent predictors and, thereafter, dropping the least important variables from the model, one by one, until all the remaining independent predictors in the model become significant.

IMPORTANT FORMULAS

Pearson correlation

$$r_{x,y} = \frac{cov(x, y)}{\sqrt{\sigma_x \times \sigma_y}}$$

$$r_{x,y} = \frac{n\sum xy - \sum x \sum y}{\sqrt{\left[n\sum x^2 - \left(\sum x\right)^2\right] \times \left[n\sum y^2 - \left(\sum y\right)^2\right]}}$$

Partial correlation

First order

$$r_{12.3} = \frac{r_{12} - r_{13}r_{23}}{\sqrt{1 - r_{13}^2}\sqrt{1 - r_{23}^2}}$$

Third order

$$r_{12.345} = \frac{r_{12.34} - r_{15.34}r_{25.34}}{\sqrt{1 - r_{15.34}^2}\sqrt{1 - r_{25.34}^2}}$$

Generalized formula

$$r_{12.345\ldots n} = \frac{r_{12.34\ldots n-1} - r_{1n.345\ldots n-1}r_{2n.345\ldots n-1}}{\sqrt{1 - r_{1n.345\ldots n-1}^2}\sqrt{1 - r_{2n.345\ldots n-1}^2}}$$ Multiple correlation

With two independent variables

$$R_{1.23} = \sqrt{\frac{r_{12}^2 + r_{13}^2 - 2r_{12}r_{13}r_{23}}{1 - r_{23}^2}}$$

Generalized formula

$$R_{1.234\ldots n} = \sqrt{1 - (1 - r_{12}^2)(1 - r_{13.2}^2)(1 - r_{14.23}^2)\,\cdots\,(1 - r_{1n.234\ldots n-1}^2)}$$

With three independent variables

$$R_{1.234} = \sqrt{1-(1-r_{12}^2)(1-r_{13.2}^2)(1-r_{14.23}^2)}$$

Simple regression equations

Population regression equation

$$\hat{y} = \beta_0 + \beta_1 x$$

Model for any particular population score

$$y_i = \beta_0 + \beta_1 x_i + \varepsilon_i$$

Sample regression equation

$$\hat{y} = b_0 + b_1 x$$

Model for any particular sample score

$$y_i = b_0 + b_1 x_i + \varepsilon_i$$

Sum of squared deviation of scores from their estimated values

$$S^2 = \sum_{i=1}^{n} (y_i - \hat{y}_i)^2$$

Normal equations

$$b_1 \sum_{i=1}^{n} x_i + nb_0 = \sum_{i=1}^{n} y_i$$

$$b_1 \sum_{i=1}^{n} x_i^2 + b_0 \sum_{i=1}^{n} x_i = \sum_{i=1}^{n} x_i y_i$$

Regression constant

$$b_0 = \frac{\sum y \sum x^2 - \sum x \sum xy}{n\sum x^2 - (\sum x)^2}$$

Regression coefficient

$$b_1 = \frac{n\sum xy - \sum x \sum y}{n\sum x^2 - \left(\sum x\right)^2}$$

Sum of squares *xx*

$$\text{SS}_{xx} = \sum (x-\bar{x})^2 = \sum x^2 - \frac{1}{n}\left(\sum x\right)^2$$

Sum of squares xy

$$\begin{aligned} SS_{xy} &= \sum (x-\bar{x})(y-\bar{y}) \\ &= \sum xy - \frac{1}{n}\left(\sum x\right)\left(\sum y\right) \end{aligned}$$

Equation of regression line (deviation form)

$$\hat{y} - \bar{y} = b_1(x - \bar{x})$$

Regression constant

$$b_0 = \frac{\sum y}{n} - b_1\frac{\sum x}{n}$$

Regression coefficient

$$b_1 = r\frac{\sigma_y}{\sigma_x}$$

$$b_1 = \frac{SS_{xy}}{SS_{xx}}$$

$$b_1 = \frac{\sum xy - \frac{1}{n}\left(\sum x\right)\left(\sum y\right)}{\sum x^2 - \frac{\left(\sum x\right)^2}{n}}$$

Regression model

$$\text{TSS} = \text{SSR} + \text{SSE}$$

Total sum of squares

$$\text{TSS} = \sum (y - \bar{y})^2$$

Sum of squares due to regression

$$\text{SSR} = \sum (\hat{y} - \bar{y})^2$$

Sum of squares due to error (residual)

$$\text{SSE} = \sum (y - \hat{y})^2$$

Standard error of estimate

In simple regression,

$$\sigma_{\text{est}} = \sqrt{\frac{\text{SSE}}{n-2}} = \sqrt{\frac{\sum (y - \hat{y})^2}{n-2}}$$

In multiple regression,

$$\sigma_{\text{est}} = \sqrt{\frac{\text{SSE}}{n-c-1}} = \sqrt{\frac{\sum (y-\hat{y})^2}{n-c-1}}$$

Standard error of the regression coefficient

$$\text{SE}(b_1) = \frac{\sqrt{\frac{\sum (y-\hat{y})^2}{n-2}}}{\sqrt{\sum (x-\bar{x})^2}}$$

$$= \frac{\sqrt{\frac{\sum (y-\hat{y})^2}{n-2}}}{\sqrt{\sum x^2 - \frac{\left(\sum x\right)^2}{n}}}$$

t-Ratio for testing the significance of the regression coefficient

$$t = \frac{b_1 - \beta_1}{\text{SE}(b_1)}$$

Relationship between F and t

$$F = t^2$$

F-ratio for model testing

$$F = \frac{\text{MSR}}{\text{MSE}}$$

Mean sum of squares due to regression

$$\text{MSR} = \text{SSR}/c$$

Mean sum of squares due to residuals

$$\text{MSE} = \text{SSE}/(n-c-1)$$

Coefficient of determination R^2

$$R^2 = \frac{\text{SSR}}{\text{SS}_{yy}} = \frac{\sum (\hat{y}-\bar{y})^2}{\sum y^2 - \frac{\left(\sum y\right)^2}{n}}$$

$$R^2 = 1 - \frac{\text{SSE}}{\text{SS}_{yy}} = 1 - \frac{\sum (y - \hat{y})^2}{\sum y^2 - \frac{\left(\sum y\right)^2}{n}}$$

$$\text{Adjusted } R^2 = 1 - \frac{\text{SSE}/(n - c - 1)}{\text{TSS}/(n - 1)}$$

Multiple regression equations

Population regression equation

$$\hat{y} = \beta_0 + \beta_1 x_1 + \beta_2 x_2 + \ldots + \beta_c x_c$$

Sample regression equation

$$\hat{y} = b_0 + b_1 x_1 + b_2 x_2 + \ldots + b_c x_c$$

Model for any particular sample score

$$y_i = b_0 + b_1 x_1 + b_2 x_2 + \ldots + b_c x_c + \varepsilon_i$$

Regression equation with two predictors

$$\hat{y} = b_0 + b_1 x_1 + b_2 x_2$$

Regression equation in standard score form

$$z_y = r_{y1.2} z_1 + r_{y2.1} z_2$$

F-test for comparing two R^2 with different predictors

$$F = \frac{(R_2^2 - R_1^2)/(c_2 - c_1)}{(1 - R_2^2)/(n - c_2 - 1)}$$

CHAPTER EXERCISE

1. Are the correlation coefficient and covariance the same? Explain.
2. Describe the procedure for testing the significance of the correlation coefficient by using the t-test.
3. What happens to the correlation coefficient if the origin and scale are changed?

4. Describe the situation where partial correlation is used. Explain its limitations.
5. Discuss the utility of R^2 square.
6. What is a suppression variable?
7. Explain the law of diminishing returns.
8. What is the importance of residuals in regression analysis?
9. What are the assumptions in regression analysis?
10. Describe the standard error of estimate.
11. What are the ways and means of testing the regression model?
12. What is the difference between standardized and unstandardized regression coefficients? Explain their uses.
13. What is the difference between R^2 square and adjusted R^2?
14. What are the different approaches in doing regression analysis?
15. Find the value of the correlation coefficient for the following data.

X	Y
4	16
12	18
18	8
8	12
6	16
20	14
22	10

16. Compute the value of the correlation coefficient for the following data. Test the significance of the coefficient at 5% level.

X	Y
102	250
85	125
110	180
75	170
70	165
82	190

17. The performance levels of 10 students on statistics test (x) and IQ test (y) are given below:

Statistics (x)	IQ (y)
20	80
15	90
25	100
22	95
18	85
16	75
15	70
20	65
26	90
28	80

Calculate the product-moment correlation coefficient and test its significance at 5% level.

18. Show that there is no effect of the change of origin and scale on the correlation coefficient with the help of an example.
19. The data obtained on 10 soccer players in a McDonald Soccer test along with their weights are given below. Find the correlation between these two variables.

McDonald Soccer Test Scores	Weights (in kg)
17	62
18	64
20	60
15	56
16	57
19	58
14	45
12	57
15	51
18	61

20. The following are the measurements on resting respiratory rate (x) and fat percentage (y) obtained on 10 athletes. Compute the correlation coefficient between u and v, where u is obtained by subtracting 14 from x and v is obtained by subtracting 13 from y.

Resting Respiratory Rate (x)	Fat Percentage (y)
13	11
15	13
16	13
17	14
15	14
14	13
16	15
17	14
12	12
14	15

21. In order to investigate the relationship between upper arm girth (x) and calf girth (y), measurements were made on college boys. The data are shown below. Compute the coefficient of correlation and test its significance at 5% level.

Arm Girth (X)	Calf Girth (Y)
30	41
28	40
31	42
28	41
30	43
29	45
31	44

22. The following data were obtained on women athletes to know the relationship between positive and negative breath-holding capacity. Use the data to determine the correlation between them.

Positive Breath-Holding Capacity	Negative Breath-Holding Capacity
41	30
44	24
46	25
45	26
32	25
47	30
54	28
56	27
57	28
55	30

23. Following are the data of height, arm length, and thigh girth. Compute r for each pair of data and determine for which pair of variables the correlation is maximum.

Height (cm) X	Arm Length (cm) Y	Thigh Girth (cm) Z
190	83	60
186	78	35
192	84	59
185	79	58
190	82	59

24. Compute partial correlations $r_{12.3}$, $r_{13.2}$, and $r_{23.1}$ by using the zero-order correlations mentioned in the following correlation matrix.

Correlation Matrix

	x_1	x_2	x_3
x_1	1	0.5	0.3
x_2		1	0.2
x_3			1

25. Determine the multiple correlations $R_{1.23}$ and $R_{23.1}$ by using the correlation matrix in question 24.

26. The following correlation matrix shows the correlations among different physical performance parameters obtained on 50 athletes. Compute $r_{13.2}$, $r_{23.1}$, and $r_{23.14}$. Interpret your findings.

Correlation Matrix

	x_1	x_2	x_3	x_4
x_1	1	0.3	0.6	0.7
x_2		1	0.5	0.4
x_3			1	0.8

x_1: Height x_2: Pull Ups x_3: Sit-Ups x_4: Back strength

27. From the correlation matrix shown in the question 26, find the value of $R_{2.13}$ and $R_{3.12}$.
28. The following correlation matrix shows the correlations among selected physical parameters measured on athletes. Compute $R_{1.23}$, $R_{2.13}$, and $R_{2.134}$ and interpret your findings.

Correlation Matrix

	x_1	x_2	x_3	x_4
x_1	1	0.6	0.3	0.8
x_2		1	0.7	0.5
x_3			1	0.4

x_1: Shuttle run x_2: Standing broad jump x_3: Height x_4: 50 Yard dash

29. In a relationship study conducted on soccer players, the following correlation matrix was obtained.

Correlation Matrix

	x_1	x_2	x_3
x_1	1	0.60	0.55
x_2		1	0.25
x_3			1

x_1: Accuracy x_2: Flexibility x_3: Leg strength

Compute the following correlations and interpret your findings.

i. $r_{12.3}$, $r_{13.2}$, and $r_{23.1}$

ii. $R_{1.23}$, $R_{2.13}$, and $R_{3.12}$

30. Draw the scatter plot for following data and determine whether there is a linear or curvilinear relationship between x and y by drawing the trend line.

x:	2	6	4	8	7	12
y:	12	16	14	20	15	22

31. In a correlation study on 20 volleyball players, the following statistics were obtained.

	Height in cm (x)	Playing Ability in Numbers (y)
Mean	165	7.2
SD	0.5	0.8
r	0.6	

Construct regression equations of y on x by computing b_0 and b_1. Explain the meaning of b_1. Find the playing ability score in the following cases:

y = ? if x = 160 cm

y = ? if x = 170 cm

z_y = ? if z_x = 1.6

32. The age (x) and height (y) of 50 children were noted and the following statistics were computed on it.

	Age in Years (x)	Height in Feet (y)
Mean	15	5.1
SD	2	0.3
r	0.8	

Develop a regression equation for estimating height on the basis of age. What would the height be if the age is 12.5 years?

33. In estimating the lean body weight (y) on the basis of height (x), a regression equation needs to be developed. If the value of standardized regression coefficient (β) is 0.6, what would be the value of the unstandardized regression coefficient (b_1) where the standard deviations of lean body weight and height are 8 lbs and 0.15 ft, respectively?
34. The regression equation of y on x_1 and x_2 is given by

$$y = 8 + 2.8\,x_1 + 3.6\,x_2$$

If $\sigma_y = 8$, $\sigma_{x_1} = 2.5$, and $\sigma_{x_2} = 0.9$, what would be the value of β_1 and β_2?
35. Develop a regression line for estimating y and find the largest and smallest residuals.

x:	10	8	7	5	6	2
y:	8	6	12	16	18	20

36. Following are the data on age in years (x) and systolic blood pressure in mm Hg (y). Obtain the regression equation of y on x and estimate the systolic blood pressure when the age is 62 years. Interpret the meaning of the regression coefficient obtained in this equation.

x:	55	40	65	38	62	46	55	49	35
y:	146	125	160	128	148	128	150	145	115

37. The following data were obtained on fat percentage (y) and body weight (x) in kilograms on six boxers:

y:	11	10	13	14	12	15
x:	85	75	87	84	82	77

Find the regression line for estimating the fat% on the basis of body weight. Estimate the fat% if the body weight is equal to 86 kg.
38. The following are the data on height in feet (x) and weight in lbs (y) of a group of girls. Develop a regression equation for estimating weight on the basis of the height and compute the residuals also. Interpret the regression coefficient obtained in the equation and graph the residual plot.

x:	5.1	5.2	5.3	5.2	5.6	5.5	5.6	5.8
y:	95	98	105	110	108	100	99	110

39. Develop the regression equation for the following data, compute the residuals, and graph a residual plot. Do these data violate any of the assumptions of regression analysis?

x:	2	3	4	6	8	9
y:	4	10	14	32	65	90

40. In a study, arm length (y) and forearm length (x) of the athletes were measured in centimeters. The data are shown below. Develop a regression equation for estimating the arm length if the forearm length is known. Also find the arm length if the forearm length of an athlete is 44 cm.

y:	62	58	60	55	52	56	57	52
x:	40	36	38	32	33	32	34	35

Compute the standard error of estimate and interpret you findings.

41. In a study, six college students were tested for their fat percentage (x) and resting respiratory rate in breaths/min (y). The data so obtained are shown below:

Fat% x	Resting Respiratory Rate in Breaths/min y
11	13
13	15
13	16
14	17
13	14
12	12

Construct a regression line to estimate the resting respiratory rate from fat percentage and do the following:

i. Interpret the regression coefficient.
ii. Find the residuals and graph the residual plot.
iii. Compute the standard error of estimate.
iv. Compute R^2 and explain its meaning.

42. Develop the regression equation for estimating the value of y on the basis of x. Compute the standard error of estimate and interpret its meaning. What is the value of y if x is 15?

x:	12	16	18	19	20	22
y:	25	35	22	16	28	32

43. In a regression analysis, the following regression equation was obtained for estimating the arm length (y) on the basis of height (x) of a college student.

$$y = 0.25\,x + 18.5$$

If the standard deviation of arm length and height were 1.8 cm and 5 cm, respectively, then what would be the value of R^2? Interpret the findings.

44. From the following set of data, develop the regression line for estimating y on the basis of x, compute R^2, and explain its meaning. Also compute adjusted R^2.

x:	1	2	3	4	5	6
y:	9	8	11	12	10	13

45. Following are the ages of the wife (x) and husband (y). Develop a regression equation for estimating the husband's age on the basis of the wife's age. Find the age of husband, if the wife's age is 22. Also compute the standard error of estimate and R^2 and interpret their meaning. Test whether the regression model is significant at 5% level.

x:	25	32	45	36	26	38	42
y:	28	33	48	42	26	45	44

ANSWERS

Check Your Progress

1. F	13. F	25. F	37. F	49. F	61. T	73. T
2. F	14. T	26. F	38. T	50. T	62. F	74. T
3. T	15. F	27. F	39. F	51. F	63. T	75. F
4. F	16. T	28. T	40. F	52. T	64. T	76. F
5. T	17. F	29. F	41. F	53. F	65. T	77. F
6. F	18. T	30. T	42. T	54. T	66. T	78. F
7. F	19. T	31. F	43. F	55. T	67. F	79. F
8. T	20. T	32. F	44. F	56. T	68. T	80. T
9. T	21. F	33. F	45. T	57. T	69. F	
10. T	22. T	34. T	46. T	58. F	70. T	
11. F	23. T	35. T	47. F	59. T	71. T	
12. F	24. F	36. F	48. T	60. F	72. F	

Practice Exercise

1. The dataset in *A* and *C* are curvilinear, whereas in *B*, *D*, and *E*, they are linear.
2. $r = 1$
3. $r = -1$
4. r_{xy} and r_{uv} are the same and are equal to 1.
5. $r = 0.76$
6. $r_{12.3} = 0.54$
7. $R_{1.23} = 0.87$
8. $r_{13.2} = -0.17$ and $r_{23.1} = 0.51$
9. $R_{3.12} = 0.61$
10. a.

	Abdomen	Suprailiac	Fat
Abdomen	1	0.891	0.852
Suprailiac		1	0.744
Fat			1

b. Abdomen skinfold is the best predictor for fat%. The correlation between the predictors is 0.891.

c. $R = 0.853$

d. The multiple correlation is higher than both the independent correlations, that is, between fat and abdomen (0.852) as well as between fat and suprailiac (0.744).

e. $R^2 = 0.73$. Since the multiple correlation obtained with two predictors (abdomen and suprailiac), that is, 0.853, is higher in comparison to the correlation between fat and abdomen (0.852), it can be said that there is a marginal improvement by using both the predictors.

11. 72.3%
12. 88.36%
13. Residuals: 3.83, 0.99, −2.23, −3.37, −2.43, −0.57, 3.37
    Residuals are normally distributed but not linear, and the assumptions of homoscedasticity and independence do not hold true.
14. $y = 1.152X + 0.391$
    Residuals: 0.935, −0.196, −1.630, −0.413, −0.674, 1.978
15. $\sigma_{est} = 8.54$, residuals are normally distributed but linear. The assumptions of homoscedasticity and independence do not hold true.
16. a. SD of error of estimate = 0.866
    b. Standardized regression coefficient = 0.910
    c. $R^2 = 0.829$, Adj $R^2 = 0.786$
    d. $t = 4.397$, which is significant at 5% level

17. a. There are three predictor variables.
   b. The model is significant because the F-value in the ANOVA is significant.
   c. Since t-ratios for the nutritional status and fitness index are significant, these are only two variables that contribute significantly to the model in estimating the job satisfaction of the employees.
   d. $\hat{y}$ (Job satisfaction) = 4.04 (Nutritional status) + 3.43 (Fitness status) + 0.25 (hygiene status).

   Interpretation of regression coefficient:

      i. By an increase of one unit in the nutritional status of an employee, his job satisfaction increases by 4.04 units, provided all other variables are held constant.
      ii. By increasing one unit of fitness index, job satisfaction increases by 3.43 units, provided all other variables are held constant.
      iii. Since the t-value of hygiene status is not significant, it does not contribute anything to the model.

   e. Fitness index is the most useful predictor because its standardized regression coefficient (0.785) is the largest among the three predictors.
   f. The standardized regression coefficients are used to compare the relative importance of the predictor variables in the model.
   g. The standard error of estimate is 4.56. If error is normally distributed, then approximately 68% of the residuals (error in predicting job satisfaction) would be within ±4.56 units, 95% within $\pm 2 \times 4.56$ (=9.12) units, and 99% within $\pm 3 \times 4.56$(=13.68) units.
   h.

$$R^2 = \frac{\text{SSR}}{\text{TSS}} = \frac{785.882}{868.875} = 0.904$$

   i. The adjusted R^2 is 0.833. This indicates that 83.3% variability in job satisfaction is explained by all three predictors in the model. The R^2 is significant because the F-ratio is significant.
   j. Only two predictor variables, that is, nutritional status and fitness index, should be used to develop the regression model for predicting job satisfaction. The regression analysis should be rerun by using the stepwise regression method.

Chapter Exercise

15. $r = -0.596$
16. $r = 0.47$, not significant at 5% level

17. $r = 0.396$, not significant at 5% level
19. $r = 0.587$
20. $r = 0.602$
21. $r = 0.426$, not significant at 5% level
22. $r = 0.396$
23. Correlation Matrix

	X	Y	Z
X	1		
Y	0.96	1	
Z	0.53	0.73	1

24. $r_{12.3} = 0.47$, $r_{13.2} = 0.23$, and $r_{23.1} = 0.06$
25. $R_{1.23} = 0.54$ and $R_{2.31} = 0.50$
26. $r_{13.2} = 0.54$, $r_{23.1} = 0.42$, and $R_{23.14} = 0.42$
27. $R_{2.13} = 0.5$ and $R_{3.12} = 0.68$
28. $\mathrm{R}_{1.23} = 0.62$, $\mathrm{R}_{2.13} = 0.81$, and $\mathrm{R}_{2.134} = 0.82$
29.
    i. $r_{12.3} = 0.57$, $r_{13.2} = 0.52$, and $r_{23.1} = -0.12$
    ii. $R_{1.23} = 0.73$, $R_{2.13} = 0.61$, and $R_{3.12} = 0.56$
30. X and s are linearly related.
31.

$$Y = -8.64 + 0.096X$$

    i. $Y = 6.72$
    ii. $y = 0.48$
    iii. $z_y = 0.96$
32. $Y = 3.3 + 0.12X$, for age = 12.5 years, height = 4.8 ft
33. Unstandardized regression coefficient (b) = 32.
34. $\beta_1 = 0.875$ and $\beta_2 = 0.405$
35.

$$Y = 24.64 - 1.79X$$

Largest residual = 4.32; smallest residual = 0.11
36. $Y = 73.68 + 1.31X$, for age 62 years, the estimated blood pressure would be approximately 155.
37. $Y = 8.099 + 0.05X$, for body weight 86 kg, the fat percentage is 12.40 approximately.
38.

$$Y = 46.48 + 10.47X$$

Residuals: −4.877 −2.924 3.029 9.076 2.888 −4.065 −6.112 2.794

39.

$$Y = -27.81 + 11.93X$$

Residuals: 7.95 2.02 −5.91 −11.77 −2.63 10.44

The linearity assumption is violated.

40.

$$Y = 23.91 + 0.93X$$

For forearm length of 44 cm, the estimated arm length would be 64.83 cm.
Standard error of estimate: 2.51 cm.

41.

i. $Y = -4.5 + 1.5X$
ii. Residuals: 1 0 1 0.5 −1 −1.5
iii. Standard error of estimate = 1.17 breaths/min.
iv. $R^2 = 0.686$

42.

$$Y = 24.48 + 0.104X$$

For $x = 15$, the estimated value of y is 26.04
Standard error of estimate: 7.69

43. $R^2 = 0.83$

44.

$$Y = 7.8 + 0.77X$$

$$R^2 = 0.595$$

$$\text{Adjusted } R^2 = 0.494$$

45.

$$Y = -0.97 + 1.12X$$

If the wife's age is 22 years, then the estimated age of the husband would be 23.7 years.
Standard error of estimate = 2.61
$R^2 = 0.93$.
The regression model is significant at 5% level.

FURTHER READING

1. Aldrich J. Correlations genuine and spurious in Pearson and Yule. Statistical Science 1995;10(4):364–376. DOI: 10.1214/ss/1177009870JSTOR 2246135.
2. Aldrich J. Fisher and regression. Statistical Science 2005;20(4):401–417. DOI: 10.1214/088342305000000331JSTOR 20061201.
3. Allison PD. Multiple Regression: A Primer. USA: Pine Forge Press; 1998. ISBN 978-0-7619-8533-4.
4. Armstrong JS. Illusions in regression analysis. International Journal of Forecasting 2012(forthcoming).
5. Baba K, Ritei S, Masaaki S. Partial correlation and conditional correlation as measures of conditional independence. Australian and New Zealand Journal of Statistics 2004;46(4):657–664. DOI: 10.1111/j.1467-842X.2004.00360.x.
6. Black Ken. Business Statistics For Contemporary Decision Making. 5th ed. New Delhi: Wiley-India; 2011.
7. Cohen J. Statistical Power Analysis for the Behavioral Sciences. 2nd ed. USA: Lawrence Erlbaum Associations, Incoporated; 1998. ISBN 978-0-8058-0283-2.
8. Cohen J, Cohen P, West SG, Aiken LS. Applied Multiple Regression/Correlation Analysis for the Behavioral Sciences. 2nd ed. Hillsdale, NJ: Lawrence Erlbaum Associates; 2003.
9. Cook RD, Weisberg S. Residuals and Influence in Regression. Repr ed. New York: Chapman and Hall; 1982. ISBN 041224280X. Accessed 2013 Feb 23.
10. Copas JB. Regression, prediction and shrinkage. Journal of Royal Statistical Society: Series B 1983;45:311–354.
11. Crown WH. Statistical Models for the Social and Behavioral Sciences: Multiple Regression and Limited-Dependent Variable Models. 1998. ISBN 0275953165.
12. Croxton FE. Applied General Statistics. 3rd ed. USA: Prentice Hall; 1967. ISBN 978-0-13-040378-0.
13. Dowdy S, Wearden S. Statistics for Research. USA: Wiley ISBN 0-471-08602-9; 1983. p 230.
14. Draper N, Smith H. Applied Regression Analysis. 2nd ed. New York: John Wiley & Sons, Inc.; 1981.
15. Draper NR, Smith H. Applied Regression Analysis. USA: Wiley-Interscience; 1998. ISBN 0-471-17082-2.
16. Edwards AL. Multiple Regression and the Analysis of Variance and Covariance. USA: David A Edwards / Tristee; 1985. ISBN 978-0-7167-1704-1.
17. Fisher RA. The goodness of fit of regression formulae, and the distribution of regression coefficients. Journal of Royal Statistical Society 1922;85(4):597–612. DOI: 10.2307/2341124JSTOR 2341124.
18. Francis DP, Coats AJ, Gibson D. How high can a correlation coefficient be? International Journal of Cardiology 1999;69:185–199. DOI: 10.1016/S0167-5273(99) 00028-5.
19. Pedhazur EJ. Multiple Regression in Behavioral Research. USA: Holt Rinehart & Winston INC; 1973. ISBN 978-0-03-086211-3.
20. Gayen AK. The frequency distribution of the product moment correlation coefficient in random samples of any size draw from nonnormal universes. Biometrika 1951;38:219–247. DOI: 10.1093/biomet/38.1-2.219.

21. Gordon D. Beat the Sports Books. New York: Cardoza; 2005. ISBN 978-1-5804-2174-4.
22. Hazewinkel M. Encyclopaedia of Mathematics, Supplement I. Netherlands: Springer; 2010. ISBN 978-90-481-4896-7.
23. Hocking RR. The analysis and selection of variables in linear regression. Biometrics 1976;32.
24. Hurvich CM, Tsai CL. The impact of model selection on inference in linear regression. American Statistician 1990;44:214–217.
25. Rodgers JL, Nicewander WA. Thirteen ways to look at the correlation coefficient. The American Statistician 1988;42(1):59–66.
26. Kenney JF, Keeping ES. Linear Regression and Correlation." Ch. 15 in Mathematics of Statistics. 3rd ed. Pt. 1. Princeton, NJ: Van Nostrand; 1962. p 252–285.
27. Nikolić D, Muresan RC, Feng W, Singer W. Scaled correlation analysis: a better way to compute a cross-correlogram. European Journal of Neuroscience 2012:1–21. DOI: 10.1111/j.1460-9568.2011.07987.x http://www.danko-nikolic.com/wp-content/uploads/2012/03/Scaled-correlation-analysis.pdf.
28. Pearson K, Yule GU, Blanchard N, Lee A. The Law of Ancestral Heredity. Biometrika (Biometrika Trust) 1903;2(2):211–236. DOI: 10.1093/biomet/2.2.211.JSTOR 2331683.
29. Dennis Cook R, Weisberg S. Criticism and influence analysis in regression. Sociological Methodology 1982;13:313–361.
30. Rao CR. Linear Statistical Inference and its Applications. 2nd ed. New York: John Wiley & Sons, Inc.; 1973.
31. Rencher AC, Pun FC. Inflation of R^2 in best subset regression. Technometrics 1980;22:49–54.
32. Richard AB. Regression Analysis: A Constructive Critique. USA: Sage Publications; 2004.
33. Roecker EB. Prediction error and its estimation for subset—selected models. Technometrics 1991;33:459–468.
34. Fisher RA. Statistical Methods for Research Workers. 14th ed. UK: Oliver and Boyd; 1970. ISBN 0-05-002170-5.
35. Stavrianopoulos K.. Achievement Goals as Predictors of Metacognitive Knowledge Monitoring and Academic Help-Seeking Behavior Among College Students. Unpublished Doctoral Dissertation. New York: University of Fordham; 2005.
36. Wilkinson L, Dallal GE. Tests of significance in forward selection regression with an F-to enter stopping rule. Technometrics 1981;23:377–380.
37. Yule GU. On the theory of correlation. Journal of Royal Statistical Society (Blackwell Publishing) 1897;60(4):812–54. DOI: 10.2307/2979746JSTOR 2979746.

10

STATISTICAL TESTS FOR NONPARAMETRIC DATA

10.1 INTRODUCTION

All parametric statistical tests used for testing hypothesis in small or large samples are based on the assumption that the population from which the sample has been drawn follows a normal distribution. Besides the assumption of normality, other assumptions are also required in using these tests for hypothesis testing. For instance, in using the *t*-test for two independent groups, it is assumed that the population variances are equal. Similarly, in using the paired *t*-test, the pair differences $(y_i - x_i)$ are assumed to be independent and normally distributed. If assumptions for these tests are not fulfilled, these parametric tests result in wrong conclusions as their power in testing the hypothesis decreases. The effect is more serious in the case of a small sample. In other words, under the breakdown of these assumptions, the probability of rejecting the null hypothesis decreases when it is false.

Even after these assumptions are fulfilled, these parametric tests are valid only when the observations are measured at least on an interval scale. What happens if the observations are obtained on either nominal or ordinal scale? In that situation, these parametric tests are not valid for testing of hypothesis. In all such situations where the normality assumption fails, assumptions required for parametric tests break down, or if the data are measured on the nominal or ordinal scale, nonparametric tests are used to test the hypothesis in the inferential study. Since the assumptions of nonparametric tests are weak and the population distribution is

Statistics for Exercise Science and Health with Microsoft® Office Excel®, First Edition. J. P. Verma.

not required to be normal, the nonparametric tests are sometimes also referred to as *distribution-free* tests. In parametric tests, the hypothesis concerning the mean is tested, whereas in the nonparametric tests, the hypothesis concerning the median is tested for its significance. In parametric tests, hypotheses concerning parameters such as the mean, proportion, and variance are tested, whereas in nonparametric tests, hypotheses that do not involve any parameter are tested. In nonparametric tests, the test statistic is computed on the basis of some of the characteristics of the data, such as signs of the measurements, order relations, or category frequencies. For this reason, subjectivity in the measurement does not alter them.

Many situations arise in exercise science and health research where the data are obtained either on the ordinal or nominal scale. For instance, assessment of pleasure after an exercise program, playing ability, or mental health produces data on the ordinal scale. Similarly, measurement of sportsmen's anxiety, motivation, achievement, and so on can be obtained by classifying them into low or high categories, giving rise to nominal data. In all such situations, nonparametric tests are well suited for hypothesis testing. The procedure for hypothesis testing by using nonparametric tests is similar to that for parametric testing except in the construction of the hypothesis and computation of the test statistic. For most of the parametric tests, there exists an alternative nonparametric test. For instance, as an alternative to the parametric two-sample *t*-test for independent groups, the nonparametric Mann–Whitney test can be used, and for the two-sample paired *t*-test, the Wilcoxon matched-pairs signed-ranks test is an alternative nonparametric test. Similarly, for one-way ANOVA in parametric tests, there is a similar nonparametric test known as the Kruskal–Wallis test.

10.2 MERITS AND DEMERITS OF NONPARAMETRIC TESTS

The advantage of using nonparametric tests is that they are easy to apply and depend on fewer assumptions. At the same time, outliers do not affect the test statistic much. Nonparametric tests may be, and often are, more powerful in detecting population differences than parametric tests, when certain assumptions are not satisfied. Moreover, these tests are the only alternative when the observations are obtained on either the nominal or ordinal scale. In this chapter, some of the most widely used nonparametric tests, including the chi-square test, are discussed in detail.

> **FACTS TO KNOW**
>
> Nonparametric tests do not assume the distribution of the population to be normal

10.3 CHI-SQUARE TEST

The chi-square test is used in investigating the nature of categorical data. It can be used in drawing conclusions in many inferential studies. This test is most widely used by researchers. The chi-square test is used to test whether a sample has been drawn from a population having a specific distribution. Consider a study in which choosing the match practice sport, the students' preferences were in the ratio of 5:2:3 toward cricket, basketball, and soccer, respectively, in a college. The college authority may want to know whether this distribution still holds true on the basis of the responses from a sample of students selected randomly. Further, in most parametric tests, it is assumed that the distribution of the population is normal. In order to test this assumption, the chi-square test can be used. The chi-square statistic is denoted by the Greek letter χ^2 and is pronounced as "kye." It is computed by the following formula:

$$\chi^2 = \sum \frac{(f_o - f_e)^2}{f_e} \tag{10.1}$$

where

f_o = observed frequency and f_e = expected frequency

The χ^2 statistic mentioned in Equation (10.1) follows a chi-square distribution with $(r - 1)$ degrees of freedom, where r is the number of categories. The chi-square test is used for data measured on a nominal scale. In testing the hypothesis, the chi-square statistic is computed on the basis of frequencies instead of scores. If a cell frequency is less than 5, then Yates' correction is applied while computing chi-square.

10.3.1 Application of Chi-Square Test

There are many applications of the chi-square test but the following two most widely used applications are discussed in detail in this chapter.

1. Testing the goodness of fit
2. Testing the independence of attributes.

10.3.2 Assumptions in Chi-Square Test

While applying the chi-square test for testing hypothesis either in the goodness of fit or independence of attributes, the following assumptions are made:

a. The sample has been drawn randomly from the population.
b. All the observations are independent of each other.
c. The sum of the observed frequencies is equal to the sum of the expected frequencies.
d. The chi-square statistic has been computed on the basis of frequencies instead of scores.

e. The expected frequency in each category is not less than 5.
f. The sample is sufficiently large.

10.3.3 Testing Goodness of Fit

In testing goodness of fit, an experimenter is interested in testing whether the observed sample frequencies are similar to those in a theoretical probability distribution. In other words, the purpose of testing is to see whether the sample has been obtained from a population that follows a particular frequency distribution. For instance, consider a situation in which the past history of a university shows that three subjects such as sport psychology, sport physiology, and sport biomechanics are equally popular among the students. This hypothesis can be tested by taking a random sample of the students and taking their preference about the subject. If the response frequencies for their preference are 60:40:50 toward sport psychology, sport physiology, and sport biomechanics, respectively, the chi-square test may be used to test whether the difference between the observed frequencies and expected frequencies (50:50:50) for their preference is significant. If the chi-square is not significant, then the fit is good, otherwise it is not. Thus, in testing the goodness of fit, the experimenter's interest is not to reject the null hypothesis in order to say that the fit is good. Another useful application of goodness of fit is to test the normality of data, which is one of the main assumptions in using a parametric test in testing of hypothesis. Thus, by using the chi-square test, one can test the normality of a population on the basis of a random sample drawn from it.

In testing the goodness of fit, a test statistic χ^2 is computed to test the null hypothesis of no difference between the observed and expected frequencies. The significant value of χ^2 with $(r - 1)$ degrees of freedom and at any given α-level of significance, $(\chi^2_{\alpha,k-1})$ can be obtained from Table A.11 in the Appendix. The degrees of freedom are calculated as $(r - 1)$, where r is the number of categories. If calculated χ^2 is greater than $\chi^2_{\alpha,k-1}$, the null hypothesis is rejected and one may conclude that the fit is not good. On the other hand, if the chi-square is not significant, one may infer that the fit is good and there is perfect conformity between the observed and expected frequencies. The detailed procedure has been shown in the following solved examples.

Example 10.1 The following table gives the number of injured athletes reporting to a college physiotherapy center during various days of the week. Test whether the injuries are uniformly distributed over the week at the significance level 0.05.

Days	Mon	Tue	Wed	Thu	Fri	Sat
No of Injuries	18	14	10	8	20	2

TABLE 10.1 Computation of Chi-Square

Days	f_o	f_e	$(f_o - f_e)$	$(f_o - f_e)^2$	$\frac{(f_o - f_e)^2}{f_e}$
Mon	18	12	6	36	3.00
Tue	14	12	2	4	0.33
Wed	10	12	−2	4	0.33
Thur	8	12	−4	16	1.33
Fri	20	12	8	64	5.33
Sat	2	12	−10	100	8.33
		$\sum f_o = 72$			18.65

Solution:

Hypothesis: To test whether injuries are uniformly distributed, the following hypotheses need to be tested.

H_0: Injuries are uniformly distributed over the week.

H_1: Injuries are not uniformly distributed over the week.

Level of significance: 0.05

Test statistic: Since this is the case of testing the goodness of fit, the chi-square shall be used as test statistic to test the null hypothesis. Under the null hypothesis, the expected frequencies of injuries on each day would be obtained by dividing the sum of the observed frequencies by 6. The computation of expected frequencies and terms involved in computing the chi-square are shown in Table 10.1:

$$\chi^2 = \sum \frac{(f_o - f_e)^2}{f_e} = 18.65$$

From Table A.11 in the Appendix, $\chi^2_{0.05,5}$ is 11.07. The degree of freedom is obtained as $(r - 1) = 5$, where r is the number of groups.

Since calculated value of $\chi^2(= 18.65)$ is greater than 11.07, H_0 may be rejected at the significance level 0.05.

Inference: Since H_0 has been rejected, it may be concluded that the injuries are not uniformly distributed throughout the week.

Example 10.2 In an experiment, the popularity of three sports was investigated in a college. Following are the frequencies of responses of the students toward their preference of sport. Each subject was allowed to give only one option.

Sports:	Soccer	Basketball	Cricket
Frequency	20	60	40

TABLE 10.2 Computation of Chi-Square

Sports	f_o	f_e	$(f_o - f_e)^2$	$\frac{(f_o - f_e)^2}{f_e}$
Soccer	20	40	400	10
Basketball	60	40	400	10
Cricket	40	40	0	0
	$\sum f_o = 120$			

Test whether all three sports are equally popular in the college at the significance level 0.05?

Solution:

Hypothesis: To test whether all three sports are equally popular in the college, the following hypotheses shall be tested.

H_0: All three sports are equally popular.

H_1: Popularity of at least one sport differs.

Level of significance: 0.05

Test statistic: Since in this example, goodness of fit is required to be tested, the chi-square shall be used as a test statistic to test the null hypothesis. Under the null hypothesis, the expected frequency for each sport would be 40. This is obtained by dividing the sum of the observed frequencies (120) by the number of groups (3) (Table 10.2).

$$\chi^2 = \sum \frac{(f_o - f_e)^2}{f_e} = 10 + 10 + 0 = 20$$

Here, the degrees of freedom for χ^2 is 2 ($= r - 1$). From Table A.11 in the Appendix, $\chi^2_{0.05,2}$ is 5.99. Since the calculated value of $\chi^2 (= 20)$ is greater than 5.99, H_0 may be rejected at the significance level 0.05.

Inference: Since H_0 has been rejected, it may be concluded that all three sports, namely, soccer, basketball, and cricket are not equally popular in the college.

10.3.4 Test for Independence of Attributes

Another application of the chi-square is to test the independence of two attributes. For instance, it may be interesting to test whether any association exists between the gender and their attitude toward sports. The attitude may be classified as positive or negative. Here, sex and attitude are the two attributes on the basis of which the subjects in the sample can be classified in a 2 × 2 table known as the *contingency* table. The chi-square test can be applied even if the frequencies are classified in an $m \times n$ table, where m and n may be any integers, but it is more efficient when used in a 2 × 2 contingency table. Thus, the chi-square can be used to test the association between the two categorical variables having two or more categories.

FACTS TO KNOW

While testing the independence of attributes, the significance of chi-square indicates that the levels of one attribute differ across the levels of another attribute

Let us see how to compute the chi-square in a 2 × 2 contingency table and test its significance. Later its computation and test of significance shall be discussed for a generalized case by means of an example. Consider the two attributes A and B representing academic and sports performance, respectively, both being dichotomous in nature. The frequencies of the subjects possessing these attributes can be shown in the 2 × 2 contingency table (Table 10.3). The symbol "*a*" represents the frequency of subjects having high performance in academics as well as sports, whereas "*d*" represents the frequency of subjects having low performance in academics as well as sports. On the other hand, the symbol "*b*" represents the frequency of subjects having high academic and low sports performance, whereas "*c*" represents the frequency of the subjects having low academic and high sports performance. Here, the null hypothesis of no association between the two attributes A and B is required to be tested.

Under the null hypothesis that the attributes are independent, the expected cell frequency for each cell is calculated as follows:

$$a_e = \frac{(a+b)\times(a+c)}{N}$$

$$b_e = \frac{(a+b)\times(b+d)}{N}$$

$$c_e = \frac{(c+d)\times(a+c)}{N}$$

$$d_e = \frac{(c+d)\times(b+d)}{N}$$

TABLE 10.3 Observed Frequencies (f_o)

		Sports (B)		
		High	Low	Total
Academic (A)	High	a	b	$a+b$
	Low	c	d	$c+d$
	Total	$a+c$	$b+d$	N

TABLE 10.4 Expected Frequencies (f_e)

		Sports (B)	
		High	Low
Academic (A)	High	a_e	b_e
	Low	c_e	d_e

The statistic chi-square (χ^2) can be calculated using the following formula:

$$\chi^2 = \sum\sum \frac{(f_o - f_e)^2}{f_e} \tag{10.2}$$

where f_o and f_e are the observed and expected frequencies as shown in Tables 10.3 and 10.4, respectively. The chi-square statistic as shown in Equation (10.2) follows chi-square distribution with $(r - 1) \times (c - 1)$ degrees of freedom.

The chi-square statistic can also be computed directly by the following formula without computing the expected frequencies:

$$\chi^2 = \frac{N(ad - bc)^2}{(a + b)(c + d)(a + c)(b + d)} \tag{10.3}$$

where a, b, c, and d are the observed frequencies as shown in Table 10.3.

The critical value of chi-square with $(r - 1) \times (c - 1)$ degrees of freedom and at α significance level ($\chi^2_{\alpha,(r-1)(k-1)}$) can be seen from the chi-distribution Table A.11 in the Appendix. The procedure for testing the independence of attributes can be easily understood by seeing Examples 10.3 and 10.4.

10.3.5 Yates' Correction

One of the assumptions in using the chi-square is that none of the expected cell frequencies should be less than 5. Generally, in a situation where this happens, concerned cell is merged with a nearby cell to make the expected frequencies more than 5 and then the analysis is done as usual. But in the case of the 2 × 2 contingency table, if the cells are merged, then the chi-square is obtained with 0 degree of freedom, which is meaningless. In such cases, a correction for continuity, which is known as *Yates' correction*, was suggested by F. Yates (1934). In applying this correction, 0.5 is subtracted from each difference of the observed and expected cell frequencies. Thus, the formula for chi-square (χ^2) with Yates' correction becomes

$$\chi^2 = \sum\sum \frac{(f_o - f_e - 0.5)^2}{f_e} \tag{10.4}$$

Example 10.3 The following table shows the response of male and female students toward sports participation. Test whether gender is associated with the response toward sports participation.

Gender	Play Sports	Do Not Play Sports
Male	55	20
Female	20	30

Solution:

Hypothesis: To test the association between gender and preference toward playing sports, the following hypotheses need to be tested.

H_0: There is no association between gender and sports participation.

H_1: There is an association between gender and sports participation.

Level of significance: 0.05

Test statistic: To test the association between the two attributes, the chi-square given below shall be used as the test statistic.

$$\chi^2 = \sum \frac{(f_o - f_e)^2}{f_e}$$

The expected frequency for each cell has been calculated by dividing the product of the marginal row and column totals associated with the cell by the total of all the frequencies N in Table 10.5. The expected frequencies so obtained are shown in Table 10.6.

$$\text{Calculated } \chi^2 = \sum \frac{(f_o - f_e)^2}{f_e} = \frac{(55-45)^2}{45} + \frac{(20-30)^2}{30}$$

$$+ \frac{(20-30)^2}{30} + \frac{(30-20)^2}{20}$$

$$= \frac{100}{45} + \frac{100}{30} + \frac{100}{30} + \frac{100}{20} = 13.89$$

$$\text{d.f.} = (r-1)(c-1) = (2-1)(2-1) = 1$$

TABLE 10.5 Observed Frequencies (f_o)

Gender	Play Sports	Do Not Play Sports	Total
Male	55	20	75
Female	20	30	50
Total	75	50	$N = 125$

TABLE 10.6 Expected Frequencies (f_e)

Gender	Play Sports	Do Not Play Sports
Male	$\frac{75 \times 75}{125} = 45$	$\frac{50 \times 75}{125} = 30$
Female	$\frac{75 \times 50}{125} = 30$	$\frac{50 \times 50}{125} = 20$

From Table A.11 in the Appendix, $\chi^2_{.05,1} = 3.84$. Since the calculated χ^2 is greater than 3.84, the null hypothesis of no association between gender and sports participation may be rejected at the significance level 0.05.

Inference: Since the null hypothesis has been rejected, it may therefore be concluded that there is an association between the gender and sports participation.

Example 10.4 Forty-five men and 45 women athletes were asked to respond to the question, "Should athletes prohibit themselves from smoking?" Each athlete answered by saying "Yes," "No," or "Undecided." The response frequencies so obtained are shown in Table 10.7. Test whether there is a genuine gender difference in their responses at the significance level 0.05. Further, compute contingency coefficient also.

Solution: Here, it is required to test whether the response pattern of men and women is different on the issue "Should athletes prohibit themselves from smoking?" This hypothesis shall be verified by testing the following null hypothesis.

Hypotheses:

H_0: There is no association between gender and response pattern.
H_1: There is an association between gender and response pattern.

Level of significance: 0.05

Test statistic: Since it is required to test the null hypothesis of no association between the gender and response, the following chi-square statistic shall be used as a test statistic.

TABLE 10.7 Observed Frequencies

Gender	Response (f_o)			Total
	Yes	No	Undecided	
Men	15	25	5	45
Women	30	10	5	45
Total	45	35	10	$N = 90$

TABLE 10.8 Expected Frequencies

	Response (f_e)		
Gender	Yes	No	Undecided
Men	$\frac{45 \times 45}{90} = 22.5$	$\frac{45 \times 35}{90} = 17.5$	$\frac{45 \times 10}{90} = 5$
Women	$\frac{45 \times 45}{90} = 22.5$	$\frac{45 \times 35}{90} = 17.5$	$\frac{45 \times 10}{90} = 5$

$$\chi^2 = \sum \frac{(f_o - f_e)^2}{f_e}$$

The expected frequencies in Table 10.7 need to be calculated for computing the chi-square. These frequencies have been obtained in Table 10.8 for each cell by dividing the product of the marginal row and column totals associated with each cell by the total of all the frequencies N.

$$\text{Calculated } \chi^2 = \sum \frac{(f_o - f_e)^2}{f_e} = \frac{(15-22.5)^2}{22.5} + \frac{(25-17.5)^2}{17.5} + \frac{(5-5)^2}{5}$$

$$= \frac{(30-22.5)^2}{22.5} + \frac{(10-17.5)^2}{17.5} + \frac{(5-5)^2}{5} = 11.42$$

$$df = (r-1)(c-1) = (2-1)(3-1) = 2$$

From Table A.11 in the Appendix, the value of $\chi^2_{.05,2}$ is 5.99. Since the calculated χ^2 (=11.42) is greater than 5.99, the null hypothesis of no association between gender and the response pattern on the issue "Should athletes prohibit themselves from smoking?" is rejected at the significance level 0.05.

Inference: Since the null hypothesis has been rejected, it may be inferred that the response patterns of males and females differ. It is worth noting that we tested the hypothesis of no association but we ended up in saying that the response patterns of males and females differ.

10.3.6 Additive Property of Chi-Square

The sum of chi-squares is also a chi-square with degrees of freedom combined. This property is useful in comparing the responses of two groups on a construct that is further divided into many variables. For example, the state anxiety questionnaire consists of many questions segregated into different dimensions. The responses of undergraduate and postgraduate students to each question can be compared by using the chi-square. Further, all these chi-squares together add up to a new chi-square with degrees of freedom combined that compares the attitude of two groups on state anxiety. The following example shall explain the fact more clearly.

TABLE 10.9 Responses of the Students

Innovation in Coaching			Agree	Disagree	Undecided
Q.1	Coaches should develop a useful philosophy of their own	UG	8	2	10
		PG	12	2	6
Q.2	A good coach should experiment on his trainees	UG	9	8	3
		PG	4	15	1
Q.3	The training pattern should be changed frequently for better results	UG	8	10	2
		PG	5	12	3
Q.4	Psychological treatments can be done in a better way by a coach than a psychologist	UG	10	5	5
		PG	14	4	2
Q.5	There should be different coaches at different times in order to avoid boredom	UG	9	6	5
		PG	9	8	4

Example 10.5 A study was conducted on 40 college students to compare the attitude of male postgraduate and undergraduate students on the issue of innovation in coaching. The responses of the students so obtained are shown in Table 10.9.

Solution: The objectives of this study are twofold. Firstly, it is required to compare the attitude of undergraduate and postgraduate students on each question, which explains different dimensions of innovation; secondly, it is required to compare the attitude of both the groups on innovation in coaching as a whole. To achieve these objectives, the following hypotheses need to be tested.

Hypotheses:

H_0: There is no association between the levels of students and their response.
H_1: There is an association between the levels of students and their response.

Level of significance: 0.05

Test statistic: Since association between two attributes needs to be tested, the following chi-square statistic shall be used as a test statistic.

$$\chi^2 = \sum \frac{(f_o - f_e)^2}{f_e}$$

The expected frequency against each observed frequency has been computed by dividing the product of the marginal row and column totals associated with each cell by the total of all the frequencies N. For instance, the expected

TABLE 10.10 Observed and Expected Frequencies for the Data on Innovation in Coaching

Questions		f_o A	f_o D	f_o U	f_o T	f_e A	f_e D	f_e U	Chi-Square
Q.1 Coaches should develop a useful philosophy of their own	UG	8	2	10	20	10	2	8	1.8
	PG	12	2	6	20	10	2	8	
	T	20	4	16	$N=40$				
Q.2 A good coach should experiment on his trainees	UG	9	8	3	20	6.5	11.5	2	5.05
	PG	4	15	1	20	6.5	11.5	2	
	T	13	23	4	$N=40$				
Q.3 The training pattern should be changed frequently for better results	UG	8	10	2	20	6.5	11	2.5	1.07
	PG	5	12	3	20	6.5	11	2.5	
	T	13	22	5	$N=40$				
Q.4 Psychological treatments can be done in a better way by a coach than a psychologist	UG	10	5	5	20	12	4.5	3.5	2.06
	PG	14	4	2	20	12	4.5	3.5	
	T	24	9	7	$N=40$				
Q.5 There should be different coaches at different times in order to avoid boredom	UG	9	6	5	20	8.5	7	4.5	0.46
	PG	8	8	4	20	8.5	7	4.5	
	T	17	14	9	$N=40$				

A: Agree, D: Disagree, U: Undecided, T: Total, UG: Undergraduate, PG: Postgraduate

frequencies against all the observed frequencies for the first question shall be as follows:

Question 1: The six expected frequencies are as follows.

$$\frac{20 \times 20}{40} = 10, \quad \frac{20 \times 4}{40} = 2, \quad \frac{20 \times 16}{40} = 8$$
$$\frac{20 \times 20}{40} = 10, \quad \frac{20 \times 4}{40} = 2, \quad \frac{20 \times 16}{40} = 8$$

The observed and expected frequencies are shown in Table 10.10.

Computation of chi-square for testing the null hypothesis in each question

$$\text{Question 1}: \chi^2 = \frac{(8-10)^2}{10} + \frac{(2-2)^2}{2} + \frac{(10-8)^2}{8} + \frac{(12-10)^2}{10}$$
$$+ \frac{(2-2)^2}{2} + \frac{(6-8)^2}{8} = 1.8$$

$$\text{Question 2}: \chi^2 = \frac{(9-6.5)^2}{6.5} + \frac{(8-11.5)^2}{11.5} + \frac{(3-2)^2}{2} + \frac{(4-6.5)^2}{6.5}$$

$$+\frac{(15-11.5)^2}{11.5} + \frac{(1-2)^2}{2} = 5.05$$

$$\text{Question 3}: \chi^2 = \frac{(8-6.5)^2}{6.5} + \frac{(10-11)^2}{11} + \frac{(2-2.5)^2}{2.5} + \frac{(5-6.5)^2}{6.5}$$

$$+\frac{(12-11)^2}{11} + \frac{(3-2.5)^2}{2.5} = 1.07$$

$$\text{Question 4}: \chi^2 = \frac{(10-12)^2}{12} + \frac{(5-4.5)^2}{4.5} + \frac{(5-3.5)^2}{3.5} + \frac{(14-12)^2}{12}$$

$$+\frac{(4-4.5)^2}{4.5} + \frac{(2-3.5)^2}{3.5} = 2.06$$

$$\text{Question 5}: \chi^2 = \frac{(9-8.5)^2}{8.5} + \frac{(6-7)^2}{7} + \frac{(5-4.5)^2}{4.5} + \frac{(8-8.5)^2}{8.5}$$

$$+\frac{(8-7)^2}{7} + \frac{(4-4.5)^2}{4.5} = 0.46$$

$$\text{Total } \chi^2 = 1.8 + 5.05 + 1.07 + 2.06 + 0.46 = 10.44$$

df for each question $= (r-1)(c-1) = (2-1)(3-1) = 2$,

$$\chi^2_{0.05,2} = 5.99$$

df for all the five questions combined $= 5 \times 2 = 10$,

$$\chi^2_{0.05,10} = 18.31$$

Since the calculated χ^2 is not greater than 5.99 for any of the questions, H_0 may not be rejected in all the five questions individually. Further combined χ^2 (=10.44) is also less than 18.31, H_0 may also not be rejected with respect to innovation in coaching.

Inference: It may be concluded that there is no association between the levels of students and response on each of the five questions on innovation. In other words, the response patterns of undergraduate and postgraduate students are not different on each of the five questions independently. Further, it may be inferred that the response of undergraduate and postgraduate students also do not differ on the issue of innovation in coaching in general.

Check Your Progress

Note: Tick the correct answer by using the sign (√).

	True	False
1. The *t*-test can be used for independent as well as dependent samples.	-	-
2. Nonparametric test should be used when the population distribution is not normal.	-	-
3. In parametric tests, the test statistic can be constructed on the basis of ranks.	-	-
4. If the observations are obtained on the ordinal or nominal scale, then some of the parametric tests can be used only in some very specific situations.	-	-
5. Nonparametric tests can be used for parametric data but the reverse is not true.	-	-
6. One should avoid using parametric tests especially if the sample is small and the related assumptions do not hold.	-	-
7. To use parametric tests, the data must be at least on an interval scale.	-	-
8. In using the *t*-test, the assumption of normality for the population distribution is not required.	-	-
9. Nonparametric tests cannot be applied if their assumptions do not hold.	-	-
10. The test statistic in nonparametric tests is constructed on the basis of signs or ranks.	-	-
11. The nonparametric tests are also known as distribution-free tests.	-	-
12. In comparing the playing ability between the two soccer teams, parametric and nonparametric tests are equally effective.	-	-
13. If assumptions of a parametric test are not fulfilled, then its power decreases.	-	-
14. Whether the sample is large or small, a parametric test should only be used if the distribution is normal.	-	-
15. Nonparametric tests are severely affected by outliers.	-	-
16. Both parametric and nonparametric tests can be used for nonparametric data.	-	-

17. Parametric tests should not be used if the data are not normally distributed. - -
18. Parametric tests are always more precise in comparison to nonparametric tests, provided their related assumptions are satisfied. - -
19. Parametric tests are affected by outliers. - -

10.4 RUNS TEST

> **FACTS TO KNOW**
>
> Nonparametric tests can be efficiently used for metric data as well if the assumptions required for parametric tests are not satisfied

The runs test is used to investigate the random occurrence of events in a sample drawn from a population. Drawing a random sample is one of the preconditions for any decision-making process in statistical inference. The runs test can be used to test whether a sample has been randomly drawn from the population or not. This test is based on the runs obtained in the sample. A run is a sequence of events occurring successively in the series. For instance, in tossing a coin seven times, if the outcome is *TTHHHTT*, then this sample consists of three runs, *TT*, *HHH*, and *TT*. In case the sample is a set of scores, then the runs are made of "+" or "−" signs that appear successively in the sample. Each observation is denoted by a "+" sign if it is greater than the previous score and a "−" sign if it is less than the previous score. If the number of runs is few, it indicates that the scores are grouped in a definite order and the scores are not random in nature, whereas a large number of runs indicates that the sample selection is affected by systematic cyclical fluctuations. In a runs test, we test the following hypotheses:

H_0: Sample values come in a random order.
H_1: Sample values come in a nonrandom order.

The null hypothesis in a runs test is tested by using the test statistic "r" in case of a small sample and "z" in case of a large sample. The sample is said to be large if both n_1 and n_2 are greater than 20, where n_1 is the number of the first type of event (or sign) and n_2 is the number of the second type of event (or sign) in the sample.

10.4.1 Test Statistic

In case of a small sample, the number of total runs "r" is the test statistic obtained by counting both the types of runs appearing in the sample. If the sample consists of occurrence of two events, say male (M) and female (F), then the test statistic "r" shall be obtained by counting the number of M and F runs. Similarly, if the sample consists of the scores, then the test statistic "r" is counted by adding the total number of "+" sign runs and the total number of "−"sign runs. If the observation is equal to its preceding observation, then denote it by zero and delete it while counting the number of runs.

10.4.2 Critical Value

The critical value for the test statistic "r" is obtained from Table A.12 in the Appendix corresponding to samples of sizes n_1 and n_2 and at an α significance level. This table provides two critical values, namely, $r_{\text{c\_lower}}$ and $r_{\text{c\_upper}}$.

10.4.3 Decision Rule

The decision rule below is followed in testing the null hypothesis: If $r_{\text{c\_lower}} < r < r_{\text{c\_upper}}$, do not reject the null hypothesis and if r is either less than $r_{\text{c\_lower}}$ or greater than $r_{\text{c\_upper}}$, reject the null hypothesis.

10.4.4 Large Sample Size

In case of large samples, that is, when n_1 and n_2 are both greater than 20, then the test statistic is obtained by the following z-statistic

$$Z = \frac{r - \text{Mean}(r)}{\text{SD}(r)} \tag{10.5}$$

where r is the total number of runs and

$$\text{Mean}(r) = \frac{2n_1 n_2}{n_1 + n_2} + 1 \tag{10.6}$$

$$\text{SD}(r) = \sqrt{\frac{2n_1 n_2(2n_1 n_2 - n_1 - n_2)}{(n_1 + n_2)^2(n_1 + n_2 - 1)}} \tag{10.7}$$

This z-statistic follows the standard normal distribution and is compared with the tabulated value of z at a particular significance level for testing the null hypothesis.

Example 10.6 In a soccer match, the arrival of boys and girls at the ticket window was observed in the following sequence:

BGG B G B B G B G G G B G G G B B G B G G G B BGG

Can it be concluded that the arrival of spectators was not biased with respect to gender? Test your hypothesis at 5% level.

Solution:

Hypothesis: The hypotheses that are required to be tested are as follows:

H_0: The arrival of boys and girls is random.
H_1: The arrival of boys and girls is not random.

Level of significance: 0.05

Test statistic: Since the sample sizes of both the groups, that is, n_1 and n_2, are less than 20, the total number of runs (r) will be used as the test statistic.

Computation or runs Given that

n_1 = number of boys in the sample = 11

n_2 = number of girls in the sample = 16

The number of runs existing in the sample can be counted by breaking it:

B	*GG*	*B*	*G*	*BB*	*G*	*B*	*GGG*	*B*	*GGG*	*BB*	*G*	*B*	*GGG*	*BB*	*GG*
1	2	3	4	5	6	7	8	9	10	11	12	13	14	15	16

Since there are 16 consecutive sequences of B and G,

$$r = \text{number of total runs} = 16$$

From Table A.12 in the Appendix, the lowest and highest critical values of the runs (r_c) for n_1=11 and n_2=16 are 8 and 20.

Since observed number of runs r (=16) lies in between 8 and 20, the null hypothesis H_0 is not rejected at 5% level.

Inference: Since the null hypothesis has not been rejected, it may be concluded that the arrival of boys and girls in the soccer match is random in nature.

Example 10.7 A random group of athletes from the university was tested for their high jump performance, which is shown below. Can it be concluded that the sample has been drawn in a random fashion? Test your hypothesis at 5% level.

High Jump Performance in Meters

1.4	1.5	1.3	1.2	1.5	1.45	1.5	1.42	1.41	1.52	1.56	1.43	1.41	1.40	1.8	1.9	1.6
1.5	1.45	1.5	1.6	1.5	1.45	1.8	1.6	1.7	1.6	1.5	1.9	1.5	1.45	1.42	1.7	1.6
1.7	1.8	1.5	1.8	1.82	1.85	1.7	1.72	1.8	1.82	1.6						

Solution:

Hypotheses: The following hypotheses are required to be tested:

H_0: The high jump performance is random in nature.

H_1: The high jump performance is not random in nature.

Level of significance: 0.05

Test statistic: Since the sample sizes of both the groups, that is, n_1 (number of + sign) and n_2 (number of − sign) are more than 20, the following z-statistic shall be used as the test statistic.

$$Z = \frac{r - \text{Mean}(r)}{\text{SD}(r)}$$

where r is the number of runs and

$$\text{Mean }(r) = \frac{2n_1n_2}{n_1 + n_2} + 1$$

$$\text{SD }(r) = \sqrt{\frac{2n_1n_2(2n_1n_2 - n_1 - n_2)}{(n_1 + n_2)^2(n_1 + n_2 - 1)}}$$

Computation of runs and z-statistic If a score is larger than the previous score, it is given a + sign and if it is smaller than the previous score, it is given a − sign. The first score has been given a − sign.

1.4	1.5	1.3	1.2	1.5	1.45	1.5	1.42	1.41	1.52	1.56	1.43	1.41	1.40	1.8	1.9	1.6
−	+	−	−	+	−	+	−	−	+	+	−	−	−	+	+	−
1.5	1.45	1.5	1.6	1.5	1.45	1.8	1.6	1.7	1.6	1.5	1.9	1.5	1.45	1.42	1.7	1.6
−	−	+	+	−	−	+	−	+	−	−	+	−	−	−	+	−
1.7	1.8	1.5	1.8	1.82	1.85	1.7	1.72	1.8	1.82	1.6						
+	+	−	+	+	+	−	+	+	+	−						

The runs have been made by keeping the consecutive signs "+" and "−" together. Thus, the total number of runs is as follows:

−	+	− −	+	−	+	− −	++	− − −	++	− − −	+ +	− −	+	−
1	2	3	4	5	6	7	8	9	10	11	12	13	14	15
+	− −	+	− − −	+	−	++	−	+++	−	+++	−			
16	17	18	19	20	21	22	23	24	25	26	27			

Here,

$$n_1 = \text{number of "−" signs} = 24, \quad n_2 = \text{number of "+" signs} = 21$$

$$r = \text{total number of runs} = 27, \qquad N = n_1 + n_2 = 45$$

$$\text{Mean }(r) = \frac{2n_1n_2}{n_1+n_2} + 1 = \frac{2\times 24\times 21}{24+21} + 1 = 23.4$$

$$\text{SD }(r) = \sqrt{\frac{2n_1n_2(2n_1n_2 - n_1 - n_2)}{(n_1+n_2)^2(n_1+n_2-1)}}$$

$$= \sqrt{\frac{2\times 24\times 21(2\times 24\times 21 - 24 - 21)}{(24+21)^2\times(24+21-1)}}$$

$$= \sqrt{\frac{970704}{89100}} = 10.895$$

Substituting the values, we get

$$Z = \frac{27 - 23.4}{10.895} = 0.330$$

From Table A.4 in the Appendix, the critical value of z at 5% level is 1.96. Since calculated value of z is less than 1.96, the null hypothesis may not be rejected.

Inference: Since the null hypothesis has not been rejected, it may be concluded that the performance in high jump is random in nature.

Check Your Progress

Note: Tick the correct answer by using the sign ($\surd$).

	True	False
20. The chi-square test is used to test whether the observed frequencies match the theoretical frequencies.	-	-
21. If the chi-square is significant, then the fit is good.	-	-
22. Chi-square cannot be used if the observations are numerical scores rather than frequencies.	-	-
23. One of the assumptions of the chi-square is that all the observations are independent of each other.	-	-
24. Normality assumption cannot be tested by the goodness-of-fit test.	-	-
25. If you add two chi-squares, the resultant shall be a chi-square.	-	-

26. In a small sample, the total number of runs "*r*" is the test statistic.	-	-
27. In testing the goodness of fit, the degrees of freedom for the chi-square is $(r-1)(c-1)$.	-	-
28. When the number of + and – signs is less than 20, the *z*-test can be used in a runs test.	-	-
29. The chi-square test is more efficient if it is used for the data in a 2 × 2 contingency table.	-	-
30. In applying the runs test, if the number of runs is between the two critical values, it indicates that the sample has not been randomly drawn.	-	-
31. Chi-square can be computed if the scores are given in the form of percentages.	-	-
32. The runs test can be used when the data are in the form of scores.	-	-
33. The degree of freedom of chi-square in testing the independence of attributes is obtained by $(r-1)$.	-	-
34. The chi-square can be computed if the observations are measured on an ordinal scale.	-	-
35. Yates' correction is used if the expected frequency for any of the cells is less than 5.	-	-
36. Whether a sample has been drawn randomly or not can be tested by using the runs test.	-	-
37. The chi-square test can be used even if the number of categories in both the attributes is not the same.	-	-
38. In *HTHTHT*, there are 2 runs.	-	-

PRACTICE EXERCISE

1. Use the chi-square test to determine whether the distribution of observed and expected frequencies in the preference of different sports given below is the same. Test your hypothesis at $\alpha = 0.05$.

Sport	Cricket	Basketball	Gymnastics	Swimming	Tennis
f_o	50	40	45	30	25
f_e	40	45	50	40	15

2. Use the following contingency table to test whether IQ is independent of sports achievement. Let $\alpha = 0.01$.

		Sports achievement	
		High	Low
IQ	High	40	20
	Low	15	25

3. On the basis of the following contingency table, can it be concluded that the response of males and females is significantly different on the statement "Male coaches are more creative than female coaches?" Let $\alpha = 0.01$.

		Response		
		Agree	Undecided	Disagree
Gender	Boys	30	5	25
	Girls	40	15	5

4. Following are the heights of students in a sample. Test whether the sample has been drawn randomly or not. Let $\alpha = 0.01$.

5.6 5.8 5.5 5.6 5.9 5.4 5.6 5.7 5.8 5.4 5.5 5.3

5. A sample of 55 persons was tested on minimum muscular fitness test. Twelve persons could not qualify in the test. The sequence of successful and unsuccessful candidates is given below, where S represents success and F, failure.

S S S S F S S S S S S S S F S S S S S S S F S F S S S S S S S
S S F F S S S S S S S S S F F S S S F F S S F S F S

With a two-tailed test and $\alpha = 0.05$, what conclusion can be drawn about the randomness of the sample?

10.5 MANN–WHITNEY *U*-TEST FOR TWO SAMPLES

The Mann–Whitney *U*-test is used for comparing two independent samples. In using this test, no assumption is required about the distribution of the population from which the samples have been drawn. In using the Mann–Whitney test, the intention of the researcher is to test whether the two samples come from the same population or not. This test can be used for parametric as well as nonparametric data, and therefore it is considered to be the most powerful nonparametric test. It can be used more efficiently as an alternative to the t-test in case one wishes to avoid assumptions such as equality of variance and normality of the population distribution. To use this test, the data must be at least on the ordinal scale and samples must be randomly drawn. In using the Mann–Whitney test, the following hypotheses are tested:

FACTS TO KNOW

In using the Mann–Whitney test, if the value of the U-statistic is less than its critical value, the null hypothesis is rejected

H_0: The two samples come from the same population.
H_1: The two samples come from different populations.

In case of a small sample, the null hypothesis is tested by using the test statistic U, whereas the z-statistic is used in case of a large sample. The test statistic U is computed on the basis of ranks rather than scores. The sample is said to be large if the sizes of the samples, n_1 and n_2, are greater than 10.

10.5.1 Test Statistic

In case of a small sample, the test statistic U is computed by following the procedure explained in the following:

a. Combine the scores of both the groups and arrange them in ascending order.
b. Assign ranks to each and every score in the combined data set.
c. Find R_1 and R_2, where R_1 is the total of all the ranks received by all the scores in the first group and R_2 is the total of all the ranks received by all the scores in the second group.
d. Compute the values of U_1 and U_2 by using the following formula:

$$U_1 = n_1 n_2 + \frac{n_1(n_1+1)}{2} - R_1 \tag{10.8}$$

and

$$U_2 = n_1 n_2 + \frac{n_2(n_2+1)}{2} - R_2 \tag{10.9}$$

$$U_2 \text{ can also be calculated by } U_2 = n_1 n_2 - U_1 \tag{10.10}$$

e. The test statistic U shall be the minimum of U_1 and U_2.

10.5.2 Critical Value

In a small sample (n_1 and n_2 both are less than 10), the test statistic U shall be compared with the tabulated value U_c obtained from Table A.13 in the Appendix for the sample sizes n_1 and n_2 to test the hypothesis.

10.5.3 Decision Rule

If the value of calculated U is less than the critical value U_c, reject the null hypothesis, otherwise accept it.

10.5.4 Large Sample Size

In case of a large sample, that is, when n_1 and n_2 are both greater than 10, the following z-statistic is used to test the null hypothesis.

$$Z = \frac{U - \mu_U}{\sigma_U} \tag{10.11}$$

where

$$\mu_U = \frac{n_1 n_2}{2} \tag{10.12}$$

and

$$\sigma_U = \sqrt{\frac{n_1 n_2 (n_1 + n_2 + 1)}{12}} \tag{10.13}$$

This z-statistic follows the standard normal distribution and is compared with the tabulated value of z at a particular significance level for testing the null hypothesis.

Example 10.8 Following are the data on the arm length of badminton players and gymnasts measured in inches. Is there sufficient evidence in the data to determine whether the arm length of badminton players is significantly greater than that of the gymnasts? Apply the Mann–Whitney U-test to draw your conclusion at 5% level.

Arm Length in Inches

Badminton (B)	Gymnasts (G)
32.8	31.2
31.6	30.8
33.2	32.4
32	31
32.8	32.1
32	30
33.6	31.3
30.1	

TABLE 10.11 Combined Scores of Both the Groups and Their Ranks

Scores (1)	Group (2)	Rank (3)
30	G	1
30.1	G	2
30.8	G	3
31	G	4
31.2	G	5
31.3	G	6
31.6	B	7
32	B	8.5
32	B	8.5
32.1	G	10
32.4	G	11
32.8	B	12.5
32.8	B	12.5
33.2	B	14
33.6	B	15

Solution:

Hypotheses: The hypotheses that are required to be tested are as follows:

H_0: Arm lengths of badminton players and gymnasts are the same.

H_1: Arm lengths of badminton players and gymnasts are not the same.

Level of Significance: 0.05

Test Statistic: Since the sample sizes in both the groups, that is, n_1 and n_2, are less than 10, the U-statistic shall be used as the test statistic.

Computation of U-statistic All the scores have been arranged in ascending order after combining the scores of both the groups. These arranged scores are shown in Table 10.11. In column 1, the combined scores have been shown, whereas column 2 indicates the group to which the corresponding score belongs. Column 3 shows the ranks of the scores in the combined group. In case of a tie, an average rank has been assigned to each of the tied scores.

Adding the ranks of all the scores in the badminton (B) and gymnastics (G) groups as shown in Table 10.11, we get

$$R_1 = \text{Sum of the ranks of all the scores in the badminton group}$$
$$= 7 + 8.5 + 8.5 + 12.5 + 12.5 + 14 + 15 = 78.0$$

$$R_2 = \text{Sum of the ranks of all the scores in the gymnastics group}$$
$$= 1 + 2 + 3 + 4 + 5 + 6 + 10 + 11 = 42$$

Here,

n_1 = number of scores in the badminton group = 7

n_2 = number of scores in the gymnastics group = 8

$$U_1 = n_1 n_2 + \frac{n_1(n_1+1)}{2} - R_1 = 7 \times 8 + \frac{7 \times (7+1)}{2} - 78 = 6$$

$$U_2 = n_1 n_2 + \frac{n_2(n_2+1)}{2} - R_2 = 7 \times 8 + \frac{8 \times (8+1)}{2} - 42 = 50$$

Since smaller of the two values U_1 and U_2 is the value of the test statistic U, here the value of the test statistic is

$$U = 6$$

From Table A.13 in the Appendix, the critical value of U for $n_1 = 7$ and $n_2 = 8$ at the significance level 0.05 is 10. Since calculated value of U (=6) is less than the critical value 10, the null hypothesis is rejected.

Inference: Since the null hypothesis has been rejected, it may therefore be concluded that the arm length of badminton and gymnastics players differs significantly.

Example 10.9 Two random samples of volleyball players and athletes were drawn to compare their performance on agility. The subjects were tested for their performance on 4 × 100 m distance and their timings were noted. These timings are shown in the following table. Can it be concluded that the timings of volleyball players differ significantly from that of athletes? Apply the Mann–Whitney U-test to test your hypothesis at 5% level.

Performance on Agility in Seconds

Volleyball (V)	Athletics (A)
10.45	9.35
11.55	9.56
11.67	8.66
10.93	9.16
11.89	9.13
12.2	11.28
12.1	10.32
11.89	11.37
10.23	10.97
10.47	10.55
10.52	10.56

Solution:

Hypotheses: The hypotheses that are required to be tested here are as follows:

H_0: The agility of the volleyball and athletic groups is the same.

H_1: The agility of the volleyball and athletic groups differs.

Level of Significance: 0.05

Test Statistic: Since both the sample sizes are greater than 10 (n_1=11, n_2=11), the sample can be considered to be large and, in this case, the following z-statistic shall be used as the test statistic to test the above null hypothesis:

$$Z = \frac{U - \mu_U}{\sigma_U}$$

where

$$\mu_U = \frac{n_1 n_2}{2}$$

and

$$\sigma_U = \sqrt{\frac{n_1 n_2 (n_1 + n_2 + 1)}{12}}$$

Computation of U and z-Statistic The values of R_1 and R_2 shall be computed first to compute the values of U_1 and U_2, respectively. All the scores have been arranged in the ascending order after combining the scores of both the groups. These arranged scores are shown in Table 10.12. In column 1, the combined scores have been shown, whereas column 2 indicates the group to which the corresponding score belongs. Column 3 shows the ranks of the scores in the combined group. In case of tie, an average rank has been assigned to each of the tied scores.

Adding the ranks of all the scores in the volleyball (V) and athletics (A) groups in Table 10.12, we get

$$R_1 = \text{Sum of the ranks of all the scores in the volleyball group}$$
$$= 6 + 8 + 9 + 10 + 13 + 17 + 18 + 19.5 + 19.5 + 21 + 22 = 163$$
$$R_2 = \text{Sum of the ranks of all the scores in the athletics group}$$
$$= 1 + 2 + 3 + 4 + 5 + 7 + 11 + 12 + 14 + 15 + 16 = 90$$

Here,

$$n_1 = \text{number of scores in the volleyball group} = 11$$
$$n_2 = \text{number of scores in the athletics group} = 11$$
$$U_1 = n_1 n_2 + \frac{n_1(n_1 + 1)}{2} - R_1 = 11 \times 11 + \frac{11 \times (11 + 1)}{2} - 163 = 24$$
$$U_2 = n_1 n_2 - U_1 = 11 \times 11 - 24 = 97$$

TABLE 10.12 Combined Scores of Both the Samples and Their Ranks

Scores (1)	Group (2)	Rank (3)
8.66	A	1
9.13	A	2
9.16	A	3
9.35	A	4
9.56	A	5
10.23	V	6
10.32	A	7
10.45	V	8
10.47	V	9
10.52	V	10
10.55	A	11
10.56	A	12
10.93	V	13
10.97	A	14
11.28	A	15
11.37	A	16
11.55	V	17
11.67	V	18
11.89	V	19.5
11.89	V	19.5
12.1	V	21
12.2	V	22

Since the two-tailed test has been used to test the hypothesis, either of the values U_1 or U_2 can be taken as the value of the Mann–Whitney statistic U.

$$U = 24$$

$$\mu_U = \frac{n_1 n_2}{2} = \frac{11 \times 11}{2} = 60.5$$

and

$$\sigma_U = \sqrt{\frac{11 \times 11(11 + 11 + 1)}{12}} = 15.23$$

$$z = \frac{24 - 60.5}{15.23} = -2.397$$

$$\Rightarrow |z| = 2.397$$

The critical value of z at 5% level is equal to 1.96. Since the calculated value of z_1 (=2.397) is greater than 1.96, the null hypothesis is rejected.

Inference: Since the null hypothesis has been rejected, it may therefore be concluded that the volleyball and athletics groups differ significantly on agility.

10.6 WILCOXON MATCHED-PAIRS SIGNED-RANKS TEST

> **FACTS TO KNOW**
>
> In using the Wilcoxon matched-pairs signed-ranks test if the value of the T-statistic is less than its critical value, the null hypothesis is rejected

This test is used to compare two groups when the data in some sense are paired and we wish to test whether the members of a pair differ. In other words, this test is suitable when the groups are related to each other. When observations are measured data, the signed-ranks test is more efficient because it takes into account the magnitude of the observed differences. This test is useful if the response of a treatment is to be tested for its significance by comparing initial and final group data. For a large sample, this test is almost as sensitive as the t-test. For small numbers with unknown distributions, this test is even more sensitive than the Student t-test. Since one can rarely be sure that scores are normally distributed, this test may be preferred over the t-test. In the Wilcoxon matched-pairs signed-ranks test, we test the following hypotheses:

H_0: No difference exists between the initial and final groups' scores.
H_1: Significant difference exists between the initial and groups' scores.

The null hypothesis in the Wilcoxon matched-pairs signed-ranks test is tested by using the test statistic T in the case of a small sample and z in the case of a large sample. The sample is said to be large if the sample size is more than 15.

10.6.1 Test Statistic

In the case of a small sample, the statistic T is used as the test statistic. This statistic is computed by using the procedure explained in the following steps:

a. Compute the difference of scores for each subject.
b. Rank these difference scores regardless of whether the difference is positive or negative. If the difference is zero, ignore it and reduce the value of n accordingly. Rank these differences from the smallest to the largest, with a rank of 1 assigned to the smallest difference. If a difference is negative, the rank is given a negative sign.
c. In case of a tie, assign an average rank to all the tied scores.
d. Obtain $T+$ and $T-$ by adding all the positive and negative ranks, respectively.
e. The minimum of $T+$ and $T-$ will give the value of the test statistic T.

10.6.2 Critical Value

The critical value T_c for the test statistic T is obtained from Table A.14 in the appendix against the sample size n.

10.6.3 Decision Rule

If the value of the test statistic T is equal to or smaller than the critical value T_c, reject the null hypothesis, otherwise accept it.

10.6.4 Large Sample Size

In case of a large sample, that is, $n > 15$, the test statistic is obtained by the following z-statistic:

$$z = \frac{T - \mu_T}{\sigma_T} \tag{10.14}$$

where T is the total of ranks for either + or − differences, whichever is less in magnitude,

$$\mu_T = \frac{n(n+1)}{4} \tag{10.15}$$

and

$$\sigma_T = \sqrt{\frac{n(n+1)(2n+1)}{24}} \tag{10.16}$$

This z-statistic follows the standard normal distribution and is compared with the tabulated value of z at a particular significance level for testing the null hypothesis.

Example 10.10 Following are the weights of the subjects before and after a circuit training program. Apply the Wilcoxon matched-pairs signed-ranks test to determine whether the initial weights of the subjects are higher than the weights measured after the circuit training program. Test your hypothesis at 5% level by assuming that the underlying distributions are symmetrical.

Weights in lbs

Circuit training program	
Pre-test	Post-test
140	135
148	144
156	149
145	146
137	138
164	155
158	149
150	148
154	157

TABLE 10.13 Computation in Wilcoxon Matched-Pairs Signed-Ranks Test

	Circuit training program			
Pair (1)	Pre-test (2)	Post-test (3)	*d* (4)	Rank (5)
1	140	135	+5	+6
2	148	144	+4	+5
3	156	149	+7	+7
4	145	146	−1	−1.5
5	137	138	−1	−1.5
6	164	155	+9	+8.5
7	158	149	+9	+8.5
8	150	148	+2	+3
9	154	157	−3	− 4

Solution:

Hypotheses: The hypotheses that are required to be tested are as follows:

$$H_0\colon M_d = 0$$

$$H_1\colon M_d > 0.$$

Level of Significance: 0.05

Test Statistic: Since the sample size is less than 15, the statistic T shall be used as a test statistic for testing the above null hypothesis.

Computation of the T-statistic In Table 10.13, the difference (d) has been computed for each subject in column 4. These difference scores have been ranked regardless of whether the difference is positive or negative. These differences have been ranked from smallest to largest, with a rank of 1 assigned to the smallest difference. If a difference is negative, the rank is given a negative sign. In case of a tie, an average rank has been assigned to each of the tied scores.

The sums of positive ranks and negative ranks have been represented by $T+$ and $T-$, respectively. The minimum of $T+$ and $T-$ will give the value of the test statistic T.

Since

$$T = \text{minimum of } (T+, T-)$$

$$T+ = \text{Sum of the positive ranks} = 6 + 5 + 7 + 8.5 + 8.5 + 3 = 38$$

$$T- = \text{Sum of the negative ranks} = 1.5 + 1.5 + 4 = 7$$

$$T = \text{minimum of } (38, 7) = 7$$

From Table A.14 in the Appendix, the critical value of test statistic T for $n = 9$ in the one-tailed test at the significance level 0.05 is 8. Since the value of the test statistic T (=7) is smaller than the critical value 8, the null hypothesis is rejected.

Inference: Since the null hypothesis has been rejected, it may be concluded on the basis of the given sampled data that the weights of the subjects after the circuit training program were significantly lower than their weights before the program. In other words, the circuit training program was useful in reducing the weights of the participants in general.

Example 10.11 An exercise scientist introduced a fitness program in an industry. Seventeen executives were given this program schedule for 4 weeks to test its effectiveness in improving their wellness. The subject's wellness was tested before and after the program as shown in the following table. Can it be concluded that the wellness scores differ significantly in the post- and pre-test groups? Test your hypothesis at 5% level assuming that the underlying distributions are symmetrical.

	Wellness scores																
Pre-test	35	32	25	22	39	42	32	36	41	44	28	26	33	35	38	37	40
Post-test	25	29	26	24	31	38	31	30	36	38	29	25	31	29	32	39	42

Solution:

Hypotheses: The hypotheses that need to be tested are as follows:

$$H_0\colon M_{\mathrm{d}} = 0.$$

$$H_1\colon M_{\mathrm{d}} \neq 0.$$

Level of Significance: 0.05

Test Statistic: Since the sample size is greater than 15, the following z-statistic shall be used as a test statistic for testing the null hypothesis.

$$z = \frac{T - \mu_{\mathrm{T}}}{\sigma_{\mathrm{T}}}$$

where T is the total of the ranks for either + or − differences, whichever is less in magnitude and

$$\mu_{\mathrm{T}} = \frac{n(n+1)}{4}$$

and

$$\sigma_{\mathrm{T}} = \sqrt{\frac{n(n+1)(2n+1)}{24}}$$

Computation of T- and z-statistic In Table 10.14, the difference (d) has been computed for each subject in column 4. These difference scores have

TABLE 10.14 Computation in Wilcoxon Matched-Pairs Signed-Ranks Test

	Anxiety Scores			
Pair (1)	Pre-test (2)	Post-test (3)	*d* (4)	Rank (5)
1	35	25	+10	+17
2	32	29	+3	+7
3	25	26	−1	−2.5
4	22	24	−2	−5.5
5	39	31	+8	+16
6	42	38	+4	+8.5
7	32	31	+1	+2.5
8	36	30	+6	+13
9	41	36	+5	+10
10	44	38	+6	+13
11	28	29	−1	−2.5
12	26	25	+1	+2.5
13	33	31	+2	+5.5
14	35	29	+6	+13
15	38	32	+6	+13
16	37	39	−6	−13
17	40	42	−4	−8.5

been ranked regardless of whether the difference is positive or negative. These differences have been ranked from the smallest to the largest, with a rank of 1 assigned to the smallest difference. If a difference is negative, the rank is given a negative sign. In case of a tie, an average rank has been assigned to each of the difference scores.

The sums of the positive ranks and negative ranks have been represented by $T+$ and $T-$, respectively. The minimum of $T+$ and $T-$ will give the value of the test statistic T.

Since

$$T = \text{minimum of } \ (T+, T-)$$

$$T+ = \text{Sum of the positive ranks}$$

$$= 17 + 7 + 16 + 8.5 + 2.5 + 13 + 10 + 13 + 2.5 + 5.5 + 13 + 13$$

$$= 121.0$$

$$T- = \text{Sum of the negative ranks}$$

$$= 2.5 + 5.5 + 2.5 + 13 + 8.5 = 32.0$$

$$T = \text{minimum of } (32, 121) = 32$$

$$\mu_{\text{T}} = \frac{n(n+1)}{4} = \frac{17(17+1)}{4} = 76.5$$

$$\sigma_T = \sqrt{\frac{n(n+1)(2n+1)}{24}} = \sqrt{\frac{17(17+1)(2\times 17+1)}{24}} = 21.12$$

$$Z = \frac{T-\mu_T}{\sigma_T} = \frac{32-76.5}{21.12} = 2.11$$

The critical value of z at 5% level is 1.96 (Table A.4 in the Appendix). Since the calculated value of z (=2.11) is greater than 1.96, the null hypothesis is rejected.

Inference: Since the null hypothesis has been rejected, it may therefore be concluded on the basis of the given sample that the wellness scores differ before and after introduction of the exercise program in the industry.

10.7 KRUSKAL–WALLIS TEST (ONE-WAY ANOVA FOR NONPARAMETRIC DATA)

The Kruskal–Wallis test is an alternative to the one-way ANOVA in nonparametric testing. It is used to compare more than two samples simultaneously and decide whether they belong to the same population or not. Consider a study in which an experimenter is interested in comparing the style of play among three universities dominant in cricketing activities. Three random samples of cricket players may be randomly drawn from these three universities and their style of play may be judged by experienced judges who would rank these players. Under this situation, the Kruskal–Wallis test may be applied to compare their performance. This test is used when the data obtained are measured at least on the ordinal scale. The Kruskal–Wallis test can be used for parametric data as well if the assumptions for applying the ANOVA do not hold. In using this test, we are interested in testing the following hypotheses:

H_0: All three groups are equal.

H_1: All three groups are not equal.

The null hypothesis above is tested by using the test statistic H, which is computed on the basis of ranks rather than scores.

10.7.1 Test Statistic

The test statistic H in the Kruskal–Wallis test is computed by using formula (10.17):

$$H = \frac{12}{n(n+1)}\sum_{i=1}^{k}\frac{R_i^2}{n_i} - 3(n+1) \tag{10.17}$$

where

K = number of groups

n_i = number of scores in the ith group.
n = total number of scores in all the groups
R_i = total of ranks of all the scores in the ith group.

The test statistic H can be computed by using the procedure explained in the following steps:

1. Pool the scores of all the groups and assign them combined ranks. Give the lowest score the rank 1 and the highest score the rank n. In case of a tie, assign an average rank to all the tied scores.
2. Add the ranks of all the scores in each group and denote it by R_i. Thus, R_i is the total of the ranks of all the scores in the ith group.
3. Compute the H-statistic by formula (10.17).
4. The statistic H follows a chi-square distribution (χ^2) with $(k - 1)$ degrees of freedom.

10.7.2 Critical Value

Since the statistic H follows a chi-square distribution, the critical value of χ^2 with $n - 1$ degrees of freedom and at significance level α may be obtained from Table A.11 in the Appendix.

10.7.3 Decision Rule

If the value of the test statistic H is greater than the critical value $\chi^2_{\alpha,k-1}$, reject the null hypothesis, otherwise do not reject it.

Example 10.12 The data on vital capacity (in liters) obtained on players selected randomly in different sports groups are shown in Table 10.15. Apply the Kruskal–Wallis test to determine whether the vital capacity of all four groups differ from each other. Assume $\alpha = 0.05$.

TABLE 10.15 Data on Vital Capacity

Athletics	Gymnastics	Swimming	Basketball
3.7	3.9	4.1	4.9
3.5	4.1	4.2	4.8
3.4	4.2	4.3	4.9
3.6	3	4.3	4.8
3.7	2.9	3.9	4.8
3.8	4.1	5.1	
4.2	5.2		
4			

Solution:

Hypotheses: The following hypotheses are required to be tested:

H_0: The vital capacity of all four sports groups is the same.
H_1: The vital capacity of at least one group differs.

Level of Significance: 0.05

Test Statistic: In comparing these four groups, the Kruskal–Wallis test shall be used in which the following H-statistic shall be used as the test statistic:

$$H = \frac{12}{n(n+1)} \sum_{i=1}^{k} \frac{R_i^2}{n_i} - 3(n+1)$$

where n is the total number of scores in all four samples and R_i is the sum of the ranks of all the scores in the ith group, where the ranks have been assigned by combining the scores of all four groups.

The statistic H follows a chi-square distribution with $k - 1$ degrees of freedom.

Computation of H-Statistic To compute rank total (R_i) of each group, the scores in all four groups have been pooled first and then combined ranks have been allotted to all the scores. The lowest score has been given rank 1 and in case of a tie, an average rank has been assigned to each of the tied scores.

The ranks of combined data are shown in Table 10.16. Column 2 indicates the score of all four groups combined in ascending order. Column 3 indicates the group to which the corresponding score belongs and column 4 shows the ranks of the scores in the combined group.

The total of the ranks acquired by the scores in each group shall be obtained by using the ranks obtained in Table 10.16.

R_1 = Sum of the ranks of all the scores in the athletics group (A)

$= 3 + 4 + 5 + 6.5 + 6.5 + 8 = 33$

R_2 = Sum of the ranks of all the scores in the gymnastics group (G)

$= 1 + 2 + 9.5 + 13 + 16 = 41.5$

R_3 = Sum of the ranks of all the scores in the swimming group (S)

$= 9.5 + 11 + 13 + 13 + 16 + 16 + 18.5 + 18.5 = 115.5$

R_4 = Sum of the ranks of all the scores in the basketball group (B)

$= 21 + 21 + 21 + 23.5 + 23.5 + 25 + 26 = 161$

Here, k = number of groups $= 4$, $n_1 = 6$, $n_2 = 5$, $n_3 = 8$, and $n_4 = 7$, and $n = 6 + 5 + 8 + 7 = 26$.

TABLE 10.16 Combined Scores of All the Groups and Their Ranks

Sr.No. (1)	Scores (2)	Group (3)	Rank (4)
1	2.9	G	1
2	3	G	2
3	3.4	A	3
4	3.5	A	4
5	3.6	A	5
6	3.7	A	6.5
7	3.7	A	6.5
8	3.8	A	8
9	3.9	G	9.5
10	3.9	S	9.5
11	4	S	11
12	4.1	G	13
13	4.1	S	13
14	4.1	S	13
15	4.2	G	16
16	4.2	S	16
17	4.2	S	16
18	4.3	S	18.5
19	4.3	S	18.5
20	4.8	B	21
21	4.8	B	21
22	4.8	B	21
23	4.9	B	23.5
24	4.9	B	23.5
25	5.1	B	25
26	5.2	B	26
A: Athletics	G: Gymnastics	S: Swimming	B: Basketball

Substituting the values,

$$H = \frac{12}{n(n+1)} \sum_{i=1}^{k} \frac{R_i^2}{n_i} - 3(n+1)$$

$$= \frac{12}{26 \times (26+1)} \left(\frac{33^2}{6} + \frac{41.5^2}{5} + \frac{115.5^2}{8} + \frac{161^2}{7} \right) - 3 \times (26+1)$$

$$= 100.79 - 81 = 19.79$$

Since the statistic H follows a χ^2 distribution, by using Table A.11 in the Appendix, the tabulated value of χ^2 with 3(=k – 1) degrees of freedom and at the significance level 0.05 is 7.815. Since the calculated value of H is greater than 7.815, the null hypothesis is rejected.

Inference: Since the null hypothesis has been rejected, it may be inferred that on the basis of the given sample vital, capacity in the four groups is not same.

10.8 THE FRIEDMAN TEST

> **FACTS TO KNOW**
>
> The H-statistic in the Kruskal–Wallis test and the F_r statistic in the Friedman test, both follow the chi-square distribution

The Friedman test is also known as the two-way ANOVA for ranks. This test is used in a situation where repeated measures are obtained on the same set of subjects. In using this test, we try to detect differences in treatments across multiple test attempts. For instance, if the effect of three different intensities of aerobic exercises is to be seen on the pleasurable state of the participants, the same set of subjects may be tested under different treatment conditions. Since it is believed that age will have an impact on the pleasurable state under different treatment conditions, therefore the subjects may be randomly selected from different age groups. The advantage of such a design is to control the error due to the subjects and reduce the experimental error by blocking. In this above example, age is the blocking variable. Since pleasurable state cannot be measured objectively, the response of the participants measured on some scale may be ranked. Thus, the data in this design may be obtained in the form of ranks; further, all the data are related to each other as they have been obtained on the same subjects. Hence, the independence assumption also fails due to which the Kruskal–Wallis test cannot be applied. Thus, in such situations, the Friedman test can be efficiently used to compare the responses of the subjects under different treatment conditions. In using this test, it is assumed that the variables under study are continuous in nature and are measured at least on an ordinal scale. The Friedman test is used when the assumptions of normality and homogeneity of variances are not met. In this test, we compare three or more groups. Here, we test the following hypotheses:

H_0: All k samples are from the same population or from populations with equal medians.

H_1: All samples are not from the same population. They differ in their median values.

The null hypothesis is tested by using the test statistic F_r, which is computed on the basis of ranks rather than scores.

10.8.1 Test Statistic

The test statistic F_r in the Friedman test is computed by using the formula mentioned in (10.18):

$$F_r = \frac{12}{nk(k+1)} \sum_{i=1}^{k} R_i^2 - 3n(k+1) \tag{10.18}$$

where

$n =$ number of subjects
$k =$ number of treatments
$R_i =$ sum of the ranks of all the scores in the ith treatment group

The test statistic F_r can be computed by using the procedure explained in the following steps:

1. Assign ranks to all the scores obtained under all the treatment conditions for each subject separately. Give the lowest score the rank 1 and, in case of a tie, assign an average rank to all the tied scores.
2. Add the ranks of all the scores in each of the three treatment groups. Thus, R_i is the sum of the ranks of all the scores in the ith treatment group.
3. Substitute these values in formula (10.18) to get the value of test statistic F_r.

The test statistic F_r follows the chi-square distribution with $k - 1$ degrees of freedom.

10.8.2 Critical Value

Since the test statistic F_r follows the chi-square distribution, the critical value in this test is obtained by referring to Table A.11 in the Appendix for $k - 1$ degrees of freedom and an α level of significance.

10.8.3 Decision Rule

If the value of test statistic F_r is greater than the critical value, reject the null hypothesis, otherwise do not reject it.

Example 10.13 A study was conducted to see the effect of music on the perceived pleasure while performing an exercise session. Ten subjects were selected for the study. These subjects were exposed to a 20 min exercise session with the same intensity under all three treatment conditions, without music, with aerobic music, and with instrumental music, in a random order. At the end of each run, subjects were asked to record how pleasurable the exercise session was on a scale

TABLE 10.17 Responses on Comfort Level During Different Treatment Conditions

Clients	No music	Aerobic music	Instrumental music
1	8	6	4
2	7	5	3
3	6	4	5
4	5	5	3
5	7	6	2
6	6	5	2
7	5	3	1
8	6	5	4
9	5	4	5
10	6	5	2

of 1 to 10, with 1 being extremely uncomfortable and 10 being extremely comfortable. The responses so obtained are shown in Table 10.17. Apply Friedman test to determine if there are differences between the music types on perceived pleasure while performing the exercise session. Test your hypothesis at 5% level.

Solution:

Hypotheses: The hypotheses that are required to be tested are as follows:

H_0: The comfort level in all three treatment conditions is equally good.

H_1: The comfort level in at least one treatment condition differs.

Level of Significance: 0.05

Test statistic: This is a repeated measure design where each subject was tested under all three treatment conditions; hence, Friedman test shall be applied to test the above null hypothesis. The statistic F_r as given below shall be used as the test statistic:

$$F_r = \frac{12}{nk(k+1)} \sum_{i=1}^{k} R_i^2 - 3n(k+1)$$

where

$R_i =$ total of ranks in the ith group after ranking the response of each subject under all three treatment conditions separately.

$n =$ number of subjects in the study

$k =$ number of treatment conditions

Computation of F_r The responses under each treatment condition have been ranked for each subject separately. The response scores of all

TABLE 10.18a Responses on Comfort Level under All Three Treatment Conditions

	Treatment Conditions		
Subjects	No Music	Aerobic Music	Instrumental Music
1	8	6	4
2	7	5	3
3	6	4	5
4	5	5	3
5	7	6	2
6	6	5	2
7	4	3	5
8	6	5	4
9	5	4	5
10	6	5	2

TABLE 10.18b Ranks of the Responses under All Three Treatment Conditions

	Treatment conditions		
Subjects	No music	Aerobic music	Instrumental music
1	3	2	1
2	3	2	1
3	3	1	2
4	2.5	2.5	1
5	3	2	1
6	3	2	1
7	2	1	3
8	3	2	1
9	2.5	1	2.5
10	3	2	1
	$R_1 = 28$	$R_2 = 17.5$	$R_3 = 14.5$

the subjects in each of the three treatment conditions have been shown in Table 10.18a, whereas their ranks have been shown in Table 10.18b.

For instance, the response of the first subject under each of the three treatment conditions are 8, 6, and 4 (as shown in Table 10.18a); therefore, their ranks would be 3, 2, and 1 as shown in Table 10.18b. In case of a tie, an average rank has been given to each of the tied scores. Adding the ranks in each of the treatment conditions, we get the values of R_1, R_2, and R_3.

Here,

$$R_1 = 28, \quad R_2 = 17.5, \quad R_3 = 14.5$$

$$n = \text{number of subjects} = 10$$

k = number of groups = 3

$$F_r = \frac{12}{nk\,(k+1)} \sum_{i=1}^{k} R_i^2 - 3n(k+1)$$

$$= \frac{12}{10 \times 3(3+1)}(28^2 + 17.5^2 + 14.5^2) - 3 \times 10(3+1)$$

$$= 130.05 - 120 = 10.05$$

From Table A.11 in the Appendix, the critical value of chi-square at 5% level with $k - 1 = 2$ degrees of freedom is 5.991. Since the calculated value of F_r (=10.05) is greater than 5.991, the null hypothesis is rejected.

Inference: Since the null hypothesis has been rejected, it may be concluded on the basis of the given sample that all three treatment conditions were not equally enjoyable.

Check Your Progress

Note: Tick the correct answer by using the sign (√).

	True	False
39. While applying the Mann–Whitney test, the ranks are assigned by combining the scores of both the groups.	-	-
40. The mean of the Mann–Whitney test statistic U is given by $n_1 \times n_2/2$.	-	-
41. The Wilcoxon matched-pairs signed-ranks test is an alternative to the two-sample t-test.	-	-
42. The Mann–Whitney test can also be used if the data are data is measured on a nominal scale measured on a nominal scale.	-	-
43. The mean of the Wilcoxon T-statistic is obtained by $n(n + 1)/2$.	-	-
44. The Kruskal–Wallis test and the Mann–Whitney test will give the same result in the case of two samples.	-	-
45. The Mann–Whitney test is equivalent to the two-sample t-test for independent groups.	-	-
46. In the Wilcoxon matched-pairs test, if the value of test statistic T is equal to or smaller than the critical value T_c, the null hypothesis is rejected.	-	-
47. The Kruskal–Wallis test is used if three or more groups are compared.	-	-

48. If the value of calculated U is less than the critical value U_c, do not reject the null hypothesis.
49. In the Kruskal–Wallis test, if the test statistic H is significant, it indicates that the samples have been drawn from the same population.
50. In the Mann–Whitney test, the z-statistic can be used to test the hypothesis if $n_1, n_2 > 10$.
51. The Friedman test is used to compare the response of the same subjects in three different treatment conditions.
52. The Mann–Whitney test can be used for paired samples if the sample is large.
53. The Friedman test is used when the assumptions of homogeneity of variances are not met.
54. In the Mann–Whitney test, we compare the medians of two groups rather than the means.
55. The Friedman test is used when the samples are independent.
56. In the Mann–Whitney test, U_2 can be computed by $n_1n_2+U_1$.
57. In the Friedman test, the test statistic F_r follows chi-square distribution with $k-1$ degrees of freedom.

PRACTICE EXERCISE

6. Following are the data on the graceful movement of gymnasts from two different universities, who were assessed them on a 10-point scale. Use the Mann–Whitney U-test to investigate whether there is a significant difference between the values of these two groups. Let $\alpha = 0.05$.

Data on Graceful Movement of Gymnasts from Two Different Universities

University A	6	8	5	8	7	9	7	5	7
University B	6	5	7	4	6	7	3	2	4

7. Use Wilcoxon matched-pairs signed-ranks test and $\alpha = 0.01$ to analyze the effect of exercise on the mood of clients in a health club on the basis of the following data.

Data on Mood of the Participants Before and After an Exercise Program

Before	13	14	17	16	21	18	11	12	13
After	18	16	15	19	15	19	18	16	14

8. Use the Kruskal–Wallis test to determine whether there is a significant difference in the following groups of data. Use $\alpha = 0.05$.

Data on Motivation Obtained on Basketball Players at Three Different Levels

State:	34	23	27	31	22	21	19		
National:	32	28	29	30	18	22	26	28	
International:	42	44	41	36	28	39	37	36	31

9. Use the following set of data to test whether there exists any significant difference among the following observations on dribbling accuracy obtained by testing the subjects under four different treatment conditions. Let $\alpha = 0.01$.

Data on Dribbling Accuracy under Different Treatment Conditions

		Treatments			
		1	2	3	4
Block (IQ)	1	5	8	6	9
	2	8	6	9	6
	3	5	3	9	12
	4	8	6	7	11
	5	5	7	9	6

10.9 COMPUTING WITH EXCEL

10.9.1 Computing Chi-Square with Excel

Excel does not provide the solution for all those statistical tests where the data are not normally distributed. Thus, nonparametric tests cannot be directly applied by using Excel. However, some of their functionalities can be used to apply the chi-square test for goodness of fit. The procedure involved in it can be understood by considering Example 10.14.

Example 10.14 Before starting a triangular 1-day cricket series among India, Pakistan, and Sri Lanka, a poll was conducted on college students regarding their preference toward a particular team winning the title. Their responses are shown below.

Teams	Observed frequencies (f_o)
India	50
Pakistan	45
Sri Lanka	25

Can it be concluded on the basis of the data that the winning preferences are the same for all the teams? Test your hypothesis at 5% level.

Solution: The chi-square test can be applied to test the goodness of fit by using the following steps:

1. Type the observed frequency in one of the rows and the expected frequency in another row, as shown in Figure 10.1. Here, the expected frequency for each cell would be obtained by dividing the total of all the observed frequencies (120) by the number of categories (3). Place the curser on any cell where you would like to get the value of the test and click the **Formulas** and then **Insert Function** as shown in Figure 10.1. You get the next screen as shown in the Figure 10.2, for selecting the command for the chi-square test.
2. Choose the category **Statistical** and then scroll and choose the command **CHITEST** as shown in Figure 10.2. Click **OK** to get the next screen as shown in Figure 10.3.
3. In Figure 10.3, define the range of observed frequency as *B*2:*D*2 and that of expected frequency as *B*3:*D*3.
4. Click **OK** in Figure 10.3 to get the *p*-value as shown in Figure 10.4. Since the *p*-value is less than 0.05, the chi-square is significant and the null hypothesis of equal preference of winning is rejected.

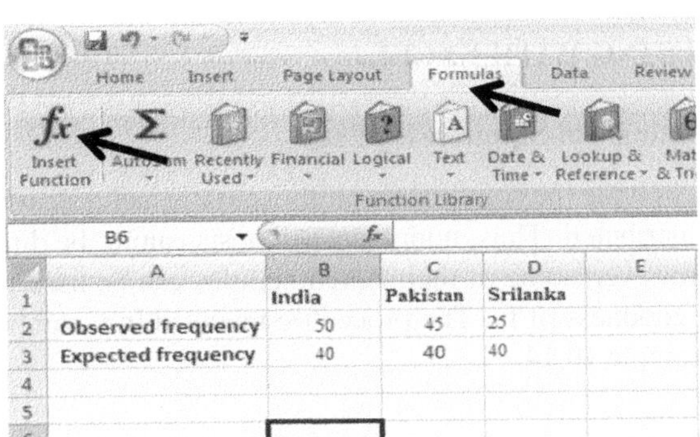

Figure 10.1 Data entry format for the chi-square test.

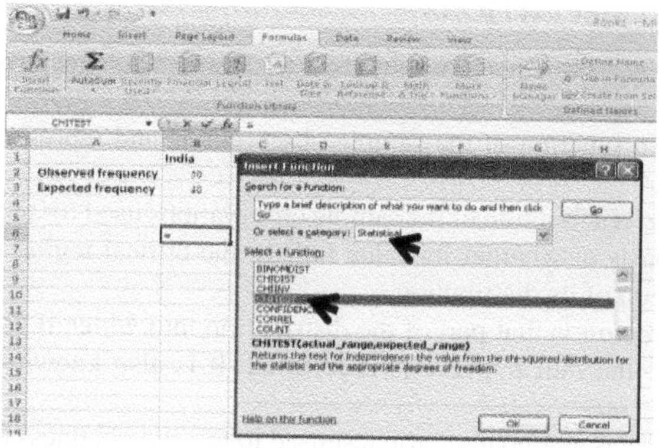

Figure 10.2 Choosing commands for the chi-square test.

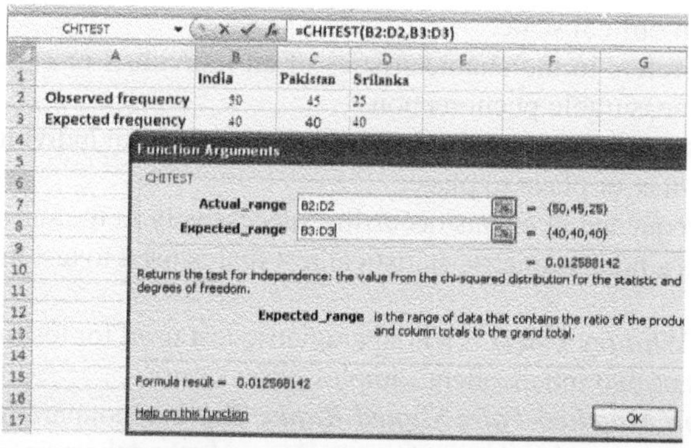

Figure 10.3 Defining the range of data.

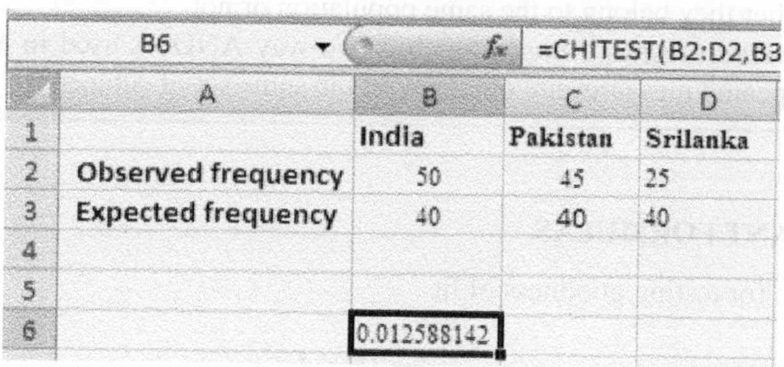

Figure 10.4 p-Value for testing the significance of chi-square.

IMPORTANT DEFINITIONS

A ***parameter*** is a statistical constant used to define the characteristics of a population.
A ***statistic*** is a function of the sample observations and represents the sample characteristics.
A ***test statistic*** is a function of the sample observations used for testing a hypothesis on the basis of whether its value falls in the critical region or in the nonrejection region of its distribution.
A ***rejection region*** is that part of the distribution into which if the value of test statistic falls, the null hypothesis is rejected. It is also known as the *critical region.*
The ***chi-square*** is a nonparametric test used to test the goodness of fit and independence of attributes.
Parametric data are those data that are measured either on interval or on ratio scale.
Nonparametric data can be defined as those data that are measured either on a nominal or on ordinal scale.
An ***attribute*** refers to the characteristics of an individual or experimental unit and is not a measurable phenomenon.
A ***variable*** is a phenomenon that keeps on changing from individual to individual, time to time, or place to place.
A ***runs*** is a sequence of events occurring successively in the series.
A ***runs test*** is a nonparametric statistical test that is used to test the randomness of the data.
The ***Mann–Whitney U-test*** is a nonparametric test used for testing whether the observations of two independent samples differ or not.
The ***Wilcoxon Matched-Pairs Signed-Ranks Test*** is a nonparametric test used for comparing two related samples to assess whether there is any significant difference between their mean ranks.
The ***Kruskal–Wallis test*** is a nonparametric alternative to the parametric one-way ANOVA and is used to compare three or more samples simultaneously to test whether they belong to the same population or not.
This ***Friedman test*** is a nonparametric two-way ANOVA used in a situation where repeated measures are obtained on the same set of subjects.

IMPORTANT FORMULAS

Chi-square for testing goodness of fit

$$\chi^2 = \sum \frac{(f_o - f_e)^2}{f_e}$$

Degrees of freedom = $r - 1$
Chi-square test for independence

$$\chi^2 = \sum\sum \frac{(f_o - f_e)^2}{f_e}$$

Degrees of freedom = $(r - 1)(c - 1)$
Alternate method of computing chi-square

$$\chi^2 = \frac{N(ad - bc)^2}{(a+b)(c+d)(a+c)(b+d)}$$

Degrees of freedom = $(r - 1)(c - 1)$
Chi-square with Yates' correction

$$\chi^2 = \sum\sum \frac{(f_o - f_e - 0.5)^2}{f_e}$$

Runs test for large sample ($n_1, n_2 > 20$)

$$\text{Test statistic } Z = \frac{r - \text{Mean}(r)}{\text{SD}(r)}$$

Mean and SD of run (r)

$$\text{Mean}(r) = \frac{2n_1n_2}{n_1 + n_2} + 1$$

$$\text{SD}(r) = \sqrt{\frac{2n_1n_2(2n_1n_2 - n_1 - n_2)}{(n_1 + n_2)^2(n_1 + n_2 - 1)}}$$

Mann–Whitney U-test

$$U_1 = n_1n_2 + \frac{n_1(n_1 + 1)}{2} - R_1$$

$$U_2 = n_1n_2 + \frac{n_2(n_2 + 1)}{2} - R_2 \quad U_2 = n_1n_2 - U_1$$

$$U = \text{Min } (U_1, U_2)$$

Mann–Whitney test for large sample ($n_1, n_2 > 10$)

$$\text{Test statistic } Z = \frac{U - \mu_U}{\sigma_U}$$

Mean and SD of *U*-statistic

$$\mu_U = \frac{n_1 n_2}{2}$$

$$\sigma_U = \sqrt{\frac{n_1 n_2 (n_1 + n_2 + 1)}{12}}$$

Wilcoxon matched-pairs signed-ranks test
For large sample ($n > 15$)

$$\text{Test statistic } z = \frac{T - \mu_T}{\sigma_T}$$

Mean and SD of the *T*-statistic

$$\mu_T = \frac{n(n+1)}{4}$$

$$\sigma_T = \sqrt{\frac{n(n+1)(2n+1)}{24}}$$

Kruskal–Wallis test

$$H = \frac{12}{n(n+1)} \sum_{i=1}^{k} \frac{R_i^2}{n_i} - 3(n+1)$$

The Friedman test

$$F_r = \frac{12}{nk(k+1)} \sum_{i=1}^{k} R_i^2 - 3n(k+1)$$

KEY TERMS

chi-square test
Friedman test
goodness of fit
independence of attributes
Kruskal–Wallis test
Mann–Whitney test
nonparametric tests
runs test
Wilcoxon matched-pairs
Yates' correction

CHAPTER EXERCISE

1. Discuss the differences between parametric and nonparametric tests.
2. Discuss the assumptions used in the chi-square test.

3. Explain different applications of the chi-square.
4. How can the randomness of a sample be tested? Explain the procedure.
5. What is the alternative to the two-sample *t*-test for independent samples in nonparametric testing? Explain the procedure for using such a test.
6. Write short notes on the following:
   a. Wilcoxon Matched-Pairs Signed-Ranks test
   b. Kruskal–Wallis test
   c. The Friedman test
7. On the basis of the past record in a college, the popularity of four different sports, namely, cricket, swimming, gymnastics, and judo was found to be in the proportion of 4:2:2:2. A random sample of the students drawn from the college was investigated by noting their preference toward a particular sport out of the four sports. The responses obtained are shown in the following table.

   Preferences of Students Toward Different Sports

Sport	Observed Frequency (f_o)
Cricket	200
Swimming	140
Gymnastics	145
Judo	115

   On the basis of these data, can it be concluded that the same response pattern still holds true? Test your hypothesis at 5% level.
8. A study was conducted to investigate the relationship between socioeconomic status and the attitude of the people toward various issues of lifestyle parameters. The subject's responses on one such statement, that is, "Brisk walking for half an hour a day improves work efficiency" were recorded as shown in the following table.

   Responses on "Brisk Walking for Half an Hour a Day Improves The Work Efficiency"

		Response				
		SA	A	UD	D	SD
Socioeconomic status	High	25	10	5	12	5
	Low	22	6	3	25	2

   SA: Strongly Agree, A: Agree, UD: Undecided, D: Disagree, SD: Strongly disagree

Is the data sufficient to draw the conclusion at 5% level that there is a significant difference in the response patterns of the subjects belonging to high and low socioeconomic status groups on the issue.

9. Test the following sequence of events by using the runs test at 5% level to determine whether the occurrence of events is random in nature.

A B A B A A B A B B B A B A B B A B A A B

10. Following is the sequence of the boys and girls entering the counseling cell of a university. Can it be concluded that the arrival of boys and girls is random in nature? Test your hypothesis by using the runs test at 5% level.

M M M F F M M F M F F M M F F F M F M M F F
F M M F M F F M M F M M F F

11. A sample of 55 persons was tested on minimum muscular fitness test. Twelve persons could not qualify in the test. The sequence of successful and unsuccessful candidates is given below, where S represents a success and F represents a failure.

S S S S F S S S S S S S F S S S S S S S F S F S S S S S
S S S S F F S S S S S S S S F F S S S F F S S F S F S

With a two-tailed test and $\alpha = 0.05$, what conclusion can be drawn about the randomness of the sample?

12. A study was conducted in a college to know the response of the students to the question of "whether the students should be allowed to use their mobiles in the class." Out of 70 students interviewed, 40 believed that the mobile should not be allowed as it disturbs the class. The sequence of responses to this question is given below, with Y denoting the response Yes for using the mobile and N denoting No. Use the runs test to test your hypothesis at 5% level as to whether the responses are random in nature.

N N Y Y Y N Y N N N Y Y Y Y N N Y N N Y N N Y Y
Y N N N N Y N Y Y Y N N Y Y N Y N N Y Y Y N N Y
Y N Y Y Y N N N N N N Y N N N N Y N N N N N

13. Use the Mann–Whitney U-test for the following data to determine whether there is a significant difference between the values of group A and group B. Test your hypothesis at 5% level.

Group A	Group B
89	56
78	45
86	75
68	72
65	55
73	68
75	45
83	67

14. Following are the number of sit-ups performed by the athletes and volleyball players in 1 min. Compare the scores of these two groups by using the Mann–Whitney test. Test your hypothesis at 5% level.

Scores on Sit-Ups

Athletics	Volleyball
65	45
56	44
68	56
58	62
59	61
55	44
61	58
56	54
67	

15. Two random samples of sportsmen and nonsportsmen were tested for their resting heart rate (in beats/min). The data so obtained are shown in the following table. Are the data sufficient to conclude that the resting heart rate of sportsmen is in general lower than that of nonsportsmen? Test your hypothesis by using the Mann–Whitney U-test at 5% level.

Heart Rate in beats/min

Sportsmen	Nonsportsmen
60	72
62	71
58	69
59	65
62	63
61	70

59	74
57	72
58	71
58	63
65	68
64	

16. An experiment was planned to compare the impact of low and medium intensity workouts on cardiorespiratory endurance. These two levels of treatment (low and medium intensity workouts) were randomly allocated to the subjects. After administering the treatment, their cardiorespiratory endurance was tested by means of VO_2 max. These values are shown in the following table. Use the Mann–Whitney U-test to determine whether the VO_2 max is greater in the medium intensity group in comparison to that of the low intensity. Use level of significance 0.05.

VO_2 Max in ml.kg.min-1

Aerobic Workout	
Medium Intensity	Low Intensity
65	62
66	56
60	55
61	62
59	62
63	55
55	56
54	57
59	48
63	49
58	
68	

17. A gym instructor wanted to know the impact of a fitness schedule on the fat percentage of male clients. A study was planned in which 12 men were randomly selected. Their fat percentage was measured before they joined the gym. After a 12-week schedule, they were again tested for their fat percentage. The data obtained are shown below. On the basis of the data, can it be concluded that the fat percentage of the clients has significantly reduced as a result of the fitness schedule? Use the Wilcoxon matched-pairs signed-ranks test to verify your hypothesis at 5% level, assuming that the underlying distributions are symmetrical.

Fat% Before and After the Program

Pre-test	Post-test
26	22
18	17
29	26
18	19
16	17
18	17
19	16
18	17
21	20
22	22
24	21
19	20

18. A coach has developed a strengthening program for his clients. In order to test its effectiveness on back strength, a random sample of 11 subjects is chosen and their back strength is measured in lbs. These subjects are given the strengthening program for 4 weeks, and after that their back strength is again tested. The data so obtained are shown below. Apply the Wilcoxon matched-pairs signed-ranks test to verify your hypothesis that strengthening program is effective in enhancing back strength. Test your hypothesis at 5% level assuming that the underlying distributions are symmetrical.

Back Strength (in lbs) Before and After the Program

Pre-test	Post-test
380	418
390	420
310	341
320	352
340	352
410	363
390	420.2
310	330
350	341
360	352
390	385
340	330

19. A volleyball coach developed a circuit training program that was administered to 16 volleyball players for 6 weeks. Their performance on standing

broad jump was noted before and after the program. Use a Wilcoxon matched-pairs signed-ranks test to determine whether the standing broad jump performances in the post-test are significantly higher than the scores in the pre-test. Test your hypothesis at the significance level 0.10, assuming that the underlying distributions are symmetrical.

Scores on Standing Broad Jump (in Meters)

Pre-test	Post-test
2.2	2.5
1.9	2.8
2.8	2.8
2.9	2.8
2.7	2.6
2.0	2.1
1.8	1.9
1.9	1.9
1.8	1.8
1.7	1.8
1.5	1.8
1.9	2.1
1.8	2.2
1.7	1.6
1.6	1.8
1.4	1.7

20. Following are the IQ scores obtained on three different populations. Use the Kruskal–Wallis test to determine whether all the three groups come from different populations. Assume $\alpha = 0.05$.

IQ Scores

Group A	Group B	Group C
95	101	110
102	105	120
98	90	102
85	89	105
95	99	132
97	113	
105		

21. Following are the lean body weight (in lbs) obtained on randomly selected sample of students in different match practice groups. Apply the

Kruskal–Wallis test to investigate whether all three groups come from different populations. Assume $\alpha = 0.05$.

Scores on Lean Body Weight (in lbs)

Match Practice Groups		
Swimming	Badminton	Yoga
138	151	140
136	149	142
141	152	144
142	156	148
140	159	141
139	158	143
150	149	
157		

22. By using the data given below test whether there is a significant difference between treatment levels. Test your hypothesis at the significance level 0.05.

Treatment

		1	2	3	4	5
Block	1	12	16	18	14	13
	2	10	23	16	15	14
	3	16	28	19	14	16
	4	12	16	14	16	18
	5	18	22	18	16	14
	6	19	20	18	12	13

23. An educational consultant wanted to investigate whether all five institutes in the city are equally good for Ph.D. programs. Nine potential Ph.D. candidates were randomly selected and were asked to rate these institutes on a 1–5 point scale. The responses of the candidates are shown in the following table. Apply the Friedman test to investigate whether there was any significant difference between the ratings of these institutes. Test your hypothesis at 1% level.

Institute

Individual	A	B	C	D	E
1	2	1	3	5	3
2	2	1	2	4	2

3	1	2	3	3	1
4	2	3	3	5	2
5	2	2	4	4	2
6	3	4	3	5	3
7	2	1	3	4	2
8	1	2	2	5	3
9	2	3	4	4	3

ANSWERS

Check Your Progress

1. T	11. T	21. F	31. F	41. F	51. T
2. T	12. F	22. T	32. T	42. F	52. F
3. F	13. T	23. T	33. F	43. F	53. T
4. F	14. F	24. F	34. F	44. T	54. T
5. T	15. F	25. T	35. T	45. T	55. F
6. T	16. F	26. T	36. T	46. T	56. F
7. T	17. T	27. F	37. T	47. T	57. T
8. F	18. T	28. F	38. F	48. F	
9. F	19. T	29. T	39. T	49. F	
10. T	20. T	30. F	40. T	50. T	

Practice Exercise

1. $\chi^2 = 8.56$, H_0 is not rejected. The distribution of observed and expected frequencies is the same.
2. $\chi^2 = 8.24$, H_0 is rejected. The IQ and sports achievement are not independent.
3. $\chi^2 = 29.76$, H_0 is rejected. The response of boys and girls is significantly different.
4. $r = 9$, H_0 is not rejected. The sample has been randomly drawn.
5. $|Z| = 0.306$, H_0 is not rejected. The given sample is random in nature.
6. $U = 15$, H_0 is rejected. The graceful movement of gymnasts differs significantly in the two universities.
7. $T = 11.5$, H_0 is not rejected. The exercise program does not affect the mood of the participants.
8. $H = 12.5$, H_0 is rejected. The motivation level of the basketball players differs at the three different levels.
9. $F_r = 3.66$, H_0 is not rejected. No difference exists between the four treatment groups in relation to dribbling accuracy.

Chapter Exercise

7. $\chi^2 = 15.42$, the same response pattern still holds true.
8. $\chi^2 = 6.21$, null hypothesis is not rejected. The response patterns of both the groups are the same.
9. The null hypothesis is not rejected. Occurrence of events is random in nature.
10. The null hypothesis is not rejected. Arrival of boys and girls is random in nature.
11. $Z = 2.3$, the null hypothesis is rejected. The sample is not random.
12. $Z = 1.51$, the null hypothesis is not rejected. The sample is random.
13. $U = 8$, the null hypothesis is rejected. There is a significant difference between groups A and B.
14. $U = 17$, the null hypothesis is not rejected. There is no difference in the sit-ups performance between the athletic and volleyball groups.
15. $Z = 3.78$, the null hypothesis is rejected. The heart rate of sportsmen is in general lower than that of nonsportsmen.
16. $Z = 1.98$, the null hypothesis is rejected. Cardiorespiratory endurance of the medium intensity group is better than that of the low intensity group.
17. $T = 12$, the null hypothesis is rejected. Fat% has significantly reduced as a result of the fitness schedule.
18. $T = 22$, the null hypothesis is not rejected. The strengthening program is not effective.
19. $Z = 2.45$, the null hypothesis is rejected. Standing broad jump is higher in the post-test.
20. $H = 10.80$, the null hypothesis is rejected. The IQs of all three groups are not the same.
21. $H = 14.36$, the null hypothesis is rejected. All three groups differ in their lean body weights.
22. $F_r = 10.67$, the null hypothesis is rejected. All the treatments are not equally effective.
23. $F_r = 20.89$, the null hypothesis is rejected. The ratings of all the institutes are not the same.

FURTHER READING

1. Bagdonavicius V, Kruopis J, Nikulin MS. Nonparametric Tests for Complete Data. London&Hoboken: ISTE&Wiley; 2011. ISBN 978-1-84821-269-5.

2. Bagdonavicius V, Nikulin MS. Chi-square goodness-of-fit test for right censored data. The International Journal of Applied Mathematics and Statistics 2011:30–50[full citation needed].

3. Corder GW, Foreman DI. Nonparametric Statistics for Non-Statisticians: A Step-by-Step Approach. New York: John Wiley & Sons, Inc.; 2009. ISBN 978-0-470-45461-9.

4. Friedman M. The use of ranks to avoid the assumption of normality implicit in the analysis of variance. Journal of the American Statistical Association (American Statistical Association) 1937;32(200):675–701. DOI: 10.2307/2279372.JSTOR 2279372.
5. Friedman M. A correction: the use of ranks to avoid the assumption of normality implicit in the analysis of variance. Journal of the American Statistical Association (American Statistical Association) 1939;34(205):109. DOI: 10.2307/2279169.JSTOR 2279169.
6. Friedman M. A comparison of alternative tests of significance for the problem of m rankings. The Annals of Mathematical Statistics 1940;11(1):86–92. DOI: 10.1214/aoms/1177731944. JSTOR 2235971.
7. Gibbons JD, Chakraborti S. Nonparametric Statistical Inference. 4th ed. USA: CRC; 2003. ISBN 0-8247-4052-1.
8. Greenwood PE, Nikulin MS. A Guide to Chi-Squared Testing. New York: John Wiley & Sons, Inc.; 1996. ISBN 0-471-55779-X.
9. Hollander M, Wolfe DA. Nonparametric Statistics. New York: John Wiley & Sons, Inc.; 1973.
10. John RT. An Introduction to Error Analysis. USA: University Science Books; 1997. p 268.
11. Nikulin MS. Chi-squared test for normality. Proceedings of the International Vilnius Conference on Probability Theory and Mathematical Statistics 1973;2:119–122.
12. Siegel S, Castellan NJ. Nonparametric Statistics for the Behavioral Sciences. 2nd ed. New York: McGraw–Hill; 1988.
13. Siegel S, Castellan NJ Jr. Nonparametric Statistics for the Behavioral Sciences. 2nd ed. New York: McGraw-Hill; 1988.
14. Spurrier JD. On the null distribution of the Kruskal–Wallis statistic. Journal of Nonparametric Statistics 2003;15(6):685–691.
15. Srivastava TN, Shailaja R. Statistics for Management. New Delhi: Tata McGraw Hill; 2010.
16. Wald-Wolfowitz (or Runs) test for randomness. Accessed from http://support.sas.com/kb/33/092.html on Nov 2014; 2008.
17. Wasserman L. All of Nonparametric Statistics. USA: Springer; 2006. ISBN 0-387-25145-5.
18. Wilson EB, Hilferty MM. The distribution of chi-squared. Proc. Natl. Acad. Sci. USA 1931;17(12):684–688.
19. Wilcoxon F. Individual comparisons by ranking methods. Biometrics Bulletin 1945;1(6):80–83.
20. Yates F. Contingency table involving small numbers and the $\chi 2$ test. Supplement to the Journal of the Royal Statistical Society 1934;1(2):217–235JSTOR 2983604.

11

MEASURING ASSOCIATIONS IN NONPARAMETRIC DATA

11.1 INTRODUCTION

The product-moment correlation method discussed in Chapter 9 can be used only in a situation when both the variables are measured either on an interval or a ratio scale. However, if any one or both the variables are nonparametric, this correlation cannot be used. Many situations in exercise science and health research may arise where the variables are either measured on a nominal or ordinal scale. In all such situations, the product-moment correlation cannot be used to measure the magnitude of the relationship. Let us consider a situation where an investigator wants to find an association between the height and playing ability of volleyball players. Since heights are measured on a ratio scale, they are parametric data, whereas playing ability is obtained by the judges' rankings (ordinal), which are nonparametric data. Since both these variables should be parameters, the product-moment correlation cannot be used, rather a nonparametric correlation method known as rank correlation may be used in this situation to measure the relationship. Since the computation of rank correlation requires both variables to be on the ordinal scale, after converting the scores of height into their (ordinal data) ranks, rank correlation can be used. The reader should note that it is possible to convert ratio data into ordinal data but the reverse is not possible.

If the relationship between two variables needs to be investigated, where one of them is parametric (interval or ratio) and the other is nominal (dichotomous), neither the product-moment correlation nor the rank order correlation can be applied.

Statistics for Exercise Science and Health with Microsoft® Office Excel®, First Edition. J. P. Verma.

In such situations, the bi-serial correlation is computed to measure the relationship. Let us consider a situation where a researcher is interested in determining the relationship between the flexibility and minimum muscular fitness of high school girls. Here, flexibility can be measured by using the sit and reach test that results in ratio data (parametric), whereas the minimum muscular fitness test results in dichotomous (nonparametric) data as the subject can be classified as either pass or fail. In this situation, the bi-serial correlation is an appropriate measure of relationship.

Yet another situation may arise in research where both the variables are measured on the nominal scale (classificatory data); in that situation, nonparametric correlations such as the tetrachoric correlation, phi coefficient, or contingency coefficient may be used. This chapter deals with different types of nonparametric correlations, which are frequently used in the area of exercise science. Figure 11.1 shows different types of nonparametric correlations that can be used in different situations.

11.2 RANK CORRELATION (MEASURE OF ASSOCIATION BETWEEN RANKED DATA)

Rank correlation is used to find the linear correlation between two variables where scores are in rank order. It is represented by the Greek letter ρ (rho) and is computed as

$$\rho = 1 - \frac{6\sum d_i^2}{n(n^2 - 1)} \tag{11.1}$$

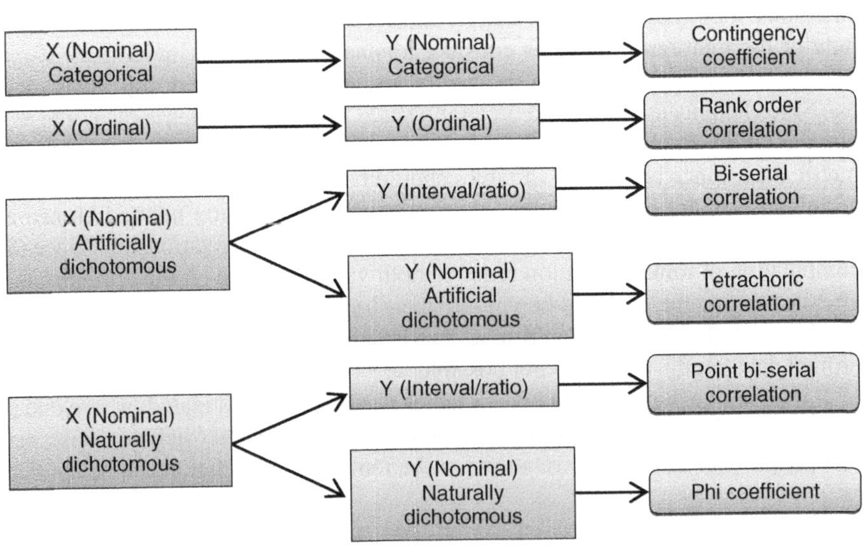

Figure 11.1 Nonparametric correlations suitable in different situations.

where d_i is the difference between the ranks of Y_i and X_i and n is the sample size. Rank correlation is also known as *Spearman's rank correlation* because it is named after Spearman, who developed it.

Rank correlation is used either in a situation where the product-moment correlation coefficient cannot be used due to violation of assumption or in a situation where the scores cannot be objectively measured and the assessment is made on the basis of individual ranks. For instance, playing ability in basketball and passing accuracy in soccer can only be judged on the basis of judges' ranking as no objective criteria are available to assess these performances. In a situation like this, the relationship between such variables can be measured only through rank correlation. If scores on one variable are in ranks and that of the other are measured quantitatively, the rank correlation is obtained by converting the quantitative data into their ranks. Further, if both the variables are in score form, rank correlation can be obtained by converting these scores into their corresponding ranks.

Rank correlation (ρ) is a nonparametric statistic. Rank indicates only the position of the subjects or items in the series and no weight is given for differences between adjacent scores. For example, individuals with scores 16, 34, 56, and 58 on a test would be ranked as 1, 2, 3, and 4, although the differences between the first and second, second and third, and third and fourth scores are 18, 22, and 2, respectively. While converting scores into ranks, the rank 1 should be given to the lowest score and the highest score should be given the highest rank. In case of a tie among the scores, an average rank is allotted to all the scores having the same magnitude. Average rank is computed by first giving an individual rank arbitrarily as if they are different scores in decreasing or increasing order and then taking the average of all these ranks. For example, suppose the scores are 3, 2, 9, 15, 9, 10, and 12. Rank 1 would be assigned to score 2, rank 2 would be assigned to score 3. Now, the next score is 9, which is repeated twice, let us see how the rank is allotted to these two scores. Arbitrarily, score 9 that comes first in the series may be given rank 3 and score 9 that comes later in the series may be given rank 4. Since both these scores are same, we take the average of the ranks 3 and 4, which is 3.5. Thus, rank 3.5 is allotted to both the scores 9. A similar procedure is followed in assigning the ranks if a score in the series is repeated more than twice.

The limits of rank correlation are -1 and $+1$, that is, $-1 \leq \rho \leq 1$. If the rank correlation is $+1$, then it indicates that there is a perfect positive linear correlation between the ranks of both the variables. Similarly, if the rank correlation is -1, it shows that there is a perfect negative linear correlation between the ranks of the two variables, whereas zero indicates no correlation between the ranks.

11.2.1 Assumptions

Unlike product-moment correlation, rank correlation does not have any assumption. In fact, when parametric data do not follow the assumptions of normality, homoscedasticity, and linearity, then rank correlation should be used instead of product-moment correlation. However, in that situation, the data need to be converted into ranks.

11.2.2 Testing Significance

The rank correlation can be tested for its significance by using the following t-statistic:

$$t = \rho\sqrt{\frac{n-2}{1-\rho^2}} \qquad (11.2)$$

> **FACTS TO KNOW**
>
> Test of significance for rank correlation is similar to that of product moment correlation

where ρ is the sample rank correlation and n is the sample size. This t-statistic follows a t-distribution with $n-2$ degrees of freedom. By using this t-statistic, the following hypotheses are tested:

$$H_0: \overline{\rho} = 0$$

$$H_1: \overline{\rho} \neq 0$$

where $\overline{\rho}$ is the rank correlation in the population. If the calculated value of t is greater than or equal to the tabulated value of t at some level of significance and $n-2$ degrees of freedom, the null hypothesis may be rejected, otherwise it is failed to be rejected.

Alternate Method The significance of the rank correlation can also be tested directly by using the significance value of r mentioned in Table A.8 in the Appendix. For given degrees of freedom and levels of significance, the values of correlation required for the significance are listed in that table. For instance, if a rank correlation of 0.54 is obtained from a sample of size 25, then the value of rank correlation required for its significance at 23 degrees of freedom and 0.05 level of significance from Table A.8 is 0.396. Since the observed rank correlation (0.54) is greater than 0.396, the null hypothesis may be rejected and one can say that the rank correlation is significant at 5% level.

11.2.3 Merits and Demerits

Rank correlation is very easy to compute and can be used in a situation where either the scores are in rank order or in a situation where one or more assumptions for using the product-moment correlation fails. Since rank correlation is computed on the basis of the ranks of two variables, it is not affected by outliers unlike the product-moment correlation coefficient. As with the product-moment correlation coefficient, rank correlation also does not explain the cause-and-effect relationship. Rank correlation is less reliable than the product-moment correlation coefficient.

TABLE 11.1 Computation of Rank Correlation

Dribbling Score (x)	Passing Score (y)	R_x	R_y	$D = R_x - R_y$	D^2
15	16	7	8	−1	1
13	10	5	3	2	4
12	8	3.5	1	2.5	6.25
14	12	6	5	1	1
16	10	8	3	5	25
11	14	2	7	−5	25
10	13	1	6	−5	25
12	10	3.5	3	0.5	0.25
					$\sum D^2 = 87.50$

Rank correlation has a high standard error due to which it cannot be used in regression analysis.

Example 11.1 In a study, the judges' marks were obtained on the dribbling performance and passing accuracy on some of the players during a basketball match. Calculate the rank correlation between the two parameters for the data shown in Table 11.1.

Solution: Since the scores awarded by the judges are subjective in nature and it is required to compute the rank correlation, these scores shall be converted into their ranks first. The lowest score has been given rank 1, and in case of tie among the scores the average rank has been given to each score having the same magnitude. Since in dribbling, the score 12 is repeated two times, an average rank 3.5 (average of 3 and 4) has been assigned to both the scores. Similarly, in passing scores, 10 is repeated thrice, hence an average rank of 3 (average of 2, 3, and 4) has been assigned to all three scores.

$$\rho = 1 - \frac{6\sum D^2}{N(N^2 - 1)}$$

$$= 1 - \frac{6 \times 87.50}{8(64 - 1)}$$

$$= 1 - 1.04$$

$$= -0.04$$

Example 11.2 Ten volleyball players were assessed for their playing ability by a qualified judge. These players were ranked according their performance (rank 1

TABLE 11.2 Computation of Rank Correlation

Playing Ability (x)	Height (y)	R_x	R_y	$D = R_x - R_y$	D^2
5	165	5	5	0	0
7	180	7	10	−3	9
8	172	8	8.5	−0.5	0.25
6	165	6	5	1	1
9	166	9	7	2	4
4	172	4	8.5	−4.5	20.25
1	150	1	2	−1	1
10	163	10	3	7	49
3	165	3	5	−2	4
2	145	2	1	1	1
					$\sum D^2 = 89.50$

refers to the lowest performance). Along with the playing ability, the heights of these players were also measured. The data so obtained are shown in Table 11.2. Compute the rank correlation and test its significance.

Solution: To compute the rank correlation, the height scores will have to be converted into ranks. Here, the score 165 is repeated three times; hence, an average rank 5 (average of 4, 5, and 6) has been assigned to these three scores. Similarly, the score 172 is repeated twice; hence, it has been assigned an average rank 8.5 (average of 8 and 9). After computing these ranks, the difference (D) of ranks for each individual and D^2 have been computed for each subject.

$$\rho = 1 - \frac{6\sum D^2}{N(N^2 - 1)}$$

$$= 1 - \frac{6 \times 89.5}{10(100 - 1)}$$

$$= 1 - 0.54$$

$$= 0.46$$

The value of rank correlation required for significance with 8 (=10 − 2) degrees of freedom and 0.05 level of significance can be seen from Table A.8 in the Appendix, which is equal to 0.632. Since the calculated rank correlation of 0.46 is smaller than 0.632, it is insignificant and therefore it may be concluded that the there is no association between the height and playing ability of the volleyball players.

Example 11.3 Twelve soccer players were tested on their playing ability by three judges. Average marks (out of 50) awarded by the three judges were taken

TABLE 11.3 Computation of Rank Correlation

Playing Ability (x)	McDonald Test (y)	R_x	R_y	$D = R_x - R_y$	D^2
30	16	8	5	3	9
32	18	11.5	9	2.5	6.25
29	17	6	6.5	−0.5	0.25
25	17	1	6.5	−5.5	30.25
30	13	8	2	6	36
27	19	3.5	11	−7.5	56.25
28	14	5	3	2	4
27	15	3.5	4	−0.5	0.25
30	12	8	1	7	49
26	18	2	9	−7	49
31	20	10	12	−2	4
32	18	11.5	9	2.5	6.25
					$\sum D^2 = 250.50$

as the performance score. These players were also tested on the McDonald Soccer test. The performances of these players so obtained are shown in Table 11.3. Compute the rank correlation and test its significance at 5% level.

Solution: In playing ability, scores 32 and 27 are repeated twice; hence, average ranks 1.5 and 9.5, respectively, have been given to them, whereas score 30 is repeated thrice, the average rank of 5 has been given to each of the 30 score. Similarly, in the McDonald test, score 17 is repeated twice, hence an average rank of 6.5 has been given to both the scores of 17; similarly, score 18 is repeated thrice, so all three scores of 18 have been given an average rank of 9.

After converting the scores into their ranks in both the variables, the difference of these ranks (D) and D^2 have been computed for each subject. These computations are shown in Table 11.3.

$$\rho = 1 - \frac{6\sum D^2}{N(N^2 - 1)}$$

$$= 1 - \frac{6 \times 250.5}{12(144 - 1)}$$

$$= 1 - 0.88$$

$$= 0.12$$

11.2.4 Test of Significance

To test the significance of rank correlation, the following hypotheses need to be tested:

$$H_0: \bar{\rho} = 0$$
$$H_1: \bar{\rho} \neq 0$$

Under the null hypothesis, the following t-statistic follows the t-distribution with $n - 2$ degrees of freedom.

$$t = \rho\sqrt{\frac{n-2}{1-\rho^2}}$$

Here, $\rho = 0.12$, $n = 12$

$$t = 0.12\sqrt{\frac{12-2}{1-0.12^2}}$$
$$= 0.38$$

From Table A.7 in the Appendix, the value of $t_{0.05}(10)$ is 2.228. Since the value of calculated t (=0.38) is less than 2.228, the null hypothesis is not rejected. It may therefore be concluded that there is no relationship between the playing ability and McDonald test performance.

11.3 BI-SERIAL CORRELATION (MEASURE OF ASSOCIATION BETWEEN A DICHOTOMOUS AND A CONTINUOUS VARIABLE)

> **FACTS TO KNOW**
>
> A naturally dichotomous variable is nominal in nature, whereas an artificially dichotomous variable is measured on the metric scale but it can be classified into two categories owing to certain criteria

Bi-serial correlation is used to measure the relationship between two variables where one variable is parametric and the other is artificially dichotomous in nature. A variable is said to be artificially dichotomous if the criteria of classification are decided by the researcher. For instance, variables such as high and low fitness, pass and fail, high and low IQ, high and low intensity training program, and high and low cardiorespiratory endurance are examples of artificially dichotomous variables. In fact, these variables are continuous but their measurement for some reason is reduced to two categories. This reduction into two categories may be a consequence of the only way in which the data can be obtained, for example, the variable may be the performance on a physical efficiency test assessed in terms of pass or fail. We can well assume a continuous scale along which individuals differ with respect to performance required to pass the test, for example, if the performance is above a certain value, one is declared as having passed, and those whose performance is below that value are considered to have failed.

On the other hand, a variable is said to be naturally dichotomous if it is decided by the nature of the individual or item. For example, variables such as a student's status (undergraduate, postgraduate), gender (male, female), and answer (true, false) are examples of naturally dichotomous variables.

The principle upon which the formula of bi-serial correlation is based is that with zero correlation, there would be no difference between the means of the continuous variable, and the larger the difference between the means, the larger the correlation. Bi-serial correlation is denoted by r_b and is computed by the formula

$$r_b = \frac{\overline{x}_p - \overline{x}_q}{s_t} \times \frac{pq}{u} \tag{11.3}$$

where

$\overline{x}_p$ = mean of the variable x (parametric) for the first group in the dichotomous variable

$\overline{x}_q$ = mean of the variable x (parametric) for the second group in the dichotomous variable

p = proportion of the frequency in the first group of the dichotomous variable

q = proportion of the frequency in the second group of the dichotomous variable

s_t = standard deviation of the variable x for all the cases in the dichotomous variable

u = ordinate of the standard normal curve at the point cutting off a tail of that distribution with area equal to q

In order to compute u, Table A.6 in the Appendix is used. The value of u is the ordinate corresponding to the larger area (p) or the smaller area (q).

The bi-serial correlation provides an estimate of the product-moment correlation coefficient. The limits of bi-serial correlation are in the range from −1 to +1. However, the value of bi-serial correlation may exceed 1 in case of a bimodal distribution.

11.3.1 Assumptions

Bi-serial correlation should not be used if p or q is larger than 0.9. In that case, it does not give a correct picture of the relationship. Computing bi-serial correlation requires one of the variables to be essentially dichotomous.

11.3.2 Testing Significance

Bi-serial correlation can be tested for its significance by using the following test statistic:

$$t = \frac{r_b}{\sigma_{r_b}} \tag{11.4}$$

where σ_{r_b} is the standard error of the bi-serial correlation and is given by

$$\sigma_{r_b} = \frac{\sqrt{pq}}{u\sqrt{n}} \tag{11.5}$$

The t-statistic shown in (11.4) follows a t-distribution with $(n - 2)$ degrees of freedom and can be used to test the following hypotheses:

$$H_0: \bar{r}_b = 0$$

$$H_1: \bar{r}_b \neq 0$$

where $\bar{r}_b$ is the population bi-serial correlation. The significance of the t-value can be tested by comparing its value with the tabulated value of t obtained from Table A.7 in the Appendix for $n - 2$ degrees of freedom and at any desired level of significance.

11.3.3 Merits and Demerits

The bi-serial correlation provides an estimate of the product-moment correlation coefficient in a situation where one of the variables is parametric and the other is artificially dichotomous. Significant bi-serial correlation indicates that the group means differ in the two categories of the dichotomous variable. For example, if the bi-serial correlation is significant between the height and minimum muscular fitness test, then it can be interpreted that the height of the subjects in passing and failing minimum muscular fitness groups differs significantly. Thus, by computing the bi-serial correlation, comparison can be made between the two groups of the dichotomous variable.

The bi-serial correlation is always less reliable in comparison to the product-moment correlation coefficient. The standard error of the bi-serial correlation is quite large in comparison to that of the product-moment correlation coefficient calculated for the same sample owing to which it is not used in regression analysis.

11.4 POINT BI-SERIAL CORRELATION (MEASURE OF CORRELATION BETWEEN A TRUE DICHOTOMOUS VARIABLE AND A CONTINUOUS VARIABLE)

The point bi-serial correlation is used to compute the correlation coefficient between two variables one of which is parametric and the other is naturally dichotomous. As mentioned earlier, the naturally dichotomous variable is the one that can be classified into either of two categories by looking at the nature of an individual or item. For instance, gender is a naturally dichotomous variable because the subject can be classified into male or female category on the basis of the nature of an individual and not because of any criteria set by the researcher. The point bi-serial correlation is mathematically equivalent to the product-moment correlation coefficient. It is denoted by r_{pb} and is computed as

$$r_{pb} = \frac{\bar{x}_p - \bar{x}_q}{s_t} \times \sqrt{pq} \tag{11.6}$$

where

$\bar{x}_p$ = mean of the variable x (parametric) for the first group in the dichotomous variable

$\bar{x}_q$ = mean of the variable x (parametric) for the second group in the dichotomous variable

p = proportion of the frequency in the first group of the dichotomous variable

q = proportion of the frequency in the second group of the dichotomous variable

s_t = standard deviation of the variable x for all the cases in the dichotomous variable

The limits, assumptions, and merits and demerits of the point bi-serial correlation are similar to those of the bi-serial correlation. The only difference between the point bi-serial correlation and bi-serial correlation is that the former is computed when the dichotomous variable is a naturally dichotomous variable instead of an artificially dichotomous variable. Further, bi-serial correlation is the estimate of the product-moment correlation, whereas point bi-serial correlation is mathematically equivalent to the product-moment correlation coefficient.

11.4.1 Testing Significance

Since the point bi-serial correlation is mathematically equivalent to the product-moment correlation coefficient, the procedure for testing its significance is equivalent to that of the product-moment correlation coefficient. The reader may refer to Chapter 9 for testing the significance of the correlation coefficient.

Example 11.4 An experiment was conducted to test the relationship between minimum muscular strength (measured by the cross Webber test) and leg length of college students. The responses so obtained are shown in Table 11.4, where f_1 and f_2 represent the frequencies of the pass and fail groups, respectively. Test the significance of the bi-serial correlation at 5% level.

Solution: The bi-serial correlation between the minimum muscular strength test and leg length shall be computed by using the following formula:

TABLE 11.4 Computation of Mean and Standard Deviation

Leg Length class Interval	Minimum Muscular Strength Test									
	Pass Group			Fail Group			Total			
	f_1	d	f_1d	f_2	d	f_2d	f_t	d	f_td	f_td^2
74–75	6	−5	−30	2	−5	−10	8	−5	−40	200
76–77	8	−4	−32	1	−4	−4	9	−4	−36	144
78–79	4	−3	−12	3	−3	−9	7	−3	−21	63
80–81	5	−2	−10	2	−2	−4	7	−2	−14	28
82–83	3	−1	−3	1	−1	−1	4	−1	−4	4
84–85	2	0	0	4	0	0	6	0	0	0
86–87	1	1	1	6	1	6	7	1	7	7
88–89	2	2	4	4	2	8	6	2	12	24
90–91	1	3	3	6	3	18	7	3	21	63
92–93	1	4	4	3	4	12	4	4	16	64
Total	33		−75	32		16	65		−59	597

$$r_b = \frac{\bar{x}_p - \bar{x}_q}{s_t} \times \frac{pq}{u}$$

To compute the bi-serial correlation, it is required to find the means of the pass and fail groups along with standard deviation of the combined group. These computations have been shown in Table 11.4.

Here, the assumed mean (AM) is 84.5 and width of the class interval (i) is 2.

$$\bar{x}_p = \text{AM} + \frac{\sum f_1 d}{\sum f_1} \times i = 84.5 + \frac{(-75)}{33} \times 2 = 79.95$$

$$\bar{x}_q = \text{AM} + \frac{\sum f_2 d}{\sum f_2} \times i = 84.5 + \frac{16}{32} \times 2 = 85.50$$

$$S_t = i \times \sqrt{\frac{1}{\sum f_t} \sum f_t d^2 - \left(\frac{\sum f_t d}{\sum f_t}\right)^2} = 5 \times \sqrt{\frac{1}{65} \times 597 - \left(\frac{-59}{65}\right)^2}$$

$$= 2 \times \sqrt{9.185 - 0.824} = 5.783$$

Here,

$$p = \frac{33}{65} = 0.5076$$

and

$$q = \frac{32}{65} = 0.4923$$

Since the larger of the two proportions (area) is 0.5076, from Table A.6 in the Appendix, the value of the ordinate u corresponding to the area 0.5076 is 0.3988.

$$\text{Therefore, } r_b = \frac{\overline{x}_p - \overline{x}_q}{s_t} \times \frac{pq}{u}$$

$$= \frac{79.95 - 85.5}{5.783} \times \frac{0.5076 \times 0.4923}{0.3988}$$

$$= -\frac{5.55}{5.783} \times \frac{0.2499}{0.3988}$$

$$= -0.6013$$

11.4.2 Testing the Significance of r_b

After finding the value of bi-serial correlation, it is required to be tested for its significance. The following hypotheses need to be tested at 5% level.

Hypotheses:

$$H_0: \overline{r}_b = 0$$

$$H_1: \overline{r}_b \neq 0$$

Level of Significance: 0.05

Test Statistic: To test the significance of bi-serial correlation, the following t-statistic shall be used as the test statistic:

$$t = \frac{r_b}{\sigma_{r_b}}$$

where

$$\sigma_{r_b} = \frac{\sqrt{pq}}{u\sqrt{n}}$$

Here, $p = 0.5076$, $q = 0.4923$, $u = 0.3988$, $n = \sum f_t = 65$, and $r_b = -0.6013$

Substituting these values,

$$\sigma_{r_b} = \frac{\sqrt{0.5076 \times 0.4923}}{0.3988 \times \sqrt{65}} = \frac{0.4999}{3.2152} = 0.1555$$

Thus,

$$t = \frac{-0.6013}{0.1555} = -3.87$$

or

$$|t| = 3.87$$

From Table A.7 in the Appendix, the tabulated value of t at 5% level and $n-2$ degrees of freedom is as follows:

$$t_{0.05}(65-2) = t_{0.05}(63) = 2.00$$

Since the calculated value of t (=3.87) is greater than 2.00, the null hypothesis may be rejected at 5% level.

Inference: Since the null hypothesis has been rejected, it may be concluded that there is a significant association between minimum muscular strength and leg length of the college students.

Check Your Progress

Note: Tick the correct answer by using the sign (√).

	True	False
1. For an artificially dichotomous variable, the classification is done on the basis of the subject's characteristics.	-	-
2. Rank correlation can be computed even if one of the variables is measured on an interval scale and the other is measured on a nominal scale.	-	-
3. Bi-serial correlation may exceed 1 in many situations.	-	-
4. As a convention, in computing rank correlation, the lowest score is given rank 1.	-	-
5. Rank correlation should be used if measurement of the variables can be made objectively.	-	-
6. The bi-serial correlation provides an estimate of the product-moment correlation coefficient.	-	-
7. Fitness status is a naturally dichotomous variable.	-	-
8. In computing rank correlation, it hardly matters if rank 1 is given to the lowest or highest score.	-	-
9. Rank correlation does not explain the cause-and-effect relationship.	-	-
10. Bi-serial correlation is used for computing association when one of the variables is continuous and the other is categorical.	-	-
11. If one of the variables is measured on a ratio scale and the other is naturally dichotomous, bi-serial correlation is used.	-	-

12.	Bi-serial correlation is used when one of the variables is measured on an interval scale and the other is artificially dichotomous.	-	-
13.	In computing rank correlation, the data should follow the assumption of homoscedasticity.	-	-
14.	In computing the bi-serial correlation, the dichotomous variable is in fact continuous but its measurement for some reason is reduced to two categories.	-	-
15.	Gender is a naturally dichotomous variable.	-	-
16.	Bi-serial correlation can be used if p or q is larger than 0.9.	-	-
17.	If the bi-serial correlation is significant, it indicates that the group means differ in the two categories of the dichotomous variable.	-	-
18.	The rank correlation can be tested for its significance by using the t-test.	-	-
19.	The bi-serial correlation is more reliable than the product-moment correlation coefficient.	-	-
20.	The degree of freedom for the t-test in testing the significance of rank correlation is $n-1$.	-	-
21.	The point bi-serial correlation is mathematically equivalent to the product-moment correlation coefficient.	-	-
22.	The rank correlation should be computed when both the variables are parametric but the assumptions about the distribution are not satisfied.	-	-
23.	The procedures used for testing the significance of the point bi-serial correlation and product-moment correlation coefficient are not the same.	-	-

11.5 TETRACHORIC CORRELATION (MEASURE OF ASSOCIATION BETWEEN DICHOTOMOUS VARIABLES)

Tetrachoric correlation is used to measure the correlation coefficient in a situation where both the variables x and y are continuous but are treated as dichotomous.

The criterion for classification is either set by the researcher or suggested by some theoretical construct. In other words, tetrachoric correlation is used in a situation when both the variables are artificially dichotomous. Under the condition of continuity and linearity, tetrachoric correlation is numerically equivalent to the product-moment correlation coefficient and may be regarded as an approximation to it. The tetrachoric correlation is represented by r_t and is calculated by the formula

$$r_t = \cos\left(\frac{180\sqrt{bc}}{\sqrt{ad} + \sqrt{bc}}\right) \tag{11.7}$$

where a, b, c, and d are the cell frequencies. To understand the procedure for computing r_t, consider an experiment to find an association between flexibility and performance in gymnastics. A sample of N subjects is tested for their performance in flexibility and gymnastics performance. The researcher may decide the criteria for classifying a subject into high and low categories on flexibility and gymnastics performance. Such classification can be made by using the principle of normality. The subject above $\bar{x} + S$ may be classified into the higher category and below $\bar{x} - S$ may be classified into the lower category. The frequencies of different categories may be arranged as shown in Table 11.5.

The tetrachoric correlation can be calculated by substituting the values of the cell frequencies a, b, c, and d in formula 11.7. It is obvious that in case of a perfect positive correlation, all cases would be distributed among the frequencies "a" and "d." If the cell frequencies "b" and "c"are zero, the value of r_t will be equal to cos 0, which is equal to 1.

Similarly, in case of perfect negative correlation, all the cell frequencies would be distributed among the frequencies "b" and "c." In that case, the cell frequencies "a" and "d" will be zero and the value of r_t will be equal to cos 180, which is equal to −1. On the other hand, in case of zero correlation, all the frequencies would be proportionately distributed in all four cells and this will give rise to cos 90, which is equal to 0. Since the value of the cosine function ranges from −1 to +1, the tetrachoric correlation (r_t) also lies between −1 and +1, that is,

$$-1 \leq r_t \leq +1$$

TABLE 11.5 Classification of Subjects According to High and Low Flexibility and Gymnastics Performance

		Gymnastics Performance		
		High	Low	Total
Flexibility	High	a	b	$a + b$
	Low	c	d	$c + d$
	Total	$a + c$	$b + d$	$N = a + b + c + d$

11.5.1 Assumptions

One of the main assumptions of tetrachoric correlation is that both variables are continuous and normally distributed. Another assumption in using the tetrachoric correlation is that both variables should be linearly related.

11.5.2 Testing Significance

The significance of tetratchoric correlation can be tested by testing the following hypotheses:

$$H_0: \bar{r}_t = 0 \ [\bar{r}_t \text{ represents the population tetrachoric correlation}]$$
$$H_1: \bar{r}_t \neq 0$$

To test the null hypothesis, the following t-statistic is used as the test statistic:

$$t = \frac{r_t}{\sigma_{r_t}} \tag{11.8}$$

This t-statistic follows the t-distribution with $n - 2$ degrees of freedom. σ_{r_t} is the standard error of the tetrachoric correlation (r_t) and is computed by the formula

$$\sigma_{r_t} = \frac{\sqrt{pqp'q'}}{uu'\sqrt{N}} \tag{11.9}$$

Here, p and q are the proportions of the subjects in high and low categories of the flexibility and p' and q' are the proportions of the subjects in high and low categories of the gymnastics performance. The values of p, q, p', and q' are computed as follows:

$$p = \frac{a+b}{N} \text{ and } q = \frac{c+d}{N}$$
$$p' = \frac{a+c}{N} \text{ and } q' = \frac{b+d}{N}$$

The significance of the t-statistic as mentioned in (11.8) can be tested by comparing its value with that of the tabulated value of t obtained from Table A.7 in the Appendix for $n - 2$ degrees of freedom and at any given level of significance.

11.5.3 Merits and Demerits

The cosine formula used for computing tetrachoric correlation gives a very close approximation to r_t only when both the variables are dichotomized at their medians. The tetratchoric correlation is less reliable in comparison to the product-moment correlation, and for this reason, it is not used in regression analysis. Tetrachoric correlation should not be used if any of the cell frequencies is 0 because in that case, the data become curvilinear.

The tetrachoric correlation is more reliable under the following three conditions:

a. The sample size N is large.
b. The value of r_t is large.
c. The divisions in both the dichotomous variables into two categories are near their medians.

Example 11.5 A basketball coach wanted to investigate the association between IQ and the playing ability of basketball players. Players were classified into high and low IQ groups. In each of the IQ groups, they were again classified into high and low playing ability groups. The classification results so obtained are shown in Table 11.6. Calculate the tetrachoric correlation and test its significance at 5% level.

Solution: First the tetrachoric correlation shall be computed and then its significance will be tested by using the t-test.

Step 1: *Computation of tetrachoric correlation*

$$r_t = \cos\left(\frac{180\sqrt{bc}}{\sqrt{ad}+\sqrt{bc}}\right)$$

$$= \cos\left(\frac{180\sqrt{10\times 20}}{\sqrt{40\times 30}+\sqrt{10\times 20}}\right)$$

$$= \cos\ 52.18$$

$$= 0.62 \qquad \text{(from Table A.1 in the Appendix)}$$

Step 2: *Test of significance* To test the significance of the tetrachoric correlation calculated above, the following hypotheses shall be tested.

TABLE 11.6 Classification of Players on the Basis of IQ and Playing Ability

		Playing Ability		
		High	Low	Total
IQ	High	40 (a)	10 (b)	50
	Low	20 (c)	30 (d)	50
	Total	60	40	$N = 100$

Hypotheses:

$$H_0 : \bar{r}_t = 0$$

$$H_1 : \bar{r}_t \neq 0 \qquad (\bar{r}_t \text{ is the tetrachoric correlation in the population})$$

Level of Significance: 0.05

Test Statistic: The significance of tetrachoric correlation shall be tested by using the following test statistic:

$$t = \frac{r_t}{\sigma_{r_t}}$$

where σ_{r_t} is the standard error of r_t and is computed by using the formula

$$\sigma_{r_t} = \frac{\sqrt{pqp'q'}}{uu'\sqrt{N}}$$

p and q are the proportions of the high and low IQ groups, whereas p' and q' are the proportions of the high and low playing ability groups.

Thus,

$$p = \frac{50}{100} = 0.5 \text{ and } q = \frac{50}{100} = 0.5, \qquad u = 0.399$$

$$p' = \frac{60}{100} = 0.60 \text{ and } q' = \frac{40}{100} = 0.40, \qquad u' = 0.386$$

The values of u and u' have been obtained from Table A.6 in the Appendix corresponding to the larger area.

Substituting these values, we get

$$\sigma_{r_t} = \frac{\sqrt{pqp'q'}}{uu'\sqrt{N}}$$

$$= \frac{\sqrt{0.5 \times 0.5 \times 0.6 \times 0.4}}{0.399 \times 0.386 \times \sqrt{100}}$$

$$= 0.159$$

Thus,

$$t = \frac{r_t}{\sigma_{r_t}}$$

$$= \frac{0.62}{0.159}$$

$$= 3.899$$

From Table A.7 in the Appendix, the value $t_{0.05}(100-2) = t_{0.05}(98) = 1.987$. Since the value of t (=3.899) is greater than 1.987, the null hypothesis may be rejected at 5% level.

Inference: Since the null hypothesis has been rejected, it may be concluded that the obtained value of tetrachoric correlation is significant. In other words, IQ is significantly associated with the playing ability of the basketball players.

Example 11.6 A sample of 240 students of class IX in a school was asked to perform pull-ups and curl-ups. The student who could do one successful pull-up was declared to have passed, otherwise was declared failed. In the same way, the curl-ups performance was also tested. The data so obtained are shown in Table 11.7. Compute the tetrachoric correlation and test its significance at the significance level 0.05.

Solution:

Step 1: *Computation of tetrachoric correlation* The tetrachoric correlation shall be computed first and then its significance will be tested by using the t-test.

$$r_t = \cos\left(\frac{180\sqrt{bc}}{\sqrt{ad}+\sqrt{bc}}\right)$$

$$= \cos\left(\frac{180\sqrt{50\times 30}}{\sqrt{100\times 60}+\sqrt{50\times 30}}\right)$$

$$= \cos 60$$

$$= 0.50 \text{ [from Table A.1 in the Appendix]}$$

Step 2: *Test of significance* To test the significance of the tetrachoric correlation, the following hypotheses shall be tested.

TABLE 11.7 Data on Pull-Ups and Curl-Ups Performance

		Pull-Ups		
		Pass	Fail	Total
Curl-ups	Pass	100 (a)	50 (b)	150
	Fail	30 (c)	60 (d)	90
	Total	130	110	$N = 240$

Hypotheses:

$$H_0: \bar{r}_t = 0$$

$$H_0: \bar{r}_t \neq 0 \qquad (\bar{r}_t \text{ is the tetrachoric correlation in the population})$$

Level of Significance: 0.05

Test Statistic: The significance of the tetrachoric correlation shall be tested by using the following test statistic:

$$t = \frac{r_t}{\sigma_{r_t}}$$

where σ_{r_t} is the standard error of r_t and is computed by using the formula

$$\sigma_{r_t} = \frac{\sqrt{pqp'q'}}{uu'\sqrt{N}}$$

p and q are the proportions of pass and fail groups in curl-ups, whereas p' and q' are the proportions of pass and fail groups in pull-ups.

$$p = \frac{150}{240} = 0.63 \text{ and } q = \frac{90}{240} = 0.37 \qquad u = 0.37$$

$$p' = \frac{130}{240} = 0.54 \text{ and } q' = \frac{110}{240} = 0.46, \quad u' = 0.378$$

The values of u and u' have been obtained from Table A.6 in the Appendix corresponding to the larger area. Substituting these values, we get

$$\sigma_{r_t} = \frac{\sqrt{pqp'q'}}{uu'\sqrt{N}}$$

$$= \frac{\sqrt{0.63 \times 0.37 \times 0.54 \times 0.46}}{0.378 \times 0.397 \times \sqrt{240}}$$

$$= 0.10$$

Thus,

$$t = \frac{r_t}{\sigma_{r_t}}$$

$$= \frac{0.50}{0.10}$$

$$= 5$$

From Table A.7 in the Appendix, the value of $t_{0.05}(240-2) = t_{0.05}(238) = 1.97$. Since the value of t (=5) is greater than 1.97, the null hypothesis may be rejected at 5% level.

Inference: Since the null hypothesis has been rejected, it may be inferred that the performance on curl-ups and pull-ups is associated with each other.

11.6 PHI COEFFICIENT (MEASURE OF ASSOCIATION BETWEEN NATURALLY DICHOTOMOUS VARIABLES)

The phi coefficient is used as a measure of correlation in a situation when both variables are naturally dichotomous, that is, when the two classes are distinctly separated on the basis of some traits. Variables of this kind are male versus female, swimmer and gymnasts, undergraduate versus postgraduate students, and so on. The phi coefficient can also be used to study the relationship between any two artificially dichotomous variables. In other words, even if the variables are quantitative in nature and owing to certain criteria their measurement has been reduced to two types of classification, the phi coefficient can still be used to assess the association between these variables. The phi coefficient is denoted by r_ϕ and is computed by the following formula:

$$r_\phi = \frac{ad - bc}{\sqrt{(a+b)(c+d)(a+c)(b+d)}} \tag{11.10}$$

where a, b, c, and d are the cell frequencies. The phi coefficient is a particular case of the product-moment correlation. The value of the product-moment correlation coefficient and phi coefficient will be same if integers 1 and 0 are assigned to represent the two categories of each variable, and the product-moment correlation coefficient is calculated in the usual way.

Consider an experiment in which the experimenter is interested in finding the association between gender and smoking. A sample of N subjects may be classified on the basis of gender and smoking trait. The frequencies of different categories may be arranged as shown in Table 11.8.

These frequencies may be substituted in formula (11.10) to compute the value of the phi coefficient.

The limits of the phi coefficient are −1 and +1. These limits can be obtained only when the two variables are evenly divided, that is, $p = q = p' = q' = 0.5$, otherwise only one of the limits −1 or +1 may be attained but not the both. Here, p and q are the proportions of the subjects in two categories of the first variable and p' and q' are the proportions of the subjects in two categories of the second variable as shown below:

$$p = \frac{a+b}{N} \text{ and } q = \frac{c+d}{N}$$

TABLE 11.8 Classification of Subjects According to Gender and Smoking Trait

		Smoking Trait		
		Smoker	Nonsmoker	Total
Gender	Male	a	b	$a+b$
	Female	c	d	$c+d$
	Total	$a+c$	$b+d$	$N=a+b+c+d$

$$p' = \frac{a+c}{N} \text{ and } q' = \frac{b+d}{N}$$

11.6.1 Assumptions

One of the main assumptions in computing the phi coefficient is that both variables should be naturally dichotomous. Because the phi coefficient is determined by the chi-square statistic, the assumptions of the chi-square test for two independent samples also apply here. The observations must be independent and should be in the form of frequencies and not scores.

11.6.2 Testing Significance

The significance of the phi coefficient can be investigated by testing the following hypotheses:

$$H_0\colon \bar{r}_\phi = 0 \text{ (represents the population phi coefficient)}$$

$$H_0\colon \bar{r}_\phi \neq 0$$

To test the null hypothesis, the following chi-square χ^2 statistic is used as a test statistic.

$$\chi^2 = N \times r_\phi^2 \tag{11.11}$$

This χ^2 statistic follows the χ^2 distribution with one degree of freedom. The significance of the χ^2 statistic as mentioned in (11.11) can be tested by comparing its value with that of the tabulated value of χ^2 obtained from Table A.11 in the Appendix for one degree of freedom and at any given level of significance.

11.6.3 Merits and Demerits

The phi coefficient can also be used in a situation where both the variables are artificially dichotomous. The values of the phi coefficient and product-moment correlation become identical if integers 1 and 0 are assigned to represent the two categories of each variable. Both the limits of the phi coefficient, that is, −1 and +1 can only be attained if both the variables are evenly divided in both the categories.

TABLE 11.9 Classification of Students on the Basis of Gender and Color of Eyes

		Eye Color		
		Black	Brown	Total
Gender	Male	80 (*a*)	20 (*b*)	100
	Female	70 (*c*)	30 (*d*)	100
	Total	150	50	$N = 200$

Example 11.7 In a randomly selected sample of male and female students, the color of their eyes was noted. Calculate the phi coefficient for the data shown in Table 11.9.

Solution: The phi coefficient shall be computed by using the following formula:

$$r_\phi = \frac{ad - bc}{\sqrt{(a+b)(c+d)(a+c)(b+d)}}$$

$$r_\phi = \frac{80 \times 30 - 20 \times 70}{\sqrt{(80+20)(70+30)(80+70)(20+30)}}$$

$$= \frac{2400 - 1400}{\sqrt{100 \times 100 \times 150 \times 50}}$$

$$= \frac{1}{5\sqrt{3}}$$

$$= 0.115$$

Example 11.8 A questionnaire measuring IQ was administered on the students of exercise science. Calculate the phi coefficient to test the significance of association between gender and IQ for the data shown in Table 11.10.

TABLE 11.10 Classification of Students on the Basis of Gender and IQ

		IQ		
		High	Low	Total
Gender	Male	15 (*a*)	25 (*b*)	40
	Female	30 (*c*)	10 (*d*)	40
	Total	45	35	$N = 80$

Solution:

Step 1: *Computing phi coefficient* The computation of phi coefficient shall be done by using the following formula:

$$r_\phi = \frac{ad - bc}{\sqrt{(a+b)(c+d)(a+c)(b+d)}}$$

$$r_\phi = \frac{15 \times 10 - 25 \times 30}{\sqrt{(15+25)(30+10)(15+30)(25+10)}}$$

$$= \frac{150 - 750}{\sqrt{40 \times 40 \times 45 \times 35}}$$

$$= -\frac{600}{600\sqrt{7}}$$

$$= -0.378$$

Step 2: *To test the significance of* r_ϕ To test the significance of r_ϕ, the following hypotheses shall be tested

Hypotheses:

$$H_0: \bar{r}_\phi = 0$$

(there is no association between gender and IQ in the population)

$$H_0: \bar{r}_\phi \neq 0$$

(there is an association between gender and IQ in the population)

Level of significance: 0.05

Test statistic: To test the significance of the phi coefficient, the following chi-square is used as a test statistic.

$$\chi^2 = N \times r_\phi^2$$

Since $r_\phi = -0.378$ and $N = 80$,

$$\chi^2 = 80 \times (-0.378)^2$$

$$= 11.43$$

From Table A.11 in the Appendix, tabulated $\chi^2_{0.05,1} = 3.84$ [degrees of freedom $= (r-1)(c-1) = 1$]. Since the calculated value of χ^2 (=11.43) is greater than 3.84, the null hypothesis may be rejected at 5% level.

Inference: Since the null hypothesis has been rejected, it may be concluded on the basis of the sampled data that gender is significantly associated with IQ.

TABLE 11.11 Response of Male and Female "Should Sports Be Given More Priority in the School Curriculum?"

		Response		
		Yes	No	Total
Gender	Male	60 (a)	20 (b)	80
	Female	15 (c)	45 (d)	60
	Total	75	65	N = 140

Example 11.9 In a survey, 140 men and women were asked to give their views on "Should sports be given more priority in the school curriculum?" They were asked to give their response in the form of either "Yes" or "No." Responses so obtained are shown in Table 11.11. On the basis of the information, can it be inferred that the response is gender based? Test your hypothesis at 5% level.

Solution:

$$r_\phi = \frac{ad - bc}{\sqrt{(a+b)(c+d)(a+c)(b+d)}}$$

$$= \frac{60 \times 45 - 20 \times 15}{\sqrt{(60+20)(15+45)(60+15)(20+45)}}$$

$$= \frac{2400}{\sqrt{80 \times 60 \times 75 \times 65}}$$

$$= \frac{2400}{4837.35}$$

$$= 0.496$$

11.7 CONTINGENCY COEFFICIENT (MEASURE OF ASSOCIATION BETWEEN CATEGORICAL VARIABLES)

The contingency coefficient is a nonparametric statistic that is used to compute the magnitude of association between any two categorical variables. The contingency coefficient is used in a situation where the chi-square is used to test the association between any two categorical variables. Here, the variables may be categorized in more than two categories as well, but the contingency coefficient gives a more accurate estimate of the association in a situation where both the variables are dichotomous. Thus, the contingency coefficient can be used to measure the association between any two variables that have been classified into $m \times n$ categories where m and n may have the same or different values. The contingency coefficient is also known as the *Pearson contingency coefficient*; it is denoted by C and is computed as

$$C = \sqrt{\frac{\chi^2}{N + \chi^2}} \tag{11.12}$$

where χ^2 is the chi-square statistic, the computation of which has been discussed in detail in Chapter 10. The significance of the contingency coefficient can be tested by using the χ^2 statistic, which is computed by the following formula:

$$\chi^2 = \sum \frac{(f_o - f_e)^2}{f_e} \tag{11.13}$$

where f_o and f_e are the observed and expected frequencies, respectively.

11.7.1 Merits and Demerits

Through the contingency coefficient, an objective assessment of association between the two attributes can be made and therefore it is free from bias. It does not require any strong assumptions about the sampling distribution. It assumes the discrete categorization of data into groups. Testing the significance of the contingency coefficient is not affected by the ordering and arranging of rows and columns. The degree of freedom is determined by the number of rows/columns.

Check Your Progress

Note: Tick the correct answer by using the sign (√).

	True	False
24. Tetrachoric correlation is suitable if both the variables are artificially dichotomous.	-	-
25. The value of cos 180 is 1.	-	-
26. The degrees of freedom of t for testing the significance of the tetrachoric correlation is $n-2$.	-	-
27. The tetratchoric correlation is more reliable than product-moment correlation.	-	-

28. The degrees of freedom of the chi-square for testing the significance of the phi coefficient is 2.	-	-
29. The phi coefficient and product-moment correlation become identical if the integers 1 and 0 are assigned to represent the two categories of each variable.	-	-
30. The tetrachoric correlation is more reliable if the divisions in both the dichotomous variables in the two categories are close to their means.	-	-
31. The phi coefficient is used when both the variables are naturally dichotomous.	-	-
32. The phi coefficient may achieve both the limits -1 and $+1$ if the variables are not evenly divided.	-	-
33. The contingency coefficient is free from bias.	-	-
34. Tetrachoric correlation should not be used if any of the cell frequencies is 0.	-	-
35. The phi coefficient is computed by using the chi-square.	-	-
36. Under certain assumptions, the tetrachoric correlation is numerically equivalent to the product-moment correlation coefficient.	-	-
37. The chi-square is used to test the significance of the phi coefficient.	-	-
38. In certain situations, the value of the tetrachoric correlation may exceed 1.	-	-
39. The phi coefficient can be computed even if the samples are not independent.	-	-
40. In computing the tetrachoric correlation, the assumption of linearity is not important.	-	-
41. Testing the significance of the contingency coefficient is affected by the ordering of rows and columns.	-	-
42. Computing the tetrachoric correlation assumes that both variables are continuous and normally distributed.	-	-
43. The contingency coefficient is used when the chi-square is used for testing the significance of association between two attributes.	-	-

PRACTICE EXERCISE

1. The ranking of 10 athletes on reaction time (X) and on 100 m performance (Y) are given below. Find the rank correlation and test its significance at 1% level.

$R(X)$	3	5	4	8	7	10	2	6	1	9
$R(Y)$	6	4	8	9	1	2	3	10	5	7

2. The following table shows frequencies of athletes belonging to high and low sports performance and academic achievement groups. Compute the tetrachoric correlation and test its significance at 5% level.

Classification of the Athletes According to Their Sports Performance and Academic Achievement

		Academic Achievement	
		High	Low
Sports Performance	High	20	45
	Low	55	35

3. A sample of 100 families was selected to know the attitude of the father and mother toward their daughter's participation in outdoor sports. Respondents were asked to answer either "yes" or "no." Compute the contingency coefficient to find the magnitude of association between the gender of the parent and their response. Test the significance of this contingency coefficient at 5% level.

Frequency of the Responses to the Question
"Do You Like Your Daughter to Participate in Outdoor Sports ?"

		Responses	
		Yes	No
Parent	Father	70	30
	Mother	20	80

Example 11.10 A study was conducted to compare the attitude of male and female subjects toward coaching of their daughter by a male coach. The observations so obtained are shown in Table 11.12. Compute the contingency coefficient

TABLE 11.12 Observed Frequencies

	Response (f_o)			
Gender	Yes	No	Undecided	Total
Male	65	20	15	100
Female	25	45	5	75
Total	90	65	20	$N = 175$

between gender and attitude, test its significance, and draw your conclusion at 5% level.

Solution: It is required to compute the contingency coefficient to find the magnitude of association between the gender and response. Further, the significance of this coefficient needs to be tested. To do so, the chi-square shall be computed first because the contingency coefficient is computed on the basis of the chi-square.

Computation of contingency coefficient Since we know that

$$C = \sqrt{\frac{\chi^2}{N + \chi^2}}$$

let us first compute chi-square

$$\chi^2 = \sum \frac{(f_o - f_e)^2}{f_e}$$

The expected frequencies have been calculated in each cell by dividing the product of marginal row and column totals associated with the cell by the total of all the frequencies N. These expected frequencies are shown in Table 11.13.

TABLE 11.13 Expected Frequencies

	Response (f_e)		
Gender	Yes	No	Undecided
Male	$\frac{100 \times 90}{175} = 51.43$	$\frac{100 \times 65}{175} = 37.14$	$\frac{100 \times 20}{175} = 11.43$
Female	$\frac{75 \times 90}{175} = 38.57$	$\frac{75 \times 65}{175} = 27.86$	$\frac{75 \times 20}{175} = 8.57$

$$\text{Calculated } \chi^2 = \sum \frac{(f_o - f_e)^2}{f_e} = \frac{(65-51.43)^2}{51.43} + \frac{(20-37.14)^2}{37.14} + \frac{(15-11.43)^2}{11.43}$$

$$= \frac{(25-38.57)^2}{38.57} + \frac{(45-27.86)^2}{27.86} + \frac{(5-8.57)^2}{8.57}$$

$$= 3.58 + 7.91 + 1.12 + 4.77 + 10.54 + 1.49$$

$$= 29.41$$

Substituting the value of chi-square, the contingency coefficient becomes

$$C = \sqrt{\frac{29.41}{175 + 29.41}}$$

$$= 0.14$$

Now that the magnitude of association between the two attributes has been computed as 0.14, the next task is to test whether this association is significant. This will be done by testing the significance of chi-square. Here, following hypotheses shall be tested:

Hypotheses:

H_0: There is no association between gender and response
H_1: There is no association between gender and response

Level of significance: 0.05

Test statistic: To test the above null hypothesis, it is required to test whether the computed value of chi-square, that is, 29.41 is significant at 5% level.

$$\text{df} = (r-1)(c-1) = (2-1)(3-1) = 2$$

From Table A.11 in the Appendix, the value of $\chi^2_{0.05,2}$ is 5.99. Since the calculated χ^2 (=29.41) is greater than 5.99, the null hypothesis of no association between gender and response (toward coaching of their daughter by a male coach) is rejected at the significance level 0.05.

Inference: Since the null hypothesis has been rejected, it may be inferred that the contingency coefficient is significant and there is a significant association between gender and response. In other words, the response patterns of males and females differ. Thus, it may be concluded that the males and females think differently about the issue as to whether their daughter should be coached by a male coach. Here, we tested the hypothesis of no association but we ended up in saying that the response patterns of males and females differ.

11.8 COMPUTING WITH EXCEL

11.8.1 Computing Rank Correlation with Excel

Excel does not provide the facility of applying nonparametric tests using the Analysis ToolPak. However, by using its computing facility, different nonparametric tests can be solved. One such example of rank correlation has been discussed here in which the solution has been obtained by using the computing facility of Excel.

Example 11.11 Following are the ranks of 14 college students on heights and fat percentage. Compute the rank correlation between the two variables.

Data on ranks obtained on height and fat percentage:

Sr. No.	Height	Fat%
1	1	6
2	2.5	9
3	2.5	13
4	4	7
5	5	10
6	6.5	12
7	6.5	3.5
8	8	1
9	10	11
10	10	2
11	10	8
12	12.5	14
13	12.5	3.5
14	14	5

Solution: The following steps are involved in computing rank correlation by using Excel:

a. Type the ranks of both the variables in any two columns of the Excel sheet as shown in Figure 11.2. The rank correlation can be computed by using the following formula:

$$\rho = 1 - \frac{6\sum D^2}{N(N^2 - 1)}$$

where D is the difference in the ranks of each individual and N is the sample size.

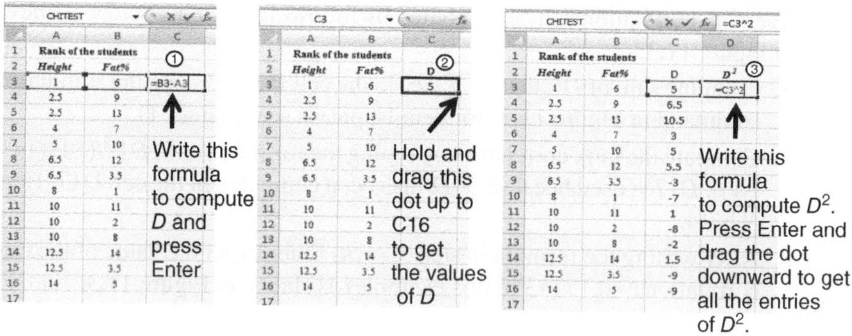

Figure 11.2 Steps in computing D and D^2.

b. Compute the values D and D^2 by following the following steps as shown in the Figure 11.2.
   1. Write the formula $=B3 - A3$ in the cell C3.
   2. After writing the formula in step 1, press the Enter key to get the value of D as 5 in step 2.
   3. In step 2, hold and drag the dot of the cell containing the value 5 downward to get the other values of the D as shown in step 3. Similarly, use the formula $=C3\text{^}2$ in cell D3 in step 3, and after pressing the Enter key, drag the dot downward to get the values of D^2 in the column. The values of D^2 so obtained are shown in Figure 11.3.

   The computation of the rank correlation has been shown in Figure 11.2 in the following sequence.

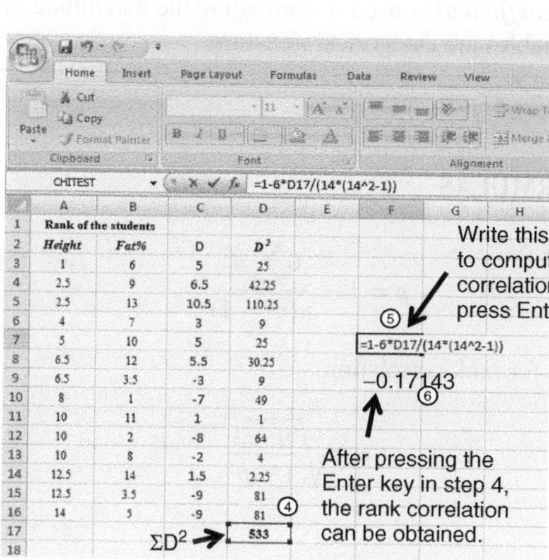

Figure 11.3 Computing rank correlation by using the formula.

c. The rank correlation can be computed by following the steps below as shown in Figure 11.3.
   4. Compute sum of D^2, that is, $\sum D^2$, in the cell D17 by using the summation command in Figure 11.3 (for details, please see Chapter 1).
   5. Compute the rank correlation by typing the formula =1-6**D*17/(14*(14^2 −1)). *D*17 is used because $\sum D^2$ has been computed in the cell D17. Here, *N* is 14.
   6. After writing the formula in step 5, press Enter to get the value of the rank correlation (−0.17143 in this example) as shown in Figure 11.3.

IMPORTANT DEFINITIONS

Rank correlation is a method of computing correlation when both the variables are measured on the ordinal scale.
Bi-serial correlation is a method of computing correlation in a situation where one of the variables is measured either on an interval or a ratio scale and the other is artificially dichotomous.
Point bi-serial correlation is a correlation method used for finding the magnitude of the relationship between two variables when one of them is measured either on an interval or a ratio scale and the other is naturally dichotomous.
Tetrachoric correlation is a method of computing correlation used in a situation when both the variables are artificially dichotomous.
The ***phi coefficient*** is a method of computing correlation in a situation when both the variables are naturally dichotomous.
The ***contingency coefficient*** is used in computing the magnitude of correlation when both the variables are categorical in nature.

IMPORTANT FORMULAS

Rank correlation

$$\rho = 1 - \frac{6\sum d_i^2}{n(n^2 - 1)}$$

Test of significance for rank correlation

$$t = \rho\sqrt{\frac{n-2}{1-\rho^2}}$$

Bi-serial correlation

$$r_{\text{b}} = \frac{\bar{x}_p - \bar{x}_q}{s_t} \times \frac{pq}{u}$$

Testing the significance of bi-serial correlation

$$t = \frac{r_{\text{b}}}{\sigma_{r_{\text{b}}}}, \text{ where } \sigma_{r_{\text{b}}} = \frac{\sqrt{pq}}{u\sqrt{n}}$$

Point bi-serial correlation

$$r_{\text{pb}} = \frac{\bar{x}_p - \bar{x}_q}{s_t} \times \sqrt{pq}$$

Tetrachoric correlation

$$r_{\text{t}} = \cos\left(\frac{180\sqrt{bc}}{\sqrt{ad} + \sqrt{bc}}\right)$$

Testing the significance of the tetrachoric correlation

$$t = \frac{r_t}{\sigma_{r_t}}, \text{ where } \sigma_{r_t} = \frac{\sqrt{pqp'q'}}{uu'\sqrt{N}}$$

Phi coefficient

$$r_{\phi} = \frac{ad - bc}{\sqrt{(a+b)(c+d)(a+c)(b+d)}}$$

Testing the significance of the phi coefficient

$$\chi^2 = N \times r_{\phi}^2$$

Contingency coefficient

$$C = \sqrt{\frac{\chi^2}{N + \chi^2}}$$

Testing the significance of the contingency coefficient

$$\chi^2 = \sum \frac{(f_o - f_e)^2}{f_e}$$

KEY TERMS

bi-serial correlation
contingency coefficient
phi coefficient
point bi-serial correlation
rank correlation
tetrachoric correlation

CHAPTER EXERCISE

1. What is the difference between product-moment correlation and rank correlation?
2. Distinguish between bi-serial correlation and point bi-serial correlation. What are they used for? Explain any one application where these tests can be used.
3. How will you test the significance of bi-serial correlation?
4. Discuss the situations where the tetrachoric correlation and phi coefficient can be used.
5. What do you mean by the contingency coefficient? How it is computed?
6. Following are the data on playing ability and the heights obtained on basketball players. The playing ability was assessed by the judges in terms of ranks and heights were measured in feet. Compute the rank correlation between them and test its significance at 5% level.

Playing Ability	Height (ft.)
1	5.7
2	6.4
3	6.4
4	6.3
5	6.3
6	6.4
7	5.8
8	6.1
9	5.9
10	6
11	6.2
12	6.3

7. The data on lean body weight and vital capacity obtained on college athletes have been shown in the following table. The lean body weight has been measured in pounds and vital capacity in liters. Compute the rank correlation and test whether it is significant at 5% level.

Lean Body Weight (in lbs)	Vital Capacity (in liters)
154.5	3.8
149.6	3.9
140.8	4.0
157.3	4.0
154.0	4.2
151.8	4.0
160.6	3.9
147.4	3.8
136.4	3.7
158.4	3.6
160.6	4.1
154.0	4.3
136.4	3.7

8. Explain the difference between product-moment correlation and rank correlation coefficient.
9. The performance of 10 students on a statistics test (x) and an IQ test (y) is given below:

x: 10	14	10	16	13	16	24	10	22
y: 30	40	44	45	30	32	40	35	39

Calculate the product-moment correlation and rank correlation. Do these two coefficients differ? Explain.

10. The IQ scores obtained on the boys and girls in a sample are shown in the following table. Compute the point bi-serial correlation and test its significance at 5% level.

IQ Scores	Boys	Girls
101–105	3	–
106–110	6	3
111–115	8	4
116–120	20	6
121–125	12	8
126–130	16	25
131–135	10	19
136–140	6	8
141–145	5	6
146–150	–	1

11. One hundred and eighty subjects who appeared in a junior research fellow (JRF) examination were tested for their numerical aptitude. The marks on their numerical aptitude and the results in the JRF examination are shown in the following table in the class interval form. Compute the bi-serial correlation.

Frequency Distribution of the Scores on the Numerical Aptitude of the Subjects in the Pass and Fail Categories

	Results of JRF	
Numerical Aptitude (CI)	Pass (f_1)	Fail (f_2)
10–15	2	5
15–20	3	7
20–25	1	11
25–30	2	9
30–35	4	8
35–40	10	6
40–45	16	2
45–50	8	1

12. Following are the lifestyle scores of male and female subjects obtained in a study to investigate whether any significant relationship exists between lifestyle and gender.

Frequency Distribution of the Lifestyle Scores of Male and Female Subjects

Lifestyle Score (CI)	Male (f_1)	Female (f_2)
25–30	2	7
31–35	4	4
36–40	4	10
41–45	12	6
46–50	10	8
51–55	14	3
56–60	6	6
61–65	8	2

Compute the point bi-serial correlation. Can it be concluded that there is a significant relationship between the gender and lifestyle of a person? Test your hypothesis at 5% level.

13. To understand the relationship between anxiety and gymnastics performance, 120 gymnasts were classified according to their performance. In each performance group, they were further classified into high and low anxiety groups. These frequencies are shown in the following table. Compute the tetrachoric correlation and test its significance at 1% level. Can it be concluded that the gymnastics performance is significantly associated with the anxiety of the gymnast?

Classification of Gymnasts According to Their Performance in Gymnastics and Anxiety

		Gymnastics Performance	
		High	Low
Anxiety	High	20	40
	Low	35	25

14. In order to know the relationship between gender and fitness performance, a group of male and female subjects was classified on the basis of their performance on a fitness test. Compute the phi coefficient and test its significance at 5% level.

Classification of the Male and Female Subjects According to Their Performance on the Fitness Test

		Fitness Test	
		Pass	Fail
Gender	Male	24	14
	Female	16	26

15. A random sample of athletes was asked about their preference for a male or female coach. Following are the responses.

Responses of the Athletes About Their Preferences

		Preference	
		Favoring Male Coach	Favoring Female Coach
Gender of Athletes	Male	75	5
	Female	50	30

Test the hypothesis that there is no association between the gender of athletes and their preference about the gender of the coach. Test your hypothesis at 5% level and compute the contingency coefficient.

16. To assess the association between sports and dermatoglyphic patterns, three groups of sportsmen, namely, athletes, swimmers, and cyclists were selected. These sportsmen were observed for their patterns on the ring finger of the right hand. Can it be concluded that there is a significant association between sports and dermatoglyphic pattern on the ring finger? Test your hypothesis at 5% level of significance.

Frequencies of the Dermatoglyphic Pattern on the Ring Finger of Right Hand

	Pattern		
	Loops	Whorls	Arch
Athletes	60	30	10
Swimmers	40	55	5
Cyclists	30	45	25

ANSWERS

Check Your Progress

1. F	12. T	23. F	34. T
2. F	13. F	24. T	35. T
3. F	14. T	25. F	36. T
4. T	15. T	26. T	37. T
5. F	16. F	27. F	38. F
6. T	17. T	28. F	39. F
7. F	18. T	29. T	40. F
8. T	19. F	30. F	41. F
9. T	20. F	31. T	42. T
10. F	21. T	32. F	43. T
11. F	22. T	33. T	

Practice Exercise

1. $\rho = (0.006)$
2. $r_t = -0.46$, $t = 3.62$, H_0 rejected, there is a significant association between sports performance and academic achievement.
3. $C = 0.4489$, $\chi^2 = 50.475$, null hypothesis rejected, there is a significant association between gender of the parent and their response.

Chapter Exercise

6. $\rho = -0.05$
7. $\rho = 0.29$, rank correlation is not significant.
9. $r = 0.276$ and $\rho = 0.313$
10. $r_{pbi} = -0.28$
11. $r_{bi} = 0.64$
12. $r_{pbi} = 0.28$
13. $r_t = -0.39$. This tetrachoric correlation is significant at 5% level; gymnastics performance is significantly associated with anxiety.
14. $r_\phi = 0.25$, $\chi^2 = 5$, r_ϕ is significant.
15. $C = 0.35$
16. $\chi^2 = 34.33$. There is a significant association between sports and dermatoglyphic pattern on ring finger.

FURTHER READING

1. Choi SC. Test of equality of dependent correlations. Biometrika 1977;64(3):645–647.
2. Davenport E, El-Sanhury N. Phi/Phimax: review and synthesis. Educational and Psychological Measurement 1991;51:821–828.

3. Ferguson GA. Statistical analysis in psychology and education. New York: McGraw-Hill; 1966.
4. Guilford J. Psychometric Methods. New York: McGraw-Hill Book Company, Inc.; 1936.
5. Guilford JP, Fruchter B. Fundamental Statistics in Psychology and Education. 5th ed. New York: McGraw-Hill; 1973.
6. Kendall MG. Rank Correlation Methods. London: Griffin; 1970. ISBN 0-85264-199-0.
7. Linacre J. The Expected Value of a Point-Biserial (or Similar) Correlation. Rasch Measurement Transactions 2008;22(1):1154.
8. Maritz JS. Distribution-Free Statistical Methods. UK: Chapman & Hall. ISBN 0-412-15940-4; 1981. p 217.
9. Michell J. Measurement scales and statistics: a clash of paradigms. Psychological Bulletin 1986;3:398–407.
10. More Correlation Coefficients - Accessed from http://www.andrews.edu/~calkins/math/edrm611/edrm13.htm#POINTB; on February 2013.
11. Spearman C. The proof and measurement of association between two things. American Journal of Psychology 1904;15:72–101.
12. Yule G U, Kendall M G. An Introduction to the Theory of Statistics. 14th(5th Impression 1968) ed. London: Charles Griffin & Co; 1950. p 268.

12

DEVELOPING NORMS FOR ASSESSING PERFORMANCE

12.1 INTRODUCTION

Norms are developed to assess an individual's performance in test items. This helps a layperson to understand where an individual stands in a group on a particular trait. For instance, if a college athlete performs the 100 m event in 12.1 s, it is difficult to understand his level of competency in the sprinting event. Similarly, if the flexibility score of a college woman is 6 in. in the sit and reach test, it is difficult to understand where she stands in her group. If these performances can somehow be converted into a comparable score on a standard scale, then one can easily understand the level of competency of the individual. For example, instead of saying that the athlete's performance in the 100 m sprint is 12.1 s, if it is shown in terms of marks, say 70 (out of 100), one can get better idea about the athlete's performance. Similarly, if the flexibility of the college women is reported in terms of marks, say 65 (out of 100), instead of 6 in. on the sit and reach test, then this is better understood by the layperson.

There are two objectives for which norms are developed. The first objective is to compare the performance of an individual with that of another in the same population. Such norms are based on the concept of ranks. The percentile scale is used to construct these types of norms. Percentile norms are helpful in assessing the position of an athlete on different test items such as explosive strength, muscular strength, flexibility, muscular endurance, and so on. Such norms are population specific and, hence, can be used only for those populations for which it has been developed. Further, these norms cannot be used in comparing the performance of

Statistics for Exercise Science and Health with Microsoft® Office Excel®, First Edition. J. P. Verma.

an athlete in two test items having different units. However, by clubbing the percentiles, another scale can be developed, which can assign an individual a single number depending on his or her performance in a particular test item. Such a scale is known as the *stanine scale*.

The second objective of developing norms is to assess an individual's performance in two different test items having different units. The Z-scale can be developed to do this job. As the Z-score is free from units, it can be used to compare the performance of an individual in two different test items having different units. The Z-scale ranges from −3 to +3 for all practical purposes and consists of almost all cases in that range as such, an individual's performance may be expressed in positive as well as negative scores. At times, these negative scores on the Z-scale may be confusing to a layperson. For instance, if an individual's performance in cardiorespiratory endurance is −0.02, one may not understand where the person's performance stands. However, a researcher may interpret that the performance is just less than the average. To solve this problem, the *T*-scale may be used, where the performance can be assessed on a scale ranging from 0 to 100, which can be easily understood by people in general.

Another problem a researcher faces in developing a scale in the area of exercise science and health research is that improvement in performance is not linear in nature. In other words, the same amount of improvement in performance at the top level requires a lot more effort than that at a lower level. For this reason, it is required to develop a scale that is based on difficulty rating. A detailed procedure has been discussed to develop such scales in this chapter.

In this chapter, scaling procedures such as the percentile scale, stanine scale, Z-scale, *T*-scale, and the scale based on difficulty ratings have been discussed in detail.

12.2 PERCENTILES

Percentiles are used by the researcher as an indicator of performance in assessing most physical and physiological parameters. Percentiles tell us how an athlete relates to a larger group. In most test and measurement books, you will find that the standards of various tests are reported in terms of percentiles. The criterion for selection is usually based on percentiles. A candidate would be admitted to an exercise science program only if he/she is above 50% of those taking certain standardized tests.

A given percentile indicates the percentage of scores below that point. For instance, if the percentile score of a college athlete on vertical jump performance is 65, this indicates that the athlete's performance is above 65% of the college athletes in the population. The percentile simply indicates the positional value of the candidate in the group. It does not tell the actual worth of an individual on the test item. It is used to compare the performance of any two individuals in any test item in the population. There are 100 percentile points in the percentile scale, and it is assumed that each percentile point has 1% of the population scores.

Usually percentiles are computed on decile points, namely, P_0, P_{10}, P_{20}, P_{30}, …, P_{100}. The points P_1 and P_{99} are the limits that include all scores in the sample. Percentiles are similar to the quartiles and the median. While percentiles divide the distribution into 100 equal parts, the quartile divides it into four equal parts, and the median into two equal parts. Thus, the quartiles and the median can be expressed in terms of percentiles. The first and third quartiles can be represented by P_{25} and P_{75}, respectively, whereas the median can be represented by P_{50}.

The percentile is a nonstandard scale and does not assume the population to be normally distributed.

> **FACTS TO KNOW**
>
> Percentile is a nonstandard scale and does not assume the population to be normally distributed

The percentile scale is based on the assumption that the distribution of scores is rectangular in shape, that is, the difference between a rank of 10 and a rank of 20 is the same as the difference between a rank of 50 and a rank of 60. Since the distribution of raw scores is rarely rectangular in research studies, one should use this scale with caution.

The xth percentile is represented by P_x and can be computed by formulas (12.1) and (12.2) in case of ungrouped and grouped data, respectively.

For ungrouped data

$$P_x = \left(\frac{x}{100} \times N\right)^{\text{th}} \text{score} \qquad (12.1)$$

where N is the size of the data.

For grouped data

$$P_x = \text{LL} + \frac{\frac{x \times N}{100} - F}{f} \times i \qquad (12.2)$$

where

LL = lower limit of the xth percentile class
N = frequency total
F = cumulative frequency of the class interval just before the xth percentile class
f = frequency of the xth percentile class
i = size of the class interval

12.2.1 Merits and Demerits of the Percentile Scale

One of the main advantages of using percentiles is how easy it is to understand and interpret. One can easily make out where an individual stands on a particular test item in the population. The percentile can easily be calculated irrespective of the shape of the distribution of scores in the sample.

The percentile scale does have limitations as well. Since percentiles are positional values, mathematical calculations such as the mean and standard deviation cannot be made. For this reason, it cannot be used in advanced statistical computations. Percentiles cannot be used to compare the performance of an individual in two different test items because the samples may have different distributions. Since the percentile follows a rectangular distribution and, in rectangular distributions, all scores have equal frequency, it is assumed that each percentile has 1% of the population. Most behavioral parameters are supposed to be normal, and hence the use of percentiles is restricted to knowing the relative standing of an individual only on a particular test item in the group. Further, percentiles are clustered at the center and spread out at extremes, and therefore it becomes disadvantageous for good athletes if they are used for the assessment of their performance.

Example 12.1 In an experiment, VO_{2max} was measured in ml/(kg min), which is shown below. Compute P_{45} and P_{85}.

VO_{2max} : 28 29 53 45 42 39 32 34 39 41 32 49 52 56 45 42 59 56
28 29 32 32 34 39 39 41 42 42 45 45 49 52 53 56 56 59

Solution: The first step in computing percentiles is to arrange the scores in ascending order.

28 29 32 32 34 39 39 41 42 42 45 45 49 52 53 56 56 59

Given that $N = 18$,

$$P_{45} = \frac{45}{100} \times 18 = \text{the 8.1th score} = 41.1$$

Similarly,

$$P_{85} = \frac{85}{100} \times 18 = \text{the 15.3th score} = 53.9$$

Example 12.2 Calculate P_{40} and P_{75} for the pull-ups scores as shown in the following table and draw your conclusions.

Pull-Ups Scores Arranged in Class Intervals

CI	18–20	15–17	12–14	9–11	6–8	3–5	0–2
f	3	4	15	6	16	14	12

Solution:

Computation of P_{40}

To compute the two percentiles, the cumulative frequencies have been computed in Table 12.1. For finding the value of P_{40}, it is required to

TABLE 12.1 Computation for P_{40} and P_{75} for Pull-Ups Score

	Class Interval (CI)	Frequency (f)	Cum. Freq. (F)
	0–2	12	12
	3–5	14	26
P_{40} class →	6–8	16	42
	9–11	6	48
P_{75} class →	12–14	15	63
	15–17	4	67
	18–20	3	70
		$\Sigma f = 70$	

compute $\frac{40 \times n}{100}$ so that the class interval in which P_{40} is supposed to lie can be located. Here, $n = 70$ and therefore

$$\frac{40 \times n}{100} = 28$$

The value of P_{40} shall lie in the class interval whose cumulative frequency includes 28. The class interval 6–8 is the P_{40} class because its cumulative frequency includes 28. After identifying the class interval, the value of P_{40} can be computed by using the following formula:

$$P_{40} = \text{LL} + \frac{\frac{40n}{100} - F}{f} \times i$$

For P_{40}, LL = 5.5, $n = 70$, $F = 26$, $f = 16$, and $i = 3$. Substituting these values,

$$P_{40} = \text{LL} + \frac{\frac{40n}{100} - F}{f} \times i$$

$$= 5.5 + \frac{\frac{40 \times 70}{100} - 26}{16} \times 3$$

$$= 5.875$$

Computation of P_{75}

For computing P_{75}, $n = 70$ and $\frac{75 \times n}{100} = 52.5$.

The class interval 12–14 is P_{75} class because its cumulative frequency includes 52.5.

For P_{75}, LL = 11.5, $n = 70$, $F = 48$, $f = 15$, and $i = 3$. Substituting these values,

$$P_{75} = \text{LL} + \frac{\frac{75 \times n}{100} - F}{f} \times i$$

$$= 11.5 + \frac{\frac{75 \times 70}{100} - 48}{15} \times 3$$

$$= 12.4$$

12.2.2 Percentile Rank

Percentile rank refers to the exact position of an individual's performance in a group. It can be defined as the proportion of scores in a population that a specific score is greater than or equal to. For example, if the vertical jump performance of an athlete is 1.8 m and this performance is greater than or equal to the performance of 92% of the athletes tested for vertical jump performance, then the percentile rank of the athlete would be 92. Percentile ranks are always expressed in whole numbers. If the percentile rank is obtained as a fraction, it is rounded off to the nearest whole number. The percentile rank cannot be 0 or 100. The lowest score is at the first percentile rank, whereas the highest score is at the 99th percentile. Since the percentile rank is a positional value, no mathematical computation can be performed on it. The percentile rank P_r of an individual having the test score X can be computed by using formula (12.3):

$$P_r = \frac{\text{CF} + 0.5 \times f}{n} \times 100 \quad (12.3)$$

where

CF = number of scores below X
F = number of times the score X occurs in the dataset
n = number of scores in the dataset

Example 12.3 If following are the scores on calf flexibility measured on athletes, compute the percentile rank of the athlete having calf flexibility 11.

Calf Flexibility:	12	11	10	8	9	6	12	11	7	5	6

Solution: Given

Total number of scores = n = 11

Number of times the score 11 occurs in the dataset = f = 2

Number of scores below 11 = CF = 7

Substituting these values in Equation (12.3),

$$P_r = \frac{\text{CF} + 0.5 \times f}{n} \times 100 = \frac{7 + 0.5 \times 2}{11} \times 100 = 72.7 \approx 73$$

Thus, the percentile rank of an athlete whose calf flexibility is 11 is 73.

12.3 Z-SCALE

The Z-scale is based on the assumption that the scores are normally distributed in the sample. Since most behavioral parameters are normally distributed, this scale may be more suitable to assess the performance of an individual in a particular test item. The Z-scale is based on the Z-score, which is obtained by applying the following transformation to the data:

$$z = \frac{x - \bar{x}}{s} \tag{12.4}$$

If the distribution of X is normal, then the distribution of Z will follow the standard normal distribution with mean 0 and variance 1. In fact, the Z-score tells us how many standard deviations above or below the mean an individual score is. The Z-scale is stretched from −3 to +3. Thus, on this scale, one can obtain positive as well as negative values. According to the properties of the normal distribution, 99.73% of the total area of the curve falls within the 3σ limits, and therefore it is expected that if the performance is measured on the Z-scale, the performance of most of the subjects would be within the range −3 to +3. Since the Z-score is free from units, it can be used to compare the performance of an athlete in two different test items having different units. For instance, on the Z-scale, if the performance of an athlete in 100 m is 0.24, whereas his performance in long jump is 0.35, then one can draw the conclusion that the athlete's performance in long jump is better in comparison to the performance in 100 m. However, this comparison is possible only if the distribution of scores in both the samples is normal. For instance, if the distribution of scores on 100 m in the sample is positively skewed and that on long jump is negatively skewed, then this comparison will give misleading results. The Z-scale can be constructed by using formula (12.4). On the Z-scale, the mean always lies at 0.

12.3.1 Merits and Demerits of Z-Scale

The distribution of percentiles is rectangular in nature, whereas most of the variables are normally distributed. This problem can be overcome by using the Z-scale. Since standard scores Z are measured on an interval scale, various statistics such as the mean and standard

FACTS TO KNOW

The Z- and T-scales assume that the distribution of the population is normal deviation can be computed on these scores. The Z-scale can be used to assess the performance of an individual. Since the Z-score is free from units, it can be used to compare the performance of an athlete on two different test items having different units.

Since Z-scores can assume positive as well as negative values, they are not easily understood. Most people prefer not to deal with negative numbers. In using negative values, mathematical error is more common. At the same time, students do not like their scores to be presented in negative numbers. For instance, if an athlete's performance on a shuttle run is expressed as −0.12, it is confusing to the general audience as well as to the athlete, whereas a researcher can understand that the performance is close to an average one.

12.4 *T*-SCALE

The problem in using the Z-scale is that the scores are represented in decimal fractions along with positive and negative signs. Therefore, if the performance is indicated in terms of Z-scores, they are difficult to interpret. To overcome this problem, the *T*-scale can be used. The *T*-score is obtained by using the following transformation for Z-scores.

$$T = 50 + 10 \times Z \tag{12.5}$$

The *T*-score is simply a transformation of the Z-score and has mean 50 and standard deviation 10. *T*-scores are always expressed in whole numbers and are nonnegative. If the computed value of the *T*-score is a fraction, it is rounded off to the nearest whole number. As with Z-scores, the distribution of *T*-scores also depends on the sample distribution and any bump in the sample is reflected in the transformation.

Since *T*-scores do not contain fractions or negative signs, they are used more frequently than Z-scores in developing norms. *T*-scores are based on the assumption that the scores in the sample are normally distributed, and therefore the normal curve area property holds true. Thus, almost all scores (99.73%) will fall within the three sigma limits if the *T*-scale is used to develop the norms for any test item. On this scale, everybody would get at least 20 marks, whereas it is difficult to get more than 80 marks, which is logically not correct. For instance, if the norms are developed on muscular strength, then nobody's performance can be less than 20 marks and nobody would get more than 80 marks on this test item, which is logically not correct. A comparison of Z- and *T*-scales can be seen in Figure 12.1.

12.5 STANINE SCALE

The stanine scale is based on the stanine score, which is another kind of standard score that is used in research studies. Just as with Z-scores and *T*-scores, a stanine score is also a way of assessing the subject's competency in a referenced group. The

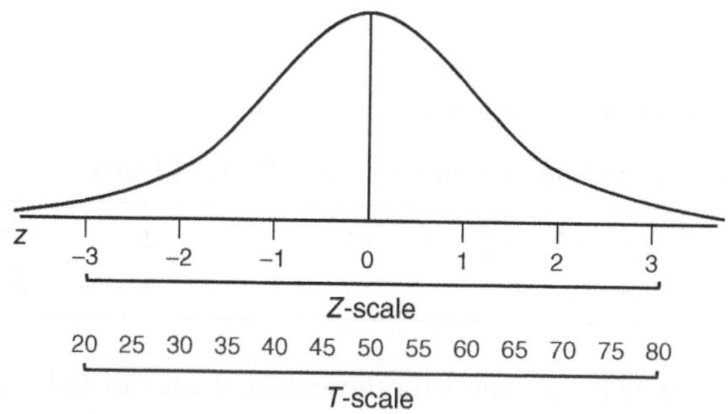

Figure 12.1 Comparison of *Z*- and *T*-scales.

stanine scores tell us whether a subject's performance is near the group mean or at a significant distance from the group mean. Stanine scores may be used to compare an athlete's performance in a certain test item with the standard of a national reference sample. Stanine scores divide the distribution of results into nine categories. A stanine score can be any number between 1 and 9 (inclusive). The stanine score is the percentage of subjects who will receive any given stanine. On a stanine scale, 4% of the total subjects are in stanine 1, 7% in stanine 2, 12% in stanine 3, 17% in stanine 4, 20% in stanine 5, 17% in stanine 6, 12% in stanine 7, 7% in stanine 8, and 4% in stanine 9. The distribution of percentage of subjects has been shown graphically in Figure 12.2

Usually, an athlete is said to have an average performance if his stanine score on any test item is a 4, 5, or 6. Stanine scores of 7 or 8 normally indicate above average performance, whereas a stanine score of 9 is normally considered as outstanding performance. On the other hand, a stanine score of 2 or 3 usually indicates below average, while a stanine score of 1 indicates a very low performance. The main difference between the *Z*-scores, *T*-scores, and stanine scores is the way these standard scores are represented. The stanine scores are always represented in single digits and can assume any number from 1 to 9. On the other hand, *Z*-scores are represented in terms of fractions with positive or negative signs, whereas the *T*-scores are represented in terms of two-digit whole numbers.

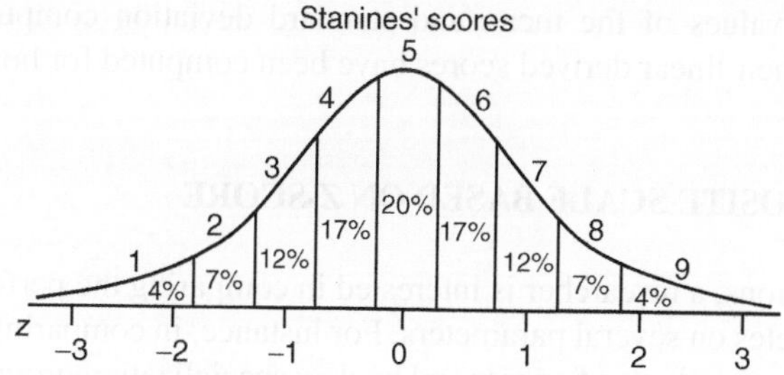

Figure 12.2 Stanine scores with percent of scores in each stanine.

Example 12.4 A sample of 10 students was tested for their performance on pull-ups and 50 yard dash. Compute the Z-scores and transform them to T-scores for both the sets of data shown in the following table.

Performance of Students on Pull-Ups and 50 Yard Dash

Pull-ups	14	13	12	7	12	7	4	7	5	4
50-yard dash	6.4	6.2	6.1	6.5	6.7	6.4	8	5.8	7.1	7.4

Solution: To compute the Z-scores for these data, the mean and standard deviation of both these variables shall be computed first. After computing these statistics, the z shall be computed by using the following formula:

$$z = \frac{x - \bar{x}}{s}$$

and the T-scores can be obtained by using the following transformation:

$$T = 50 + 10 \times Z$$

These computations have been shown in Table 12.2. Here, $n = 10$

$$\bar{x}_1 = \frac{\sum x_1}{n} = \frac{85}{10} = 8.5$$

$$\bar{x}_2 = \frac{\sum x_2}{n} = \frac{66.6}{10} = 6.66$$

$$s_1 = \sqrt{\frac{1}{n}\sum x_1^2 - \left(\frac{\sum x_1}{n}\right)^2} = \sqrt{\frac{857}{10} - \left(\frac{85}{10}\right)^2} = 3.67$$

$$s_2 = \sqrt{\frac{1}{n}\sum x_2^2 - \left(\frac{\sum x_2}{n}\right)^2} = \sqrt{\frac{447.52}{10} - \left(\frac{66.6}{10}\right)^2} = 0.63$$

By using the values of the mean and standard deviation computed above, the Z-scores and their linear derived scores have been computed for both the variables in Table 12.2.

12.6 COMPOSITE SCALE BASED ON Z-SCORE

In many situations, a researcher is interested in comparing the performance of two groups of athletes on several parameters. For instance, in comparing health-related fitness of college students of soccer and hockey specialization groups, one needs to combine the performance in each test item of the health-related fitness for each

TABLE 12.2 Computing Z-Scores and Transformed Linear Scores

Pull-Ups (in Seconds) x_1	$Z_1 = \frac{x_1 - \bar{x}_1}{s_1}$	$T_1 = 50 + 10 \times Z_1$	50 yard dash (in Numbers) x_2	$Z_2 = \frac{x_2 - \bar{x}_2}{s_2}$	$T_2 = 50 + 10 \times Z_2$
14	1.50	65	6.4	−0.41	45.9
13	1.23	62.3	6.2	−0.73	42.7
12	0.95	59.5	6.1	−0.89	41.1
7	−0.41	45.9	6.5	−0.25	47.5
12	0.95	59.5	6.7	0.06	50.6
7	−0.41	45.9	6.4	−0.41	45.9
4	−1.23	37.7	8.0	2.13	71.3
7	−0.41	45.9	5.8	−1.37	36.3
5	−0.95	40.5	7.1	0.70	57.0
4	−1.23	37.7	7.4	1.17	61.7
$\sum x_1 = 85$			$\sum x_2 = 66.6$		
$\sum x_1^2 = 857$			$\sum x_2^2 = 447.52$		

individual in both the groups. This is done by first converting the original performance into the standard score in each of the test items and then adding these standard scores to give rise to what we call the *composite scores*. Thus, composite scores of the two groups of students can be compared either by using the *Z*- or *T*-test as the case may be.

12.6.1 Conditions for Using Z-Score

In order to compare the composite scores in these two groups, the following two assumptions must be satisfied.

a. The variance of each trait in both the groups must be same.
b. The distribution in terms of skewness and kurtosis must be nearly equal for each trait in both the groups.

Check Your Progress

Note: Tick the correct answer by using the sign (√).

	True	False
1. The distribution of percentiles is normal.	-	-
2. Stanine scores can only be represented as a single-digit numbers.	-	-

3. If the performance of an athlete on vertical jump, measured on the *Z*-scale is −0.05, it is considered to be very poor.	-	-
4. The *T*-scale is based on the assumption that the distribution of the sample observations is normal.	-	-
5. The men and standard deviation of *Z*-scores are 1 and 0, respectively.	-	-
6. Percentiles tell us about the relative positioning as well as the level of competency.	-	-
7. Stanine scores cannot be represented as fractions.	-	-
8. If the percentile scores of an athlete on 100 m and shot put are 65, then the athlete is equally competent in both the events.	-	-
9. The *Z*-score follows the standard normal distribution.	-	-
10. If the performance of a college girl on flexibility is 2.2 on the *Z*-scale, it is considered to be very good.	-	-
11. If the performance is measured on *T*-scale, one can get a score of 95.	-	-
12. The percentile rank can never be 0 or 100.	-	-
13. It is assumed that each percentile point has 1% of the population scores.	-	-
14. Statistical calculations such as the mean and standard deviation can be done on *Z*-scores.	-	-
15. *T*-scores are obtained by applying any transformation to the *Z*-scores.	-	-
16. If the percentile rank of an athlete on the long jump event is 75, it simply indicates that the performance of 75% of the athlete is above this performance.	-	-
17. It is difficult to obtain higher scale values on the *T*-scale.	-	-
18. A stanine score 5 contains 20% of the population.	-	-
19. Quartiles are nothing but percentiles.	-	-
20. Since percentiles are scores, the mean and standard deviation can be calculated.	-	-
21. A stanine score of 5 is considered to be average, 6 good, and 4 poor.	-	-
22. Percentiles are based on the assumption that the distribution of scores in the sample is rectangular.	-	-
23. Composite scores of *Z* can be obtained by adding the *Z*-scores of all the variables.	-	-

PRACTICE EXERCISE

1. Following are the scores in the 40 m dash timings (in seconds). Compute P_{55} and P_{65}.

40 m dash:	5.70	5.90	5.80	6.00	6.10	5.85	6.15	6.05	6.2

2. Compute the percentile rank for the push-ups scores 22 and 26 by using the following data on push-ups obtained on school girls.

Push-Ups:	23	26	30	19	26	25	28	24	20

3. Compute the *Z*-scores and *T*-scores for the following data of standing long jump (in inches) obtained on college boys by assuming that the mean=84 and SD=2.

Standing long jump:	78	82	80	79	90	85

4. Compute composite scores for the data shown in the following table by using both *Z*- and *T*- scales.

Data on Different Push-Ups and Sit-Ups

	Push-Ups (in No.)	Sit-Ups (in No.)
	8	36
	12	40
	15	45
	10	42
	14	35
Population mean	11	41
Population SD	1.5	2

Example 12.5 The data on different structural measures obtained on the women basketball players are shown in Table 12.3. Compute the composite scores in terms of *Z* for each subject. Also compute the composite scores in terms of *T* by converting the scores of all the variables into their linear derived form.

Solution: To find composite scores, the *Z*-scores for all the variables shall be computed. The composite *Z*-scores shall be computed by adding these *Z*-scores of all the variables for each subject. In order to compute composite *T*-scores, the *Z*-scores

TABLE 12.3 Computation of Composite Scores in Terms of Z and T

	Ponderal Index			Crural Index			Body Fat			Composite Score	
Sr. No.	x_1	$z_1 = \frac{x_1 - \bar{x}_1}{s_1}$	$T_l = 50 + 10 \times Z_1$	x_2	$z_2 = \frac{x_2 - \bar{x}_2}{s_2}$	$T_2 = 50 + 10 \times Z_2$	x_3	$z_3 = \frac{x_3 - \bar{x}_3}{s_3}$	$T_3 = 50 + 10 \times Z_3$	Z	T
1	43.28	−0.93	40.7	0.93	−1	40	35	1.95	69.5	0.02	150.2
2	46.13	1.73	67.3	0.98	0.67	56.7	25.4	−0.38	46.2	2.02	170.2
3	44.16	−0.11	48.9	0.94	−0.67	43.3	25.7	−0.31	46.9	−1.09	139.1
4	44.65	0.35	53.5	0.97	0.33	53.3	23.2	−0.92	40.8	−0.24	147.6
5	43.2	−1.01	39.9	1	1.33	63.3	25.6	−0.34	46.6	−0.02	149.8
	$\sum x_1 = 221.42$			$\sum x_2 = 4.82$			$\sum x_3 = 134.9$				
	$\sum x_1^2 = 9811.10$			$\sum x_2^2 = 4.65$			$\sum x_3^2 = 3724.25$				

for all the variables will be converted into their linear form by using the following transformation:

$$T = 50 + 10 \times Z$$

where Z is the standard score and T is its linear derived score.

Since the mean and standard deviation have not been given, these statistics shall be computed first for all the variables. After computing Z-scores for all the variables, the composite scores shall be computed by adding these Z-scores. The composite T-scores shall be computed by adding all the T-scores for each variable. The computation has been shown in Table 12.3. Here, $n = 5$.

$$\bar{x}_1 = \frac{\sum x_1}{n} = \frac{221.42}{5} = 44.28$$

$$\bar{x}_2 = \frac{\sum x_2}{n} = \frac{4.82}{5} = 0.96$$

$$\bar{x}_3 = \frac{\sum x_3}{n} = \frac{134.9}{5} = 26.98$$

$$s_1 = \sqrt{\frac{1}{n}\sum x_1^2 - \left(\frac{\sum x_1}{n}\right)^2} = \sqrt{\frac{9811.1}{5} - \left(\frac{221.42}{5}\right)^2} = 1.07$$

$$s_2 = \sqrt{\frac{1}{n}\sum x_2^2 - \left(\frac{\sum x_2}{n}\right)^2} = \sqrt{\frac{4.65}{5} - \left(\frac{4.82}{5}\right)^2} = 0.03$$

$$s_3 = \sqrt{\frac{1}{n}\sum x_3^2 - \left(\frac{\sum x_3}{n}\right)^2} = \sqrt{\frac{3724.25}{5} - \left(\frac{134.9}{5}\right)^2} = 4.11$$

12.7 SCALING OF RATINGS IN TERMS OF THE NORMAL CURVE

In many sports, such as basketball, hockey, and soccer, playing ability cannot be measured objectively. In such situations, judges rate or rank the sportsperson on the basis of their performance. Suppose that two judges rate a group of sportspersons and that the frequency distributions of ratings for the two judges are known. The problem is how to assign weights to these ratings so that the ratings of the two judges may be compared or combined. The procedure discussed in Example 12.6 can be used to assign weights to the ratings given by the judges. This procedure can be used by the researcher in developing the key of a questionnaire by giving proper weights to the responses for each question on the basis of the respondent's response in a pilot study. In using this method, it is assumed that the ratings follow a normal distribution. This procedure is known as the *weighted scale method*.

TABLE 12.4 Computation of Weighted Scale for the Data on Game Performance of College Basketball Players

	Rating	*A*	*B*	*C*	*D*	*E*
1.	Area covered by the rating $\varphi(x_2) - \varphi(x_1)$	0.09	0.20	0.41	0.23	0.07
2.	Area below the rating $\varphi(x_1)$	0.91	0.71	0.30	0.07	0
3.	Lower limit of the grade x_1	1.341	0.553	−0.525	−1.475	$-\infty$
4.	Upper limit of the grade x_2	$+\infty$	1.341	0.553	−0.525	−1.475
5.	Ordinate at the lower limit $\psi(x_1)$	0.1624	0.3424	0.3476	0.1342	0
6.	Ordinate at the upper limit $\psi(x_2)$	0	0.1624	0.3424	0.3476	0.1342
7.	Scale value $\dfrac{\psi(x_1) - \psi(x_2)}{\varphi(x_2) - \varphi(x_1)}$	1.80	0.889	0.013	−0.93	−1.92
8.	Transforming the weights by subtracting −1.92	$3.72 \approx 4$	$2.82 \approx 3$	$1.93 \approx 2$	$0.99 \approx 1$	$0 \approx 0$
9.	Multiplying the values in row (8) by 10	$37.2 \approx 37$	$28.2 \approx 28$	$19.3 \approx 19$	$9.9 \approx 10$	$0 \approx 0$

Example 12.6 A group of 100 college basketball players was rated by an expert coach on a five-point scale, namely, A, B, C, D, and E with respect to their game performance. The rank A denoted the highest performance, whereas E was the lowest. The results are shown in the table below. Calculate the weights attached to each grade.

Rating of Basketball Players on the Basis of Their Playing Ability

Rating	A	B	C	D	E
Frequency	9	20	41	23	7

Solution: It is assumed that the playing ability is normally distributed. Under this assumption, the scale values for different grades can be obtained by following the procedure discussed in the following steps. The computation has been shown in Table 12.4.

Step 1: In the first row, areas covered by the ratings have been obtained by converting the frequency into its percentage. Here, x_1 and x_2 are the ranges of performance for a particular rating, whereas $\varphi(x_1)$ and $\varphi(x_2)$ are the areas below x_1 and x_2, respectively, in the standard normal curve area table.

$$\text{For trait } A,\quad \text{area covered} = \frac{9}{100} = 0.09$$

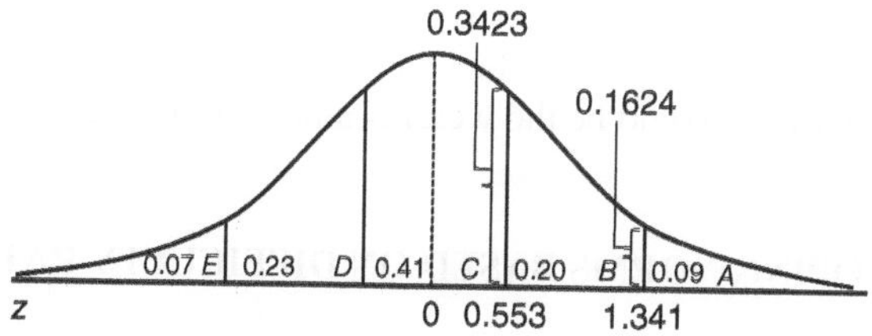

Figure 12.3 Normal curve showing the area attached to each grade and its limits.

and

$$\text{for trait } B, \ \text{area covered} = \frac{20}{100} = 0.2$$

Step 2: In second row, the area below each rating is computed by subtracting the cumulative entry of the first row from 1. For example,

$$\text{Area below } A = 1 - 0.09 = 0.91$$
$$\text{Area below } B = 1 - (0.09 + 0.20) = 0.71$$
$$\text{Area below } C = 1 - (0.9 + 0.20 + 0.41) = 0.30$$

Step 3: In the third row, the lower limit of all the grades has been obtained by using the normal curve area table (see Figure 12.3).

Step 4: Similarly, in the fourth row, the upper limit of all the grades has been obtained by using the normal curve area table (see Figure 12.3).

Step 5: By using the normal curve ordinate table (Table A.5 in the Appendix), the ordinate of each grade at the lower limit has been obtained for each grade.

Step 6: In row 6, by using the same ordinate table, the ordinate of each trait at the higher limit has been obtained.

Step 7: In row 7, scale values have been obtained by dividing the difference of the entries in the fifth and sixth rows by the corresponding entry in row 1 for each grade. For example:

$$\text{Scale value for } A = \frac{0.1624 - 0}{0.09} = 1.80$$

$$\text{Scale value for } B = \frac{0.3423 - 0.1624}{0.20} = 0.899$$

$$\text{Scale value for } C = \frac{0.3476 - 0.3424}{0.41} = 0.013$$

Step 8: Finally, in row 8, the scale values have been obtained by subtracting the least scale value of row 7 from each of the entries of row 7. In this case, the least value is −1.92; thus, −1.92 has been subtracted from each of the entries of row 7. This has been in order to do away with the negative sign as well as to assign 0 to the least efficient grade.

Step 9: Further, in row 9, a new scale value has been obtained by multiplying the corresponding scale values in row 8 by a constant 10. The values so obtained in row 9 would be the weights attached to the corresponding rating.

12.8 DEVELOPING NORMS BASED ON DIFFICULTY RATINGS

None of the scales (Z, T, or stanine) discussed so far is suitable in assessing the actual worth of an athlete's performance in sports. This is so because the marking pattern on these scales is not based on difficulty ratings. More effort is required to improve the performance at a higher level in comparison to the same degree of improvement at a lower level. Thus, an athlete should be rewarded more for improvement at a higher level in comparison to that at a lower level for the same degree of improvement. The procedure discussed above can be extended to decide weights for each performance, which shall facilitate the development of norms based on difficulty ratings. The detailed procedure for developing norms based on difficulty ratings can be seen in Example 12.7.

Example 12.7 Two hundred male athletes of the 15–16 year age group from different sports schools were tested for their performance on push-ups. The performance in the form of frequencies so obtained is listed in the following table. Construct a scale based on difficulty ratings for push-up performance based on the following information.

Push-Up Performance of Athletes Along with Their Frequencies

Push-ups	8	10	12	14	16	18	20	22	24	26	28	30	32	34	36
Frequency	4	12	8	18	16	20	20	22	16	16	20	12	8	4	4

Solution: Computation of scale values corresponding to push-up performance has been shown in Table 12.5. The following steps shall be used to develop the scale based on difficulty ratings.

Steps

1. Entries in the first row are the performance of push-ups in the given problem.
2. In the second row, the frequency for each grade has been converted into its percentage. These entries denote the area, $\varphi(x_2) - \varphi(x_1)$ in the normal curve covered by the performance.
3. In the third row, the area below each performance has been computed by subtracting the cumulative entries of the second row from 1. For example,

$$\text{Area below } A = 1 - 0.02 = 0.98$$

TABLE 12.5 Computation of Scale Values for the Performance of Push-Ups

		A	B	C	D	E	F	G	H	I	J	K	L	M	N	O
1.	Performance	36	34	32	30	28	26	24	22	20	18	16	14	12	10	8
2.	Area covered by the performance $\varphi(x_2) - \varphi(x_1)$	0.02	0.02	0.04	0.06	0.10	0.08	0.08	0.11	0.10	0.10	0.08	0.09	0.04	0.06	0.02
3.	Area below the performance $\varphi(x_1)$	0.98	0.96	0.92	0.86	0.76	0.68	0.60	0.49	0.39	0.29	0.21	0.12	0.08	0.02	00
4.	Lower limit of the push-ups (x_1)	2.05	1.75	1.41	1.08	0.71	0.47	0.25	−0.03	−0.28	−0.55	−0.81	−1.18	−1.41	−2.05	−∞
5.	Upper limit of the push-ups (x_2)	∞	2.05	1.75	1.41	1.08	0.71	0.47	0.25	−0.03	−0.28	−0.55	−0.81	−1.18	−1.41	−2.05
6.	Ordinate at the lower limit $\psi(x_1)$	0.049	0.086	0.148	0.223	0.310	0.357	0.387	0.399	0.384	0.343	0.287	0.199	0.148	0.049	0
7.	Ordinate at the upper limit $\psi(x_2)$	0	0.049	0.086	0.148	0.223	0.310	0.357	0.387	0.399	0.384	0.343	0.287	0.199	0.148	0.049
8.	Scale value $\dfrac{\psi(x_1) - \psi(x_2)}{\varphi(x_2) - \varphi(x_1)}$	2.45	1.85	1.55	1.25	0.87	0.59	0.38	0.11	−0.15	−0.41	−0.70	−0.98	−1.28	−1.65	−2.45
9.	Linear transformed scores	74.5	68.5	65.5	62.5	58.7	55.9	53.8	51.1	48.5	45.9	43.0	40.2	37.2	33.5	25.5
10.	Cumulative score	764.29	689.79	621.29	555.79	493.29	434.59	378.71	324.96	273.87	225.37	179.47	136.47	96.25	59.00	25.50
11.	Scale values (SV)	100	90.25	81.29	72.72	64.54	56.86	49.5	42.52	35.83	29.49	23.48	17.86	12.59	7.72	3.34
12.	Scale values (rounded off)	100	90	81	73	65	57	50	43	36	29	23	18	13	8	3

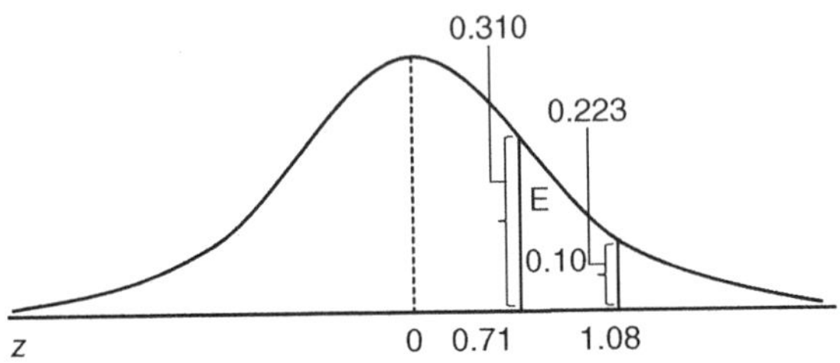

Figure 12.4 Normal curve showing the limits of grade *E* and the area attached to it.

$$\text{Area below } B = 1 - (0.02 + 0.02) = 0.96$$

$$\text{Area below } C = 1 - (0.02 + 0.02 + 0.04) = 0.92$$

4. In the fourth row, the lower limit of all the performances has been obtained by using the normal curve area table (see Figure 12.4 in which the lower limit of the area E is shown). Here, corresponding to each entry in the third row, the z-value has been computed.
5. Similarly, in the fifth row the upper limit of all the performances has been obtained by using the normal curve area table (see Figure 12.4 in which upper limit of the area E is shown). In this row, the first entry would be infinity and the other entries would be same as those in row 4, starting from the first entry onward. For example,
   Upper limit of $D = 1.41$, which is the same as the entry in the fourth row for grade C.

   Remark In case of the event where a lesser value indicates better performance, performance score are written in reverse order in the first row. For instance, in the case of the 100 m event, the shortest timing would come first and the longest timing would come last. The other steps are exactly the same.

6. In the sixth row, the value of the ordinate for each performance corresponding to the z-entry in the fourth row has been obtained by using the ordinate table of the normal distribution (Table A.5 in the Appendix).
7. In the seventh row, the ordinate values corresponding to the z-entries in row 5 have been obtained by using Table A.5. (Entries in this row are nothing but the diagonal entries in the sixth row.)
8. In the eighth row, the scale values have been obtained by dividing the difference of entries in the sixth and seventh rows by the corresponding entries in row 2.
9. In the ninth row, the scale values obtained in the eighth row have been converted into the corresponding linear derived form by using the formula:

$$Z_L = 10 \times Z + 50$$

10. In row 10, the linear scale values are added in a cumulative manner.
11. In the 11th row, each entry has been obtained by dividing the corresponding entry of the 10th row by the highest cumulative total, multiplied by 100. For example,

$$\text{For column } A = \frac{764.29}{764.29} \times 100 = 100$$

$$\text{For column } D = \frac{555.79}{764.29} \times 100 = 72.2$$

12. Finally, in the 12th row, the scale values (SVs) have been obtained by rounding off the entries in the 11th row.

12.9 COMPUTING WITH EXCEL

12.9.1 Computing *Z*- and *T*-scores with Excel

The Excel computing facility can be used to construct different types of scales. Here, the method of computing *Z*- and *T*-scale values shall be discussed by using Excel features by means of the following example.

Example 12.8 A sample of 15 male college students was tested for their lean body weight (in lbs). The data so obtained are shown below. Compute the *Z*- and *T*-scores for the lean body weight.

Scores of the Male Students on Lean Body Weight (in lbs)

151.58	126.28	138.16	148.28	151.58	146.52	141.46
128.75	160.38	139.92	143.22	156.86	144.76	

Solution: The following steps are involved in computing *Z*- and *T*-scores using Excel:

a. Type the data in any column of the Excel sheet as shown in Figure 12.5. The *Z*-scores can be computed by the following formula:

$$z = \frac{x - \bar{x}}{s}$$

and the *T*-scores can be computed by using the following formula:

$$T = 50 + 10 \times z$$

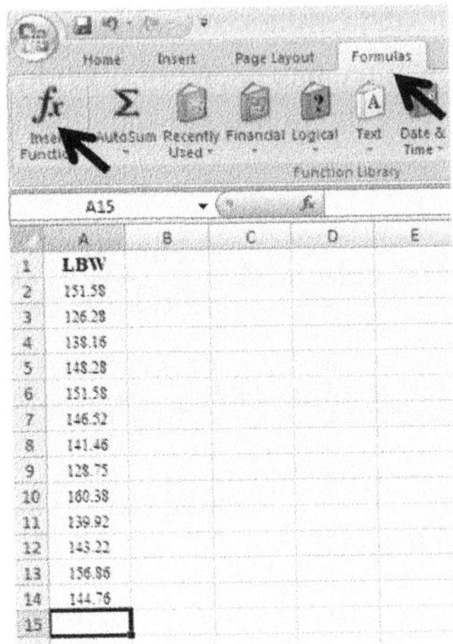

Figure 12.5 Data entry format for computing *Z*- and *T*-scores.

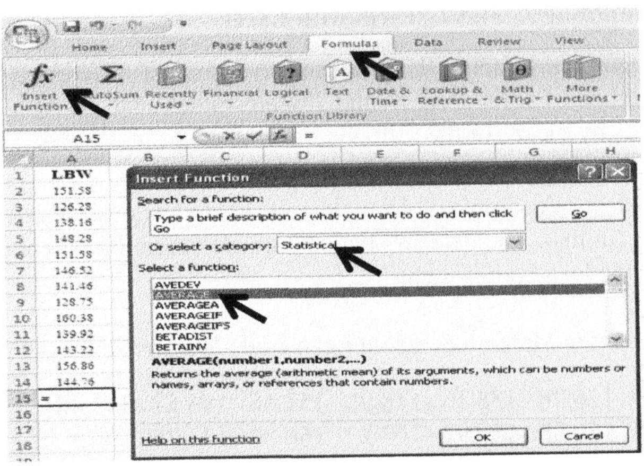

Figure 12.6 Choosing commands for the mean.

b. Compute the mean and standard deviation of the scores following the steps below:

   1. Place the cursor on the cell below the score (in this case, it is *A*15) and click **Formulas** and then **Insert Function** as shown in the Figure 12.5.
   2. Upon clicking the **Insert Function**, you will get the screen as shown in Figure 12.6. Do the following on the screen.
   3. Choose the category **Statistical** and choose the command **Average** by scrolling to find the value of the mean and click **OK** to get the next screen as shown in Figure 12.7.
   4. In Figure 12.7, define the range of data as *A*2:*A*14 and click **OK** to get the value of the mean at the location *A*15 as shown in Figure 12.8.

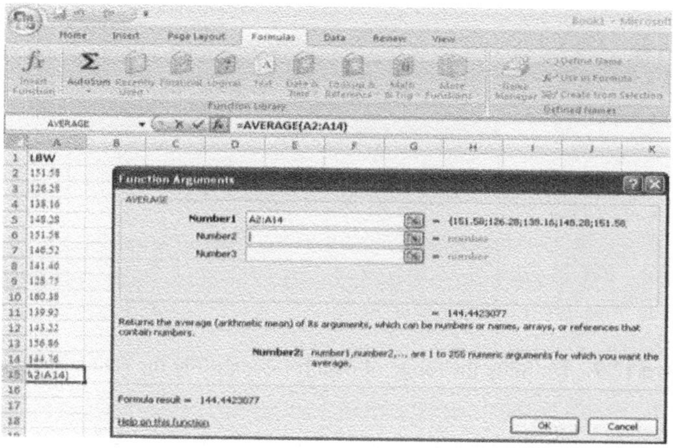

Figure 12.7 Defining the range of data for the mean.

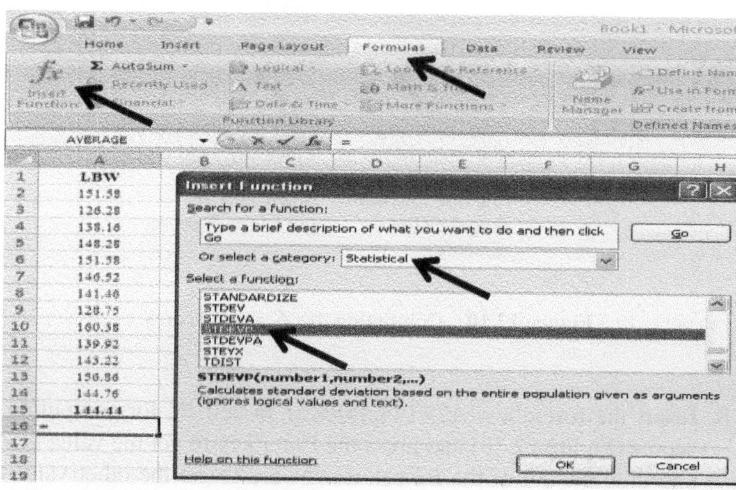

Figure 12.8 Choosing commands for the standard deviation.

5. On the screen shown in Figure 12.8, click the cursor at the location *A*16 (where you want to get the value of the standard deviation).
6. Click **Insert Function** and choose the category **Statistical**. Scroll down and choose the command **STDEVP** for computing the standard deviation. Click **OK** to get the screen as shown in Figure 12.9 to define the range of the data.
7. Define the range of data as *A*2:*A*14 (Figure 12.9) and click **OK** to get the value of the standard deviation at the location *A*16 as shown in Figure 12.10.

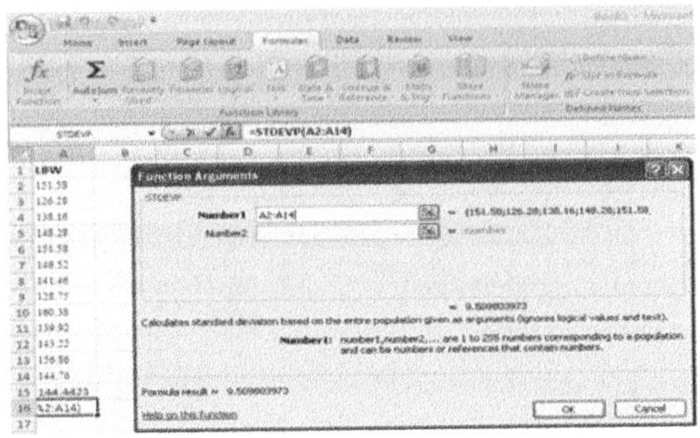

Figure 12.9 Defining the range of data for computing the standard deviation.

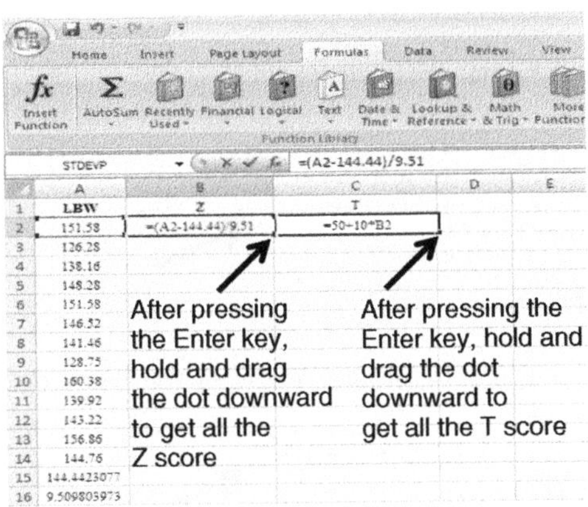

Figure 12.10 Computing the Z- and T-scores.

8. Insert the formula =($A2-144.44$)/9.51 in cell $B2$ for computing the Z-scores (Figure 12.10) and press the Enter key to get the value of Z. Hold and drag the dot of the $B2$ cell downward to get the other values of the Z-scores as shown in Figure 12.11. Here, the values of the mean and standard deviation, 144.44 and 9.51, respectively, have been obtained by rounding off.
9. Once all the Z-values are generated by the above process, insert the formula =50+10*$B2$ in the cell $C2$ for computing the T-scores. After typing the formula, press the Enter key. Hold and drag the dot of the cell $C2$ downward to generate other values of the T-scores as shown in Figure 12.11.
10. After applying the formulas for the Z- and T-scores, the values obtained are shown in Figure 12.11.

The output shown in Figure 12.11 can be formatted by formatting the cell entries of different columns (Readers are advised to see the procedure

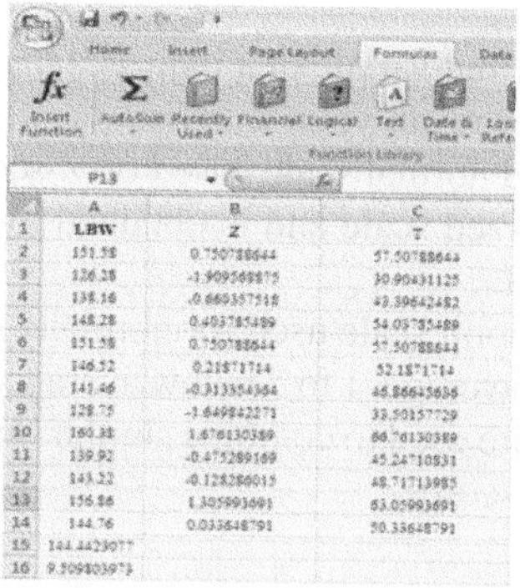

Figure 12.11 Output showing the values of the *Z*- and *T*-scores.

TABLE 12.6 *Z*- and *T*-Scores

LBW	*Z*-scores	*T*-scores
151.58	0.75	57.51
126.28	−1.91	30.90
138.16	−0.66	43.40
148.28	0.40	54.04
151.58	0.75	57.51
146.52	0.22	52.19
141.46	−0.31	46.87
128.75	−1.65	33.50
160.38	1.68	66.76
139.92	−0.48	45.25
143.22	−0.13	48.72
156.86	1.31	63.06
144.76	0.03	50.34

Mean = 144.44 SD = 9.51 LBW = Lean body weight

discussed in Chapter 1 in this regard). After formatting and giving a heading to the mean and standard deviation, the final result will appear as shown in Table 12.6.

IMPORTANT DEFINITIONS

A ***percentile*** indicates the percentage of scores below that point.
A ***percentile rank*** can be defined as the proportion of scores in a population that a specific score is greater than or equal to.

Z-score is a standard normal variate that indicates the number of standard deviations above or below the mean your score is.
The ***Z-scale*** is a standard normal scale based on Z-scores.
The ***T-scale*** is a normalized scale and is obtained by multiplying the Z-scores by 10 and adding 50 to it.
Stanine scale is a nine-point scale used for normally distributed data where the score 4 to 6 refers to the average, 1 to 3 below average, and 7 to 9 above average.
Composite score is a score used to combine similar kinds of data by adding their corresponding standard scores.

IMPORTANT FORMULAS

Percentile

Ungrouped data

$$P_x = \frac{x}{100} \times N$$

Grouped data

$$P_x = \mathrm{LL} + \frac{\frac{x \times N}{100} - F}{f} \times i$$

Percentile rank

$$P_r = \frac{\mathrm{CF} + 0.5 \times f}{n} \times 100$$

Z-score

$$z = \frac{x - \bar{x}}{s}$$

Mean

$$\bar{x} = \frac{\sum x}{n}$$

Standard deviation

$$s = \sqrt{\frac{1}{n}\sum x^2 - \left(\frac{\sum x}{n}\right)^2}$$

T-score

$$T = 50 + 10 \times z$$

KEY TERMS

T-scale	stanine scale	percentile rank
Z-scale	weighted scale	percentiles
composite score	norms	

CHAPTER EXERCISE

1. What is the percentile scale used for?
2. Explain percentile rank. How is it computed?
3. What is the difference between *Z*- and *T*-scales?
4. Write a short note on the stanine scale. How are the scores distributed in the stanine scale?
5. In what situation a composite scale is constructed? Explain by means of an example.
6. Compute P_{45} and P_{85} by using the following data on static abdominal endurance (in seconds) measured on schoolboys.

   Static Abdominal Endurance: 130 125 95 105 135 120 125 110 105 115

7. Compute the percentile rank for the weight 120 lb on the basis of the data shown below.

   Weight: 110 123 128 132 115 98 95 105 99 120 132 120 112 114 120

8. Following are the height (in cms) of the boys in a school. Compute percentile rank for a score of 155 cm. Also compute P_{35} and P_{65}.

   Height: 156 158 155 165 166 170 165 150 155 165 155

9. Following are the data on push-ups obtained on schoolboys in a study. Compute P_{42}, P_{56}, and P_{74} and interpret your findings.

Data on Push-Ups Organized in Class Interval Form

Class Interval:	20–22	23–25	26–28	29–31	32–34	35–37	38–40	41–43
Frequency:	6	4	8	6	12	9	7	3

10. In a study, wrist flexibility was measured on 130 college women. Compute percentiles at the decile points.

Scores on Women Flexibility (in Degrees) Arranged in Class Interval Form

Class interval:	41–42	43–44	45–46	47–48	49–50	51–52	53–54	55–56	57–58	59–60
Frequency:	6	12	8	20	18	28	12	11	8	7

11. A sample of schoolboys was tested on a 12-min run test. The distance covered (in meters) by the subjects are shown below. Compute the 40th and 65th percentiles and interpret your findings.

Performance of School Boys on 12-min Run Test (in Meters)

Class interval:	1890–1930	1930–1970	1970–2010	2010–2050	2050–2090	2090–2130
Frequency:	25	32	10	50	20	5

12. The mean and standard deviation for the data on pull-ups for schoolgirls are 25 and 2, respectively, compute the *Z*- and *T*-scores for the following data.

Pull-Ups (X):	22	19	24	28	30	31	26	27

13. Compute composite scores with *Z*- and *T*-scales by using the information in the following table.

Data on Different Physical Parameters

	Push-Ups (in No.)	Pull-Ups (in No.)	Vertical Jump (in Meter)
	20	8	1.30
	25	9	1.15
	28	7	1.20
	29	6	1.45
	27	5	1.00
	26	8	1.35
	25	7	1.25
Population mean	26	7	1.25
Population SD	2	1.5	0.10

14. By using the following data on flexibility (in cms) obtained on college women, categorize the scores into their stanine scores.

30 31 30.5 40 42 41.5 35.5 36.5 32.5 33.5 31 31.5 37 36 34 33
37.5 34.5 36.5 34 39 40.5 41 40 37 36 35.5 38.5

15. A researcher wanted to construct a scale for the 100 m dash based on difficulty ratings. He selected 125 boys randomly from the schools and their 100 m

performance was measured. The performance obtained is shown in the following table. Construct the scale based on their difficulty ratings.

Performance of the School Boys on 100 m Dash

100 m dash	12.2	12.4	12.6	12.8	13.0	13.2	13.4	13.6	13.8	14.0
Frequency	2	5	11	16	19	17	20	11	8	6

ANSWERS

Check Your Progress

1. F	5. F	9. T	13. T	17. T	21. F
2. T	6. F	10. T	14. T	18. T	22. T
3. F	7. T	11. F	15. F	19. T	23. T
4. T	8. F	12. T	16. F	20. F	

Practice Exercise

1. $P_{55} = 5.995$, $P_{65} = 6.043$
2. $P_{22} = 22.22$, $P_{26} = 66.67$
3.

X	*Z*-score	*T*-score
78	−3	20
82	−1	40
80	−2	30
79	−2.5	25
90	3	80
85	0.5	55

4.

Push-Ups	*Z*	*T*	Sit-Ups	*Z*	*T*	Composite *Z*	Composite *T*
8.00	−2.00	30.00	36.00	−2.50	25.00	−4.50	55.00
12.00	0.67	56.67	40.00	−0.50	45.00	0.17	101.67
15.00	2.67	76.67	45.00	2.00	70.00	4.67	146.67
10.00	−0.67	43.33	42.00	0.50	55.00	−0.17	98.33
14.00	2.00	70.00	35.00	−3.00	20.00	−1.00	90.00

Chapter Exercise

6. $P_{45} = 112.5$, $P_{85} = 77.5$
7. Percentile rank of the weight 120 lbs score is 63.3.

8. Percentile rank = 22.73, $P_{35} = 155$, and $P_{65} = 165$.
9. $P_{42} = 31.05$, $P_{56} = 33.2$, $P_{74} = 36.07$.
10.

P_{10}	43.67
P_{20}	46.5
P_{30}	47.8
P_{40}	49.17
P_{50}	50.57
P_{60}	51.5
P_{70}	52.43
P_{80}	54.5
P_{90}	56.86

11. P_{40}=1969.75, P_{65}=2030.24
12.

Pull-Ups (*X*):	22	19	24	28	30	31	26	27
Z:	−1.5	−3	−0.5	1.5	2.5	3	0.5	1
T:	35	20	45	65	75	80	55	60

13. Composite Score: −1.83 −0.17 0.5 2.83 −3.33 1.67 −0.5

14.

Flexibility score:	30	30.5–31	31–32.5	33–34.5	35.5–36.5	37–39	40–40.5	41–41.5	42
Stanine scores:	1	2	3	4	5	6	7	8	9

FURTHER READING

1. Engineering Statistics Handbook: Percentile. NIST. June 2012.
2. Carroll SR, Carroll DJ. Statistics made simple for school leaders: Data-Driven decision making. Scarecrow Education, Inc.: Oxford, UK 2002.
3. Cronbach LJ. Essentials of Psychological Testing. 3rd ed. New York: Harper & Row; 1970.
4. Duda JL, Whitehead J. Measurement of goal perspectives in the physical domain. In: Duda JL, editor. Advances in Sport and Exercise Psychology Measurement. Morgantown, WV: Fitness Information Technology; 1998. p 21–48. (ISBN: 978-1-885693-11-2)
5. Eidleman GJ. Z-scores – a guide to failure prediction. The CPA Journal Online 1995.
6. Glaser R. Instructional technology and the measurement of learning outcomes. American Psychologist 1963;18:510–522.
7. Lane, D. Percentiles. Accessed 2007 Sep 15; XXXX.

8. Midgley C, Kaplan A, Middleton M, Maehr ML, Urdan T, Anderman LH, Anderman E, Roeser R. The development and validation of scales assessing students' achievement goal orientations. Contemporary and Educational Psychology 1998;23:113–131.
9. Mertler CA. Using standardized test data to guide instruction and intervention. College Park, MD: ERIC Clearinghouse on Assessment and Evaluation 2002.
10. Schoonjans F, De Bacquer D, Schmid P. Estimation of population percentiles. Epidemiology 2011;22(5):750–751. DOI: 10.1097/EDE.0b013e318225c1de.
11. Sprinthall RC. Basic Statistical Analysis. 7th copyright 2003 ed. Pearson Education Group; XXXX.
12. Thorndike RL. Applied Psychometrics. Boston, MA: Houghton Mifflin; 1982.
13. Verma JP, Ghufran M. Statistics for Psychology: A Comprehensive Text. New Delhi: Tata McGraw Hill Education; 2012.

APPENDIX

TABLE A.1 Trigonometric Function

Angle (in degree)	Sin	Cos	Tan	Angle (in degree)
0	0	1	0	0
1	0.0174	0.9998	0.0175	1
2	0.0349	0.9994	0.0349	2
3	0.0523	0.9986	0.0524	3
4	0.0698	0.9976	0.0699	4
5	0.0872	0.9962	0.0875	5
6	0.1045	0.9945	0.1051	6
7	0.1219	0.9926	0.1228	7
8	0.1392	0.9903	0.1405	8
9	0.1564	0.9877	0.1584	9
10	0.1736	0.9848	0.1763	10
11	0.1908	0.9816	0.1944	11
12	0.2079	0.9781	0.2126	12
13	0.2249	0.9744	0.2309	13
14	0.2419	0.9703	0.2493	14
15	0.2588	0.9659	0.2679	15
16	0.2756	0.9613	0.2867	16
17	0.2924	0.9563	0.3057	17
18	0.3090	0.9511	0.3249	18

(continued)

Statistics for Exercise Science and Health with Microsoft® Office Excel®, First Edition. J. P. Verma.

TABLE A.1 *(Continued)*

Angle (in degree)	Sin	Cos	Tan	Angle (in degree)
19	0.3256	0.9455	0.3443	19
20	0.3420	0.9397	0.3640	20
21	0.3584	0.9336	0.3839	21
22	0.3746	0.9272	0.4040	22
23	0.3907	0.9205	0.4245	23
24	0.4067	0.9135	0.4452	24
25	0.4226	0.9063	0.4663	25
26	0.4384	0.8988	0.4877	26
27	0.4540	0.8910	0.5095	27
28	0.4695	0.8829	0.5317	28
29	0.4848	0.8746	0.5543	29
30	0.5000	0.8660	0.5773	30
31	0.5150	0.8571	0.6009	31
32	0.5299	0.8480	0.6249	32
33	0.5446	0.8387	0.6494	33
34	0.5592	0.8290	0.6745	34
35	0.5736	0.8191	0.7002	35
36	0.5878	0.8090	0.7265	36
37	0.6018	0.7986	0.7535	37
38	0.6157	0.7880	0.7813	38
39	0.6293	0.7772	0.8098	39
40	0.6428	0.7660	0.8391	40
41	0.6561	0.7547	0.8693	41
42	0.6691	0.7431	0.9004	42
43	0.6820	0.7314	0.9325	43
44	0.6947	0.7193	0.9657	44
45	0.7071	0.7071	1	45
46	0.7193	0.6947	1.0355	46
47	0.7314	0.6820	1.0724	47
48	0.7431	0.6691	1.1106	48
49	0.7547	0.6561	1.1504	49
50	0.7660	0.6428	1.1918	50
51	0.7772	0.6293	1.2349	51
52	0.7880	0.6157	1.2799	52
53	0.7986	0.6018	1.3270	53
54	0.809	0.5878	1.3764	54
55	0.8191	0.5736	1.4281	55
56	0.829	0.5592	1.4826	56
57	0.8387	0.5446	1.5399	57
58	0.848	0.5299	1.6003	58
59	0.8571	0.515	1.6643	59
60	0.866	0.5	1.7321	60

(continued)

TABLE A.1 ***(Continued)***

Angle (in degree)	Sin	Cos	Tan	Angle (in degree)
61	0.8746	0.4848	1.8040	61
62	0.8829	0.4695	1.8907	62
63	0.8910	0.454	1.9626	63
64	0.8988	0.4384	2.0503	64
65	0.9063	0.4226	2.1445	65
66	0.9135	0.4067	2.2460	66
67	0.9205	0.3907	2.3559	67
68	0.9272	0.3746	2.4751	68
69	0.9336	0.3584	2.6051	69
70	0.9397	0.342	2.7475	70
71	0.9455	0.3256	2.9042	71
72	0.9511	0.309	3.0777	72
73	0.9563	0.2924	3.2709	73
74	0.9613	0.2756	3.4874	74
75	0.9659	0.2588	3.7321	75
76	0.9703	0.2419	4.0108	76
77	0.9744	0.2249	4.3315	77
78	0.9781	0.2079	4.7046	78
79	0.9816	0.1908	5.1446	79
80	0.9848	0.1736	5.6713	80
81	0.9877	0.1564	6.3138	81
82	0.9903	0.1392	7.1154	82
83	0.9926	0.1219	8.1443	83
84	0.9945	0.1045	9.5144	84
85	0.9962	0.0872	11.430	85
86	0.9976	0.0698	14.301	86
87	0.9986	0.0523	19.081	87
88	0.9994	0.0349	28.636	88
89	0.9998	0.0174	57.290	89
90	1	0	∞	90

TABLE A.2 Binomial Probability Distribution

$N = 3$

	Probability								
x	0.1	0.2	0.3	0.4	0.5	0.6	0.7	0.8	0.9
0	0.729	0.512	0.343	0.216	0.125	0.064	0.027	0.008	0.001
1	0.243	0.384	0.441	0.432	0.375	0.288	0.189	0.096	0.027
2	0.027	0.096	0.189	0.288	0.375	0.432	0.441	0.384	0.243
3	0.001	0.008	0.027	0.064	0.125	0.216	0.343	0.512	0.729

$N = 4$

	Probability								
x	0.1	0.2	0.3	0.4	0.5	0.6	0.7	0.8	0.9
0	0.6561	0.4096	0.2401	0.1296	0.0625	0.0256	0.0081	0.0016	0.0001
1	0.2916	0.4096	0.4116	0.3456	0.2500	0.1536	0.0756	0.0256	0.0036
2	0.0486	0.1536	0.2646	0.3456	0.3750	0.3456	0.2646	0.1536	0.0486
3	0.0036	0.0256	0.0756	0.1536	0.2500	0.3456	0.4116	0.4096	0.2916
4	0.0001	0.0016	0.0081	0.0256	0.0625	0.1296	0.2401	0.4096	0.6561

$N = 5$

	Probability								
x	0.1	0.2	0.3	0.4	0.5	0.6	0.7	0.8	0.9
0	0.59049	0.32768	0.16807	0.07776	0.03125	0.01024	0.00243	0.00032	0.00001
1	0.32805	0.40960	0.36015	0.25920	0.15625	0.07680	0.02835	0.00640	0.00045
2	0.07290	0.20480	0.30870	0.34560	0.31250	0.23040	0.13230	0.05120	0.00810
3	0.00810	0.05120	0.13230	0.23040	0.31250	0.34560	0.30870	0.20480	0.07290
4	0.00045	0.00640	0.02835	0.07680	0.15625	0.25920	0.36015	0.40960	0.32805
5	0.00001	0.00032	0.00243	0.01024	0.03125	0.07776	0.16807	0.32768	0.59049

$N = 6$

	Probability								
x	0.1	0.2	0.3	0.4	0.5	0.6	0.7	0.8	0.9
0	0.53144	0.26214	0.11765	0.04666	0.01562	0.00410	0.00073	0.00006	0.00000
1	0.35429	0.39322	0.30253	0.18662	0.09375	0.03686	0.01021	0.00154	0.00005
2	0.09842	0.24576	0.32414	0.31104	0.23438	0.13824	0.05954	0.01536	0.00122
3	0.01458	0.08192	0.18522	0.27648	0.31250	0.27648	0.18522	0.08192	0.01458
4	0.00122	0.01536	0.05954	0.13824	0.23438	0.31104	0.32414	0.24576	0.09842
5	0.00005	0.00154	0.01021	0.03686	0.09375	0.18662	0.30253	0.39322	0.35429
6	0.00000	0.00006	0.00073	0.00410	0.01562	0.04666	0.11765	0.26214	0.53144

$N = 7$

	Probability								
x	0.1	0.2	0.3	0.4	0.5	0.6	0.7	0.8	0.9
0	0.47830	0.20972	0.08235	0.02799	0.00781	0.00164	0.00022	0.00001	0.00000
1	0.37201	0.36700	0.24706	0.13064	0.05469	0.01720	0.00357	0.00036	0.00001
2	0.12400	0.27525	0.31765	0.26127	0.16406	0.07741	0.02500	0.00430	0.00017
3	0.02296	0.11469	0.22689	0.29030	0.27344	0.19354	0.09724	0.02867	0.00255
4	0.00255	0.02867	0.09724	0.19354	0.27344	0.29030	0.22689	0.11469	0.02296
5	0.00017	0.00430	0.02500	0.07741	0.16406	0.26127	0.31765	0.27525	0.12400
6	0.00001	0.00036	0.00357	0.01720	0.05469	0.13064	0.24706	0.36700	0.37201
7	0.00000	0.00001	0.00022	0.00164	0.00781	0.02799	0.08235	0.20972	0.47830

(continued)

TABLE A.2 (*Continued*)

$N = 8$

	Probability								
x	0.1	0.2	0.3	0.4	0.5	0.6	0.7	0.8	0.9
0	0.43047	0.16777	0.05765	0.01680	0.00391	0.00066	0.00007	0.00000	0.00000
1	0.38264	0.33554	0.19765	0.08958	0.03125	0.00786	0.00122	0.00008	0.00000
2	0.14880	0.29360	0.29648	0.20902	0.10938	0.04129	0.01000	0.00115	0.00002
3	0.03307	0.14680	0.25412	0.27869	0.21875	0.12386	0.04668	0.00918	0.00041
4	0.00459	0.04588	0.13614	0.23224	0.27344	0.23224	0.13614	0.04588	0.00459
5	0.00041	0.00918	0.04668	0.12386	0.21875	0.27869	0.25412	0.14680	0.03307
6	0.00002	0.00115	0.01000	0.04129	0.10938	0.20902	0.29648	0.29360	0.14880
7	0.00000	0.00008	0.00122	0.00786	0.03125	0.08958	0.19765	0.33554	0.38264
8	0.00000	0.00000	0.00007	0.00066	0.00391	0.01680	0.05765	0.16777	0.43047

$N = 9$

	Probability								
x	0.1	0.2	0.3	0.4	0.5	0.6	0.7	0.8	0.9
0	0.38742	0.13422	0.04035	0.01008	0.00195	0.00026	0.00002	0.00000	0.00000
1	0.38742	0.30199	0.15565	0.06047	0.01758	0.00354	0.00041	0.00002	0.00000
2	0.17219	0.30199	0.26683	0.16124	0.07031	0.02123	0.00386	0.00029	0.00000
3	0.04464	0.17616	0.26683	0.25082	0.16406	0.07432	0.02100	0.00275	0.00006
4	0.00744	0.06606	0.17153	0.25082	0.24609	0.16722	0.07351	0.01652	0.00083
5	0.00083	0.01652	0.07351	0.16722	0.24609	0.25082	0.17153	0.06606	0.00744
6	0.00006	0.00275	0.02100	0.07432	0.16406	0.25082	0.26683	0.17616	0.04464
7	0.00000	0.00029	0.00386	0.02123	0.07031	0.16124	0.26683	0.30199	0.17219
8	0.00000	0.00002	0.00041	0.00354	0.01758	0.06047	0.15565	0.30199	0.38742
9	0.00000	0.00000	0.00002	0.00026	0.00195	0.01008	0.04035	0.13422	0.38742

$N = 10$

	Probability								
x	0.1	0.2	0.3	0.4	0.5	0.6	0.7	0.8	0.9
0	0.34868	0.10737	0.02825	0.00605	0.00098	0.00010	0.00001	0.00000	0.00000
1	0.38742	0.26844	0.12106	0.04031	0.00977	0.00157	0.00014	0.00000	0.00000
2	0.19371	0.30199	0.23347	0.12093	0.04395	0.01062	0.00145	0.00007	0.00000
3	0.05740	0.20133	0.26683	0.21499	0.11719	0.04247	0.00900	0.00079	0.00001
4	0.01116	0.08808	0.20012	0.25082	0.20508	0.11148	0.03676	0.00551	0.00014
5	0.00149	0.02642	0.10292	0.20066	0.24609	0.20066	0.10292	0.02642	0.00149
6	0.00014	0.00551	0.03676	0.11148	0.20508	0.25082	0.20012	0.08808	0.01116
7	0.00001	0.00079	0.00900	0.04247	0.11719	0.21499	0.26683	0.20133	0.05740
8	0.00000	0.00007	0.00145	0.01062	0.04395	0.12093	0.23347	0.30199	0.19371
9	0.00000	0.00000	0.00014	0.00157	0.00977	0.04031	0.12106	0.26844	0.38742
10	0.00000	0.00000	0.00001	0.00010	0.00098	0.00605	0.02825	0.10737	0.34868

(*continued*)

TABLE A.2 (*Continued*)

N = 11

	Probability								
x	0.1	0.2	0.3	0.4	0.5	0.6	0.7	0.8	0.9
0	0.31381	0.08590	0.01977	0.00363	0.00049	0.00004	0.00000	0.00000	0.00000
1	0.38355	0.23622	0.09322	0.02661	0.00537	0.00069	0.00005	0.00000	0.00000
2	0.21308	0.29528	0.19975	0.08868	0.02686	0.00519	0.00053	0.00002	0.00000
3	0.07103	0.22146	0.25682	0.17737	0.08057	0.02336	0.00371	0.00022	0.00000
4	0.01578	0.11073	0.22013	0.23649	0.16113	0.07007	0.01733	0.00173	0.00002
5	0.00246	0.03876	0.13208	0.22072	0.22559	0.14715	0.05661	0.00969	0.00027
6	0.00027	0.00969	0.05661	0.14715	0.22559	0.22072	0.13208	0.03876	0.00246
7	0.00002	0.00173	0.01733	0.07007	0.16113	0.23649	0.22013	0.11073	0.01578
8	0.00000	0.00022	0.00371	0.02336	0.08057	0.17737	0.25682	0.22146	0.07103
9	0.00000	0.00002	0.00053	0.00519	0.02686	0.08868	0.19975	0.29528	0.21308
10	0.00000	0.00000	0.00005	0.00069	0.00537	0.02661	0.09322	0.23622	0.38355
11	0.00000	0.00000	0.00000	0.00004	0.00049	0.00363	0.01977	0.08590	0.31381

N = 12

	Probability								
x	0.1	0.2	0.3	0.4	0.5	0.6	0.7	0.8	0.9
0	0.28243	0.06872	0.01384	0.00218	0.00024	0.00002	0.00000	0.00000	0.00000
1	0.37657	0.20616	0.07118	0.01741	0.00293	0.00030	0.00001	0.00000	0.00000
2	0.23013	0.28347	0.16779	0.06385	0.01611	0.00249	0.00019	0.00000	0.00000
3	0.08523	0.23622	0.23970	0.14189	0.05371	0.01246	0.00149	0.00006	0.00000
4	0.02131	0.13288	0.23114	0.21284	0.12085	0.04204	0.00780	0.00052	0.00000
5	0.00379	0.05315	0.15850	0.22703	0.19336	0.10090	0.02911	0.00332	0.00005
6	0.00049	0.01550	0.07925	0.17658	0.22559	0.17658	0.07925	0.01550	0.00049
7	0.00005	0.00332	0.02911	0.10090	0.19336	0.22703	0.15850	0.05315	0.00379
8	0.00000	0.00052	0.00780	0.04204	0.12085	0.21284	0.23114	0.13288	0.02131
9	0.00000	0.00006	0.00149	0.01246	0.05371	0.14189	0.23970	0.23622	0.08523
10	0.00000	0.00000	0.00019	0.00249	0.01611	0.06385	0.16779	0.28347	0.23013
11	0.00000	0.00000	0.00001	0.00030	0.00293	0.01741	0.07118	0.20616	0.37657
12	0.00000	0.00000	0.00000	0.00002	0.00024	0.00218	0.01384	0.06872	0.28243

N = 13

	Probability								
x	0.1	0.2	0.3	0.4	0.5	0.6	0.7	0.8	0.9
0	0.25419	0.05498	0.00969	0.00131	0.00012	0.00001	0.00000	0.00000	0.00000
1	0.36716	0.17867	0.05398	0.01132	0.00159	0.00013	0.00000	0.00000	0.00000
2	0.24477	0.26801	0.13881	0.04528	0.00952	0.00118	0.00007	0.00000	0.00000
3	0.09972	0.24567	0.21813	0.11068	0.03491	0.00648	0.00058	0.00001	0.00000
4	0.02770	0.15355	0.23371	0.18446	0.08728	0.02429	0.00338	0.00015	0.00000
5	0.00554	0.06910	0.18029	0.22135	0.15710	0.06559	0.01419	0.00108	0.00001
6	0.00082	0.02303	0.10302	0.19676	0.20947	0.13117	0.04415	0.00576	0.00009
7	0.00009	0.00576	0.04415	0.13117	0.20947	0.19676	0.10302	0.02303	0.00082
8	0.00001	0.00108	0.01419	0.06559	0.15710	0.22135	0.18029	0.06910	0.00554
9	0.00000	0.00015	0.00338	0.02429	0.08728	0.18446	0.23371	0.15355	0.02770
10	0.00000	0.00001	0.00058	0.00648	0.03491	0.11068	0.21813	0.24567	0.09972
11	0.00000	0.00000	0.00007	0.00118	0.00952	0.04528	0.13881	0.26801	0.24477
12	0.00000	0.00000	0.00000	0.00013	0.00159	0.01132	0.05398	0.17867	0.36716
13	0.00000	0.00000	0.00000	0.00001	0.00012	0.00131	0.00969	0.05498	0.25419

(*continued*)

TABLE A.2 (*Continued*)

$N = 14$

	Probability								
x	0.1	0.2	0.3	0.4	0.5	0.6	0.7	0.8	0.9
0	0.22877	0.04398	0.00678	0.00078	0.00006	0.00000	0.00000	0.00000	0.00000
1	0.35586	0.15393	0.04069	0.00731	0.00085	0.00006	0.00000	0.00000	0.00000
2	0.25701	0.25014	0.11336	0.03169	0.00555	0.00055	0.00002	0.00000	0.00000
3	0.11423	0.25014	0.19433	0.08452	0.02222	0.00330	0.00022	0.00000	0.00000
4	0.03490	0.17197	0.22903	0.15495	0.06110	0.01360	0.00142	0.00004	0.00000
5	0.00776	0.08599	0.19631	0.20660	0.12219	0.04081	0.00662	0.00034	0.00000
6	0.00129	0.03224	0.12620	0.20660	0.18329	0.09182	0.02318	0.00202	0.00002
7	0.00016	0.00921	0.06181	0.15741	0.20947	0.15741	0.06181	0.00921	0.00016
8	0.00002	0.00202	0.02318	0.09182	0.18329	0.20660	0.12620	0.03224	0.00129
9	0.00000	0.00034	0.00662	0.04081	0.12219	0.20660	0.19631	0.08599	0.00776
10	0.00000	0.00004	0.00142	0.01360	0.06110	0.15495	0.22903	0.17197	0.03490
11	0.00000	0.00000	0.00022	0.00330	0.02222	0.08452	0.19433	0.25014	0.11423
12	0.00000	0.00000	0.00002	0.00055	0.00555	0.03169	0.11336	0.25014	0.25701
13	0.00000	0.00000	0.00000	0.00006	0.00085	0.00731	0.04069	0.15393	0.35586
14	0.00000	0.00000	0.00000	0.00000	0.00006	0.00078	0.00678	0.04398	0.22877

$N = 15$

	Probability								
x	0.1	0.2	0.3	0.4	0.5	0.6	0.7	0.8	0.9
0	0.20589	0.03518	0.00475	0.00047	0.00003	0.00000	0.00000	0.00000	0.00000
1	0.34315	0.13194	0.03052	0.00470	0.00046	0.00002	0.00000	0.00000	0.00000
2	0.26690	0.23090	0.09156	0.02194	0.00320	0.00025	0.00001	0.00000	0.00000
3	0.12851	0.25014	0.17004	0.06339	0.01389	0.00165	0.00008	0.00000	0.00000
4	0.04284	0.18760	0.21862	0.12678	0.04166	0.00742	0.00058	0.00001	0.00000
5	0.01047	0.10318	0.20613	0.18594	0.09164	0.02449	0.00298	0.00010	0.00000
6	0.00194	0.04299	0.14724	0.20660	0.15274	0.06121	0.01159	0.00067	0.00000
7	0.00028	0.01382	0.08113	0.17708	0.19638	0.11806	0.03477	0.00345	0.00003
8	0.00003	0.00345	0.03477	0.11806	0.19638	0.17708	0.08113	0.01382	0.00028
9	0.00000	0.00067	0.01159	0.06121	0.15274	0.20660	0.14724	0.04299	0.00194
10	0.00000	0.00010	0.00298	0.02449	0.09164	0.18594	0.20613	0.10318	0.01047
11	0.00000	0.00001	0.00058	0.00742	0.04166	0.12678	0.21862	0.18760	0.04284
12	0.00000	0.00000	0.00008	0.00165	0.01389	0.06339	0.17004	0.25014	0.12851
13	0.00000	0.00000	0.00001	0.00025	0.00320	0.02194	0.09156	0.23090	0.26690
14	0.00000	0.00000	0.00000	0.00002	0.00046	0.00470	0.03052	0.13194	0.34315
15	0.00000	0.00000	0.00000	0.00000	0.00003	0.00047	0.00475	0.03518	0.20589

TABLE A.3 Poisson Probability Distribution

	Mean (λ)									
x	0.1	0.2	0.3	0.4	0.5	0.6	0.7	0.8	0.9	1
0	0.90484	0.81873	0.74082	0.67032	0.60653	0.54881	0.49659	0.44933	0.40657	0.36788
1	0.09048	0.16375	0.22225	0.26813	0.30327	0.32929	0.34761	0.35946	0.36591	0.36788
2	0.00452	0.01637	0.03334	0.05363	0.07582	0.09879	0.12166	0.14379	0.16466	0.18394
3	0.00015	0.00109	0.00333	0.00715	0.01264	0.01976	0.02839	0.03834	0.04940	0.06131
4	0.00000	0.00005	0.00025	0.00072	0.00158	0.00296	0.00497	0.00767	0.01111	0.01533
5	0.00000	0.00000	0.00002	0.00006	0.00016	0.00036	0.00070	0.00123	0.00200	0.00307

	Mean (λ)									
x	1.1	1.2	1.3	1.4	1.5	1.6	1.7	1.8	1.9	2
0	0.33287	0.30119	0.27253	0.24660	0.22313	0.20190	0.18268	0.16530	0.14957	0.13534
1	0.36616	0.36143	0.35429	0.34524	0.33470	0.32303	0.31056	0.29754	0.28418	0.27067
2	0.20139	0.21686	0.23029	0.24167	0.25102	0.25843	0.26398	0.26778	0.26997	0.27067
3	0.07384	0.08674	0.09979	0.11278	0.12551	0.13783	0.14959	0.16067	0.17098	0.18045
4	0.02031	0.02602	0.03243	0.03947	0.04707	0.05513	0.06357	0.07230	0.08122	0.09022
5	0.00447	0.00625	0.00843	0.01105	0.01412	0.01764	0.02162	0.02603	0.03086	0.03609
6	0.00082	0.00125	0.00183	0.00258	0.00353	0.00470	0.00612	0.00781	0.00977	0.01203
7	0.00013	0.00021	0.00034	0.00052	0.00076	0.00108	0.00149	0.00201	0.00265	0.00344
8	0.00002	0.00003	0.00006	0.00009	0.00014	0.00022	0.00032	0.00045	0.00063	0.00086
9	0.00000	0.00000	0.00001	0.00001	0.00002	0.00004	0.00006	0.00009	0.00013	0.00019
10	0.00000	0.00000	0.00000	0.00000	0.00000	0.00001	0.00001	0.00002	0.00003	0.00004

	Mean (λ)									
x	2.1	2.2	2.3	2.4	2.5	2.6	2.7	2.8	2.9	3
0	0.12246	0.11080	0.10026	0.09072	0.08208	0.07427	0.06721	0.06081	0.05502	0.04979
1	0.25716	0.24377	0.23060	0.21772	0.20521	0.19311	0.18145	0.17027	0.15957	0.14936
2	0.27002	0.26814	0.26518	0.26127	0.25652	0.25104	0.24496	0.23838	0.23137	0.22404
3	0.18901	0.19664	0.20331	0.20901	0.21376	0.21757	0.22047	0.22248	0.22366	0.22404
4	0.09923	0.10815	0.11690	0.12541	0.13360	0.14142	0.14882	0.15574	0.16215	0.16803
5	0.04168	0.04759	0.05378	0.06020	0.06680	0.07354	0.08036	0.08721	0.09405	0.10082
6	0.01459	0.01745	0.02061	0.02408	0.02783	0.03187	0.03616	0.04070	0.04546	0.05041
7	0.00438	0.00548	0.00677	0.00826	0.00994	0.01184	0.01395	0.01628	0.01883	0.02160
8	0.00115	0.00151	0.00195	0.00248	0.00311	0.00385	0.00471	0.00570	0.00683	0.00810
9	0.00027	0.00037	0.00050	0.00066	0.00086	0.00111	0.00141	0.00177	0.00220	0.00270
10	0.00006	0.00008	0.00011	0.00016	0.00022	0.00029	0.00038	0.00050	0.00064	0.00081
11	0.00001	0.00002	0.00002	0.00003	0.00005	0.00007	0.00009	0.00013	0.00017	0.00022
12	0.00000	0.00000	0.00000	0.00001	0.00001	0.00001	0.00002	0.00003	0.00004	0.00006
13	0.00000	0.00000	0.00000	0.00000	0.00000	0.00000	0.00000	0.00001	0.00001	0.00001
14	0.00000	0.00000	0.00000	0.00000	0.00000	0.00000	0.00000	0.00000	0.00000	0.00000
15	0.00000	0.00000	0.00000	0.00000	0.00000	0.00000	0.00000	0.00000	0.00000	0.00000

(*continued*)

TABLE A.3 (*Continued*)

	Mean (λ)									
x	3.1	3.2	3.3	3.4	3.5	3.6	3.7	3.8	3.9	4
0	0.04505	0.04076	0.03688	0.03337	0.03020	0.02732	0.02472	0.02237	0.02024	0.01832
1	0.13965	0.13044	0.12171	0.11347	0.10569	0.09837	0.09148	0.08501	0.07894	0.07326
2	0.21646	0.20870	0.20083	0.19290	0.18496	0.17706	0.16923	0.16152	0.15394	0.14653
3	0.22368	0.22262	0.22091	0.21862	0.21579	0.21247	0.20872	0.20459	0.20012	0.19537
4	0.17335	0.17809	0.18225	0.18582	0.18881	0.19122	0.19307	0.19436	0.19512	0.19537
5	0.10748	0.11398	0.12029	0.12636	0.13217	0.13768	0.14287	0.14771	0.15219	0.15629
6	0.05553	0.06079	0.06616	0.07160	0.07710	0.08261	0.08810	0.09355	0.09893	0.10420
7	0.02459	0.02779	0.03119	0.03478	0.03855	0.04248	0.04657	0.05079	0.05512	0.05954
8	0.00953	0.01112	0.01287	0.01478	0.01687	0.01912	0.02154	0.02412	0.02687	0.02977
9	0.00328	0.00395	0.00472	0.00558	0.00656	0.00765	0.00885	0.01019	0.01164	0.01323
10	0.00102	0.00126	0.00156	0.00190	0.00230	0.00275	0.00328	0.00387	0.00454	0.00529
11	0.00029	0.00037	0.00047	0.00059	0.00073	0.00090	0.00110	0.00134	0.00161	0.00192
12	0.00007	0.00010	0.00013	0.00017	0.00021	0.00027	0.00034	0.00042	0.00052	0.00064
13	0.00002	0.00002	0.00003	0.00004	0.00006	0.00007	0.00010	0.00012	0.00016	0.00020
14	0.00000	0.00001	0.00001	0.00001	0.00001	0.00002	0.00003	0.00003	0.00004	0.00006
15	0.00000	0.00000	0.00000	0.00000	0.00000	0.00000	0.00001	0.00001	0.00001	0.00002

	Mean (λ)									
x	4.1	4.2	4.3	4.4	4.5	4.6	4.7	4.8	4.9	5
0	0.01657	0.01500	0.01357	0.01228	0.01111	0.01005	0.00910	0.00823	0.00745	0.00674
1	0.06795	0.06298	0.05834	0.05402	0.04999	0.04624	0.04275	0.03950	0.03649	0.03369
2	0.13929	0.13226	0.12544	0.11884	0.11248	0.10635	0.10046	0.09481	0.08940	0.08422
3	0.19037	0.18517	0.17980	0.17431	0.16872	0.16307	0.15738	0.15169	0.14601	0.14037
4	0.19513	0.19442	0.19328	0.19174	0.18981	0.18753	0.18493	0.18203	0.17887	0.17547
5	0.16000	0.16332	0.16622	0.16873	0.17083	0.17253	0.17383	0.17475	0.17529	0.17547
6	0.10934	0.11432	0.11913	0.12373	0.12812	0.13227	0.13617	0.13980	0.14315	0.14622
7	0.06404	0.06859	0.07318	0.07778	0.08236	0.08692	0.09143	0.09586	0.10021	0.10444
8	0.03282	0.03601	0.03933	0.04278	0.04633	0.04998	0.05371	0.05752	0.06138	0.06528
9	0.01495	0.01681	0.01879	0.02091	0.02316	0.02554	0.02805	0.03068	0.03342	0.03627
10	0.00613	0.00706	0.00808	0.00920	0.01042	0.01175	0.01318	0.01472	0.01637	0.01813
11	0.00228	0.00269	0.00316	0.00368	0.00426	0.00491	0.00563	0.00643	0.00729	0.00824
12	0.00078	0.00094	0.00113	0.00135	0.00160	0.00188	0.00221	0.00257	0.00298	0.00343
13	0.00025	0.00030	0.00037	0.00046	0.00055	0.00067	0.00080	0.00095	0.00112	0.00132
14	0.00007	0.00009	0.00011	0.00014	0.00018	0.00022	0.00027	0.00033	0.00039	0.00047
15	0.00002	0.00003	0.00003	0.00004	0.00005	0.00007	0.00008	0.00010	0.00013	0.00016

(*continued*)

TABLE A.3 (*Continued*)

	Mean (λ)									
x	5.1	5.2	5.3	5.4	5.5	5.6	5.7	5.8	5.9	6
0	0.00610	0.00552	0.00499	0.00452	0.00409	0.00370	0.00335	0.00303	0.00274	0.00248
1	0.03109	0.02869	0.02646	0.02439	0.02248	0.02071	0.01907	0.01756	0.01616	0.01487
2	0.07929	0.07458	0.07011	0.06585	0.06181	0.05798	0.05436	0.05092	0.04768	0.04462
3	0.13479	0.12928	0.12386	0.11853	0.11332	0.10823	0.10327	0.09845	0.09377	0.08924
4	0.17186	0.16806	0.16411	0.16002	0.15582	0.15153	0.14717	0.14276	0.13831	0.13385
5	0.17529	0.17479	0.17396	0.17282	0.17140	0.16971	0.16777	0.16560	0.16321	0.16062
6	0.14900	0.15148	0.15366	0.15554	0.15712	0.15840	0.15938	0.16008	0.16049	0.16062
7	0.10856	0.11253	0.11634	0.11999	0.12345	0.12672	0.12978	0.13263	0.13527	0.13768
8	0.06921	0.07314	0.07708	0.08099	0.08487	0.08870	0.09247	0.09616	0.09976	0.10326
9	0.03922	0.04226	0.04539	0.04859	0.05187	0.05519	0.05856	0.06197	0.06540	0.06884
10	0.02000	0.02198	0.02406	0.02624	0.02853	0.03091	0.03338	0.03594	0.03859	0.04130
11	0.00927	0.01039	0.01159	0.01288	0.01426	0.01573	0.01730	0.01895	0.02070	0.02253
12	0.00394	0.00450	0.00512	0.00580	0.00654	0.00734	0.00822	0.00916	0.01018	0.01126
13	0.00155	0.00180	0.00209	0.00241	0.00277	0.00316	0.00360	0.00409	0.00462	0.00520
14	0.00056	0.00067	0.00079	0.00093	0.00109	0.00127	0.00147	0.00169	0.00195	0.00223
15	0.00019	0.00023	0.00028	0.00033	0.00040	0.00047	0.00056	0.00065	0.00077	0.00089

	Mean (λ)									
x	6.1	6.2	6.3	6.4	6.5	6.6	6.7	6.8	6.9	7
0	0.00224	0.00203	0.00184	0.00166	0.00150	0.00136	0.00123	0.00111	0.00101	0.00091
1	0.01368	0.01258	0.01157	0.01063	0.00977	0.00898	0.00825	0.00757	0.00695	0.00638
2	0.04173	0.03901	0.03644	0.03403	0.03176	0.02963	0.02763	0.02575	0.02399	0.02234
3	0.08485	0.08061	0.07653	0.07259	0.06881	0.06518	0.06170	0.05837	0.05518	0.05213
4	0.12939	0.12495	0.12053	0.11615	0.11182	0.10755	0.10335	0.09923	0.09518	0.09123
5	0.15786	0.15494	0.15187	0.14867	0.14537	0.14197	0.13849	0.13495	0.13135	0.12772
6	0.16049	0.16010	0.15946	0.15859	0.15748	0.15617	0.15465	0.15294	0.15105	0.14900
7	0.13986	0.14180	0.14352	0.14499	0.14623	0.14724	0.14802	0.14857	0.14890	0.14900
8	0.10664	0.10990	0.11302	0.11599	0.11882	0.12148	0.12397	0.12628	0.12842	0.13038
9	0.07228	0.07571	0.07911	0.08248	0.08581	0.08908	0.09229	0.09541	0.09846	0.10140
10	0.04409	0.04694	0.04984	0.05279	0.05578	0.05879	0.06183	0.06488	0.06794	0.07098
11	0.02445	0.02646	0.02855	0.03071	0.03296	0.03528	0.03766	0.04011	0.04261	0.04517
12	0.01243	0.01367	0.01499	0.01638	0.01785	0.01940	0.02103	0.02273	0.02450	0.02635
13	0.00583	0.00652	0.00726	0.00806	0.00893	0.00985	0.01084	0.01189	0.01301	0.01419
14	0.00254	0.00289	0.00327	0.00369	0.00414	0.00464	0.00519	0.00577	0.00641	0.00709
15	0.00103	0.00119	0.00137	0.00157	0.00180	0.00204	0.00232	0.00262	0.00295	0.00331
16	0.00039	0.00046	0.00054	0.00063	0.00073	0.00084	0.00097	0.00111	0.00127	0.00145
17	0.00014	0.00017	0.00020	0.00024	0.00028	0.00033	0.00038	0.00045	0.00052	0.00060
18	0.00005	0.00006	0.00007	0.00008	0.00010	0.00012	0.00014	0.00017	0.00020	0.00023
19	0.00002	0.00002	0.00002	0.00003	0.00003	0.00004	0.00005	0.00006	0.00007	0.00009
20	0.00000	0.00001	0.00001	0.00001	0.00001	0.00001	0.00002	0.00002	0.00002	0.00003

(*continued*)

TABLE A.3 (*Continued*)

	Mean (λ)									
x	7.1	7.2	7.3	7.4	7.5	7.6	7.7	7.8	7.9	8
0	0.00083	0.00075	0.00068	0.00061	0.00055	0.00050	0.00045	0.00041	0.00037	0.00034
1	0.00586	0.00538	0.00493	0.00452	0.00415	0.00380	0.00349	0.00320	0.00293	0.00268
2	0.02080	0.01935	0.01800	0.01674	0.01556	0.01445	0.01342	0.01246	0.01157	0.01073
3	0.04922	0.04644	0.04380	0.04128	0.03889	0.03661	0.03446	0.03241	0.03047	0.02863
4	0.08736	0.08360	0.07993	0.07637	0.07292	0.06957	0.06633	0.06319	0.06017	0.05725
5	0.12406	0.12038	0.11670	0.11303	0.10937	0.10574	0.10214	0.09858	0.09507	0.09160
6	0.14680	0.14446	0.14199	0.13941	0.13672	0.13394	0.13108	0.12816	0.12517	0.12214
7	0.14890	0.14859	0.14807	0.14737	0.14648	0.14542	0.14419	0.14280	0.14126	0.13959
8	0.13215	0.13373	0.13512	0.13632	0.13733	0.13815	0.13878	0.13923	0.13950	0.13959
9	0.10425	0.10698	0.10960	0.11208	0.11444	0.11666	0.11874	0.12067	0.12245	0.12408
10	0.07402	0.07703	0.08000	0.08294	0.08583	0.08866	0.09143	0.09412	0.09673	0.09926
11	0.04777	0.05042	0.05309	0.05580	0.05852	0.06126	0.06400	0.06674	0.06947	0.07219
12	0.02827	0.03025	0.03230	0.03441	0.03658	0.03880	0.04107	0.04338	0.04574	0.04813
13	0.01544	0.01675	0.01814	0.01959	0.02110	0.02268	0.02432	0.02603	0.02779	0.02962
14	0.00783	0.00862	0.00946	0.01035	0.01130	0.01231	0.01338	0.01450	0.01568	0.01692
15	0.00371	0.00414	0.00460	0.00511	0.00565	0.00624	0.00687	0.00754	0.00826	0.00903
16	0.00164	0.00186	0.00210	0.00236	0.00265	0.00296	0.00330	0.00368	0.00408	0.00451
17	0.00069	0.00079	0.00090	0.00103	0.00117	0.00132	0.00150	0.00169	0.00190	0.00212
18	0.00027	0.00032	0.00037	0.00042	0.00049	0.00056	0.00064	0.00073	0.00083	0.00094
19	0.00010	0.00012	0.00014	0.00016	0.00019	0.00022	0.00026	0.00030	0.00035	0.00040
20	0.00004	0.00004	0.00005	0.00006	0.00007	0.00009	0.00010	0.00012	0.00014	0.00016

	Mean (λ)									
x	8.1	8.2	8.3	8.4	8.5	8.6	8.7	8.8	8.9	9
0	0.00030	0.00027	0.00025	0.00022	0.00020	0.00018	0.00017	0.00015	0.00014	0.00012
1	0.00246	0.00225	0.00206	0.00189	0.00173	0.00158	0.00145	0.00133	0.00121	0.00111
2	0.00996	0.00923	0.00856	0.00793	0.00735	0.00681	0.00630	0.00584	0.00540	0.00500
3	0.02689	0.02524	0.02368	0.02221	0.02083	0.01952	0.01828	0.01712	0.01602	0.01499
4	0.05444	0.05174	0.04914	0.04665	0.04425	0.04196	0.03977	0.03766	0.03566	0.03374
5	0.08820	0.08485	0.08158	0.07837	0.07523	0.07217	0.06919	0.06629	0.06347	0.06073
6	0.11907	0.11597	0.11285	0.10972	0.10658	0.10345	0.10033	0.09722	0.09414	0.09109
7	0.13778	0.13585	0.13380	0.13166	0.12942	0.12709	0.12469	0.12222	0.11970	0.11712
8	0.13950	0.13924	0.13882	0.13824	0.13751	0.13663	0.13560	0.13445	0.13316	0.13176
9	0.12555	0.12687	0.12803	0.12903	0.12987	0.13055	0.13108	0.13146	0.13168	0.13176
10	0.10170	0.10403	0.10626	0.10838	0.11039	0.11228	0.11404	0.11568	0.11720	0.11858
11	0.07488	0.07755	0.08018	0.08276	0.08530	0.08778	0.09020	0.09255	0.09482	0.09702
12	0.05055	0.05299	0.05546	0.05793	0.06042	0.06291	0.06539	0.06787	0.07033	0.07277
13	0.03149	0.03343	0.03541	0.03743	0.03951	0.04162	0.04376	0.04594	0.04815	0.05038
14	0.01822	0.01958	0.02099	0.02246	0.02399	0.02556	0.02720	0.02888	0.03061	0.03238
15	0.00984	0.01070	0.01162	0.01258	0.01359	0.01466	0.01577	0.01694	0.01816	0.01943
16	0.00498	0.00549	0.00603	0.00660	0.00722	0.00788	0.00858	0.00932	0.01010	0.01093
17	0.00237	0.00265	0.00294	0.00326	0.00361	0.00399	0.00439	0.00482	0.00529	0.00579
18	0.00107	0.00121	0.00136	0.00152	0.00170	0.00190	0.00212	0.00236	0.00261	0.00289
19	0.00046	0.00052	0.00059	0.00067	0.00076	0.00086	0.00097	0.00109	0.00122	0.00137
20	0.00018	0.00021	0.00025	0.00028	0.00032	0.00037	0.00042	0.00048	0.00055	0.00062

(*continued*)

TABLE A.3 (*Continued*)

	Mean (λ)									
x	9.1	9.2	9.3	9.4	9.5	9.6	9.7	9.8	9.9	10
0	0.00011	0.00010	0.00009	0.00008	0.00007	0.00007	0.00006	0.00006	0.00005	0.00005
1	0.00102	0.00093	0.00085	0.00078	0.00071	0.00065	0.00059	0.00054	0.00050	0.00045
2	0.00462	0.00428	0.00395	0.00365	0.00338	0.00312	0.00288	0.00266	0.00246	0.00227
3	0.01402	0.01311	0.01226	0.01145	0.01070	0.00999	0.00932	0.00870	0.00811	0.00757
4	0.03191	0.03016	0.02850	0.02691	0.02540	0.02397	0.02261	0.02131	0.02008	0.01892
5	0.05807	0.05549	0.05300	0.05059	0.04827	0.04602	0.04386	0.04177	0.03976	0.03783
6	0.08807	0.08509	0.08215	0.07926	0.07642	0.07363	0.07090	0.06822	0.06561	0.06306
7	0.11449	0.11183	0.10915	0.10644	0.10371	0.10098	0.09825	0.09551	0.09279	0.09008
8	0.13024	0.12861	0.12688	0.12506	0.12316	0.12118	0.11912	0.11700	0.11483	0.11260
9	0.13168	0.13147	0.13111	0.13062	0.13000	0.12926	0.12839	0.12740	0.12631	0.12511
10	0.11983	0.12095	0.12193	0.12279	0.12350	0.12409	0.12454	0.12486	0.12505	0.12511
11	0.09913	0.10116	0.10309	0.10493	0.10666	0.10829	0.10982	0.11124	0.11254	0.11374
12	0.07518	0.07755	0.07990	0.08219	0.08444	0.08663	0.08877	0.09084	0.09285	0.09478
13	0.05262	0.05488	0.05716	0.05943	0.06171	0.06398	0.06624	0.06848	0.07071	0.07291
14	0.03421	0.03607	0.03797	0.03990	0.04187	0.04387	0.04589	0.04794	0.05000	0.05208
15	0.02075	0.02212	0.02354	0.02501	0.02652	0.02808	0.02968	0.03132	0.03300	0.03472
16	0.01180	0.01272	0.01368	0.01469	0.01575	0.01685	0.01799	0.01918	0.02042	0.02170
17	0.00632	0.00688	0.00749	0.00812	0.00880	0.00951	0.01027	0.01106	0.01189	0.01276
18	0.00319	0.00352	0.00387	0.00424	0.00464	0.00507	0.00553	0.00602	0.00654	0.00709
19	0.00153	0.00170	0.00189	0.00210	0.00232	0.00256	0.00282	0.00311	0.00341	0.00373
20	0.00070	0.00078	0.00088	0.00099	0.00110	0.00123	0.00137	0.00152	0.00169	0.00187

TABLE A.4 The Normal Curve Area Between the Mean and a Given z Value

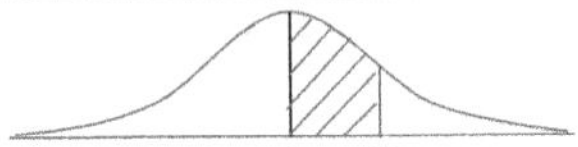

z	0.00	0.01	0.02	0.03	0.04	0.05	0.06	0.07	0.08	0.09
0.0	0.0000	0.0040	0.0080	0.0120	0.0160	0.0199	0.0239	0.0279	0.0319	0.0359
0.1	0.0398	0.0438	0.0478	0.0517	0.0557	0.0596	0.0636	0.0675	0.0714	0.0753
0.2	0.0793	0.0832	0.0871	0.0910	0.0948	0.0987	0.1026	0.1064	0.1103	0.1141
0.3	0.1179	0.1217	0.1255	0.1293	0.1331	0.1368	0.1406	0.1443	0.1480	0.1517
0.4	0.1554	0.1591	0.1628	0.1664	0.1700	0.1736	0.1772	0.1808	0.1844	0.1879
0.5	0.1915	0.1950	0.1985	0.2019	0.2054	0.2088	0.2123	0.2157	0.2190	0.2224
0.6	0.2257	0.2291	0.2324	0.2357	0.2389	0.2422	0.2454	0.2486	0.2517	0.2549
0.7	0.2580	0.2611	0.2642	0.2673	0.2704	0.2734	0.2764	0.2794	0.2823	0.2852
0.8	0.2881	0.2910	0.2939	0.2967	0.2995	0.3023	0.3051	0.3078	0.3106	0.3133
0.9	0.3159	0.3186	0.3212	0.3238	0.3264	0.3289	0.3315	0.3340	0.3365	0.3389
1.0	0.3413	0.3438	0.3461	0.3485	0.3508	0.3531	0.3554	0.3577	0.3599	0.3621
1.1	0.3643	0.3665	0.3686	0.3708	0.3729	0.3749	0.3770	0.3790	0.3810	0.3830
1.2	0.3849	0.3869	0.3888	0.3907	0.3925	0.3944	0.3962	0.3980	0.3997	0.4015
1.3	0.4032	0.4049	0.4066	0.4082	0.4099	0.4115	0.4131	0.4147	0.4162	0.4177
1.4	0.4192	0.4207	0.4222	0.4236	0.4251	0.4265	0.4279	0.4292	0.4306	0.4319
1.5	0.4332	0.4345	0.4357	0.4370	0.4382	0.4394	0.4406	0.4418	0.4429	0.4441
1.6	0.4452	0.4463	0.4474	0.4484	0.4495	0.4505	0.4515	0.4525	0.4535	0.4545
1.7	0.4554	0.4564	0.4573	0.4582	0.4591	0.4599	0.4608	0.4616	0.4625	0.4633
1.8	0.4641	0.4649	0.4656	0.4664	0.4671	0.4678	0.4686	0.4693	0.4699	0.4706
1.9	0.4713	0.4719	0.4726	0.4732	0.4738	0.4744	0.4750	0.4756	0.4761	0.4767
2.0	0.4772	0.4778	0.4783	0.4788	0.4793	0.4798	0.4803	0.4808	0.4812	0.4817
2.1	0.4821	0.4826	0.4830	0.4834	0.4838	0.4842	0.4846	0.4850	0.4854	0.4857
2.2	0.4861	0.4864	0.4868	0.4871	0.4875	0.4878	0.4881	0.4884	0.4887	0.4890
2.3	0.4893	0.4896	0.4898	0.4901	0.4904	0.4906	0.4909	0.4911	0.4913	0.4916
2.4	0.4918	0.4920	0.4922	0.4925	0.4927	0.4929	0.4931	0.4932	0.4934	0.4936
2.5	0.4938	0.4940	0.4941	0.4943	0.4945	0.4946	0.4948	0.4949	0.4951	0.4952
2.6	0.4953	0.4955	0.4956	0.4957	0.4959	0.4960	0.4961	0.4962	0.4963	0.4964
2.7	0.4965	0.4966	0.4967	0.4968	0.4969	0.4970	0.4971	0.4972	0.4973	0.4974
2.8	0.4974	0.4975	0.4976	0.4977	0.4977	0.4978	0.4979	0.4979	0.4980	0.4981
2.9	0.4981	0.4982	0.4982	0.4983	0.4984	0.4984	0.4985	0.4985	0.4986	0.4986
3.0	0.4987	0.4987	0.4987	0.4988	0.4988	0.4989	0.4989	0.4989	0.4990	0.4990

TABLE A.5 Ordinates at Different Values of z-Score in the Standard Normal Distribution

z	0	1	2	3	4	5	6	7	8	9
0.0	0.398942	0.398922	0.398862	0.398763	0.398623	0.398444	0.398225	0.397966	0.397668	0.397330
0.1	0.396953	0.396536	0.396080	0.395585	0.395052	0.394479	0.393868	0.393219	0.392531	0.391806
0.2	0.391043	0.390242	0.389404	0.388529	0.387617	0.386668	0.385683	0.384663	0.383606	0.382515
0.3	0.381388	0.380226	0.379031	0.377801	0.376537	0.375240	0.373911	0.372548	0.371154	0.369728
0.4	0.368270	0.366782	0.365263	0.363714	0.362135	0.360527	0.358890	0.357225	0.355533	0.353812
0.5	0.352065	0.350292	0.348493	0.346668	0.344818	0.342944	0.341046	0.339124	0.337180	0.335213
0.6	0.333225	0.331215	0.329184	0.327133	0.325062	0.322972	0.320864	0.318737	0.316593	0.314432
0.7	0.312254	0.310060	0.307851	0.305627	0.303389	0.301137	0.298872	0.296595	0.294305	0.292004
0.8	0.289692	0.287369	0.285036	0.282694	0.280344	0.277985	0.275618	0.273244	0.270864	0.268477
0.9	0.266085	0.263688	0.261286	0.258881	0.256471	0.254059	0.251644	0.249228	0.246809	0.244390

z	0	1	2	3	4	5	6	7	8	9
1.0	0.241971	0.239551	0.237132	0.234714	0.232297	0.229882	0.227470	0.225060	0.222653	0.220251
1.1	0.217852	0.215458	0.213069	0.210686	0.208308	0.205936	0.203571	0.201214	0.198863	0.196520
1.2	0.194186	0.191860	0.189543	0.187235	0.184937	0.182649	0.180371	0.178104	0.175847	0.173602
1.3	0.171369	0.169147	0.166937	0.164740	0.162555	0.160383	0.158225	0.156080	0.153948	0.151831
1.4	0.149727	0.147639	0.145564	0.143505	0.141460	0.139431	0.137417	0.135418	0.133435	0.131468
1.5	0.129518	0.127583	0.125665	0.123763	0.121878	0.120009	0.118157	0.116323	0.114505	0.112704
1.6	0.110921	0.109155	0.107406	0.105675	0.103961	0.102265	0.100586	0.098925	0.097282	0.095657
1.7	0.094049	0.092459	0.090887	0.089333	0.087796	0.086277	0.084776	0.083293	0.081828	0.080380
1.8	0.078950	0.077538	0.076143	0.074766	0.073407	0.072065	0.070740	0.069433	0.068144	0.066871
1.9	0.065616	0.064378	0.063157	0.061952	0.060765	0.059595	0.058441	0.057304	0.056183	0.055079

(*continued*)

TABLE A.5 (*Continued*)

z	0	1	2	3	4	5	6	7	8	9
2.0	0.053991	0.052919	0.051864	0.050824	0.049800	0.048792	0.047800	0.046823	0.045861	0.044915
2.1	0.043984	0.043067	0.042166	0.041280	0.040408	0.039550	0.038707	0.037878	0.037063	0.036262
2.2	0.035475	0.034701	0.033941	0.033194	0.032460	0.031740	0.031032	0.030337	0.029655	0.028985
2.3	0.028327	0.027682	0.027048	0.026426	0.025817	0.025218	0.024631	0.024056	0.023491	0.022937
2.4	0.022395	0.021862	0.021341	0.020829	0.020328	0.019837	0.019356	0.018885	0.018423	0.017971
2.5	0.017528	0.017095	0.016670	0.016254	0.015848	0.015449	0.015060	0.014678	0.014305	0.013940
2.6	0.013583	0.013234	0.012892	0.012558	0.012232	0.011912	0.011600	0.011295	0.010997	0.010706
2.7	0.010421	0.010143	3z98712	3z96058	3z93466	3z90936	3z88465	3z86052	3z83697	3z81398
2.8	3z79155	3z76965	3z74829	3z72744	3z70711	3z68728	3z66793	3z64907	3z63067	3z61274
2.9	3z59525	3z57821	3z56160	3z54541	3z52963	3z51426	3z49929	3z48470	3z47050	3z45666

z	0	1	2	3	4	5	6	7	8	9
3.0	3z44318	3z43007	3z41729	3z40486	3z39276	3z38098	3z36951	3z35836	3z34751	3z33695
3.1	3z32668	3z31669	3z30698	3z29754	3z28835	3z27943	3z27075	3z26231	3z25412	3z24615
3.2	3z23841	3z23089	3z22358	3z21649	3z20960	3z20290	3z19641	3z19010	3z18397	3z17803
3.3	3z17226	3z16666	3z16122	3z15595	3z15084	3z14587	3z14106	3z13639	3z13187	3z12748
3.4	3z12322	3z11910	3z11510	3z11122	3z10747	3z10383	3z10030	4z96886	4z93577	4z90372
3.5	4z87268	4z84263	4z81352	4z78534	4z75807	4z73166	4z70611	4z68138	4z65745	4z63430
3.6	4z61190	4z59024	4z56928	4z54901	4z52941	4z51046	4z49214	4z47443	4z45731	4z44077
3.7	4z42478	4z40933	4z39440	4z37998	4z36605	4z35260	4z33960	4z32705	4z31494	4z30324
3.8	4z29195	4z28105	4z27053	4z26037	4z25058	4z24113	4z23201	4z22321	4z21473	4z20655
3.9	4z19866	4z19105	4z18371	4z17664	4z16983	4z16326	4z15693	4z15083	4z14495	4z13928

(*continued*)

TABLE A.5 (*Continued*)

z	0	1	2	3	4	5	6	7	8	9
4.0	4z13383	4z12858	4z12352	4z11864	4z11395	4z10943	4z10509	4z10090	5z96870	5z92993
4.1	5z89262	5z85672	5z82218	5z78895	5z75700	5z72626	5z69670	5z66828	5z64095	5z61468
4.2	5z58943	5z56516	5z54183	5z51942	5z49788	5z47719	5z45731	5z43821	5z41988	5z40226
4.3	5z38535	5z36911	5z35353	5z33856	5z32420	5z31041	5z29719	5z28449	5z27231	5z26063
4.4	5z24942	5z23868	5z22837	5z21848	5z20900	5z19992	5z19121	5z18286	5z17486	5z16719
4.5	5z15984	5z15280	5z14605	5z13959	5z13340	5z12747	5z12180	5z11636	5z11116	5z10618
4.6	5z10141	6z96845	6z92477	6z88297	6z84298	6z80472	6z76812	6z73311	6z69962	6z66760
4.7	6z63698	6z60771	6z57972	6z55296	6z52739	6z50295	6z47960	6z45728	6z43596	6z41559
4.8	6z39613	6z37755	6z35980	6z34285	6z32667	6z31122	6z29647	6z28239	6z26895	6z25613
4.9	6z24390	6z23222	6z22108	6z21046	6z20033	6z19066	6z18144	6z17265	6z16428	6z15629
5.0	6z14867	6z14141	6z13450	6z12791	6z12162	6z11564	6z10994	6z10451	7z99339	7z94414

TABLE A.6 Standard Scores (or Deviates) and Ordinates Corresponding to Divisions of the Area under the Normal Curve into a Larger Proportion (*B*) and a Smaller Proportion (*C*)

B Larger area	*Z* Standard score	*u* Ordinate	*C* Smaller area
0.500	0.000	0.3989	0.500
0.505	0.0125	0.3989	0.495
0.510	0.0251	0.3988	0.490
0.515	0.0376	0.3987	0.485
0.520	0.0502	0.3984	0.480
0.525	0.0627	0.3982	0.475
0.530	0.0753	0.3978	0.470
0.535	0.0878	0.3974	0.465
0.540	0.1004	0.3969	0.460
0.545	0.1130	0.3964	0.455
0.550	0.1257	0.3958	0.450
0.555	0.1383	0.3951	0.445
0.560	0.1510	0.3944	0.440
0.565	0.1637	0.3936	0.435
0.570	0.1764	0.3928	0.430
0.575	0.1891	0.3919	0.425
0.580	0.2019	0.3909	0.420
0.585	0.2147	0.3899	0.415
0.590	0.2275	0.3887	0.410
0.595	0.2404	0.3876	0.405
0.600	0.2533	0.3863	0.400
0.605	0.2663	0.3850	0.395
0.610	0.2793	0.3837	0.390
0.615	0.2924	0.3822	0.385
0.620	0.3055	0.3808	0.380
0.625	0.3186	0.3792	0.375
0.630	0.3319	0.3776	0.370
0.635	0.3451	0.3759	0.365
0.640	0.3585	0.3741	0.360
0.645	0.3719	0.3723	0.355
0.650	0.3853	0.3704	0.350
0.655	0.3989	0.3684	0.345
0.660	0.4125	0.3664	0.340
0.665	0.4261	0.3643	0.335
0.670	0.4399	0.3621	0.330
0.675	0.4538	0.3599	0.325
0.680	0.4677	0.3576	0.320
0.685	0.4817	0.3552	0.315
0.690	0.4959	0.3528	0.310
0.695	0.5101	0.3503	0.305
0.700	0.5244	0.3477	0.300

(*continued*)

TABLE A.6 (*Continued*)

B Larger area	*Z* Standard score	*u* Ordinate	*C* Smaller area
0.705	0.5388	0.3450	0.295
0.710	0.5534	0.3423	0.290
0.715	0.5681	0.3395	0.285
0.720	0.5828	0.3366	0.280
0.725	0.5978	0.3337	0.275
0.730	0.6128	0.3306	0.270
0.735	0.6280	0.3275	0.265
0.740	0.6433	0.3244	0.260
0.745	0.6588	0.3211	0.255
0.750	0.6745	0.3178	0.250
0.755	0.6903	0.3144	0.245
0.760	0.7063	0.3109	0.240
0.765	0.7225	0.3073	0.235
0.770	0.7388	0.3036	0.230
0.775	0.7554	0.2999	0.225
0.780	0.7722	0.2961	0.220
0.785	0.7892	0.2922	0.215
0.790	0.8064	0.2882	0.210
0.795	0.8239	0.2841	0.205
0.800	0.8416	0.2800	0.200
0.805	0.8596	0.2757	0.195
0.810	0.8779	0.2714	0.190
0.815	0.8965	0.2669	0.185
0.820	0.9154	0.2624	0.180
0.825	0.9346	0.2578	0.175
0.830	0.9542	0.2531	0.170
0.835	0.9741	0.2482	0.165
0.840	0.9945	0.2433	0.160
0.845	1.0152	0.2383	0.155
0.850	1.0364	0.2332	0.150
0.855	1.0581	0.2279	0.145
0.860	1.0803	0.2226	0.140
0.865	1.1031	0.2171	0.135
0.870	1.1264	0.2115	0.130
0.875	1.1503	0.2059	0.125
0.880	1.1750	0.2000	0.120
0.885	1.2004	0.1941	0.115
0.890	1.2265	0.1880	0.110
0.895	1.2536	0.1818	0.105
0.900	1.2816	0.1755	0.100
0.905	1.3106	0.1690	0.095
0.910	1.3408	0.1624	0.090
0.915	1.3722	0.1556	0.085

(*continued*)

TABLE A.6 ***(Continued)***

B Larger area	*Z* Standard score	*u* Ordinate	*C* Smaller area
0.920	1.4051	0.1487	0.080
0.925	1.4395	0.1416	0.075
0.930	1.4757	0.1343	0.070
0.935	1.5141	0.1268	0.065
0.940	1.5548	0.1191	0.060
0.945	1.5982	0.1112	0.055
0.950	1.6449	0.1031	0.050
0.955	1.6954	0.0948	0.045
0.960	1.7507	0.0862	0.040
0.965	1.8119	0.0773	0.035
0.970	1.8808	0.0680	0.030
0.975	1.9600	0.0584	0.025
0.980	2.0537	0.0484	0.020
0.985	2.1701	0.0379	0.015
0.990	2.3263	0.0267	0.010
0.995	2.5758	0.0145	0.005
0.996	2.6521	0.0118	0.004
0.997	2.7478	0.0091	0.003
0.998	2.8782	0.0063	0.002
0.999	3.0902	0.0034	0.001
0.9995	3.2905	0.0018	0.0005

TABLE A.7 Critical Values of "t"

df	α for two-tailed test 0.2	0.1	0.05	0.02	0.01	0.001
1	3.078	6.314	12.71	31.82	63.66	636.62
2	1.886	2.920	4.303	6.965	9.925	31.599
3	1.638	2.353	3.182	4.541	5.841	12.924
4	1.533	2.132	2.776	3.747	4.604	8.610
5	1.476	2.015	2.571	3.365	4.032	6.869
6	1.440	1.943	2.447	3.143	3.707	5.959
7	1.415	1.895	2.365	2.998	3.499	5.408
8	1.397	1.860	2.306	2.896	3.355	5.041
9	1.383	1.833	2.262	2.821	3.25	4.781
10	1.372	1.812	2.228	2.764	3.169	4.587
11	1.363	1.796	2.201	2.718	3.106	4.437
12	1.356	1.782	2.179	2.681	3.055	4.318
13	1.350	1.771	2.160	2.65	3.012	4.221
14	1.345	1.761	2.145	2.624	2.977	4.140
15	1.341	1.753	2.131	2.602	2.947	4.073
16	1.337	1.746	2.120	2.583	2.921	4.015
17	1.333	1.740	2.110	2.567	2.898	3.965
18	1.330	1.734	2.101	2.552	2.878	3.922
19	1.328	1.729	2.093	2.539	2.861	3.883
20	1.325	1.725	2.086	2.528	2.845	3.850
21	1.323	1.721	2.080	2.518	2.831	3.819
22	1.321	1.717	2.074	2.508	2.819	3.792
23	1.319	1.714	2.069	2.500	2.807	3.768
24	1.318	1.711	2.064	2.492	2.797	3.745
25	1.316	1.708	2.060	2.485	2.787	3.725
26	1.315	1.706	2.056	2.479	2.779	3.707
27	1.314	1.703	2.052	2.473	2.771	3.690
28	1.313	1.701	2.048	2.467	2.763	3.674
29	1.311	1.699	2.045	2.462	2.756	3.659
30	1.310	1.697	2.042	2.457	2.750	3.646
40	1.303	1.684	2.021	2.423	2.704	3.551
60	1.296	1.671	2.000	2.390	2.660	3.460
80	1.292	1.664	1.990	2.374	2.639	3.416
100	1.290	1.660	1.984	2.364	2.626	3.390
1000	1.282	1.646	1.962	2.330	2.581	3.300
∞	1.282	1.645	1.960	2.326	2.576	3.291
df	0.10	0.05	0.025	0.01	0.005	0.0005
	α for one-tailed test					

TABLE A.8 Critical Values of the Correlation Coefficient

	α for two-tailed test			
df (*n* − 2)	0.10	0.05	0.02	0.01
1	0.988	0.997	0.9995	0.9999
2	0.900	0.950	0.980	0.990
3	0.805	0.878	0.934	0.959
4	0.729	0.811	0.882	0.917
5	0.669	0.754	0.833	0.874
6	0.622	0.707	0.789	0.834
7	0.582	0.666	0.750	0.798
8	0.549	0.632	0.716	0.765
9	0.521	0.602	0.685	0.735
10	0.497	0.576	0.658	0.708
11	0.476	0.553	0.634	0.684
12	0.458	0.532	0.612	0.661
13	0.441	0.514	0.592	0.641
14	0.426	0.497	0.574	0.623
15	0.412	0.482	0.558	0.606
16	0.400	0.468	0.542	0.590
17	0.389	0.456	0.528	0.575
18	0.378	0.444	0.516	0.561
19	0.369	0.433	0.503	0.549
20	0.360	0.423	0.492	0.537
21	0.352	0.413	0.482	0.526
22	0.344	0.404	0.472	0.515
23	0.337	0.396	0.462	0.505
24	0.330	0.388	0.453	0.496
25	0.323	0.381	0.445	0.487
26	0.317	0.374	0.437	0.479
27	0.311	0.367	0.430	0.471
28	0.306	0.361	0.423	0.463
29	0.301	0.355	0.416	0.456
30	0.296	0.349	0.409	0.449
35	0.275	0.325	0.381	0.418
40	0.257	0.304	0.358	0.393
45	0.243	0.288	0.338	0.372
50	0.231	0.273	0.322	0.354
60	0.211	0.250	0.295	0.325
70	0.195	0.232	0.274	0.303
80	0.183	0.217	0.256	0.283
90	0.173	0.205	0.242	0.267
100	0.164	0.195	0.230	0.254
df (*n* − 2)	0.05	0.25	0.01	0.005
	α for one-tailed test			

TABLE A.9 *F*-Table: Critical Values $\alpha = 0.05$

n_1/n_2	1	2	3	4	5	6	7	8	9	10	11	12	13	14	15	16	17	18	19	20	22	24	26	28	30	35	40	45	50	60	70	80	100	200	500	1000	>1000	n_1/n_2
3	1.13	9.55	9.28	9.12	9.01	8.94	8.89	8.85	8.81	8.79	8.76	8.74	8.73	8.71	8.7	8.69	8.68	8.67	8.67	8.66	8.65	8.64	8.63	8.62	8.62	8.6	8.59	8.59	8.58	8.57	8.57	8.56	8.55	8.54	8.53	8.53	8.54	3
4	7.71	6.94	6.59	6.39	6.26	6.16	6.09	6.04	6	5.96	5.94	5.91	5.89	5.87	5.86	5.84	5.83	5.82	5.81	5.8	5.79	5.77	5.76	5.75	5.75	5.73	5.72	5.71	5.7	5.69	5.68	5.67	5.66	5.65	5.64	5.63	5.63	4
5	6.61	5.79	5.41	5.19	5.05	4.95	4.88	4.82	4.77	4.74	4.7	4.68	4.66	4.64	4.62	4.6	4.59	4.58	4.57	4.56	4.54	4.53	4.52	4.5	4.5	4.48	4.46	4.45	4.44	4.43	4.42	4.42	4.41	4.39	4.37	4.37	4.36	5
6	5.99	5.14	4.76	4.53	4.39	4.28	4.21	4.15	4.1	4.06	4.03	4	3.98	3.96	3.94	3.92	3.91	3.9	3.88	3.87	3.86	3.84	3.83	3.82	3.81	3.79	3.77	3.76	3.75	3.74	3.73	3.72	3.71	3.69	3.68	3.67	3.67	6
7	5.59	4.74	4.35	4.12	3.97	3.87	3.79	3.73	3.68	3.64	3.6	3.57	3.55	3.53	3.51	3.49	3.48	3.47	3.46	3.44	3.43	3.41	3.4	3.39	3.38	3.36	3.34	3.33	3.32	3.3	3.29	3.29	3.27	3.25	3.24	3.23	3.23	7
8	5.32	4.46	4.07	3.84	3.69	3.58	3.5	3.44	3.39	3.35	3.31	3.28	3.26	3.24	3.22	3.2	3.19	3.17	3.16	3.15	3.13	3.12	3.1	3.09	3.08	3.06	3.04	3.03	3.02	3.01	2.99	2.99	2.97	2.95	2.94	2.93	2.93	8
9	5.12	4.26	3.86	3.63	3.48	3.37	3.29	3.23	3.18	3.14	3.1	3.07	3.05	3.03	3.01	2.99	2.97	2.96	2.95	2.94	2.92	2.9	2.89	2.87	2.86	2.84	2.83	2.81	2.8	2.79	2.78	2.77	2.76	2.73	2.72	2.71	2.71	9
10	4.96	4.1	3.71	3.48	3.33	3.22	3.14	3.07	3.02	2.98	2.94	2.91	2.89	2.86	2.85	2.83	2.81	2.8	2.79	2.77	2.75	2.74	2.72	2.71	2.7	2.68	2.66	2.65	2.64	2.62	2.61	2.6	2.59	2.56	2.55	2.54	2.54	10
11	4.84	3.98	3.59	3.36	3.2	3.09	3.01	2.95	2.9	2.85	2.82	2.79	2.76	2.74	2.72	2.7	2.69	2.67	2.66	2.65	2.63	2.61	2.59	2.58	2.57	2.55	2.53	2.52	2.51	2.49	2.48	2.47	2.46	2.43	2.42	2.41	2.41	11
12	4.75	3.89	3.49	3.26	3.11	3	2.91	2.85	2.8	2.75	2.72	2.69	2.66	2.64	2.62	2.6	2.58	2.57	2.56	2.54	2.52	2.51	2.49	2.48	2.47	2.44	2.43	2.41	2.4	2.38	2.37	2.36	2.35	2.32	2.31	2.3	2.3	12
13	4.67	3.81	3.41	3.18	3.03	2.92	2.83	2.77	2.71	2.67	2.63	2.6	2.58	2.55	2.53	2.51	2.5	2.48	2.47	2.46	2.44	2.42	2.41	2.39	2.38	2.36	2.34	2.33	2.31	2.3	2.28	2.27	2.26	2.23	2.22	2.21	2.21	13
14	4.6	3.74	3.34	3.11	2.96	2.85	2.76	2.7	2.65	2.6	2.57	2.53	2.51	2.48	2.46	2.44	2.43	2.41	2.4	2.39	2.37	2.35	2.33	2.32	2.31	2.28	2.27	2.25	2.24	2.22	2.21	2.2	2.19	2.16	2.14	2.14	2.13	14
15	4.54	3.68	3.29	3.06	2.9	2.79	2.71	2.64	2.59	2.54	2.51	2.48	2.45	2.42	2.4	2.38	2.37	2.35	2.34	2.33	2.31	2.29	2.27	2.26	2.25	2.22	2.2	2.19	2.18	2.16	2.15	2.14	2.12	2.1	2.08	2.07	2.07	15
16	4.49	3.63	3.24	3.01	2.85	2.74	2.66	2.59	2.54	2.49	2.46	2.42	2.4	2.37	2.35	2.33	2.32	2.3	2.29	2.28	2.25	2.24	2.22	2.21	2.19	2.17	2.15	2.14	2.12	2.11	2.09	2.08	2.07	2.04	2.02	2.02	2.01	16
17	4.45	3.59	3.2	2.96	2.81	2.7	2.61	2.55	2.49	2.45	2.41	2.38	2.35	2.33	2.31	2.29	2.27	2.26	2.24	2.23	2.21	2.19	2.17	2.16	2.15	2.12	2.1	2.09	2.08	2.06	2.05	2.03	2.02	1.99	1.97	1.97	1.96	17
18	4.41	3.55	3.16	2.93	2.77	2.66	2.58	2.51	2.46	2.41	2.37	2.34	2.31	2.29	2.27	2.25	2.23	2.22	2.2	2.19	2.17	2.15	2.13	2.12	2.11	2.08	2.06	2.05	2.04	2.02	2	1.99	1.98	1.95	1.93	1.92	1.92	18
19	4.38	3.52	3.13	2.9	2.74	2.63	2.54	2.48	2.42	2.38	2.34	2.31	2.28	2.26	2.23	2.21	2.2	2.18	2.17	2.16	2.13	2.11	2.1	2.08	2.07	2.05	2.03	2.01	2	1.98	1.97	1.96	1.94	1.91	1.89	1.88	1.88	19
20	4.35	3.49	3.1	2.87	2.71	2.6	2.51	2.45	2.39	2.35	2.31	2.28	2.25	2.23	2.2	2.18	2.17	2.15	2.14	2.12	2.1	2.08	2.07	2.05	2.04	2.01	1.99	1.98	1.97	1.95	1.93	1.92	1.91	1.88	1.86	1.85	1.84	20
22	4.3	3.44	3.05	2.82	2.66	2.55	2.46	2.4	2.34	2.3	2.26	2.23	2.2	2.17	2.15	2.13	2.11	2.1	2.08	2.07	2.05	2.03	2.01	2	1.98	1.96	1.94	1.92	1.91	1.89	1.88	1.86	1.85	1.82	1.8	1.79	1.78	22
24	4.26	3.4	3.01	2.78	2.62	2.51	2.42	2.36	2.3	2.25	2.22	2.18	2.15	2.13	2.11	2.09	2.07	2.05	2.04	2.03	2	1.98	1.97	1.95	1.94	1.91	1.89	1.88	1.86	1.84	1.83	1.82	1.8	1.77	1.75	1.74	1.73	24
26	4.23	3.37	2.98	2.74	2.59	2.47	2.39	2.32	2.27	2.22	2.18	2.15	2.12	2.09	2.07	2.05	2.03	2.02	2	1.99	1.97	1.95	1.93	1.91	1.9	1.87	1.85	1.84	1.82	1.8	1.79	1.78	1.76	1.73	1.71	1.7	1.69	26
28	4.2	3.34	2.95	2.71	2.56	2.45	2.36	2.29	2.24	2.19	2.15	2.12	2.09	2.06	2.04	2.02	2	1.99	1.97	1.96	1.93	1.91	1.9	1.88	1.87	1.84	1.82	1.8	1.79	1.77	1.75	1.74	1.73	1.69	1.67	1.66	1.66	28
30	4.17	3.32	2.92	2.69	2.53	2.42	2.33	2.27	2.21	2.16	2.13	2.09	2.06	2.04	2.01	1.99	1.98	1.96	1.95	1.93	1.91	1.89	1.87	1.85	1.84	1.81	1.79	1.77	1.76	1.74	1.72	1.71	1.7	1.66	1.64	1.63	1.62	30
35	4.12	3.27	2.87	2.64	2.49	2.37	2.29	2.22	2.16	2.11	2.08	2.04	2.01	1.99	1.96	1.94	1.92	1.91	1.89	1.88	1.85	1.83	1.82	1.8	1.79	1.76	1.74	1.72	1.7	1.68	1.66	1.65	1.63	1.6	1.57	1.57	1.56	35
40	4.08	3.23	2.84	2.61	2.45	2.34	2.25	2.18	2.12	2.08	2.04	2	1.97	1.95	1.92	1.9	1.89	1.87	1.85	1.84	1.81	1.79	1.77	1.76	1.74	1.72	1.69	1.67	1.66	1.64	1.62	1.61	1.59	1.55	1.53	1.52	1.51	40
45	4.06	3.2	2.81	2.58	2.42	2.31	2.22	2.15	2.1	2.05	2.01	1.97	1.94	1.92	1.89	1.87	1.86	1.84	1.82	1.81	1.78	1.76	1.74	1.73	1.71	1.68	1.66	1.64	1.63	1.6	1.59	1.57	1.55	1.51	1.49	1.48	1.47	45
50	4.03	3.18	2.79	2.56	2.4	2.29	2.2	2.13	2.07	2.03	1.99	1.95	1.92	1.89	1.87	1.85	1.83	1.81	1.8	1.78	1.76	1.74	1.72	1.7	1.69	1.66	1.63	1.61	1.6	1.58	1.56	1.54	1.52	1.48	1.46	1.45	1.44	50
60	4	3.15	2.76	2.53	2.37	2.25	2.17	2.1	2.04	1.99	1.95	1.92	1.89	1.86	1.84	1.82	1.8	1.78	1.76	1.75	1.72	1.7	1.68	1.66	1.65	1.62	1.59	1.57	1.56	1.53	1.52	1.5	1.48	1.44	1.41	1.4	1.39	60
70	3.98	3.13	2.74	2.5	2.35	2.23	2.14	2.07	2.02	1.97	1.93	1.89	1.86	1.84	1.81	1.79	1.77	1.75	1.74	1.72	1.7	1.67	1.65	1.64	1.62	1.59	1.57	1.55	1.53	1.5	1.49	1.47	1.45	1.4	1.37	1.36	1.35	70
80	3.96	3.11	2.72	2.49	2.33	2.21	2.13	2.06	2	1.95	1.91	1.88	1.84	1.82	1.79	1.77	1.75	1.73	1.72	1.7	1.68	1.65	1.63	1.62	1.6	1.57	1.54	1.52	1.51	1.48	1.46	1.45	1.43	1.38	1.35	1.34	1.33	80
100	3.94	3.09	2.7	2.46	2.31	2.19	2.1	2.03	1.97	1.93	1.89	1.85	1.82	1.79	1.77	1.75	1.73	1.71	1.69	1.68	1.65	1.63	1.61	1.59	1.57	1.54	1.52	1.49	1.48	1.45	1.43	1.41	1.39	1.34	1.31	1.3	1.28	100
200	3.89	3.04	2.65	2.42	2.26	2.14	2.06	1.98	1.93	1.88	1.84	1.8	1.77	1.74	1.72	1.69	1.67	1.66	1.64	1.62	1.6	1.57	1.55	1.53	1.52	1.48	1.46	1.43	1.41	1.39	1.36	1.35	1.32	1.26	1.22	1.21	1.19	200
500	3.86	3.01	2.62	2.39	2.23	2.12	2.03	1.96	1.9	1.85	1.81	1.77	1.74	1.71	1.69	1.66	1.64	1.62	1.61	1.59	1.56	1.54	1.52	1.5	1.48	1.45	1.42	1.4	1.38	1.35	1.32	1.3	1.28	1.21	1.16	1.14	1.12	500
1000	3.85	3	2.61	2.38	2.22	2.11	2.02	1.95	1.89	1.84	1.8	1.76	1.73	1.7	1.68	1.65	1.63	1.61	1.6	1.58	1.55	1.53	1.51	1.49	1.47	1.43	1.41	1.38	1.36	1.33	1.31	1.29	1.26	1.19	1.13	1.11	1.08	1000
>1000	1.04	3	2.61	2.37	2.21	2.1	2.01	1.94	1.88	1.83	1.79	1.75	1.72	1.69	1.67	1.64	1.62	1.61	1.59	1.57	1.54	1.52	1.5	1.48	1.46	1.42	1.4	1.37	1.35	1.32	1.3	1.28	1.25	1.17	1.11	1.08	1.03	>1000
n_1/n_2	1	2	3	4	5	6	7	8	9	10	11	12	13	14	15	16	17	18	19	20	22	24	26	28	30	35	40	45	50	60	70	80	100	200	500	1000	>1000	n_1/n_2

TABLE A.10 *F*-Table: Critical Values $\alpha = 0.01$

n_1/n_2	1	2	3	4	5	6	7	8	9	10	11	12	13	14	15	16	17	18	19	20	22	24	26	28	30	35	40	45	50	60	70	80	100	200	500	1000	>1000	n_1/n_2
3	34.12	3.82	29.46	28.71	28.24	27.91	27.67	27.49	27.35	27.23	27.13	27.05	26.98	26.92	26.87	26.83	26.79	26.75	26.72	26.69	26.64	26.6	26.56	26.53	26.5	26.45	26.41	26.38	26.35	26.32	26.29	26.27	26.24	26.18	26.15	26.13	26.15	3
4	21.2	18	16.69	15.98	15.52	15.21	14.98	14.8	14.66	14.55	14.45	14.37	14.31	14.25	14.2	14.15	14.11	14.08	14.05	14.02	13.97	13.93	13.89	13.86	13.84	13.79	13.75	13.71	13.69	13.65	13.63	13.61	13.58	13.52	13.49	13.47	13.47	4
5	16.26	13.27	12.06	11.39	1.97	1.67	1.46	1.29	1.16	1.05	9.96	9.89	9.82	9.77	9.72	9.68	9.64	9.61	9.58	9.55	9.51	9.47	9.43	9.4	9.38	9.33	9.29	9.26	9.24	9.2	9.18	9.16	9.13	9.08	9.04	9.03	9.02	5
6	13.75	1.92	9.78	9.15	8.75	8.47	8.26	8.1	7.98	7.87	7.79	7.72	7.66	7.61	7.56	7.52	7.48	7.45	7.42	7.4	7.35	7.31	7.28	7.25	7.23	7.18	7.14	7.11	7.09	7.06	7.03	7.01	6.99	6.93	6.9	6.89	6.89	6
7	12.25	9.55	8.45	7.85	7.46	7.19	6.99	6.84	6.72	6.62	6.54	6.47	6.41	6.36	6.31	6.28	6.24	6.21	6.18	6.16	6.11	6.07	6.04	6.02	5.99	5.94	5.91	5.88	5.86	5.82	5.8	5.78	5.75	5.7	5.67	5.66	5.65	7
8	11.26	8.65	7.59	7.01	6.63	6.37	6.18	6.03	5.91	5.81	5.73	5.67	5.61	5.56	5.52	5.48	5.44	5.41	5.38	5.36	5.32	5.28	5.25	5.22	5.2	5.15	5.12	5.09	5.07	5.03	5.01	4.99	4.96	4.91	4.88	4.87	4.86	8
9	1.56	8.02	6.99	6.42	6.06	5.8	5.61	5.47	5.35	5.26	5.18	5.11	5.05	5.01	4.96	4.92	4.89	4.86	4.83	4.81	4.77	4.73	4.7	4.67	4.65	4.6	4.57	4.54	4.52	4.48	4.46	4.44	4.42	4.36	4.33	4.32	4.32	9
10	1.04	7.56	6.55	5.99	5.64	5.39	5.2	5.06	4.94	4.85	4.77	4.71	4.65	4.6	4.56	4.52	4.49	4.46	4.43	4.41	4.36	4.33	4.3	4.27	4.25	4.2	4.17	4.14	4.12	4.08	4.06	4.04	4.01	3.96	3.93	3.92	3.91	10
11	9.65	7.21	6.22	5.67	5.32	5.07	4.89	4.74	4.63	4.54	4.46	4.4	4.34	4.29	4.25	4.21	4.18	4.15	4.12	4.1	4.06	4.02	3.99	3.96	3.94	3.89	3.86	3.83	3.81	3.78	3.75	3.73	3.71	3.66	3.62	3.61	3.6	11
12	9.33	6.93	5.95	5.41	5.06	4.82	4.64	4.5	4.39	4.3	4.22	4.16	4.1	4.05	4.01	3.97	3.94	3.91	3.88	3.86	3.82	3.78	3.75	3.72	3.7	3.65	3.62	3.59	3.57	3.54	3.51	3.49	3.47	3.41	3.38	3.37	3.36	12
13	9.07	6.7	5.74	5.21	4.86	4.62	4.44	4.3	4.19	4.1	4.02	3.96	3.91	3.86	3.82	3.78	3.75	3.72	3.69	3.66	3.62	3.59	3.56	3.53	3.51	3.46	3.43	3.4	3.38	3.34	3.32	3.3	3.27	3.22	3.19	3.18	3.17	13
14	8.86	6.51	5.56	5.04	4.7	4.46	4.28	4.14	4.03	3.94	3.86	3.8	3.75	3.7	3.66	3.62	3.59	3.56	3.53	3.51	3.46	3.43	3.4	3.37	3.35	3.3	3.27	3.24	3.22	3.18	3.16	3.14	3.11	3.06	3.03	3.01	3.01	14
15	8.68	6.36	5.42	4.89	4.56	4.32	4.14	4	3.89	3.8	3.73	3.67	3.61	3.56	3.52	3.49	3.45	3.42	3.4	3.37	3.33	3.29	3.26	3.24	3.21	3.17	3.13	3.1	3.08	3.05	3.02	3	2.98	2.92	2.89	2.88	2.87	15
16	8.53	6.23	5.29	4.77	4.44	4.2	4.03	3.89	3.78	3.69	3.62	3.55	3.5	3.45	3.41	3.37	3.34	3.31	3.28	3.26	3.22	3.18	3.15	3.12	3.1	3.05	3.02	2.99	2.97	2.93	2.91	2.89	2.86	2.81	2.78	2.76	2.75	16
17	8.4	6.11	5.19	4.67	4.34	4.1	3.93	3.79	3.68	3.59	3.52	3.46	3.4	3.35	3.31	3.27	3.24	3.21	3.19	3.16	3.12	3.08	3.05	3.03	3	2.96	2.92	2.89	2.87	2.83	2.81	2.79	2.76	2.71	2.68	2.66	2.65	17
18	8.29	6.01	5.09	4.58	4.25	4.01	3.84	3.71	3.6	3.51	3.43	3.37	3.32	3.27	3.23	3.19	3.16	3.13	3.1	3.08	3.03	3	2.97	2.94	2.92	2.87	2.84	2.81	2.78	2.75	2.72	2.71	2.68	2.62	2.59	2.58	2.57	18
19	8.19	5.93	5.01	4.5	4.17	3.94	3.77	3.63	3.52	3.43	3.36	3.3	3.24	3.19	3.15	3.12	3.08	3.05	3.03	3	2.96	2.92	2.89	2.87	2.84	2.8	2.76	2.73	2.71	2.67	2.65	2.63	2.6	2.55	2.51	2.5	2.49	19
20	8.1	5.85	4.94	4.43	4.1	3.87	3.7	3.56	3.46	3.37	3.29	3.23	3.18	3.13	3.09	3.05	3.02	2.99	2.96	2.94	2.9	2.86	2.83	2.8	2.78	2.73	2.69	2.67	2.64	2.61	2.58	2.56	2.54	2.48	2.44	2.43	2.42	20
22	7.95	5.72	4.82	4.31	3.99	3.76	3.59	3.45	3.35	3.26	3.18	3.12	3.07	3.02	2.98	2.94	2.91	2.88	2.85	2.83	2.78	2.75	2.72	2.69	2.67	2.62	2.58	2.55	2.53	2.5	2.47	2.45	2.42	2.36	2.33	2.32	2.31	22
24	7.82	5.61	4.72	4.22	3.9	3.67	3.5	3.36	3.26	3.17	3.09	3.03	2.98	2.93	2.89	2.85	2.82	2.79	2.76	2.74	2.7	2.66	2.63	2.6	2.58	2.53	2.49	2.46	2.44	2.4	2.38	2.36	2.33	2.27	2.24	2.22	2.21	24
26	7.72	5.53	4.64	4.14	3.82	3.59	3.42	3.29	3.18	3.09	3.02	2.96	2.9	2.86	2.82	2.78	2.75	2.72	2.69	2.66	2.62	2.58	2.55	2.53	2.5	2.45	2.42	2.39	2.36	2.33	2.3	2.28	2.25	2.19	2.16	2.14	2.13	26
28	7.64	5.45	4.57	4.07	3.75	3.53	3.36	3.23	3.12	3.03	2.96	2.9	2.84	2.79	2.75	2.72	2.68	2.65	2.63	2.6	2.56	2.52	2.49	2.46	2.44	2.39	2.35	2.32	2.3	2.26	2.24	2.22	2.19	2.13	2.09	2.08	2.07	28
30	7.56	5.39	4.51	4.02	3.7	3.47	3.3	3.17	3.07	2.98	2.91	2.84	2.79	2.74	2.7	2.66	2.63	2.6	2.57	2.55	2.51	2.47	2.44	2.41	2.39	2.34	2.3	2.27	2.25	2.21	2.18	2.16	2.13	2.07	2.03	2.02	2.01	30
35	7.42	5.27	4.4	3.91	3.59	3.37	3.2	3.07	2.96	2.88	2.8	2.74	2.69	2.64	2.6	2.56	2.53	2.5	2.47	2.44	2.4	2.36	2.33	2.31	2.28	2.23	2.19	2.16	2.14	2.1	2.07	2.05	2.02	1.96	1.92	1.9	1.89	35
40	7.31	5.18	4.31	3.83	3.51	3.29	3.12	2.99	2.89	2.8	2.73	2.66	2.61	2.56	2.52	2.48	2.45	2.42	2.39	2.37	2.33	2.29	2.26	2.23	2.2	2.15	2.11	2.08	2.06	2.02	1.99	1.97	1.94	1.87	1.83	1.82	1.81	40
45	7.23	5.11	4.25	3.77	3.45	3.23	3.07	2.94	2.83	2.74	2.67	2.61	2.55	2.51	2.46	2.43	2.39	2.36	2.34	2.31	2.27	2.23	2.2	2.17	2.14	2.09	2.05	2.02	2	1.96	1.93	1.91	1.88	1.81	1.77	1.75	1.74	45
50	7.17	5.06	4.2	3.72	3.41	3.19	3.02	2.89	2.79	2.7	2.63	2.56	2.51	2.46	2.42	2.38	2.35	2.32	2.29	2.27	2.22	2.18	2.15	2.12	2.1	2.05	2.01	1.97	1.95	1.91	1.88	1.86	1.82	1.76	1.71	1.7	1.69	50
60	7.08	4.98	4.13	3.65	3.34	3.12	2.95	2.82	2.72	2.63	2.56	2.5	2.44	2.39	2.35	2.31	2.28	2.25	2.22	2.2	2.15	2.12	2.08	2.05	2.03	1.98	1.94	1.9	1.88	1.84	1.81	1.78	1.75	1.68	1.63	1.62	1.6	60
70	7.01	4.92	4.07	3.6	3.29	3.07	2.91	2.78	2.67	2.59	2.51	2.45	2.4	2.35	2.31	2.27	2.23	2.2	2.18	2.15	2.11	2.07	2.03	2.01	1.98	1.93	1.89	1.85	1.83	1.78	1.75	1.73	1.7	1.62	1.57	1.56	1.54	70
80	6.96	4.88	4.04	3.56	3.26	3.04	2.87	2.74	2.64	2.55	2.48	2.42	2.36	2.31	2.27	2.23	2.2	2.17	2.14	2.12	2.07	2.03	2	1.97	1.94	1.89	1.85	1.82	1.79	1.75	1.71	1.69	1.65	1.58	1.53	1.51	1.5	80
100	6.9	4.82	3.98	3.51	3.21	2.99	2.82	2.69	2.59	2.5	2.43	2.37	2.31	2.27	2.22	2.19	2.15	2.12	2.09	2.07	2.02	1.98	1.95	1.92	1.89	1.84	1.8	1.76	1.74	1.69	1.66	1.63	1.6	1.52	1.47	1.45	1.43	100
200	6.76	4.71	3.88	3.41	3.11	2.89	2.73	2.6	2.5	2.41	2.34	2.27	2.22	2.17	2.13	2.09	2.06	2.03	2	1.97	1.93	1.89	1.85	1.82	1.79	1.74	1.69	1.66	1.63	1.58	1.55	1.52	1.48	1.39	1.33	1.3	1.28	200
500	6.69	4.65	3.82	3.36	3.05	2.84	2.68	2.55	2.44	2.36	2.28	2.22	2.17	2.12	2.07	2.04	2	1.97	1.94	1.92	1.87	1.83	1.79	1.76	1.74	1.68	1.63	1.6	1.57	1.52	1.48	1.45	1.41	1.31	1.23	1.2	1.17	500
1000	6.66	4.63	3.8	3.34	3.04	2.82	2.66	2.53	2.43	2.34	2.27	2.2	2.15	2.1	2.06	2.02	1.98	1.95	1.92	1.9	1.85	1.81	1.77	1.74	1.72	1.66	1.61	1.58	1.54	1.5	1.46	1.43	1.38	1.28	1.19	1.16	1.12	1000
>1000	1.04	4.61	3.78	3.32	3.02	2.8	2.64	2.51	2.41	2.32	2.25	2.19	2.13	2.08	2.04	2	1.97	1.94	1.91	1.88	1.83	1.79	1.76	1.73	1.7	1.64	1.59	1.56	1.53	1.48	1.44	1.41	1.36	1.25	1.16	1.11	1.05	>1000
n_1/n_2	1	2	3	4	5	6	7	8	9	10	11	12	13	14	15	16	17	18	19	20	22	24	26	28	30	35	40	45	50	60	70	80	100	200	500	1000	>1000	n_1/n_2

TABLE A.11 The Chi-square Table

Values of χ^2 for selected probabilities

	Area in upper tail									
df	0.995	0.99	0.975	0.95	0.90	0.10	0.05	0.025	0.01	0.005
1			0.001	0.004	0.016	2.706	3.841	5.024	6.635	7.879
2	0.010	0.020	0.051	0.103	0.211	4.605	5.991	7.378	9.210	1.597
3	0.072	0.115	0.216	0.352	0.584	6.251	7.815	9.348	11.345	12.838
4	0.207	0.297	0.484	0.711	1.064	7.779	9.488	11.143	13.277	14.860
5	0.412	0.554	0.831	1.145	1.610	9.236	11.070	12.833	15.086	16.750
6	0.676	0.872	1.237	1.635	2.204	1.645	12.592	14.449	16.812	18.548
7	0.989	1.239	1.690	2.167	2.833	12.017	14.067	16.013	18.475	2.278
8	1.344	1.646	2.180	2.733	3.490	13.362	15.507	17.535	2.090	21.955
9	1.735	2.088	2.700	3.325	4.168	14.684	16.919	19.023	21.666	23.589
10	2.156	2.558	3.247	3.940	4.865	15.987	18.307	2.483	23.209	25.188
11	2.603	3.053	3.816	4.575	5.578	17.275	19.675	21.920	24.725	26.757
12	3.074	3.571	4.404	5.226	6.304	18.549	21.026	23.337	26.217	28.300
13	3.565	4.107	5.009	5.892	7.042	19.812	22.362	24.736	27.688	29.819
14	4.075	4.660	5.629	6.571	7.790	21.064	23.685	26.119	29.141	31.319
15	4.601	5.229	6.262	7.261	8.547	22.307	24.996	27.488	3.578	32.801
16	5.142	5.812	6.908	7.962	9.312	23.542	26.296	28.845	32.000	34.267
17	5.697	6.408	7.564	8.672	1.085	24.769	27.587	3.191	33.409	35.718
18	6.265	7.015	8.231	9.390	1.865	25.989	28.869	31.526	34.805	37.156
19	6.844	7.633	8.907	1.117	11.651	27.204	3.144	32.852	36.191	38.582
20	7.434	8.260	9.591	1.851	12.443	28.412	31.410	34.170	37.566	39.997
21	8.034	8.897	1.283	11.591	13.240	29.615	32.671	35.479	38.932	41.401
22	8.643	9.542	1.982	12.338	14.041	3.813	33.924	36.781	4.289	42.796
23	9.260	1.196	11.689	13.091	14.848	32.007	35.172	38.076	41.638	44.181
24	9.886	1.856	12.401	13.848	15.659	33.196	36.415	39.364	42.980	45.559
25	1.520	11.524	13.120	14.611	16.473	34.382	37.652	4.646	44.314	46.928
26	11.160	12.198	13.844	15.379	17.292	35.563	38.885	41.923	45.642	48.290
27	11.808	12.879	14.573	16.151	18.114	36.741	4.113	43.195	46.963	49.645
28	12.461	13.565	15.308	16.928	18.939	37.916	41.337	44.461	48.278	5.993
29	13.121	14.256	16.047	17.708	19.768	39.087	42.557	45.722	49.588	52.336
30	13.787	14.953	16.791	18.493	2.599	4.256	43.773	46.979	5.892	53.672
40	2.707	22.164	24.433	26.509	29.051	51.805	55.758	59.342	63.691	66.766
50	27.991	29.707	32.357	34.764	37.689	63.167	67.505	71.420	76.154	79.490
60	35.534	37.485	4.482	43.188	46.459	74.397	79.082	83.298	88.379	91.952
70	43.275	45.442	48.758	51.739	55.329	85.527	9.531	95.023	10.425	104.215
80	51.172	53.540	57.153	6.391	64.278	96.578	101.879	106.629	112.329	116.321
90	59.196	61.754	65.647	69.126	73.291	107.565	113.145	118.136	124.116	128.299
100	67.328	7.065	74.222	77.929	82.358	118.498	124.342	129.561	135.807	14.169

TABLE A.12 Critical Values for Number of Runs *R*

Value of n_1	Value of n_2: 2	3	4	5	6	7	8	9	10	11	12	13	14	15	16	17	18	19	20
2	1	1	1	1	1	1	1	1	1	1	2	2	2	2	2	2	2	2	2
	6	6	6	6	6	6	6	6	6	6	6	6	6	6	6	6	6	6	6
3	1	1	1	1	2	2	2	2	2	2	2	2	2	3	3	3	3	3	3
	6	8	8	8	8	8	8	8	8	8	8	8	8	8	8	8	8	8	8
4	1	1	1	2	2	2	3	3	3	3	3	3	3	3	4	4	4	4	4
	6	8	9	9	9	10	10	10	10	10	10	10	10	10	10	10	10	10	10
5	1	1	2	2	3	3	3	3	3	4	4	4	4	4	4	4	5	5	5
	6	8	9	10	10	11	11	12	12	12	12	12	12	12	12	12	12	12	12
6	1	2	2	3	3	3	3	4	4	4	4	5	5	5	5	5	5	6	6
	6	8	9	10	11	12	12	13	13	13	13	14	14	14	14	14	14	14	14
7	1	2	2	3	3	3	4	4	5	5	5	5	5	6	6	6	6	6	6
	6	8	10	11	12	13	13	14	14	14	14	15	15	15	16	16	16	16	16
8	1	2	3	3	3	4	4	5	5	5	6	6	6	6	6	7	7	7	7
	6	8	10	11	12	13	14	14	15	15	16	16	16	16	17	17	17	17	17
9	1	2	3	3	4	4	5	5	5	6	6	6	7	7	7	7	8	8	8
	6	8	10	12	13	14	14	15	16	16	16	17	17	18	18	18	18	18	18
10	1	2	3	3	4	5	5	5	6	6	7	7	7	7	8	8	8	8	9
	6	8	10	12	13	14	15	16	16	17	17	18	18	18	19	19	19	20	20
11	1	2	3	4	4	5	5	6	6	7	7	7	8	8	8	9	9	9	9
	6	8	10	12	13	14	15	16	17	17	18	19	19	19	20	20	20	21	21
12	2	2	3	4	4	5	6	6	7	7	7	8	8	8	9	9	9	10	10
	6	8	10	12	13	14	16	16	17	18	19	19	20	20	21	21	21	22	22
13	2	2	3	4	5	5	6	6	7	7	8	8	9	9	9	10	10	10	10
	6	8	10	12	14	15	16	17	18	19	19	20	20	21	21	22	22	23	23
14	2	2	3	4	5	5	6	7	7	8	8	9	9	9	10	10	10	11	11
	6	8	10	12	14	15	16	17	18	19	20	20	21	22	22	23	23	23	24
15	2	3	3	4	5	6	6	7	7	8	8	9	9	10	10	11	11	11	12
	6	8	10	12	14	15	16	18	18	19	20	21	22	22	23	23	24	24	25
16	2	3	4	4	5	6	6	7	8	8	9	9	10	10	11	11	11	12	12
	6	8	10	12	14	16	17	18	19	20	21	21	22	23	23	24	25	25	25
17	2	3	4	4	5	6	7	7	8	9	9	10	10	11	11	11	12	12	13
	6	8	10	12	14	16	17	18	19	20	21	22	23	23	24	25	25	26	26
18	2	3	4	5	5	6	7	8	8	9	9	10	10	11	11	12	12	13	13
	6	8	10	12	14	16	17	18	19	20	21	22	23	24	25	25	26	26	27
19	2	3	4	5	6	6	7	8	8	9	10	10	11	11	12	12	13	13	13
	6	8	10	12	14	16	17	18	20	21	22	23	23	24	25	26	26	27	27
20	2	3	4	5	6	6	7	8	9	9	10	10	11	12	12	13	13	13	14
	6	8	10	12	14	16	17	18	20	21	22	23	24	25	25	26	27	27	28

Note: The entries in this table are the critical *R* value assuming a two-tailed test with a significance level of $\alpha = 0.05$.

Source: Adapted from Swed FS, Eisenhart C. The Annals of Mathematical Statistics 1943; 14: 83–86, with the kind permission of the publisher.

TABLE A.13 Critical Values for the Mann–Whitney U-Test

	Level of significance: 5% ($p = 0.05$) Size of the largest sample (n_2)															
	5	6	7	8	9	10	11	12	13	14	15	16	17	18	19	20
2	0	0	0	0	0	0	0	1	1	1	1	1	2	2	2	2
3	0	1	1	2	2	3	3	4	4	5	5	6	6	7	7	8
4	1	2	3	4	4	5	6	7	8	9	10	11	11	12	13	14
5	2	3	5	6	7	8	9	11	12	13	14	15	17	18	19	20
6		5	6	8	10	11	13	14	16	17	19	21	22	24	25	27
7			8	10	12	14	16	18	20	22	24	26	28	30	32	34
8				13	15	17	19	22	24	26	29	31	34	36	38	41
9					17	20	23	26	28	31	34	37	39	42	45	48
10						23	26	29	33	36	39	42	45	48	52	55
11							30	33	37	40	44	47	51	55	58	62
12								37	41	45	49	53	57	61	65	69
13									45	50	54	59	63	67	72	76
14										55	59	64	67	74	78	83
15											64	70	75	80	85	90
16												75	81	86	92	98
17													87	93	99	105
18														99	106	112
19															113	119
20																127

Source: Adapted and abridged from the Table of Auble D. 1953. Extended tables for the Mann–Whitney statistic. Bulletin of the Institute of Educational Research of Indiana University, 1, No. 2, with the kind permission of the author and the publisher.

TABLE A.14 Critical Values of T for the Wilcoxon Matched-pairs Signed-ranks Test (Small Samples)

	Level of significance for one-tail test			
	.05	.025	.01	.005
	Level of significance for two-tailed test			
n	.10	.05	.02	.01
7	3	2	0	—
8	5	4	2	0
9	8	6	3	2
10	10	8	5	3
11	13	11	7	5
12	17	14	10	7
13	21	17	13	10
14	25	21	16	13
15	30	25	20	16
16	35	30	24	20
17	41	35	28	23
18	47	40	33	28
19	53	46	38	32
20	60	52	43	38

Source: Adapted and abridged from the Table of Wilcoxon, F. (1949) *Some rapid approximate statistical procedures*. New York: American Cyanamid Company, with the kind permission of the author and publisher.

TABLE A.15 Critical Values of Studentized Range Distribution(q) for Familywise $\alpha = .05$

Denominator	Number of Groups (Treatments)							
DF	3	4	5	6	7	8	9	10
1	26.98	32.82	37.08	40.41	43.12	45.40	47.36	49.07
2	8.33	9.80	10.88	11.73	12.43	13.03	13.54	13.99
3	5.91	6.83	7.50	8.04	8.48	8.85	9.18	9.46
4	5.04	5.76	6.29	6.71	7.05	7.35	7.60	7.83
5	4.60	5.22	5.67	6.03	6.33	6.58	6.80	7.00
6	4.34	4.90	5.31	5.63	5.90	6.12	6.32	6.49
7	4.17	4.68	0.06	5.36	5.61	5.82	6.00	6.16
8	4.04	4.53	4.89	5.17	5.40	5.60	5.77	5.92
9	3.95	4.42	4.76	5.02	5.24	5.43	5.60	5.74
10	3.88	4.33	4.65	4.91	5.12	5.30	5.46	5.60
11	3.82	4.26	4.57	4.82	5.03	5.20	5.35	5.49
12	3.77	4.20	4.51	4.75	4.95	5.12	5.26	5.40
13	3.73	4.15	4.45	4.69	4.88	5.05	5.19	5.32
14	3.70	4.11	4.41	4.64	4.83	4.99	5.13	5.25
15	3.67	4.08	4.37	4.60	4.78	4.94	5.08	5.20
16	3.65	4.05	4.33	4.56	4.74	4.90	5.03	5.15
17	3.63	4.02	4.30	4.52	4.71	4.86	4.99	5.11
18	3.61	4.00	4.28	4.49	4.67	4.82	4.96	5.07
19	3.59	3.98	4.25	4.47	4.65	4.79	4.92	5.04
20	3.58	3.96	4.23	4.45	4.62	4.77	4.90	5.01
21	3.57	3.94	4.21	4.42	4.60	4.74	4.87	4.98
22	3.55	3.93	4.20	4.41	4.58	4.72	4.85	4.96
23	3.54	3.91	4.18	4.39	4.56	4.70	4.83	4.94
24	3.53	3.90	4.17	4.37	4.54	4.68	4.81	4.92
25	3.52	3.89	4.15	4.36	4.53	4.67	4.79	4.90
26	3.51	3.88	4.14	4.35	4.51	4.65	4.77	4.88
27	3.51	3.87	4.13	4.33	4.50	4.64	4.76	4.86
28	3.50	3.86	4.12	4.32	4.49	4.63	4.75	4.85
29	3.49	3.85	4.11	4.31	4.48	4.61	4.73	4.84
30	3.49	3.85	4.10	4.30	4.46	4.60	4.72	4.82
31	3.48	3.84	4.09	4.29	4.45	4.59	4.71	4.81
32	3.48	3.83	4.09	4.28	4.45	4.58	4.70	4.80
33	3.47	3.83	4.08	4.28	4.44	4.57	4.69	4.79
34	3.47	3.82	4.07	4.27	4.43	4.56	4.68	4.78
35	3.46	3.81	4.07	4.26	4.42	4.56	4.67	4.77
36	3.46	3.81	4.06	4.26	4.41	4.55	4.66	4.76
37	3.45	3.80	4.05	4.25	4.41	4.54	4.66	4.76
38	3.45	3.80	4.05	4.24	4.40	4.53	4.65	4.75
39	3.45	3.80	4.04	4.24	4.39	4.53	4.64	4.74
40	3.44	3.79	4.04	4.23	4.39	4.52	4.63	4.74
41	3.44	3.79	4.04	4.23	4.38	4.52	4.63	4.73
42	3.44	3.78	4.03	4.22	4.38	4.51	4.62	4.72
43	3.43	3.78	4.03	4.22	4.37	4.50	4.62	4.72

TABLE A.15 ***(Continued)***

Denominator DF	Number of Groups (Treatments) 3	4	5	6	7	8	9	10
44	3.43	3.78	4.02	4.21	4.37	4.50	4.61	4.71
45	3.43	3.77	4.02	4.21	4.36	4.49	4.61	4.71
46	3.43	3.77	4.02	4.21	4.36	4.49	4.60	4.70
47	3.42	3.77	4.01	4.20	4.36	4.49	4.60	4.70
48	3.42	3.76	4.01	4.20	4.35	4.48	4.59	4.69
49	3.42	3.76	4.01	4.19	4.35	4.48	4.59	4.69
50	3.42	3.76	4.00	4.19	4.34	4.47	4.58	4.68
51	3.41	3.76	4.00	4.19	4.34	4.47	4.58	4.68
52	3.41	3.75	4.00	4.18	4.34	4.47	4.58	4.67
53	3.41	3.75	3.99	4.18	4.33	4.46	4.57	4.67
54	3.41	3.75	3.99	4.18	4.33	4.46	4.57	4.67
55	3.41	3.75	3.99	4.18	4.33	4.46	4.57	4.66
56	3.41	3.75	3.99	4.17	4.33	4.45	4.56	4.66
57	3.40	3.74	3.98	4.17	4.32	4.45	4.56	4.66
58	3.40	3.74	3.98	4.17	4.32	4.45	4.56	4.65
59	3.40	3.74	3.98	4.17	4.32	4.44	4.55	4.65
60	3.40	3.74	3.98	4.16	4.31	4.44	4.55	4.65
61	3.40	3.74	3.98	4.16	4.31	4.44	4.55	4.64
62	3.40	3.73	3.97	4.16	4.31	4.44	4.55	4.64
63	3.40	3.73	3.97	4.16	4.31	4.43	4.54	4.64
64	3.39	3.73	3.97	4.16	4.31	4.43	4.54	4.64
65	3.39	3.73	3.97	4.15	4.30	4.43	4.54	4.63
66	3.39	3.73	3.97	4.15	4.30	4.43	4.54	4.63
67	3.39	3.73	3.97	4.15	4.30	4.43	4.53	4.63
68	3.39	3.73	3.96	4.15	4.30	4.42	4.53	4.63
69	3.39	3.72	3.96	4.15	4.30	4.42	4.53	4.62
70	3.39	3.72	3.96	4.14	4.29	4.42	4.53	4.62
71	3.39	3.72	3.96	4.14	4.29	4.42	4.53	4.62
72	3.38	3.72	3.96	4.14	4.29	4.42	4.52	4.62
73	3.38	3.72	3.96	4.14	4.29	4.41	4.52	4.62
74	3.38	3.72	3.95	4.14	4.29	4.41	4.52	4.61
75	3.38	3.72	3.95	4.14	4.29	4.41	4.52	4.61
76	3.38	3.72	3.95	4.14	4.28	4.41	4.52	4.61
77	3.38	3.71	3.95	4.13	4.28	4.41	4.51	4.61
78	3.38	3.71	3.95	4.13	4.28	4.41	4.51	4.61
79	3.38	3.71	3.95	4.13	4.28	4.40	4.51	4.60
80	3.38	3.71	3.95	4.13	4.28	4.40	4.51	4.60
81	3.38	3.71	3.95	4.13	4.28	4.40	4.51	4.60
82	3.38	3.71	3.95	4.13	4.28	4.40	4.51	4.60
83	3.38	3.71	3.94	4.13	4.27	4.40	4.50	4.60
84	3.37	3.71	3.94	4.13	4.27	4.40	4.50	4.60
85	3.37	3.71	3.94	4.12	4.27	4.40	4.50	4.60
86	3.37	3.71	3.94	4.12	4.27	4.39	4.50	4.59

(continued)

TABLE A.15 (*Continued*)

Denominator DF	Number of Groups (Treatments) 3	4	5	6	7	8	9	10
87	3.37	3.70	3.94	4.12	4.27	4.39	4.50	4.59
88	3.37	3.70	3.94	4.12	4.27	4.39	4.50	4.59
89	3.37	3.70	3.94	4.12	4.27	4.39	4.50	4.59
90	3.37	3.70	3.94	4.12	4.27	4.39	4.50	4.59
91	3.37	3.70	3.94	4.12	4.26	4.39	4.49	4.59
92	3.37	3.70	3.94	4.12	4.26	4.39	4.49	4.59
93	3.37	3.70	3.93	4.12	4.26	4.39	4.49	4.59
94	3.37	3.70	3.93	4.11	4.26	4.38	4.49	4.58
95	3.37	3.70	3.93	4.11	4.26	4.38	4.49	4.58
96	3.37	3.70	3.93	4.11	4.26	4.38	4.49	4.58
97	3.37	3.70	3.93	4.11	4.26	4.38	4.49	4.58
98	3.37	3.70	3.93	4.11	4.26	4.38	4.49	4.58
99	3.37	3.70	3.93	4.11	4.26	4.38	4.49	4.58
100	3.37	3.70	3.93	4.11	4.26	4.38	4.48	4.58

Source: Adapted and abridged from the Tables for Statisticians, E.S. Pearson and H.O. Hartley, Vol. 1, 3rd edition. pp. 176–77.

INDEX

Statistics for Exercise Science and Health with Microsoft® Office Excel®, First Edition. J. P. Verma.

Printed and bound by CPI Group (UK) Ltd, Croydon, CR0 4YY

16/09/2026

14963423-0006